INSULIN RESISTANCE

THE METABOLIC SYNDROME X

CONTEMPORARY ENDOCRINOLOGY

P. Michael Conn, SERIES EDITOR

19. **Human Growth Hormone:** *Basic and Clinical Research,* edited by Roy G. SMITH AND MICHAEL O. THORNER, 1999

18. **Menopause:** *Endocrinology and Management,* edited by DAVID B. SEIFER AND ELIZABETH A. KENNARD, 1999

17. **The IGF System:** *Molecular Biology, Physiology, and Clinical Applications,* edited by RON G. ROSENFELD AND CHARLES T. ROBERTS, JR. 1999

16. **Neurosteroids:** *A New Regulatory Function in the Nervous System,* edited by ETIENNE-EMILE BAULIEU, MICHAEL SCHUMACHER, AND PAUL ROBEL, 1999

15. **Autoimmune Endocrinopathies,** edited by ROBERT VOLPÉ, 1999

14. **Hormone Resistance Syndromes,** edited by J. LARRY JAMESON, 1999

13. **Hormone Replacement Therapy,** edited by A. WAYNE MEIKLE, 1999

12. **Insulin Resistance:** *The Metabolic Syndrome X,* edited by GERALD M. REAVEN AND AMI LAWS, 1999

11. **Endocrinology of Breast Cancer,** edited by ANDREA MANNI, 1999

10. **Molecular and Cellular Pediatric Endocrinology,** edited by STUART HANDWERGER, 1999

 9. **The Endocrinology of Pregnancy,** edited by FULLER W. BAZER, 1998

 8. **Gastrointestinal Endocrinology,** edited by GEORGE H. GREELEY, JR., 1999

 7. **Clinical Management of Diabetic Neuropathy,** edited by ARISTIDIS VEVES, 1998

 6. **G Proteins, Receptors, and Disease,** edited by ALLEN M. SPIEGEL, 1998

 5. **Natriuretic Peptides in Health and Disease,** edited by WILLIS K. SAMSON AND ELLIS R. LEVIN, 1997

 4. **Endocrinology of Critical Diseases,** edited by K. PATRICK OBER, 1997

 3. **Diseases of the Pituitary:** *Diagnosis and Treatment,* edited by MARGARET E. WIERMAN, 1997

 2. **Diseases of the Thyroid,** edited by LEWIS E. BRAVERMAN, 1997

 1. **Endocrinology of the Vasculature,** edited by JAMES R. SOWERS, 1996

INSULIN RESISTANCE

THE METABOLIC SYNDROME X

Edited by

GERALD M. REAVEN, MD

Shaman Pharmaceuticals, Inc., South San Francisco, CA
and Stanford University School of Medicine, Stanford, CA

AMI LAWS, MD

Stanford University School of Medicine, Stanford, CA

 HUMANA PRESS, TOTOWA, NEW JERSEY

Library of Congress Cataloging-in-Publication Data

Insulin resistance: the metabolic syndrome X/edited by Gerald M. Reaven, Ami
Laws.
      p. cm. -- (Contemporary endocrinology ; 12)
   Includes bibliographical references and index.
   ISBN 0-89603-588-3 (alk. paper)
   1. Insulin resistance. I. Reaven, Gerald M. II. Laws, Ami. III.
Series: Contemporary endocrinology (Totowa, N.J.) ; 12.
   [DNLM: 1. Insulin Resistance. WK 820 I5961 1999]
RC662.I55 1999
616.4'6207--dc21
DNLM/DL   98-36840
for Library of Congress   CIP

PREFACE

Given the dramatic impact that the introduction of insulin had on the treatment of patients with diabetes, it should not be surprising that this complicated syndrome was initially believed to be one simple disease, secondary to lack of insulin. What may be more surprising to the modern reader is that this unitarian hypothesis of diabetes was challenged within 15 years following the availability of insulin. In 1936, Himsworth published his epochal paper[1] describing a method based on the concomitant administration of oral glucose and subcutaneous insulin to quantify the ability of insulin to dispose of a glucose load in patients with diabetes. As far as we can ascertain, this represents the first time an effort was made to evaluate the possibility that resistance to insulin-mediated glucose disposal could play a role in human disease. Based upon measurements of the plasma glucose response to the combined glucose–insulin challenge in patients with diabetes, Himsworth concluded that there were at least two different types of diabetes—defined as being either insulin-sensitive or insulin-insensitive. This separation of patients with hyperglycemia into two different syndromes bears an uncanny resemblance to what we now refer to as Type 1 and Type 2 diabetes, and antedates by approximately 40 years this designation as promulgated by the National Diabetes Data Group.[2]

Unfortunately, the elegant clinical studies of Himsworth and colleagues on the pathogenesis of hyperglycemia in patients with diabetes were terminated with the advent of World War II. However, shortly after the war's end, Himsworth delivered a series of lectures summarizing the results of the studies of diabetes performed by his research group.[3] He ended his presentation by stating that "we should accustom ourselves to the idea that a primary deficiency of insulin is only one, and then not the most common, of the diabetic syndromes."

We think it safe to say that the medical profession has finally paid heed to the admonition of Himsworth, and accustomed itself to the central role that insulin resistance plays in the etiology of Type 2 diabetes. Indeed, this concept is so widely accepted that we saw no reason to address in this book the relationship between insulin resistance and Type 2 diabetes. Rather, to paraphrase Himsworth, we believe it has become time to accustom ourselves to the fact that the importance of insulin resistance in human disease far transcends its role in the etiology of Type 2 diabetes. Results of studies performed over the past decade have clearly established the fact that resistance to insulin-mediated glucose disposal and compensatory hyperinsulinemia occur frequently in the population at large, and, when present, greatly increase the risk of a series of health-related consequences.[4,5]

The goal of *Insulin Resistance: The Metabolic Syndrome X* is to summarize current understanding of the importance of this role of insulin, particularly as it relates to non-diabetic clinical syndromes. For this purpose, the book has been divided into three parts. *Part I* focuses on those factors—genetic and lifestyle—that contribute to the wide differences in insulin action that exist in the population at large. In *Part II*, attention has been directed to the pathophysiologic consequences of insulin resistance, and the efforts made to compensate for this defect in order to prevent decompensation of glucose homeostasis. *Part III* is devoted to consideration of the clinical syndromes, excluding Type 2 diabetes, related to insulin resistance.

Finally, a word about the overall approach of *Insulin Resistance:* The Metabolic Syndrome X. Every effort has been made to avoid noncritical summaries of the topics addressed. Rather, authors have been requested to present a point of view, taking advantage of their unique insights. Controversy has been encouraged, as befits a rapidly moving and changing field of inquiry. The editors can only hope that you, the reader, will enjoy both reading and learning as much from each chapter as we did. Although discussions will probably continue indefinitely about the most appropriate terms to describe the two major types of clinical diabetes, for purposes of consistency, Type 1 and Type 2 diabetes will be used throughout this volume to refer to insulin-dependent diabetes mellitus (IDDM) and non-insulin dependent diabetes (NIDDM), respectively.

REFERENCES

1. Himsworth HP. Diabetes mellitus: Its differentiation into insulin-sensitive and insulin-insensitive types. Lancet 1936;1:127-130.

2. National Data Group. Classification and diagnosis of diabetes mellitus and other categories of glucose intolerance. Diabetes 1979;28:1039-1957.

3. Himsworth HP. The syndrome of diabetes mellitus and its causes. Lancet 1949;1:465 473.

4. Reaven GM. Role of insulin resistance in human disease. Diabetes 1988;37:1595-1607.

5. Reaven GM. Syndrome X: past, present, and future. In Clinical Research in Diabetes and Obesity, (Draznin B and Rizza R, eds) Humana Press, New Jersey, pp. 357–382.

CONTENTS

Preface v

Contributors ix

Part I   **Genetic and Environmental Factors Affecting Insulin Action**

1   Genetics of Insulin Resistance 3
Michael P. Stern and Braxton D. Mitchell

2   Ethnic Variation in Insulin Resistance
and Risk of Type 2 Diabetes 19
Paul M. McKeigue

3   Fetal Effects on Insulin Resistance and Glucose Tolerance 35
Paul M. McKeigue

4   Obesity and Insulin Resistance:
Epidemiologic, Metabolic, and Molecular Aspects 51
Jean-Pierre Després and André Marette

5   The Role of Body Fat Distribution in Insulin Resistance 83
Abhimanyu Garg

6   Physical Activity and Insulin Resistance in Man 97
Flemming Dela, Kári Mikines, and Henrik Galbo

7   Insulin Resistance in Smokers and Other Long-Term Users
of Nicotine 121
Björn Eliasson and Ulf Smith

Part II   **Pathophysiology of Insulin Resistance**

8   Insulin Resistance and Inhibitors of Insulin Receptor
Tyrosine Kinase 139
*Jack F. Youngren, Ira D. Goldfine, Vincenzo Trischitta,
and Betty A. Maddux*

9   NMR Studies on the Mechanism of Insulin Resistance 159
*Gianluca Perseghin, Kitt Falk Petersen,
and Gerald I. Shulman*

10   Skeletal Muscle Insulin Resistance in Humans:
Cellular Mechanisms 179
Lawrence J. Mandarino

11   The Role of the Liver in Insulin Action and Resistance 197
Jerry Radziuk and Susan Pye

12   The Pathophysiological Consequences of Adipose Tissue
Insulin Resistance 233
Gerald M. Reaven

13   Insulin Action and Endothelial Function 247
     Alain D. Baron and Michael J. Quon

Part III   Clinical Syndromes Associated with Insulin Resistance

14   Insulin Resistance and Dyslipidemia:
     Implications for Coronary Heart Disease Risk 267
     Ami Laws

15   Insulin Resistance and Blood Pressure...281
     Ele Ferrannini

16   Microalbuminuria and Insulin Resistance 309
     Jeannie Yip and Roberto Trevisan

17   PAI-1, Obesity, and Insulin Resistance.......................................317
     *Irène Juhan-Vague, Marie-Christine Alessi,
          and Pierre E. Morange*

18   Insulin Resistance and Cardiovascular Disease 333
     Aaron R. Folsom

19   Insulin Resistance Effects on Sex Hormones and Ovulation
          in the Polycystic Ovary Syndrome...347
     John E. Nestler

     Index...367

CONTRIBUTORS

MARIE-CHRISTINE ALESSI, MD, PHD, *Laboratory of Hematology, Faculty of Medicine, CHU Timone, Marseille, France*

ALAIN D. BARON, MD, *Indiana University School of Medicine, Indianapolis, IN*

FLEMMING DELA, MD, DMSC, *Panum Institute, University of Copenhagen, Copenhagen*

JEAN-PIERRE DESPRÉS, PHD, *Lipid Research Center, CHUL Research Center, Sainte-Foy, Québec*

BJÖRN ELIASSON, MD, *Lundberg Laboratory for Diabetes Research, Sahlgrenska University Hospital, Göteberg, Sweden*

ELE FERRANNINI, MD, *CNR Institute of Clinical Physiology, Pisa, Italy*

AARON R. FOLSOM, MD, *Division of Epidemiology, School of Public Health, University of Minnesota, Minneapolis, MN*

HENRIK GALBO, MD, DMSC, *Panum Institute, University of Copenhagen, Copenhagen, Denmark*

ABHIMANYU GARG, MD, *Center for Human Nutrition, UT Southwestern Medical Center at Dallas, Dallas, TX*

IRA D. GOLDFINE, MD, *Mount Zion Medical Center, University of California, San Francisco, CA*

IRÈNE JUHAN-VAGUE, MD, PHD, *Laboratory of Hematology, Faculty of Medicine, CHU Timone, Marseille, France*

AMI LAWS, MD, *Department of Medicine, Stanford University School of Medicine, Stanford, CA*

LAWRENCE J. MANDARINO, PHD, *Division of Diabetes, Departments of Medicine and Biochemistry, University of Texas Health Science Center at San Antonio, San Antonio, TX*

BETTY A. MADDUX, BS, *Mount Zion Medical Center, University of California, San Francisco, CA*

ANDRÉ MARETTE, PHD, *Lipid Research Center, CHUL Research Center, Sainte-Foy, Québec*

PAUL M. MCKEIGUE, MB, PHD, *Department of Epidemiology and Population Health, London School of Hygiene and Tropical Medicine, London, United Kingdom*

KÁRI MIKINES, MD, DMSC, *Panum Institute, University of Copenhagen, Copenhagen, Denmark*

BRAXTON D. MITCHELL, PHD, *Department of Genetics, Southwest Foundation for Biomedical Research, San Antonio, TX*

PIERRE E. MORANGE, MD, *Laboratory of Hematology, Faculty of Medicine, CHU Timone, Marseille, France*

JOHN E. NESTLER, MD, *Division of Endocrinology and Metabolism, Department of Internal Medicine, Medical College of Virginia, Virginia Commonwealth University, Richmond, VA*

GIANLUCA PERSEGHIN, MD, *Aminoacids/Stable Isotope Laboratory and Clinical NMR Spectroscopy Unit, Department of Internal Medicine, Instituto Scientifico H San Raffaele, Milan, Italy*

KITT FALK PETERSEN, MD, *Department of Internal Medicine, Yale University School of Medicine, New Haven, CT*

SUSAN PYE, MSC, *Ottawa Civic Hospital, Ottawa, Canada*

MICHAEL J. QUON, MD, PHD, *Hypertension–Endocrine Branch, National Heart, Lung, and Blood Institute, National Institutes of Health, Bethesda, MD*

JERRY RADZIUK, PHD, MD, CM, FRCP, *Diabetes and Metabolism Research Unit, Ottawa Civic Hospital and the University of Ottawa, Ottawa, Canada*

GERALD M. REAVEN, MD, *Shaman Pharmaceuticals, Inc., South San Francisco, CA and School of Medicine, Stanford University, Stanford, CA*

ULF SMITH, MD, *Lundberg Laboratory for Diabetes Research, Sahlgrenska University Hospital, Göteberg, Sweden*

GERALD I. SHULMAN, MD, PHD, *Howard Hughes Medical Institute, Department of Internal Medicine, Yale University School of Medicine, New Haven, CT*

MICHAEL P. STERN, MD, *Division of Clinical Epidemiology, Department of Medicine, University of Texas Health Science Center, San Antonio, TX*

ROBERTO TREVISAN, MD, PHD, *Department of Clinical and Experimental Medicine, University of Padova, Italy*

VINCENZO TRISCHITTA, MD, *Divisione e Unita e Recerca di Endocrinologia, Instituto Scientifico Casa Sollievo della Sofferenza, San Giovanni Rotondo, Italy*

JEANNIE YIP, MB, *The Permanente Medical Group, Oakland, CA*

JACK F. YOUNGREN, MB, PHD, *School of Medicine and Mount Zion Medical Center, University of California, San Francisco, CA*

I

GENETIC AND ENVIRONMENTAL FACTORS AFFECTING INSULIN ACTION

1

Genetics of Insulin Resistance

Michael P. Stern, MD
and Braxton D. Mitchell, PhD

Contents

INTRODUCTION
RARE, MONOGENIC CAUSES OF INSULIN RESISTANCE
EVIDENCE FOR A GENETIC BASIS FOR COMMON FORMS
  OF INSULIN RESISTANCE
MODE OF INHERITANCE OF INSULINEMIA AND INSULIN RESISTANCE
LINKAGE OF INSULIN RESISTANCE TO CANDIDATE GENES
  AND CHROMOSOMAL REGIONS
THE INSULIN RESISTANCE SYNDROME
CONCLUSIONS
REFERENCES

INTRODUCTION

Insulin-stimulated glucose uptake varies widely between individuals. The wide range of variability has been documented by Hollenbeck and Reaven *(1)* who measured in vivo insulin sensitivity, using the euglycemic clamp technique, in a group of apparently healthy, non-obese subjects with normal glucose tolerance. After dividing the subjects into four quartiles based on their insulin sensitivity values, these investigators observed a two-and-a-half-fold difference in mean insulin sensitivity between subjects in the most sensitive compared to the least sensitive quartile. In fact, the degree of insulin resistance observed in normal individuals can equal that seen in diabetic individuals *(1)*. Thus, although it is now widely appreciated that insulin resistance precedes the development of Type 2 diabetes, it is equally important to recognize that mild or even severe insulin resistance may be found in individuals who will never develop diabetes. There is a substantial body of evidence that points to genetic factors as the source of much of this normal variation in insulin resistance.

Although this chapter will focus on the common forms of insulin resistance, we will first describe the rare, monogenic forms of this disorder, since they may hold lessons relevant to the broader topic. Following this, we will summarize the evidence that the common forms of insulin resistance also have genetic determinants. This evidence

From: *Contemporary Endocrinology: Insulin Resistance*
Edited by: G. Reaven and A. Laws © Humana Press Inc., Totowa, NJ

derives from studies that have demonstrated the familial nature of insulin resistance, including studies that have estimated heritability from twin and extended pedigree data. Next, we will review studies in which segregation analyses have been used to infer the mode of inheritance of insulin resistance. We will then summarize the current status of efforts to identify the specific genes that lead to insulin resistance. Finally, the chapter will conclude with a discussion of potential genetic influences on the constellation of traits that comprise the Insulin Resistance Syndrome (IRS).

RARE, MONOGENIC CAUSES OF INSULIN RESISTANCE

The insulin receptor gene, located on chromosome 19 (bands p13.2–13.3), contains 22 exons and is over 150,000 kilobases long. The more than 50 mutations of this gene that have been described to date *(2)* represent well-characterized, albeit rare causes of insulin resistance. These mutations have been categorized into five classes *(3)*. Class 1 mutations lead to impaired biosynthesis of the insulin receptor. They are either nonsense mutations or, more often, deletions or splicing defects. The latter two types of defects can cause shifts in the reading frame that can lead to premature termination of transcription. The result is reduced amounts of insulin receptor mRNA in the cytoplasm and reduced levels of receptor on the cell surface. (If the patient is a heterozygote, expression of the normal allele will result in cytoplasmic mRNA and receptor on the cell surface, albeit in reduced amounts.) The remaining four classes of mutations are due primarily to missense mutations that cause amino acid substitutions in the insulin receptor protein. These classes of mutations do not typically result in reduced amount of cytoplasmic mRNA. Following translation of mRNA the insulin receptor undergoes a complex series of post-translational changes as it is transported through the endoplasmic reticulum and Golgi apparatus. Class 2 mutations interfere with this process by, for example, interfering with proteolytic processing or folding of the protein chain. This impaired processing can lead to decreased amounts of receptor protein being expressed on the cell surface. By contrast, Class 3 and 4 mutations are associated with normal amounts of insulin receptor on the cell surface. In the case of Class 3 mutations, insulin binding to the receptor is impaired, and, in the case of Class 4 mutations, tyrosine kinase activity, the first step in insulin signaling, is impaired. Class 4 mutations typically act in a dominant fashion. Finally, Class 5 mutations result in accelerated degradation of the insulin receptor. Normally, the majority of receptors which are internalized after binding with insulin are recycled to the cell membrane and only a fraction are earmarked for degradation. Class 5 mutations cause a higher proportion of the internalized receptors to be degraded leading to reduced amounts of receptor on the cell surface. It should be noted that these five mechanisms are not necessarily mutually exclusive. For example, mutations which result in abnormal post-translation processing may also be associated with impaired insulin binding and/or impaired tyrosine kinase activity *(4)*.

A number of syndromes are associated with mutations of the insulin receptor gene *(5)*. Type A insulin resistance is characterized by the triad of insulin resistance, acanthosis nigricans, and hyperandrogenicity. This type of insulin resistance can also be seen in patients with the polycystic ovary syndrome *(6)*. Leprechaunism is characterized by severe insulin resistance, intrauterine growth retardation, hirsuitism, and fasting hypoglycemia. The mechanism for the hypoglycemia is obscure. Few of these patients survive beyond the first year of life. The Rabson-Mendenhall Syndrome displays, in addition to the above features, abnormalities of teeth and nails and pineal hyperplasia. Many patients with insulin receptor mutations have glucose intolerance, or in some cases frank diabetes. Often they are severely insulin resistant and, in some cases, may have insulin levels as much as 100-times normal. Those who are diabetic may require several thousand units of insulin per day. The specific syndromes, however, are not well-correlated with specific mutations. One possibility is that the particular syndrome reflects, not the specific mutation, but rather the functional severity of the insulin resistance *(3)*. For example, most cases of Leprechaunism have mutations of both insulin receptor alleles leading to severe insulin resistance. Frequently, these patients are compound heterozygotes. Patients with Type A insulin resistance, on the other hand, are usually heterozygotes with milder degrees of insulin resistance, although in some cases they too can have two abnormal alleles, in which case they are typically more severely insulin resistant. Another possible mechanism whereby different mutations could lead to different clinical syndromes is based on the concept of branching pathways, each leading to different biological effects, perhaps through involvement of different tyrosine kinase pathways. Thus, certain mutations might lead to impairment in growth (Leprechaunism) and others only to metabolic impairments (Type A insulin resistance). To date, however, there has been no direct evidence for this mechanism. Finally, the particular syndrome expressed could be influenced by the polygenic background of the patient which would differ in individual cases.

Many individuals with insulin receptor mutations are asymptomatic. This is particularly the case with heterozygotes, many of whom might never have come to medical attention had they not produced offspring who were either homozygotes or compound heterozygotes. When studied, however, the heterozygote parents of these individuals are often found to be insulin resistant and glucose intolerant. This raises the question of whether mutations of the insulin receptor gene could play a role in insulin resistance and diabetes in the general population. The incidence of Leprechaunism has been estimated to be 1 in 4×10^6 live births which corresponds to an allele frequency of 1 in 2×10^3. This allele frequency implies that one in a thousand individuals are "carriers." For various reason this figure is likely to be an underestimate *(5)*. Presumably, the frequency of heterozygotes would be even higher among patients with Type 2 diabetes. Because of the difficulty of screening for such a large and diverse number of mutations, the population frequency of insulin receptor mutations is not well established. Nevertheless, although insulin receptor mutations may make some contribution to insulin resistance and diabetes in the general population, other lines of evidence, specifically linkage studies, suggest that this contribution is not large. This topic will be discussed in greater detail in a later section of this chapter.

EVIDENCE FOR A GENETIC BASIS FOR COMMON FORMS OF INSULIN RESISTANCE

There is substantial evidence that the common forms of insulin resistance are strongly influenced by heredity. Several lines of reasoning support this concept. First, nondiabetic relatives of diabetic individuals are more insulin resistant than nondiabetic controls. Second, variability in insulin sensitivity is significantly less within families than between families, and third, a substantial heritable component to insulin resistance has been estimated from twin and extended pedigree studies. Each of these lines of evidence will now be reviewed.

Insulin Resistance in Relatives of Type 2 Diabetic Subjects

A number of studies have indicated that nondiabetic relatives of diabetic subjects are both more hyperinsulinemic and more insulin resistant than controls. An important limitation of such studies, and indeed all studies based on family resemblance (see next two sections), is that they do not distinguish between shared environment and genetic factors as the cause of the resemblance. Nevertheless, these studies have contributed to the overall impression that insulin resistance has genetic determinants. Haffner et al. *(7)* reported that fasting insulin concentrations increase in a stepwise fashion in nondiabetic Mexican Americans having zero, one, or two Type 2 diabetic parents. Since Type 2 diabetic subjects are almost invariably insulin resistant, these results imply that insulin resistance is more frequent in the offspring of individuals with Type 2 diabetes. Similar findings have also been reported in non-Hispanic Caucasians from Utah among whom nondiabetic members of pedigrees ascertained on two Type 2 diabetic siblings had higher insulin concentrations 1 hour after an oral glucose load than spouse controls *(8)*.

Direct measurements of insulin resistance, using either intravenous glucose tolerance tests, the euglycemic insulin clamp technique, or the steady state plasma glucose (SSPG) method, have also provided evidence for greater degrees of insulin resistance in relatives of Type 2 diabetic subjects. Using the intravenous glucose tolerance test, Warram et al. *(9)* showed that the fractional glucose removal rate was reduced in 155 nondiabetic offspring of two Type 2 diabetic parents compared to 186 unrelated controls, suggesting insulin resistance in the offspring. In addition, second, although not first, phase insulin secretion was higher in the offspring, a finding that is compatible with compensatory hypersecretion of insulin in response to insulin resistance.

A limitation of the study by Warram et al. *(9)* is that the fractional glucose removal rate reflects both insulin dependent and insulin independent glucose disposal, and, to a lesser extent, suppression of hepatic glucose output. Differentiation between insulin dependent and insulin independent glucose disposal can be made when intravenous glucose tolerance test data are analyzed by the minimal model method developed by Bergman et al. *(10)*. Using this technique, Osei et al. *(11)* reported that insulin sensitivity (S_I) was 45% lower in nondiabetic subjects with at least one Type 2 diabetic parent compared to controls, matched for age, sex, and body mass index, but with no family history of diabetes. The authors estimated that family history accounted for 27% of the variance in S_I. By contrast, there was no difference between offspring and controls in glucose effectiveness (S_G) which reflects insulin independent glucose disposal. On the other hand, at least one study, using the minimal model method, failed to find a difference in S_I between nondiabetic offspring of two diabetic parents and controls *(12)*.

Diminished insulin sensitivity in nondiabetic relatives of Type 2 diabetic parents has also been demonstrated using the euglycemic clamp technique. Eriksson et al. *(13)* compared insulin sensitivity in 26 nondiabetic Finns who were first-degree relatives of Type 2 diabetic subjects and 14 matched controls with no family history of diabetes. The results, presented in Fig. 1, indicate a stepwise decrease in insulin-stimulated glucose disposal as one moves from controls, to glucose tolerant first-degree relatives of diabetic subjects, to relatives with impaired glucose tolerance (IGT), to patients with frank diabetes. These decreases are almost entirely due to reductions in nonoxidative glucose disposal, which is reduced by approximately 50% in relatives of diabetic subjects both with and without IGT. Indeed, nonoxidative glucose disposal is reduced in the first-degree relatives nearly as much as in the diabetic patients themselves. By contrast, glu-

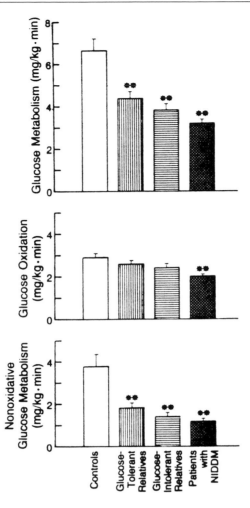

Fig. 1. Insulin-stimulated total body glucose metabolism, glucose oxidation, and nonoxidative glucose metabolism, measured by the euglycemic clamp technique, in control subjects, relatives with normal and impaired glucose tolerance, and patients with Type 2 diabetes. (From ref. *13.* Copyright © 1989 Massachusetts Medical Society. All rights reserved.)

cose oxidation is quite similar in relatives and controls, and is only modestly, albeit statistically significantly, reduced in patients with frank diabetes. In this study, insulin secretion was also evaluated using the hyperglycemic clamp technique and was found to be normal in first-degree relatives with normal glucose tolerance. In relatives with IGT first phase insulin secretion was reduced, although second phase insulin secretion remained normal.

Similar results were reported by Gulli et al. *(14)* who studied 11 nondiabetic Mexican American offspring of two Type 2 diabetic parents and 10 Mexican American controls without a family history of diabetes who were matched to the offspring on age, sex, and body weight. In this study a mild, but statistically significant impairment in insulin-stimulated glucose oxidation was noted in the offspring, but as in the previously cited study by Eriksson et al. *(13)*, the major defect was in nonoxidative glucose disposal. Compared to controls, the rate of nonoxidative glucose disposal during low- and high-dose insulin infusion rates was reduced by 88 and 45%, respectively, in the offspring. No difference was observed between offspring and controls in insulin-mediated suppression of hepatic glucose output, but insulin-mediated suppression of lipid oxidation and free fatty acid concentrations were impaired in the offspring. These latter findings indicate that the insulin resistance found in relatives of Type 2 diabetic subjects extends to at least some of the non-carbohydrate related actions of insulin. In this study first and second phase insulin secretion were assessed by the hyperglycemic clamp technique, and were found to be increased in the offspring by 44 and 35%, respectively. As previously noted, such increases are suggestive of compensatory hypersecretion of insulin in response to insulin resistance.

Another approach to evaluating islet cell function and insulin sensitivity is referred to as "continuous infusion of glucose with model assessment" or CIGMA. Using this technique O'Rahilly et al. *(15)* studied 154 nondiabetic first-degree relatives of Type 2 diabetic subjects and found that they had diminished insulin sensitivity compared to 64 controls. As in the study by Eriksson et al. *(13)*, previously cited, islet cell function was diminished in relatives with impaired glucose tolerance.

In addition to Caucasians and Mexican Americans, diminished insulin sensitivity has also been demonstrated in first degree relatives of Type 2 diabetic subjects of Chinese ethnicity. Using the SSPG method, Ho et al. *(16)* compared 25 nondiabetic offspring of at least one Type 2 diabetic parent with 25 nondiabetic controls, both of whose parents had normal glucose tolerance. Following 4-h infusions of glucose, insulin, and somatostatin (the latter to suppress endogenous insulin secretion), the offspring had higher plasma glucose levels despite having attained slightly higher insulin levels, indicating that they were significantly more insulin resistant than the controls. This population is of particular interest, since the subjects were quite lean (BMI approximately 21 kg/m^2), suggesting that the increased insulin resistance observed in relatives of diabetic individuals is not dependent on obesity.

Variability of Insulinemia and Insulin Resistance Within and Between Families

Martin et al. *(17)* studied 183 nondiabetic offspring of two diabetic parents from 105 families. Insulin sensitivity (S_I) and glucose effectiveness (S_G, i.e., insulin independent glucose disposal) were measured by the intravenous glucose tolerance technique. Family clustering was assessed by intraclass correlations, which compare the variability of a trait within families to the variability across families. A correlation near 1.0 indicates that family members tend to resemble one another with respect to the trait, whereas a correlation near zero indicates that family members are no more likely to resemble one another than they are to resemble unrelated individuals. S_I showed an intraclass correlation for siblings of 0.25 ($p = 0.013$) implying that 50% of its variability was of family origin. Adjustment for obesity and fasting insulin concentrations, which themselves showed family clustering, did not materially affect the intraclass correlation for S_I. By contrast, S_G failed to show any evidence of family clustering. In Fig. 2 families are ranked according to their midrange S_I value. It is apparent that the range of S_I values within families is less than the overall range across all families, further supporting the conclusion that family members are more likely to resemble one another than they are to resemble unrelated individuals. The authors of this study also called attention to the 10 families with the lowest S_I values at the extreme left of the graph, among whom the within-family

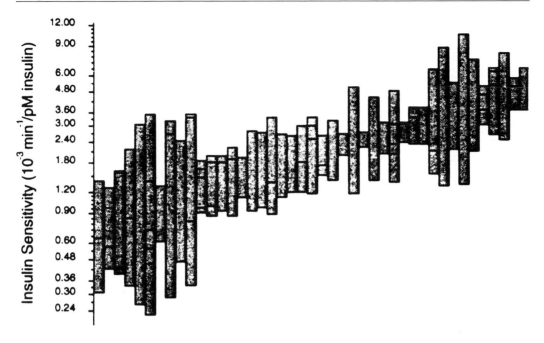

Fig. 2. Insulin sensitivity in 43 families ranked according to the midrange value of logS$_I$ within each family. It is apparent that the range of insulin sensitivities within families is narrower than across families *(17)*. (Reproduced with permission from the American Diabetes Association)

variability was greater than for most of the other families. They noted that the wide variation within the families on the left side of the graph is compatible with autosomal dominant inheritance in which some family members (affecteds) would have very low values of S$_I$, and others (unaffecteds) would have normal values. By contrast, the narrower S$_I$ range in the families on the right side of the graph would be more suggestive of polygenic inheritance.

Family clustering of insulin sensitivity, as measured by the euglycemic clamp technique, has also been demonstrated in Pima Indians *(18)*. In this study the investigators measured glucose disposal rates at both low (physiological) and high (supraphysiological) insulin infusion rates in 116 nondiabetic siblings from 45 families. The high insulin infusion rate produces maximal insulin-stimulated glucose uptake (i.e., M$_{high}$), reductions of which are thought to reflect a post-receptor defect in insulin action. The intraclass correlation for insulin action at the high infusion rate was 0.42 ($p \leq 0.0001$). A lesser degree of family clustering was observed for insulin action at the physiological infusion rate (i.e., M$_{low}$) for which the intraclass correlation was 0.26.

Estimates of Heritability of Insulinemia and Insulin Resistance

Heritability is defined as the proportion of the total phenotypic variance attributable to the additive effects of genes. Twin studies are commonly used to estimate this genetic parameter. The power of twin studies resides in the fact that monozygotic (MZ) twin pairs share all their genes while dizygotic (DZ) twin pairs share on average only one-half of their genes. Thus, the degree of phenotypic similarity between MZ twins relative to DZ twin is proportional to the extent of genetic influence on the phenotype in question. As noted above, this interpretation assumes that lifestyle and other environmental influences are similar between the two types of twins. In fact, there is evidence that MZ twins not infrequently share environments and lifestyles to a greater extent than do DZ twins. To the extent that these environmental influences can be measured, however, they can be accounted for in the estimates of heritability.

In an analysis of 278 women twin pairs, Mayer et al. *(19)* computed intraclass correlation coefficients for log fasting insulin concentration of 0.64 and 0.40 for MZ and DZ twin pairs, respectively. The corresponding heritability estimate was 47%. After accounting for age and behavioral factors, the heritability decreased to 30%, suggesting that some of the greater similarity among MZ compared to DZ twins was of environmental origin. Similar results were obtained in a study of 34 twin pairs by Narkiewicz et al. *(20)*. These investigators also observed higher variability in DZ twin pairs than in MZ twin pairs and estimated a heritability of 54% for fasting insulin and 66% for relative insulin resistance, as measured by the homeostasis model *(21)*. Neither estimate was altered substantially by adjustment for age, gender, and body mass index (BMI).

The heritability of insulin concentrations has also been estimated from pedigree data. Based on an analysis of over 900 nondiabetic individuals from 42 large, extended Mexican American pedigrees from San Antonio, TX (USA), Mitchell et al. *(22)* reported the heritability of fasting and 2-h post glucose load insulin (log transformed) to be 35 and 13%, respectively. After accounting for the variance attributable to age, sex, and other risk factors, the additive effects of genes (i.e., heritability) accounted for 39 and 16%, respectively, of the remaining variance. The estimated heritability for fasting insulin concentration was similar to those obtained from the twin studies cited above. (Heritability of 2-h insulin levels was not estimated in the twin studies.)

MODE OF INHERITANCE OF INSULINEMIA AND INSULIN RESISTANCE

The studies summarized previously provide evidence that there is a substantial genetic influence on insulinemia and insulin resistance. A key question is whether this genetic influence results principally from the action of a large number of genes, each having only a very modest effect on insulin sensitivity (i.e., polygenes), or whether it results from the action of a relatively few genes, each having a large effect. A definitive answer to this question is lacking, although there is some support for the latter possibility. For example, Bogardus et al. *(23)* reported that both insulinemia and insulin action were found to have trimodal distributions in Pima Indians. Such distributions could have been produced by single major genes having codominant effects.

Segregation analysis has also been used to study the mode of inheritance of insulinemia and insulin action. The goal of segregation analysis is to evaluate the distribution of phenotypes within families to assess whether it is consistent with the effects of a single, cosegregating locus. This type of analysis is used to detect the effects of single genes with relatively large effects on phenotypic variation, while simultaneously adjusting for the effects of age, sex, environmental influences, and polygenic background.

Segregation analyses in two different pedigree studies have provided support for single loci that have relatively large effects on insulin concentrations. Schumacher et al. *(24)* performed a complex segregation analysis of insulin concentration in 16 Caucasian families. The families were selected because at least two siblings had been previously diagnosed with Type 2 diabetes mellitus. Two hundred and seventy-one subjects with normal glucose tolerance were included in the segregation analyses. These analyses

Table 1
Genes Associated with Insulin Resistance
and/or Insulin Concentrations

Gene	Reference
Fatty acid binding protein 2 (FABP2)	(27,28)
β-3 adrenergic receptor (B3AR)	(41,47,48)
Insulin receptor substrate 1 (IRS1)	(42,49)
Angiotensin I-converting enzyme (ACE)	(43,50)
Lipoprotein lipase (LPL)	(44)
Insulin (INS)	(45)
Tumor necrosis factor alpha (TNFα)	(46)

suggested the presence of major genes for both fasting insulin concentration and insulin concentration 1 h following an oral glucose challenge. Approximately 33% of the total variance in fasting insulin could be apportioned to the major gene and an additional 11% to polygenic inheritance. In the case of 1-h insulin concentration, 48% of the variation could be apportioned to the major gene and an additional 4% to polygenic inheritance.

Several years later, Mitchell et al., (25) performed a complex segregation analysis of insulin concentrations in 42 Mexican American families from San Antonio, Texas. Unlike the Utah study, these Mexican American families were randomly ascertained, i.e., not ascertained on a specific disease phenotype. Evidence was found for a major gene influencing insulin concentrations measured two hours following an oral glucose challenge. The putative major gene accounted for 31% of the population variance in this trait.

LINKAGE OF INSULIN RESISTANCE TO CANDIDATE GENES AND CHROMOSOMAL REGIONS

Candidate Gene Studies

The number of candidate genes that could potentially influence insulin action is legion. Both the insulin signaling pathway and the processes of glucose uptake and metabolism involve numerous proteins, any one of which could have variants capable of influencing insulin sensitivity. Thus, all of the genes that code for these proteins are potential candidate genes for insulin resistance (26). Numerous association studies have been performed to evaluate whether any of the genes currently known to play a role in these processes influences insulin sensitivity. As discussed at the beginning of this chapter, a number of mutations of the insulin receptor gene have been identified which have extreme effects on insulin resistance. The frequency of these mutations, however, is thought to be low. Linkage studies utilizing highly polymorphic markers with high heterozygosity, e.g., microsatellite markers, can be used to establish linkage to a particular candidate gene across multiple pedigrees, even when different mutations of the candidate gene are segregating in the different pedigrees. Thus far, linkage studies of this type have not suggested a major role for the insulin receptor gene in producing insulin resistance in the general population.

In addition to the insulin receptor gene, a number of other candidate genes have also been reported to be associated with insulin resistance (see Table 1). For nearly all of these genes, however, no consensus has emerged regarding their relative role, if any, in producing insulin resistance. In nearly all cases, additional studies of the candidate gene polymorphisms in other populations failed to replicate the initial findings, and in some cases, significant associations were observed only in subgroups of the population (e.g., in obese individuals).

One gene for which reasonably consistent results have been reported is the fatty acid binding protein 2 (*FABP2*), which is expressed in the small intestine. This protein contains a single ligand binding site that displays a high affinity for both saturated and unsaturated long-chain fatty acids. Evidence that genetic variation at the *FABP2* locus might play a role in insulin resistance was first reported by Prochazka et al. *(27)*, who performed a sib-pair linkage analysis of insulin resistance in nondiabetic Pima Indians. Insulin resistance was assessed by euglycemic clamp in 123 pairs of nondiabetic siblings. Siblings who shared both alleles along a region of chromosome 4q26–31 had more similar fasting insulin concentrations and maximal insulin action than siblings who shared only one or no alleles in this region ($p < 0.001$). In Mexican Americans, Mitchell et al. *(28)* performed a combined segregation and linkage analysis of 2-h insulin concentration and found evidence for linkage of this trait to a microsatellite marker tightly linked to the *FABP2* locus (lod score = 2.8). The best-fitting model indicated that this locus accounted for 32% of the total phenotypic variability in 2-h insulin concentrations. A variant in the *FABP2* gene has recently been identified by Baier et al. *(29)* that appears to be associated with insulin resistance. This variant is characterized by a substitution of threonine for alanine in codon 54 of the gene. The threonine-containing variant is relatively common in the population, occurring in about 30% of both Pima Indians and Caucasians. This allele is associated in vivo with higher concentrations of fasting insulin, an increased rate of fat oxidation, and a decreased rate of insulin-stimulated glucose uptake as measured by the euglycemic clamp technique. Moreover, the threonine-containing protein has a twofold higher affinity for long-chain fatty acids than the alanine-containing protein.

In contrast to the aforementioned results, no associations were observed in three European populations (Finland, UK, and Wales) between either insulinemia or insulin resistance as assessed by the homeostasis model Matthews et al. *(21),* and a trinucleotide repeat polymorphism linked to the *FABP2* gene *(30)*. When data from the three populations were pooled, however, a significant association was noted between one of the alleles and Type 2 diabetes. It is important to emphasize that this study analyzed associations in unrelated individuals, rather than linkage in related individuals. Even if a functional variant of the *FABP2* gene contributed to insulin resistance, associations of this type would not be detected unless the marker which was tested was in linkage disequilibrium with the functional site.

Chromosomal Regions Linked to Insulin Resistance

In addition to the candidate gene approach, efforts have been made to screen the entire genome to identify chromosomal regions which may harbor genes that influence insulin resistance. These genome-wide scans make use of microsatellite markers more or less evenly spaced throughout the genome. A region on chromosome 3q23–24 has been linked to low M values and 2-h insulin concentrations in Pima Indians *(31)* and to glucose values in Mexican Americans *(32)*. In addition, a region on chromosome 7q21–25 has been linked to both fasting and 2-h insulin concentrations in Pima Indians *(31)* and a region on chromosome 1p32–22 has been linked to insulin levels and various measures of body fat in the Quebec Family Study *(33)*. The identity of the genes within these regions influencing insulin resistance is as yet not known.

THE INSULIN RESISTANCE SYNDROME

It is well established that insulin resistance clusters with a large number of other traits, among them: hyperinsulinemia, presumably a compensatory response to the insulin resistance; obesity, particularly, abdominal obesity; hypertension; and dyslipidemia of the high triglyceride, low high-density lipoprotein (HDL) cholesterol type. This cluster of traits has been referred to as the Insulin Resistance Syndrome (IRS). Although not originally described as part of the syndrome, a number of other traits also cluster with the IRS. These include microalbuminuria, small dense low-density lipoprotein (LDL) cholesterol, plasminogen activator inhibitor-1, and perhaps others. Some of this clustering may have a genetic basis, although the support for this hypothesis is indirect. Prospective studies have revealed that both insulin resistance and most, if not all, of the other elements of the IRS are predictive of future diabetes, reviewed by Stern (34). In the following sections we will discuss techniques for analyzing clusters and for assessing the extent to which the elements of clusters have common genetic determinants (pleiotropy).

Analysis of Clusters

Most analyses of the IRS have been based on pairwise correlations between various elements of the syndrome. However, more sophisticated statistical techniques such as factor analysis are also available for analyzing clusters. These techniques permit one to assess the extent to which a cluster is produced by a single underlying "factor" which ties together *all* elements of the cluster, or by two or more underlying "factors" which tie together subsets of the variables in the overall cluster. The clusters or subclusters that are identified can then be used as phenotypes in genetic analysis, including linkage analysis.

Edwards et al. (35) used factor analysis to analyze data from the Kaiser Permanente Women Twins Study. One twin was selected at random from each pair for the initial analysis and the results were subsequently confirmed on the remaining twins. Ten correlated variables were included in the analysis and these were reduced to three uncorrelated factors. The three factors each accounted for approximately 22% of the overall variance in the data. The first factor reflected primarily body fat distribution along with measures of glucose and insulin metabolism, the second, glucose and insulin metabolism plus blood pressure, and the third, primarily dyslipidemia, including LDL particle size. In a later paper, Edwards et al. (36) took advantage of the monozygotic and dizygotic twin data to estimate the heritability of these factors using three techniques: the classical approach; analysis of variance; and the maximum likelihood approach. All three factors showed statistically significant heritability. For Factor 1 the heritability estimates were 61, 14, and 71%, respectively, by the three methods. For Factor 2 the heritability estimates ranged from 57 to 92%, and for Factor 3, from 25 to 32%.

Data from the Framingham Offspring Study were also subjected to factor analysis (37), and the results were in general similar to those from the Kaiser Study, albeit with certain differences. Again three factors were identified, each accounting for between 17 and 21% of the overall variance. The first two factors were quite similar to the factors identified in the Kaiser Study, except that, along with measures of body fat distribution, dyslipidemia appeared to cluster with Factor 1 in the Framingham Study, and, unlike the Kaiser Study, blood pressure did not cluster with Factor 2. Factor 3 appeared to be primarily a blood pressure factor in the Framingham Study, rather than a dyslipidemia factor as in the Kaiser Study. In the Framingham Study the results were quite similar in men and women. Heritability of these factors are not currently available.

The results of these studies using factor analysis imply that the IRS cannot be explained by a single underlying pathological mechanism, since if it could, only a single factor would be expected *(37)*. Thus, there may be separate genetic and environmental determinants for the various factors. A possible strategy for illuminating the genetic determinants of the IRS might be to use these factors as phenotypes in a linkage study. The factor analyses previously presented were based on phenotypic correlations. In principle it would be possible to base such analyses on genetic correlations (*see* sections on "Pleiotropy" and "Quantitative Genetic Studies"). Factors derived in this way would presumably be more genetically homogeneous, and might, therefore, be more suitable for linkage analysis.

Pleiotropy

Traits may cluster together because they share either genetic or environmental determinants. If family data are available, one can attempt to distinguish between these two alternatives by disaggregating the usual phenotypic correlations into genetic correlations and environmental correlations. Pleiotropy refers to the genetic effects that arise when a single gene influences more than one trait. For example, if insulin resistance leads to compensatory hyperinsulinemia, a gene that influences insulin resistance could also influence insulinemia. Conversely, if cigaret smoking produces both emphysema and bladder cancer, a higher rate of bladder cancer among emphysema patients could result from the shared environmental exposure even if the traits had no genetic determinants in common. If traits are more highly correlated in related than unrelated individuals, particularly if the degree of correlation parallels the kinship relationships among the related individuals, pleiotropy is suggested. Conversely, if the degree of correlation between individuals is unrelated to their kinship relationships, an environmental basis for the correlation is suggested. In the next two sections we will discuss studies in which family data have been used to assess genetic and environmental correlations between various elements of the IRS. We will also discuss studies in which formal tests of pleiotropy between traits have been evaluated.

Quantitative Genetic Studies

Family and twin studies have revealed that there are strong heritable components to lipids and lipoproteins, blood pressure, and obesity *(22,38)*. In the San Antonio Family Heart Study, the additive effects of genes accounted for 35–40% of the total variability in triglyceride and total, HDL, and LDL cholesterol concentrations, 42% of the variability in BMI, and 20–30% of the variability in systolic and diastolic blood pressure *(39)*. Since genes also contribute significantly to variation in insulin concentration in this population (35 and 13% for fasting and 2-h insulin concentrations, respectively), the question of whether the same or different genes influence variation in this constellation of traits arises.

The degree of pleiotropy between genes influencing insulin concentrations and genes influencing other cardiovascular risk factors has been estimated from several different family studies. In the San Antonio Family Heart Study, Mitchell et al. *(39)* estimated the genetic correlations between insulin and other Insulin Resistance Syndrome-related traits in order to evaluate the extent to which different traits (e.g., insulin and BMI) might be influenced by the same genes. Fasting insulin concentrations were significantly genetically correlated with BMI ($r = 0.49$), with HDL cholesterol ($r = -0.36$), and with triglycerides ($r = 0.30$). These results can be interpreted as indicating that shared genes accounted for 24% of the additive genetic variance in insulin and body mass index, 13% of the additive genetic variance in insulin and HDL cholesterol, and 9% of the additive genetic variance in insulin and triglycerides. The genetic correlation of fasting insulin with both systolic and diastolic blood pressure was not significantly different from zero, providing no evidence for pleiotropy between fasting insulin and blood pressure. Parallel analyses performed using the 2-h insulin measurement similarly provided evidence for pleiotropy with body mass index, HDL cholesterol, and triglycerides, but not with blood pressure.

Major Gene Effects on IRS

Because segregation analysis suggested the presence of a major gene influencing 2-h insulin concentrations in San Antonio Family Heart Study subjects, Mitchell et al. *(39)* addressed the question of whether that particular locus had pleiotropic effects on any other traits. Using bivariate segregation analysis, they found that individuals predicted to have the allele associated with high 2-h insulin concentrations were significantly more likely to have higher levels of fasting insulin ($p = 0.02$), but, surprisingly, significantly *lower* levels of BMI ($p = 0.05$). There was no evidence for pleiotropy between 2-h insulin concentrations and any of the lipid measures or blood pressure. Thus, these analyses provided no evidence that the pleiotropy between insulin and body mass index, HDL cholesterol, and triglycerides was attributable to the 2-h insulin major gene previously detected through segregation analysis. This result does not preclude the possibility of pleiotropy between other hyperinsulinemia genes and the various IRS traits.

The contribution of genetic and environmental influences to the clustering of the metabolic factors which comprise the IRS was also examined by Hong et al. *(40)* in their study of 289 pairs of elderly twins from the Swedish Adoption/Twin Study. Unlike the study by Mitchell et al. *(39)*, these investigators estimated not only the pairwise genetic correlations between traits, but also allowed for genetic effects that could simultaneously influence more than two traits. Insulin resistance was defined by the homeostasis model *(21)*. The best fitting model included a common genetic factor that accounted for 52, 39, 11, 10, and 6% of the variability in BMI, insulin resistance, triglycerides, HDL cholesterol, and systolic blood pressure, respectively. Environmental factors also accounted for a substantial portion of the variation in these traits, and a trait-specific genetic loading also accounted for a substantial portion of the variation in triglycerides, HDL cholesterol, and systolic blood pressure.

CONCLUSIONS

Substantial evidence exists that insulin resistance is under genetic control. Many studies have confirmed that both insulinemia and insulin resistance are elevated in non-diabetic relatives of diabetic subjects. Studies of twins and extended pedigrees have generated heritability estimates of 66% for insulin resistance and 35–54% for insulinemia. Moreover, there is evidence that major genes account for at least some of this heritability. Efforts to identify these genes, however, have thus far met with limited success. Although over 50 mutations of the insulin receptor gene have been identified, these appear to be rare causes of insulin resistance. The most consistent results have been observed with the fatty acid binding protein-2 (*FABP2*) which has been linked to insulinemia and insulin resistance in several populations. Negative results, however, have also been reported for this gene. Genome scans have also been used to search for linkage of insulinemia and insulin resistance to chromosomal regions. A number of promising linkages have been reported, although, thus far, the genes responsible for these linkages have not been identified.

Insulin resistance also clusters with a number of other diabetes and cardiovascular risk factors, among them obesity, particularly central obesity, dyslipidemia, and hypertension. This clustering has been referred to as the Insulin Resistance Syndrome (IRS). Evidence for pleiotropy between various elements of the IRS has been reported indicating the existence of genes that influence two or more phenotypic features of the syndrome. These genes too remain to be identified.

REFERENCES

1. Hollenbeck C, Reaven GM. Variations in insulin-stimulated glucose uptake in healthy individuals with normal glucose tolerance. J Clin Endocrinol Metab 1987;64:1169–1173.
2. Hone J, Accili D, Al-Gazali LI, Lestringant G, Orban T, Taylor SI. Homozygosity for a new mutation (Ile^{119} → Met) in the insulin receptor gene in five sibs with familial insulin resistance. J Med Genet 1994;31:715–716.
3. Taylor SI, Cama A, Accili D, Barbetti F, Quon MJ, de la Luz Sierra M, Suzuki Y, Koller E, Levy-Toledano R, Wertheimer E et al. Mutations in the insulin receptor gene. Endocrin Rev 1992; 13:566–595.
4. Accili D, Cama A, Barbetti F, Kadowaki H, Kadowaki T, Taylor SI. Insulin resistance due to mutations of the insulin receptor gene: an overview. J Endocrinol Invest 1992;15:857–864.
5. Taylor SI. Lilly Lecture: molecular mechanisms of insulin resistance. Lessons from patients with mutations in the insulin-receptor gene. Diabetes 1992;41:1473–490.
6. Muller-Wieland D, Taub R, Tewari DS, Kriauciunas KM, Sethu S, Reddy K, Kahn CR. Insulin-receptor gene and its expression in patients with insulin resistance. Diabetes 1989;38:31–38.
7. Haffner SM, Stern MP, Hazuda HP, Mitchell BD, Patterson JK. Increased insulin concentrations in nondiabetic offspring of diabetic parents. New Eng J Med 1988;319:1297–1301.
8. Elbein SC, Maxwell TM, Schumacher MC. Insulin and glucose levels and prevalence of glucose intolerance in pedigrees with multiple diabetic siblings. Diabetes 1991;40:1024–32.
9. Warram JH, Martin BC, Krolewski AS, Soeldner JS, Kahn CR. Slow glucose removal rate and hyperinsulinemia precede the development of Type II diabetes in the offspring of diabetic parents. Ann Int Med 1990;113:909–915.
10. Bergman RN, Prager R, Volund A, Olefsky J. Equivalence of the insulin sensitivity index in man derived by the minimal model method and the euglycemic glucose clamp. J Clin Invest 1987;79:790–800.
11. Osei K, Cottrell DA, Orabella MM. Insulin sensitivity, glucose effectiveness, and body fat distribution pattern in nondiabetic offspring of patients with NIDDM. Diabetes Care 1991;14:890–896.
12. Johnston C, Ward WK, Beard JC, McKnight B, Porte D. Islet function and insulin sensitivity in nondiabetic offspring of conjugal Type 2 diabetic patients. Diabetic Med 1990;7:119–125.
13. Eriksson J, Franssila-Kallunki A, Ekstrand A, Saloranta C, Widén E, Schalin C, Groop L. Early metabolic defects in persons at increased risk for non-insulin-dependent diabetes mellitus. New Eng J Med 1989;321:337–343.
14. Gulli G, Ferrannini E, Stern M, Haffner S, DeFronzo RA. The metabolic profile of NIDDM is fully established in glucose-tolerant offspring of two Mexican-American NIDDM parents. Diabetes 1992;41:1575–1586.
15. O'Rahilly SP, Nugent Z, Rudenski AS, Hosker JP, Burnett MA, Darling P, Turner RC. Beta-cell dysfunction, rather than insulin insensitivity, is the primary defect in familial Type 2 diabetes. Lancet 1986;2:360–364.
16. Ho LT, Chang ZY, Wang JT, Li SH, Liu YF, Chen Y-DI, Reaven GM. Insulin insensitivity in offspring of parents with Type 2 diabetes mellitus. Diabetic Med 1989;7:31–34.
17. Martin BC, Warram JH, Rosner B, Rich SS, Soeldner JS, Krolewski AS. Family clustering of insulin sensitivity. Diabetes 1992;41:850–854.
18. Lillioja S, Mott DM, Zawadzki JK, Young AA, Abbott WGH, Knowler WC, Bennett PH, Moll P, Bogardus C. In vivo insulin action is familial characteristic in nondiabetic Pima Indians. Diabetes 1987;36:1329–1335.

19. Mayer EJ, Newman B, Austin MA, Zhang D, Quesenberry CP, Edwards K, Selby JV. Genetic and environmental influences on insulin levels and the insulin resistance syndrome: an analysis of women twins. Am J Epidemiol 1996;143:323–332.

20. Narkiewicz K, Chrostowska M, Kuchta G, Szczech R, Welz A, Rynkiewicz A, Lysiak-Szydlowska W, Pawlowski R, Krupa-Wojciechowska B. Genetic influences on insulinemia in normotensive twins. Am J Hypertens 1997;10(4 Pt 1):467–470.

21. Matthews DR, Hosker JP, Rudenski AS, Naylor BA, Treacher DF, Turner RC. Homeostasis model assessment: insulin resistance and β-cell function from fasting plasma glucose and insulin concentrations in man. Diabetologia 1985;28:412–419.

22. Mitchell BD, Kammerer CM, Blangero J, Mahaney MC, Rainwater DL, Dyke B, Hixson JE, Henkel RD, Sharp MR, Comuzzie AG, VandeBerg JL, Stern MP, MacCluer JW. Genetic and environmental contributions to cardiovascular risk factors in Mexican Americans: The San Antonio Family Heart Study. Circulation 1996;94:2159–2170.

23. Bogardus C, Lillioja S, Nyomba BL, Zurlo F, Swinburn B, Esposito-Del Puente A, Knowler WC, Ravussin E, Mott DM, Bennett PH. Distribution of in vivo insulin action in Pima Indians as mixture of three normal distributions. Diabetes 1989;38:1423–1432.

24. Schumacher MC, Hasstedt SJ, Hunt SC, Williams RR, Elbein SC. Major gene effect for insulin levels in familial NIDDM pedigrees. Diabetes 1992;41:416–423.

25. Mitchell BD, Kammerer CM, Hixson JE, Atwood LD, Hackleman S, Blangero J, Haffner SM, Stern MP, MacCluer JW. Evidence for a major gene affecting post-challenge insulin levels in Mexican Americans. Diabetes 1995;44:284–289.

26. Moller DE, Bjorbaek C, Vidal-Puig A. Candidate genes for insulin resistance. Diabetes Care 1996;19:396–400.

27. Prochazka M, Lillioja S, Tait JF, Knowler WC, Mott DM, Spraul M, Bennett PH, Bogardus C. Linkage of chromosomal markers on 4q with a putative gene determining maximal insulin action in Pima Indians. Diabetes 1993;42:514–519.

28. Mitchell BD, Kammerer CM, O'Connell P, Harrison CR, Manire M, Shipman P, Moyer M, Stern MP, Frazier ML. Evidence for linkage of post-challenge insulin levels with intestinal fatty acid binding protein (FABP2) in Mexican Americans. Diabetes 1995;44:1046–1053.

29. Baier LJ, Sacchettini JC, Knowler WC, Eads J, Paolisso G, Tataranni PA, Mochizuki H, Bennett PH, Bogardus C, Prochazka M. An amino acid substitution in the human intestinal fatty acid binding protein is associated with increased fatty acid binding, increased fat oxidation, and insulin resistance. J Clin Invest 1995;95:1281–1287.

30. Humphreys P, McCarthy M, Tuomilehto J, Tuomilehto-Wolf E, Stratton I, Morgan R, Rees A, Owens D, Stengard J, Nissinen A et al. Chromosome 4q locus associated with insulin resistance in Pima Indians. Studies in three European NIDDM populations. Diabetes 1994;43:800–804.

31. Pratley R, Thompson DB, Prochazka M, Baier L, Pima Diabetes Gene Group. A genome scan for linkage to quantitative traits predicting NIDDM in Pima Indians. Diabetes 1997;46(suppl 1):170A (abstract).

32. Mitchell BD, Blangero J, Cole SA, Schneider J, Stern MP, MacCluer JW, Hixson JE. Linkage of glucose levels to markers on chromosome 3q in Mexican Americans. Am J Hum Genet ;1997;61(suppl) A286 (abstract).

33. Chagnon YC, Perusse L, Lamothe M, Chagnon M, Nadeau A, Dionne FT, Gagnon J, Chung WK, Leibel RL, Bouchard C. Suggestive linkages between markers on human 1p32–p22 and body fat and insulin levels in the Quebec Family Study. Obes Res 5:115–21, 1997.

34. Stern MP. Perspectives in Diabetes. Diabetes and cardiovascular disease: the "common soil" hypothesis. Diabetes 1995;44:369–374.

35. Edwards KL, Austin MA, Newman B, Mayer E, Krauss RM, Selby JV. Multivariate analysis of the insulin resistance syndrome in women. Arterioscl Thromb 1994;14:1940–1945.

36. Edwards KL, Newman B, Mayer E, Selby JV, Krauss RM, Austin MA. Heritability of factors of the insulin resistance syndrome in women twins. Genet Epidemiol 1997;14:241–253.

37. Meigs JB, D'Agostino RB, Wilson PWF, Cupples A, Nathan DM, Singer DE. Risk variable clustering in the Insulin Resistance Syndrome. The Framingham Offspring Study. Diabetes 1997;46:1594–1600.

38. Peyser PA. Genetic epidemiology of coronary artery disease. Epidemiol Rev 1997;19:80–90.

39. Mitchell BD, Kammerer CM, Mahaney MC, Blangero J, Comuzzie AG, Atwood LD, Haffner SM, Stern MP, MacCluer JW. Genetic analysis of the IRS: pleiotropic effects of genes influencing insulin levels on lipoprotein and obesity measures. Arterioscl Thromb Vasc Biol 1996;16:281–288.

40. Hong Y, Pedersen NL, Brismar K, de Faire U. Genetic and environmental architecture of the features of the insulin-resistance syndrome. Am J Hum Genet 1997;60:143–152.

41. Widén E, Lehto M, Kannen T, Walston J, Shuldiner AR, Groop LC. Association of a polymorphism in the β_3-adrenergic-receptor-gene with features of the insulin resistance syndrome in Finns. New Eng J Med 1995;333:348–351.

42. Clausen JO, Hansen T, Bjorbaek C, Echwald SM, Urhammer SA, Rasmussen S, Andersen CB, Hansen L, Almind K, Winther K et al. Insulin resistance: interactions between obesity and a common variant of insulin receptor substrate-1. Lancet 1995;346:397–402.

43. Chiu KC, McCarthy JE. The insertion allele at the angiotensin I-converting enzyme gene locus is associated with insulin resistance. Metabolism 1997;46:395–399.

44. Cole SA, Aston CE, Hamman RF, Ferrell RE. Association of a PvuII RFLP at the lipoprotein lipase locus with fasting insulin levels in Hispanic men. Genet Epidemiol 1993;10:177–188.

45. Haneda M, Polonsky KS, Bergenstal RM, Jaspan JB, Shoelson SE, Blix PM, Chan SJ, Kwok SC, Wishner WB, Zeidler A et al. Familial hyperinsulinemia due to a structurally abnormal insulin. Definition of an emerging new clinical syndrome. N Engl J Med 1984;310:1288–1294.

46. Fernandez-Real JM, Gutierrez C, Ricart W, Casamitjana R, Fernandez-Castaner M, Vendrell J, Richart C, Soler J. The TNF-alpha gene Nco I polymorphism influences the relationship among insulin resistance, percent body fat, and increased serum leptin levels. Diabetes 1997;46:1468–1472.

47. Sakane N, Yoshida T, Umekawa T, Kondo M, Sakai Y, Takahashi T. β_3-adrenergic receptor polymorphism: a genetic marker for visceral fat obesity and the insulin resistance syndrome. Diabetologia 1997;40:200–204.

48. Urhammer SA, Clausen JO, Hansen T, Pederson O. Insulin sensitivity and body weight changes in young carriers of the codon 64 amino acid polymorphism of the β-3-adrenergic receptor gene. Diabetes 1996;45:1115–1120.

49. Zhang Y, Wat N, Stratton IM, Warren-Perry MG, Orho M, Groop L, Turner RC. UKPDS 19: Heterogeneity in NIDDM: separate contributions of IRS–1 and β3-adrenergic-receptor mutations to insulin resistance and obesity respectively with no evidence for glycogen synthase gene mutations. UK Prospective Diabetes Study. Diabetologia 1996;39:1505–1511.

50. Katsuya T, Horiuchi M, Chen YD, Koike G, Pratt RE, Dzau VJ, Reaven GM. Relations between deletion polymorphism of the angiotensin-converting enzyme gene and insulin resistance, glucose intolerance, hyperinsulinemia, and dyslipidemia. Arterioscl Thromb Vasc Biol 1995;15:779–782.

2

Ethnic Variation in Insulin Resistance and Risk of Type 2 Diabetes

Paul M. McKeigue, MB, PhD

CONTENTS

INTRODUCTION
ETHNIC VARIATION IN PREVALENCE OF DIABETES
SOUTH ASIANS
PENINSULAR ARABS
NATIVE AMERICANS AND MEXICAN-AMERICANS
NATIVE AUSTRALIANS
WEST AFRICANS
SUMMARY INTERPRETATION
REFERENCES

INTRODUCTION

Prevalence of Type 2 diabetes varies more than tenfold between high- and low-risk populations. Studies of migrants and admixed populations indicate that this ethnic variation in diabetes risk depends upon the interaction of environmental factors that influence obesity with genetic factors that influence insulin sensitivity. Although insulin resistance is common to all populations at high risk of diabetes, the disturbances of lipid metabolism and body fat pattern that accompany insulin resistance vary between these populations. In Native Americans and Pacific islanders, insulin resistance and obesity are associated with high plasma triglyceride but low plasma cholesterol levels. In Peninsular Arabs, glucose intolerance is associated with raised plasma total cholesterol and apolipoprotein B, as well as raised plasma triglyceride. In South Asians, insulin resistance is associated with high rates of coronary disease, raised plasma triglyceride, low high-density lipoprotein (HDL) cholesterol, alterations in low density lipoproteins (LDL) subfraction pattern, and central obesity. In West Africans, prevalence of diabetes and insulin resistance are almost as high as in South Asians, but plasma triglyceride levels are lower and HDL cholesterol levels are higher than in weight-matched Europeans. This favorable lipid pattern may account for the low coronary heart disease risk in men of West African descent compared with European men of similar socioeconomic status.

From: *Contemporary Endocrinology: Insulin Resistance*
Edited by: G. Reaven and A. Laws © Humana Press Inc., Totowa, NJ

Table 1
Ethnic Variation in Prevalence of Type 2 Diabetes

	Prevalence (age 30–64)	*Risk ratio (Northern Europeans = 1)*
Pima Native Americans	50%	12
Nauruans	40%	10
Native Australians	25%	6
Peninsular Arabs	25%	6
South Asians	20%	5
West Africans	12%	3
Northern Europeans	4%	1

The metabolic mechanisms underlying this ethnic variation in insulin resistance are not understood. Studies of ethnic variation in the storage and metabolism of lipids in adipocytes and muscle cells may contribute to understanding the basis of ethnic variation in insulin resistance.

ETHNIC VARIATION IN PREVALENCE OF DIABETES

Table 1 summarizes the results of studies in the World Health Organization (WHO) database of prevalence surveys based on the 1980 criteria for diabetes. Prevalence rates are highest in Pima Native Americans and Nauruan islanders, slightly lower in Native Australians and Peninsular Arabs, moderately high in South Asians and West Africans, and lowest of all in northern European populations.

Relation to Insulin Resistance and Obesity

This ethnic variation in prevalence of diabetes is paralleled by variation in insulin resistance. Mean plasma insulin levels in the fasting state or after a glucose load in nondiabetic individuals are consistently higher in populations at high risk of Type 2 diabetes than in northern Europeans. Direct measurement of insulin resistance by methods such as the euglycemic clamp or the insulin suppression test have confirmed that these ethnic differences in fasting or post-load insulin levels represent ethnic differences in insulin resistance.

Populations that have high rates of Type 2 diabetes are generally living in urban (Tables 2 and 3) societies where physical activity is low and mean energy intake is high. Where it has been possible to compare such a high-risk population with a lean, physically active low-income rural (Tables 2 and 3) population from the same ethnic group, prevalence of diabetes has generally been found to be far lower in the low-income rural population than in the high-risk urban population. Thus, for instance, prevalence of diabetes in Pima Native Americans living in Arizona is six times higher than in people from the same ethnic group living in Maycoba in rural Mexico, where the mean body mass index (BMI) is about 8 kg/m^2 less *(1)*. In the Indian state of Tamil Nadu, prevalence of diabetes is four times higher in the city of Madras than in a rural area where mean BMI is about 5 kg/m^2 less *(2)*.

Although within each high-risk population the associations of glucose intolerance and insulin resistance with raised plasma triglyceride levels, low HDL cholesterol, small dense LDL particles, hypertension and central obesity are generally in the same direction,

Table 2
Diabetes in Pima Adults in USA and Rural Mexico

	Arizona		Maycoba	
	Men	Women	Men	Women
Diabetes prevalence (%)	54	37	8	6
BMI (kg m^{-2})	30.8	35.5	24.8	25.1
Plasma cholesterol(mmol/L)	4.7	4.3	3.7	3.8

Table 3
Diabetes in Urban and Rural Tamils

	Urban		Rural	
	Men	Women	Men	Women
Diabetes prevalence (%)	8.4	7.9	2.6	1.6
BMI (kg m^{-2})	22.5	23.4	17.6	18.7
Household income (US $/month)	158	156	14	12

the balance between these disturbances of lipid and carbohydrate metabolism varies markedly between different populations at high risk of Type 2 diabetes, as reviewed in detail below. This may be relevant to understanding why some, but not all, populations at high risk of Type 2 diabetes are at high risk of coronary heart disease (CHD).

SOUTH ASIANS

Large-scale migration from South Asia to other countries has occurred during the last 160 years. The first report of high prevalence of diabetes in South Asian migrants was from Saigon in 1913 *(3)*. Table 4 summarizes the results of recent surveys in South Asian populations that have used glucose tolerance tests and WHO criteria for the diagnosis of diabetes. The prevalence rates of about 20% in men and women aged over 35 years are remarkably consistent between overseas South Asian populations *(4–9)* and urban populations in South Asia itself *(2,10,11)*. A much lower prevalence rate—3% in the age group 45–64 years—was recorded in a rural South Asian population *(2)*.

Elevated fasting and post-load insulin levels in nondiabetic South Asians compared with Europeans were first reported from South Africa *(12,13)*, and subsequently from England *(4,14)*. Table 5 summarizes the results of a large survey comparing prevalence of diabetes and associated coronary risk factors in South Asians and Europeans in London, England *(4)*. Geometric mean 2-h insulin levels are twice as high in nondiabetic South Asians as in Europeans *(4)*. A study comparing South Asians and Europeans resident in the San Francisco area has demonstrated that this ethnic difference in post-load insulin levels represents an ethnic difference in insulin resistance *(15)*. Mean steady-state plasma glucose during the insulin suppression test was approximately 60% higher in South Asians than in weight-matched Europeans. This is comparable to the difference in insulin resistance observed when patients with Type 2 diabetes are compared with weight-matched controls. As in other populations, the higher average insulin resistance in South Asians compared with Europeans is accompanied by higher mean plasma trig-

Table 4
Prevalence of Noninsulin Dependent Diabetes in South Asians

Year	Place	Age	Prevalence	Reference
South Asians overseas				
1977	Trinidad	35–69	21%	5
1983	Fiji	35–64	25%	6
1985	South Africa	30–	22%	7
1990	Singapore	40–69	25%	8
1990	Mauritius	35–64	20%	9
1991	England	40–69	19%	4
India				
1985	Urban Karnataka	45–64	29%	10
1992	Urban Madras	45–64	18%	2
1992	Rural Tamil Nadu	45–64	3%	2
1994	Pakistan			11
Prevalence in Europeans, for comparison				
1991	London	40–69	4%	4

Table 5
Mean Levels of Coronary Risk Factors in South Asians and Europeans
in the Southall Study[a]

	Men			Women	
	European	South Asian	Afro-Caribbean	European	South Asian
BMI (kg/m^2)	25.9	25.7	26.3	25.2	27.0
Waist/hip girth ratio	0.94	0.98	0.94	0.76	0.85
Median systolic BP (mmHg)	121	126	128	120	126
Diabetes prevalence	5%	20%	15%	2%	16%
2-h Insulin (mU/L)	19	41	22	21	44
Total cholesterol (mmol/L)	6.1	6.0	5.9	6.3	6.0
HDL cholesterol (mmol/L)	1.25	1.16	1.37	1.58	1.38
2 h Triglyceride (mmol/L)	1.39	1.72	0.99	1.01	1.27

[a]Adapted from ref. *4*.

lyceride levels and lower HDL cholesterol levels *(4,14)*. Between fasting and 2 h after a glucose load, plasma triglyceride levels fall less in South Asians than in Europeans; thus the ethnic differences in mean plasma triglyceride are larger at 2 h than in the fasting state *(4)*. The fall in plasma triglycerides in response to glucose challenge is likely to be a measure of the ability of insulin to suppress lipolysis in portal fat depots, as nonesterified fatty acids derived from portal fat depots are the main substrate for hepatic triglyceride synthesis. In comparison with Europeans, South Asian men and women have on average a more central distribution of body fat than Europeans, with thicker trunk skinfolds and higher mean waist-hip girth ratios (WHR) for a given level of body mass index *(4,16)*. The difference in mean waist-hip ratio between weight-matched South Asians and Europeans of the same sex is equivalent to about two-thirds of one standard deviation *(4)*.

Table 6
Mortality from CHD in South Asians Overseas

		Groups contrasted	Age	CHD mortality ratio	Reference
Singapore	1980–86	S. Asian/Chinese	30–69	3.8	17
Fiji	1980	S. Asian/Melanesian	40–59	3.0	18
Trinidad	1977–86	S. Asian/African	35–69	2.4	5
South Africa	1985	S. Asian/European	35–74	1.4	19
England	1990–93	S. Asian/European	20–69	1.5	20

Table 7
What Features of the Insulin Resistance Syndrome are Common
to all South Asian Groups at High Risk of CHD?

Common to all S. Asian populations at risk	Not common to all S. Asian populations at risk
Central obesity	High blood pressure (not Muslims)
Hyperinsulinemia	Low HDL cholesterol (not Sikhs)
High diabetes prevalence	High fasting triglyceride (not Gujarati Hindus)
High post-glucose triglyceride	

Adjusting for anthropometric measures of body fat pattern however does not fully account for the ethnic differences in diabetes prevalence and insulin levels (4).

Relationship of Coronary Risk to Insulin Resistance in South Asians

Mortality from CHD is higher in South Asians overseas than in other groups settled in the same countries (5,17–20) (Table 6). In comparison with high-risk populations such as Europeans in South Africa or England, the relative risk for CHD mortality associated with South Asian origin is about 1.4 (19,20), and in comparison with low-risk groups such as Chinese in Singapore (17) or Africans in Trinidad (5) the relative risk is about 3. In the USA, where most South Asians are recent migrants who are likely to have been selected for fitness, CHD mortality rates are no higher in South Asians than in Europeans (21). Reliable population-based coronary mortality data from South Asia are not available but prevalence surveys suggest that rates of CHD are high in urban populations but low in rural areas (22–25). In England high mortality from CHD is common to all the main groups of migrants from South Asia: Hindus from western India, Sikhs from northern India, and Muslims from Pakistan and Bangladesh (26,27). Thus, any general explanation for the high CHD risk in South Asians must invoke risk factors that are shared by all these groups.

Metabolic disturbances associated with insulin resistance have been suggested as the most likely explanation for the high CHD rates in South Asians compared with other groups (4). This is consistent with the associations of coronary heart disease with glucose intolerance, elevated insulin and triglyceride levels that have been observed in South Asians in cross-sectional (28) and case-control studies (29). In some South Asian groups who share high CHD risk, some of the risk factors associated with insulin resistance are not more unfavorably distributed than in Europeans. These comparisons are summarized in Table 7. In comparison with Europeans, South Asian Muslims do not have higher systolic and diastolic blood pressures, Sikhs do not have lower HDL cholesterol, and

Gujarati Hindus do not have higher fasting triglyceride levels. As high CHD risk is common to all these groups, it follows that the increased CHD risk in South Asians cannot be mediated mainly through raised blood pressure, low HDL cholesterol or raised fasting triglyceride. Common to all South Asian populations at high risk of CHD are central obesity, hyperinsulinemia, high diabetes prevalence and raised triglyceride levels after a glucose load (4,14).

PENINSULAR ARABS

Type 2 diabetes has become a leading cause of adult morbidity in the Arabian Peninsula (30–35). Case-control studies of myocardial infarction suggest that the excess risk associated with diabetes accounts for a high proportion of cases of coronary heart disease in the region (36–38). In three prevalence surveys, the prevalence has ranged from 14% among men and women aged 35–64 years in Oman (33) to more than 30% among men and women aged 40–69 years in Saudi Arabia and Bahrai (39,40). In Bahrainis prevalence of diabetes varied between ethnic groups: age-standardized prevalence in the age group 40–69 years was 25% in Shiite Arabs, 48% in Sunni Arabs, and 23% in Iranians (40). The higher prevalence of diabetes in Sunni Arabs compared with Shiite Arabs or Iranians was not accounted for by obesity or physical activity. As Shiite and Sunni Arabs in Bahrain are descended from different Arabian tribes, it is possible that this ethnic difference has a genetic basis.

Whereas in populations of European descent, glucose intolerance and insulin resistance are generally not associated with raised plasma total cholesterol levels (41,42), in Bahrainis and Kuwaitis glucose intolerance is strongly associated with higher average plasma levels of total cholesterol and apolipoprotein B (apoB) (40,43). This association is unexplained by adjusting for obesity. In Bahrainis, factors that predict diabetes—Sunni Arab ethnic origin and positive family history of diabetes—are associated with raised plasma cholesterol levels even in nondiabetic individuals (40). This suggests that raised cholesterol levels may precede the development of glucose intolerance, perhaps as part of a familial disturbance in Peninsular Arabs consisting of insulin resistance and raised plasma cholesterol levels.

NATIVE AMERICANS AND MEXICAN-AMERICANS

The high prevalence of diabetes in Pimas and other Native American populations has been the focus of considerable research effort. Insulin levels were first reported to be higher in nondiabetic Pimas than in Europeans in 1977 (44). In a study where insulin action was measured in 245 nondiabetic Pimas by euglycemic clamp studies, the distribution of insulin action was found to be trimodal and to fit a mixture of three normal distributions better than one or two normal distributions (45). The authors interpreted this as evidence that a single major gene might account for a high proportion of variance in insulin sensitivity among Pimas. It is not clear, however, whether European admixture was present in any of the Pimas in this study.

Mean BMI in Pimas aged 20–44 years is between 30 and 35 kg m^{-2} (46). Although mean plasma triglyceride levels are, as one would expect, higher in Pimas than in Europeans, mean plasma cholesterol levels are about 0.7 mmol/l lower (46). This is not what one would predict, since plasma cholesterol and triglyceride concentrations are positively correlated within populations. In a tracer study, the proportion of VLDL-apoB that was converted to LDL-apoB was found to be lower and the fractional catabolic rate of LDL-apoB was found to be higher in Pimas than in Europeans *(47)*. This suggests that differences in lipoprotein metabolism may underlie the low plasma cholesterol levels in Pimas. Such differences in lipid metabolism may help to explain why, when stratified by diabetes status, mortality rates from CHD are lower in Pimas than in Europeans *(48)*.

In Mexican-Americans, the proportion of Native American admixture is about 35% *(49)* and the prevalence of diabetes is approximately four times higher than in non-Hispanic Europeans. In a study where admixture of each individual was estimated from nine phenotypic markers, no relation of diabetes to Native American admixture could be estimated *(49)*. Variation in the proportion of European admixture is thought to underlie the inverse association of diabetes with socioeconomic status in Mexican-Americans *(50)*.

Post-load insulin levels are higher in Mexican-Americans than in non-Hispanic Europeans, even after adjusting for obesity *(51)*. A study using the frequently-sampled intravenous glucose tolerance test has confirmed that differences in insulin resistance underlie this ethnic difference in insulin levels *(52)*. The distribution of body fat is more central in Mexican-Americans than in Europeans *(53,54)*. As in other populations at high risk of diabetes, the higher insulin levels are accompanied by higher plasma triglyceride, lower plasma HDL cholesterol and smaller mean LDL particle size *(55)* in Mexican-Americans compared with Europeans.

Age-standardized mortality from CHD among Mexican-American men in Texas is about 20% lower than in non-Hispanic Europeans men *(56)*. In women, CHD mortality in Mexican-Americans is similar to that in non-Hispanic Europeans. A possible explanation for this effect of ethnic origin on the sex difference in CHD risk is that a reduced risk associated with Mexican-American origin is counterbalanced in Mexican-American women by the increased risk associated with obesity.

NATIVE AUSTRALIANS

Prevalence of diabetes is high in all groups of Native Australian descent that have been studied, even in relatively lean rural populations where the mean BMI is less than 23 kg/m^2 *(57,58)*. In Native Australian populations with a more urbanized lifestyle, the prevalence is around 30% in those aged over 35 years *(59)*. Plasma insulin and triglyceride levels are higher and HDL cholesterol levels are lower in Native Australians than in Europeans *(57,60)*. Post-load insulin/glucose ratios are higher in unadmixed Native Australians than in those who have European admixture *(61)*. In a study comparing Native Australians with a family history of diabetes with European controls, the basal hepatic glucose production rate was found to be higher and the rate of clearance of an oral glucose load was found to be lower in Native Australians *(62)*.

As in other populations at high risk of diabetes, average BMI is higher in Native Australian women than in European women, but not much higher in Native Australian men than in European men *(59,63)*. In a small traditionally-orientated group living in a remote area in northeastern Arnhem Land, the mean body mass index in adults was 17 kg/m^2 *(64)*. Despite this very low BMI, mean fasting insulin levels were higher than in European adults with mean BMI of 21 kg/m^2. This suggests that insulin resistance in Native Australians occurs even in very lean individuals, and is not just a complication of obesity.

Table 8
Diabetes Prevalence by WHO Criteria in Afro-Caribbeans and African-Americans

				Prevalence		
	Year	*Sex*	*Age*	*European*	*West African*	*Reference*
Trinidad	1978	M&F	35–69	6%	12%	67
USA	1980	M&F	40–64	10%	18%	66
Southall, UK	1989	M	40–64	5%	14%	4
Brent, UK	1991	M	40–64	7%	13%	68
		F		4%	18%	

Although mortality from circulatory disease is two to three times higher in Native Australians than in the general population of Australia *(65)*, it is difficult to determine whether this can be specifically attributed to risk factors associated with insulin resistance as Native Australians have high mortality from most leading causes of death.

WEST AFRICANS

Among people of West African descent settled in Europe and the Americas, prevalence of Type 2 diabetes is two to three times higher than in Europeans. Table 8 summarizes surveys in Europe and the Americas which have compared prevalence of Type 2 diabetes between West Africans and Europeans using glucose tolerance tests and WHO criteria. The ratio of diabetes prevalence in people of African descent to that in Europeans was 1.8 in the United States *(66)*, 2.4 in Trinidad *(67)* and around 3 in the UK *(4,68)*.

In men average BMI is generally similar in West Africans and Europeans of comparable socioeconomic status, but in women average BMI is generally 2 to 3 kg/m^2 higher in West Africans than in Europeans. Adjusting for obesity does not account for the excess of diabetes in West Africans compared with Europeans *(68)*. Mean fasting and post-load insulin levels are higher in West Africans than in Europeans, even after matching or adjusting for weight-for-height *(68)*. In the Insulin Resistance Atherosclerosis Study, mean insulin sensitivity measured by the frequently-sampled intravenous glucose tolerance test was found to be lower in West Africans than in Europeans *(69)*. However in a recent study where body composition and fat distribution were measured by computed tomography, mean insulin sensitivity was not significantly different between West Africans and Europeans after adjusting for body fat mass and visceral adipose tissue *(70)*.

Lipids and Coronary Risk in West Africans

Studies comparing plasma lipids in West Africans and Europeans have consistently found that West African men have lower plasma triglyceride and higher HDL cholesterol than European men *(68,71,72)*. At 2 h after a glucose load than in the fasting state, plasma triglyceride levels are about 30% lower in Afro-Caribbean than in European men (Table 5). This relatively favorable lipid pattern in West African compared with European men is maintained even in those with glucose intolerance (68,73) (Table 9). The same pattern of ethnic differences has been reported in a comparison of West African and European women in pregnancy *(74)*. In comparisons of West African and European women in older age groups, ethnic differences in plasma lipids are confounded by the ethnic difference

Table 9
Brent Study: Fasting Triglyceride and HDL Cholesterol in Men
by Ethnicity and Glucose Tolerance[a]

	European		Afro-Caribbean
Triglyceride (mmol/L)			
Normoglycemic	1.49	[c]	1.08
Glucose intolerant	1.89	[c]	1.22
HDL cholesterol (mmol/L)			
Normoglycemic	1.36	[c]	1.52
Glucose intolerant	1.25	[b]	1.51

[a]Adapted from ref. *77*.
[b]$p < 0.05$
[c]$p < 0.001$

Table 10
Southall Study: Mean Obesity Indices in Men
by Ethnicity and Glucose Tolerance

	European		South Asian		Afro-Caribbean	
	NG	GI	NG	GI	NG	GI
N	1395	111	1056	352	158	48
BMI (kg/m^2)	25.7	28.2	25.4	26.5	25.8	28.2
WHR	0.93	0.99	0.97	1.00	0.93	0.98
Waist/thigh ratio	1.60	1.71	1.65	1.71	1.52	1.60

BMI = body mass index; NG = normoglycemic; GI = glucose intolerant

in obesity. When adjusted for fat mass and visceral fat, plasma triglyceride is lower and HDL cholesterol is higher in West African than in European women *(70,75)*. The differences in triglyceride and HDL cholesterol levels between West Africans and Europeans are thus in the opposite direction to the differences that we would predict from the higher prevalence of Type 2 diabetes and lower mean insulin sensitivity in West Africans. Within populations of West African descent, however, the correlations of insulin resistance with plasma triglyceride and HDL cholesterol levels have been found to be similar to the correlations observed in Europeans *(76)*. Thus although the insulin resistance syndrome occurs within both European and West African populations, when West Africans are contrasted with Europeans there is a dissociation of insulin resistance from the disturbances of plasma lipids that usually accompany it.

In contrast with South Asians, West Africans do not, on average, have a more central of body fat than Europeans. Comparisons of body fat distribution based on waist/hip ratio are difficult to interpret because hip girth depends upon the shape and size of the pelvis and this may differ between West African and European men. Mean waist/thigh girth ratio is lower in Afro-Caribbeans than in Europeans (Table 10). After adjustment for total body fat, mean visceral adipose tissue mass measured by computed tomography has been found to be less in West African than in European women *(70)*.

In England and the Caribbean, mortality from CHD is far lower among men of West African descent than in Europeans or South Asians *(5,78)*. Although this does not apply in the US where mortality from CHD is high in African-Americans, when groups of similar socioeconomic status are compared CHD mortality in men is lower in African-Americans than in Europeans *(79)*. The favorable lipid pattern in West African men may account for the low risk of CHD in this group, despite the high prevalence of diabetes and hypertension.

In the Insulin Resistance and Atherosclerosis Study, insulin resistance measured by the frequently-sampled intravenous glucose tolerance test was correlated with carotid atherosclerosis (measured as intimal-medial thickness) in European-Americans (both Hispanic and non-Hispanic) but not in African-Americans *(80)*. A complication in the interpretation of the results was that in 15% of participants, the model yielded a zero value for insulin sensitivity. The size of the difference in predicted intimal-medial thickness at the 25th and 75th percentiles of insulin sensitivity was comparable to the size of effects associated with smoking or hypertension. Adjusting for glucose tolerance status did not fully account for the association in Whites. The lack of relation between carotid intimal-medial thickness and insulin sensitivity not in African-Americans *(80)* may reflect the lack of association between insulin resistance and hypertension in African-Americans, since hypertension is a main risk factor for atherosclerosis in the carotid arteries.

SUMMARY INTERPRETATION

Evidence from migrant studies points to genetic explanations for much of the variation in diabetes and insulin resistance between high-risk ethnic groups such as South Asians and low-risk ethnic groups such as Europeans. Prevalence of diabetes is uniformly high (around 20% in those aged over 35 years) in urban populations of South Asian descent even where migration occurred during the mid-nineteenth century *(81)*. Although it is plausible that an effect of maternal environment could persist over one or two generations after migration, it is unlikely that such an effect would persist five or six generations after migration as an exposure specific to Indians. In Singapore, for instance, a rapid transition to affluence has been shared by all three of the main ethnic groups (Chinese, Malays and Indians) but prevalence of diabetes is far higher in Indians than in Chinese *(8)*. The most compelling evidence for genetic explanations of ethnic variation comes from studies in admixed populations that show a relationship between prevalence of diabetes and markers of admixture from the high-risk population. Thus, in Nauruans and Pima Native Americans, inverse associations of diabetes with genetic markers of European admixture have been reported *(82,83)*. If differences in disease risk between genetically distant ethnic groups have a genetic basis, it is possible in principle to map the genes underlying these differences by studying populations where there has been recent admixture *(84)*.

Ethnic variation in the risk of diabetes has been attributed to the presence of a "thrifty genotype" *(85)* in populations at high risk. This term was coined by Neel, who suggested that evolutionary selection for traits that confer the ability to survive when food supplies are unreliable might select also for genes that increase the risk of diabetes when food is abundant. Evolutionary selection pressure for the ability to survive food scarcity is likely to have been especially strong among people living as hunter-gatherers or under desert conditions, as in some Native Australian or Native American populations. Neel originally suggested that hyperinsulinemia might be the primary trait, leading to increased fat storage. The studies reviewed above, however, suggest that hyperinsulinemia in high-risk ethnic groups is secondary to insulin resistance. Resistance to insulin-mediated glucose uptake, by sparing the oxidation of glucose in time of starvation, could be an advantage in time of food scarcity by minimizing the need for gluconeogenesis from protein. The tendency to deposit fat in visceral depots may itself have advantages under conditions of unreliable food supply and physically demanding work. In small isolated populations such as Nauruan islanders, genetic drift may also have contributed to variation in insulin resistance and prevalence of diabetes. The main environmental contribution to variation in diabetes risk in these high risk population appears to come from determinants of obesity. From comparisons of groups of the same ethnic origin in different environments, one can estimate that a rise in average body mass index by 2 to 3 kg/m^2 approximately doubles the prevalence of diabetes in high-risk groups such as South Asians and Native Americans.

Although the pattern of metabolic disturbances associated with insulin resistance is present in most populations that are at high risk of diabetes, the balance between these disturbances varies markedly between the various groups studied. Thus in South Asians, there is a pronounced tendency to central adiposity, raised triglyceride levels after a glucose load, and the risk of CDL is high. In West Africans, body fat has a less central distribution than in Europeans, plasma triglyceride levels after a glucose load are low and the risk of CDL is low. In Peninsular Arabs, there appears to be a familial syndrome in which obesity and insulin resistance are associated with raised plasma levels of cholesterol and apolipoprotein B. This resembles the pattern described in familial combined hyperlipidemia *(86)*. In Pima Native Americans, and to a lesser extent in Mexican-Americans, generalized adiposity and insulin resistance are accompanied by low plasma total cholesterol levels and low risk of CHD.

This general picture of ethnic variation suggests that high prevalence of diabetes and insulin resistance in the population can be compatible with either high or low risk of CHD, depending upon the extent to which disturbances of lipid metabolism are present in association with insulin resistance. Because plasma HDL cholesterol levels and the composition and size of particles in the LDL fraction are both modulated by plasma triglyceride levels *(87)*, these disturbances of lipid metabolism are likely to depend upon the extent to which insulin resistance is associated with effects on the rate of production and clearance of plasma triglyceride. Recent studies suggest that insulin resistance may depend on levels of triglyceride stores in muscle cells *(88)*—studies comparing triglyceride stores in muscle in different ethnic groups may help to establish whether this can account for ethnic variation in insulin resistance. If current efforts to clone genes that have been mapped in linkage studies of diabetes or insulin resistance in high-risk groups such as Mexican-Americans *(89)* are successful, this may revolutionize our understanding of ethnic differences in insulin resistance.

REFERENCES

1. Ravussin E, Bennett PH, Valencia ME, Schulz LO, Esparza J. Effects of a traditional life-style on obesity in Pima Indians. Diabetes Care 1994;17:1067–1074.
2. Ramachandran A, Snehalatha C, Dharmaraj D, Viswanathan M. Prevalence of glucose intolerance in Asian Indians—urban-rural difference and significance of upper-body adiposity. Diabetes Care 1992;15:1348–1355.
3. Montel MLR. Une question sur le diabete. In: Comptes rendus des travaux du Troisieme Congres Biennial tenu a Saigon, Saigon: Far Eastern Association of Tropical Medicine. 1913:522–523.
4. McKeigue PM, Shah B, Marmot MG. Relation of central obesity and insulin resistance with high diabetes prevalence and cardiovascular risk in South Asians. Lancet 1991;337:382–386.
5. Miller GJ, Beckles GLA, Maude GH, Carson DC, Alexis SD, Price SGL, Byam NTA. Ethnicity and other characteristics predictive of coronary heart disease in a developing country—principal results of the St James survey, Trinidad. Int J Epidemiol 1989;18:808–817.

6. Zimmet P, Taylor R, Ram P, King H, Sloman G, Raper LR, Hunt D. Prevalence of diabetes and impaired glucose tolerance in the biracial (Melanesian and Indian) population of Fiji: a rural-urban comparison. Am J Epidemiol 1983;118:673–688.

7. Omar MAK, Seedat MA, Dyer RB, Rajput MC, Motala AA, Joubert SM. The prevalence of diabetes mellitus in a large group of South African Indians. S Afr Med J 1985;67:924–926.

8. Hughes K, Yeo PPB, Lun KC, et al. Cardiovascular diseases in Chinese,Malays and Indians in Singapore. II. Differences in risk factor levels. J Epidemiol Community Health 1990;44:29–35.

9. Dowse GK, Gareeboo H, Zimmet P, et al. High prevalence of NIDDM and impaired glucose tolerance in Indian, Creole and Chinese Mauritians. Diabetes 1990;39:390–396.

10. Ramachandran A, Jali MV, Mohan V, Snehalatha C, Viswanathan M. High prevalence of diabetes in an urban population in south India. BMJ 1988;297:587–590.

11. Shera AS, Rafique G, Khwaja IA, Ara J, Baqai S, King H. Pakistan national diabetes survey: prevalence of glucose intolerance and associated factors in Shikarpur, Sindh Province. Diabetic Med 1995;12:1116–1121.

12. Walker ARP, Bernstein RE, Du Plessis I. Hyperinsulinaemia from glucose dose in South African Indian children. S Afr Med J 1972;46:1916.

13. Keller P, Schatz L, Jackson WPU. Immunoreactive insulin in various South African population groups. S Afr Med J 1972;46:152–157.

14. McKeigue PM, Marmot MG, Syndercombe Court YD, Cottier DE, Rahman S, Riemersma RA. Diabetes, hyperinsulinaemia and coronary risk factors in Bangladeshis in east London. Br Heart J 1988;60:390–396.

15. Laws A, Jeppesen JL, Maheux PC, Schaaf P, Chen YDI, Reaven GM. Resistance to insulin-stimulated glucose uptake and dyslipidaemia in Asian Indians. Arterioscler Thromb 1994;14:917–922.

16. McKeigue PM, Pierpoint T, Ferrie JE, Marmot MG. Relationship of glucose intolerance and hyperinsulinaemia to body fat pattern in South Asians and Europeans. Diabetologia 1992;35:785–791.

17. Hughes K, Lun KC, Yeo PPB. Cardiovascular diseases in Chinese, Malays and Indians in Singapore. I. Differences in mortality. J Epidemiol Community Health 1990;44:24–28.

18. Tuomilehto J, Ram P, Eseroma R, Taylor R, Zimmet P. Cardiovascular diseases in Fiji: analysis of mortality, morbidity and risk factors. Bull World Health Organ 1984;62:133–143.

19. Steinberg WJ, Balfe DL, Kustner HG. Decline in the ischemic heart disease mortality rates of South Africans, 1968-1985. S Afr Med J 1988;74:547–550.

20. Office of Population Censuses and Surveys. Mortality and geography: a review in the mid-1980s. The Registrar-General's decennial supplement for England and Wales, series DS no. 9. London: HMSO, 1990.

21. Wild SH, Laws A, Fortmann SP, Varady AN, Byrne CD. Mortality from coronary heart disease and stroke for six ethnic groups in California, 1985 to 1990. Ann Epidemiol 1995;5:432–439.

22. Sarvotham SG, Berry JN. Prevalence of coronary heart disease in an urban population in northern India. Circulation 1968;37:939–953.

23. Chadha SL, Radhakrishnan S, Ramachandran K, Kaul U, Gopinath N. Epidemiological study of coronary heart disease in urban population of Delhi. Indian J Med Res 1990;92:424–430.

24. Dewan BD, Malhotra KC, Gupta SP. Epidemiological study of coronary heart disease in a rural community in Haryana. Indian Heart J 1974;26:68–78.

25. Jajoo UN, Kalantri SP, Gupta OP, Jain AP, Gupta K. The prevalence of coronary heart disease in rural population from central India. J Assoc Physicians India 1988;36:689–693.

26. Balarajan R, Adelstein AM, Bulusu L, Shukla V. Patterns of mortality among migrants to England and Wales from the Indian subcontinent. BMJ 1984;289:1185–1187.

27. McKeigue PM, Marmot MG. Mortality from coronary heart disease in Asian communities in London. BMJ 1988;297:903.

28. McKeigue PM, Ferrie JE, Pierpoint T, Marmot MG. Association of early-onset coronary heart disease in South Asian men with glucose intolerance and hyperinsulinemia. Circulation 1993;87:152–161.

29. Pais P, Pogue J, Gerstein H, et al. Risk-factors for acute myocardial-infarction in indians—a case-control study. Lancet 1996;348:358–363.

30. Musaiger AO. Diabetes mellitus in Bahrain: an overview. Diabetic Med 1992;9:574–578.

31. Alzaid AA, Sobki S, De Silva V. Prevalence of microalbuminuria in Saudi Arabians with non-insulin-dependent diabetes mellitus: a clinic-based study. Diabetes Res Clin Pract 1994;26:115–120.

32. El-Mugamer IT, Ali Zayat AS, Hossain MM, Pugh RN. Diabetes, obesity and hypertension in urban and rural people of bedouin origin in the United Arab Emirates. J Trop Med Hyg 1995;98:407–415.

33. Asfour MG, Lambourne A, Soliman A, et al. High prevalence of diabetes mellitus and impaired glucose tolerance in the Sultanate of Oman: results of the 1991 national survey. Diabetic Med 1995;12:1122–1125.

34. Alwan A, King H. Diabetes in the Eastern Mediterranean (Middle East) region: the World Health Organization responds to a major public health challenge [editorial]. Diabetic Med 1995;12:1057–1058.

35. Abdella N, Khogali M, Al-Ali S, Gumaa K, Bajaj J. Known type 2 diabetes mellitus among the Kuwaiti population. A prevalence study. Acta Diabetol 1996;33:145–149.

36. Ahmed AF, Abdelsalaam SA, Mahmoud ME, Gadri MA. A case-control study of the incidence of coronary heart disease risk factors in Saudis at AlMadina Almounawarah. Saudi Med J 1993;14:146–151.

37. Al-Roomi KA, Musaiger AO, Al-Awadi AH. Lifestyle and the risk of acute myocardial infarction in a Gulf Arab population. Int J Epidemiol 1994;23:931–939.

38. Al-Owaish RA, Zack M. Risk factors associated with acute myocardial infarction in Kuwait, 1978. Int J Epidemiol 1982;11:368–371.

39. Al-Nuaim AR. Prevalence of glucose intolerance in urban and rural communities in Saudi Arabia. Diabetic Med 1997;14:595–602.

40. Al-Mahroos F, McKeigue PM. High prevalence of diabetes mellitus in Bahrainis: associations with ethnicity and raised plasma cholesterol. Diabetes Care 1998;21:936–942.

41. Walden CE, Knopp RH, Wahl PW, Beach KW, Strandness E. Sex differences in the effect of diabetes mellitus on lipoprotein triglyceride and cholesterol concentrations. N Engl J Med 1984;311:953–959.

42. Laakso M, Pyorala K, Voutilainen E, Marniemi J. Plasma insulin and serum lipids and lipoproteins in middle-aged non-insulin dependent diabetic and non-diabetic subjects. Am J Epidemiol 1987;125:611–621.

43. Al-Muhtaseb N, Al-Yusuf AR, Abdella N, Fenech F. Lipoproteins and apolipoproteins in young nonobese Arab women with NIDDM treated with insulin. Diabetes Care 1989;12:325–331.

44. Aronoff SL, Bennett PH, Gorden P, Rushforth N, Miller M. Unexplained hyperinsulinaemia in normal and "prediabetic" Pima Indians compared with normal Caucasians. An example of racial differences in insulin secretion. Diabetes 1977;26:827–840.

45. Bogardus C, Lillioja S, Swinburn B, et al. Distribution of in vivo insulin action in Pima Indians as mixture of three normal distributions. Diabetes 1989;38:1423–1432.

46. Howard BV, Davis MP, Pettitt DJ, Knowler WC, Bennett PH. Plasma and lipoprotein cholesterol and triglyceride concentrations in the Pima Indians: distributions differing from those of Caucasians. Circulation 1983;68:714–724.

47. Howard BV, Egusa G, Beltz WF, Kesaniemi YA, Grundy SM. Compensatory mechanisms governing the concentration of plasma low density lipoprotein. J Lipid Res 1986;27:11–20.

48. Nelson RG, Sievers ML, Knowler WC, et al. Low incidence of fatal coronary heart disease in Pima Indians despite high prevalence of non-insulin-dependent diabetes. Circulation 1990;81:987–995.

49. Hanis CL, Chakraborty R, Ferrell RE, Schull WJ. Individual admixture estimates: disease associations and individual risk of diabetes and gallbladder disease among Mexican-Americans in Starr County, Texas. Am J Phys Anthropol 1986;70:433–441.

50. Chakraborty R, Ferrell RE, Stern MP, Haffner SM, Hazuda HP, Rosenthal M. Relationship of prevalence of non-insulin-dependent diabetes mellitus to Amerindian admixture in the Mexican Americans of San Antonio, Texas. Genetic Epidemiol 1986;3:435–454.

51. Haffner SM, Stern MP, Hazuda HP, Pugh JA, Patterson JK. Hyperinsulinemia in a population at high risk for non-insulin-dependent diabetes mellitus. N Engl J Med 1986;315:220–224.

52. Haffner SM, Stern MP, Dunn J, Mobley M, Blackwell J, Bergman RN. Diminished insulin sensitivity and increased insulin response in nonobese, nondiabetic Mexican-Americans. Metabolism 1990;39:842–847.

53. Haffner SM, Stern MP, Hazuda HP, Rosenthal M, Knapp JA, Malina RM. Role of obesity and fat distribution in non-insulin-dependent diabetes mellitus in Mexican Americans and Non-Hispanic Whites. Diabetes Care 1986;9:153–161.

54. Haffner SM, Stern MP, Hazuda HP, Pugh J, Patterson JK. Do upper-body and centralized adiposity measure different aspects of regional body-fat distribution? Diabetes 1987;36:43–51.

55. Haffner SM, Mykkanen L, Valdez RA, Paidi M, Stern MP, Howard BV. LDL size and subclass pattern in a biethnic population. Arterioscl Thromb 1993;13:1623–1630.

56. Goff DC, Jr., Ramsey DJ, Labarthe DR, Nichaman MZ. Acute myocardial infarction and coronary heart disease mortality among Mexican Americans and non-Hispanic whites in Texas, 1980 through 1989. Ethnicity and Disease 1993;3:64–69.

57. O'Dea K, Lion RJ, Lee A, Traianedes K, Hopper JL, Rae C. Diabetes, hyperinsulinemia and hyperlipidemia in small Aboriginal community in northern Australia. Diabetes Care 1990;13:830–835.

58. Gault A, O'Dea K, Rowley KG, McLeay T, Traianedes K. Abnormal glucose-tolerance and other coronary heart disease risk factors in an isolated Aboriginal community in Central Australia. Diabetes Care 1996;19:1269–1273.

59. O'Dea K, Patel M, Kubisch D, Hopper J, Traianedes K. Obesity, diabetes, and hyperlipidemia in a central Australian aboriginal community with a long history of acculturation. Diabetes Care 1993;16:1004–1010.

60. O'Dea K, Traianedes K, Hopper JL, Larkins RG. Impaired glucose tolerance, hyperinsulinemia and hypertriglyceridemia in Australian Aborigines from the desert. Diabetes Care 1988;11:23–29.

61. Wise PH, Edwards FM, Craig RJ, Evans B, Marchland JB, Sutherland B, Thomas DW. Diabetes and associated variables in the South Australian Aboriginal. Aust NZ J Med 1976;6:191–196.

62. Proietto J, Nankervis AJ, Traianedes K, Rosella G, O'Dea K. Identification of early metabolic defects in diabetes-prone Australian aborigines. Diabetes Res Clin Pract 1992;17:217–226.

63. Guest CS, O'Dea K, Hopper JL, Larkins RG. Hyperinsulinemia and obesity in Aborigines of southeastern Australia, with comparisons from rural and urban Europid populations. Diabetes Res Clin Pract 1993;20:155–164.

64. O'Dea K, White NG, Sinclair AJ. An investigation of nutrition-related risk factors in an isolated Aboriginal community in northern Australia: advantages of a traditionally-orientated life-style. Med J Aust 1988;148:177–180.

65. Veroni M, Gracey M, Rouse I. Patterns of mortality in Western Australian Aboriginals, 1983–1989. Int J Epidemiol 1994;23:73–81.

66. Harris MI, Hadden WC, Knowler WC, Bennett PH. Prevalence of diabetes and impaired glucose tolerance and plasma glucose levels in US population aged 20-74 yr. Diabetes 1987;36:523–534.

67. Beckles GLA, Miller GJ, Kirkwood BR, Alexis SD, Carson DC, Byam NTA. High total and cardiovascular disease mortality in adults of Indian descent in Trinidad, unexplained by major coronary risk factors. Lancet 1986;1:1298–1301.

68. Chaturvedi N, McKeigue PM, Marmot MG. Resting and ambulatory blood pressure differences in Afro-Caribbeans and Europeans. Hypertension 1993;22:90–96.

69. Haffner SM, D'Agostino R, Saad MF, et al. Increased insulin resistance and insulin secretion in nondiabetic African-Americans and Hispanics compared with non-Hispanic whites. The Insulin Resistance Atherosclerosis Study. Diabetes 1996;45:742–748.

70. Albu JB, Murphy L, Frager DH, Johnson JA, Pi Sunyer FX. Visceral fat and race-dependent health risks in obese nondiabetic premenopausal women. Diabetes 1997;46:456–462.

71. Slack J, Noble N, Meade TW, North WRS. Lipid and lipoprotein concentrations in 1604 men and women in working populations in northwest London. BMJ 1977;2:353–356.

72. Morrison JA, Khoury P, Mellies M, Kelly K, Horvitz R, Glueck CJ. Lipid and lipoprotein distributions in black adults. The Cincinnati Lipid Research Clinic's Princeton School Study. JAMA 1981;245:939–942.

73. Summerson JH, Konen JC, Dignan MB. Racial differences in lipid and lipoprotein levels in diabetes. Metabolism 1992;41:851–855.

74. Koukkou E, Watts GF, Mazurkiewicz J, Lowy C. Ethnic differences in lipid and lipoprotein metabolism in pregnant women of African and Caucasian origin. J Clin Pathol 1994;47:1105–1107.

75. Conway JM, Yanovski SZ, Avila NA, Hubbard VS. Visceral adipose tissue differences in black and caucasian women. Am J Clin Nutr 1995;61:765–771.

76. Falkner B, Kushner H, Tulenko T, Sumner AE, Marsh JB. Insulin sensitivity, lipids, and blood pressure in young American blacks. Arterioscl Thromb Vasc Biol 1995;15:1798–1804.

77. Chaturvedi N, McKeigue PM, Marmot MG. Relationship of glucose intolerance to coronary risk in Afro-Caribbeans compared with Europeans. Diabetologia 1994;37:765–772.

78. Wild S, McKeigue PM. Cross-sectional analysis of mortality by country of birth in England and Wales 1970–1992. BMJ 1997;314:708–710.

79. Keil JE, Sutherland SE, Hames CG, Lackland DT, Gazes PC, Knapp RG, Tyroler HA. Coronary disease mortality and risk factors in black and white men. Results from the combined Charleston, SC, and Evans County, Georgia, heart studies. Arch Intern Med 1995;155:1521–1527.

80. Howard G, O'Leary DH, Zaccaro D, et al. Insulin sensitivity and atherosclerosis. The Insulin Resistance Atherosclerosis Study (IRAS) Investigators. Circulation 1996;93:1809–1817.

81. McKeigue PM, Miller GJ, Marmot MG. Coronary heart disease in South Asians overseas: a review. J Clin Epidemiol 1989;42:597-609.

82. Serjeantson SW, Owerbach D, Zimmet P, Nerup J, Thoma K. Genetics of diabetes in Nauru: effects of foreign admixture, HLA antigens and the insulin-gene-linked polymorphism. Diabetologia 1983;25:13–17.

83. Knowler WC, Williams RC, Pettitt DJ, Steinberg AG. Gm3;5,13,14 and type 2 diabetes mellitus: an association in American Indians with genetic admixture. Am J Hum Genet 1988;43:520–526.

84. McKeigue PM. Mapping genes that underlie ethnic differences in disease risk: methods for detecting linkage in admixed populations by conditioning on parental admixture. Am J Hum Genet 1998;63:241–251.

85. Neel JV. Diabetes mellitus: a 'thrifty' genotype rendered detrimental by 'progress'. Am J Hum Genet 1962;14:353–362.

86. Aitman TJ, Godsland IF, Farren B, Crook D, Wong HJ, Scott J. Defects of insulin action on fatty acid and carbohydrate metabolism in familial combined hyperlipidemia. Arterioscl Thromb Vasc Biol 1997;17:748–754.

87. Austin MA, King MC, Vranizan KM, Krauss RM. Atherogenic lipoprotein phenotype: a proposed genetic marker for coronary heart disease risk. Circulation 1990;82:495–506.

88. Phillips DIW, Caddy S, Ilic V, Fielding BA, Frayn KN, Borthwick AC, Taylor R. Intramuscular triglyceride and muscle insulin sensitivity: evidence for a relationship in nondiabetic subjects. Metabolism 1996;45:947–950.

89. Hanis CL, Boerwinkle E, Chakraborty R, Ellsworth DJ, Concannon P, Stirling B, Morrison VA. A genome-wide search for human non-insulin-dependent (Type 2) diabetes genes reveals a major susceptibility locus on chromosome 2. Nat Genet 1996;13:161–166.

3

Fetal Effects on Insulin Resistance and Glucose Tolerance

Paul M. McKeigue, MB, PhD

CONTENTS

SUMMARY
INTRODUCTION
DIABETES AND IMPAIRED GLUCOSE TOLERANCE
    IN RELATION TO SIZE AT BIRTH
GLUCOSE LEVELS IN YOUNG ADULTS AND CHILDREN
    IN RELATION TO SIZE AT BIRTH
INSULIN RESISTANCE AND INSULIN SECRETION
    IN RELATION TO SIZE AT BIRTH
EXPERIMENTAL STUDIES OF MALNUTRITION IN EARLY LIFE
IS THE ASSOCIATION OF REDUCED SIZE AT BIRTH WITH INSULIN
    RESISTANCE CAUSAL?
CAN IMPAIRED FETAL GROWTH ACCOUNT FOR ETHNIC DIFFERENCES
    IN PREVALENCE OF DIABETES?
SMALL BABY SYNDROME OR INSULIN RESISTANCE SYNDROME?
PHYSIOLOGICAL BASIS OF INSULIN RESISTANCE
    IN ADULTS WHO WERE SMALL AT BIRTH
CONCLUSIONS
REFERENCES

SUMMARY

Inverse associations of non-insulin-dependent diabetes (Type 2 diabetes) in adult life mellitus with size at birth were first identified in two cohorts of adults born in England, and have since been confirmed in three other populations. Other studies in children and young adults have shown that plasma glucose levels after oral glucose challenge are inversely related to birth weight. The association of glucose intolerance with reduced size at birth appears to be mediated through insulin resistance, rather than through impairment of β-cell function as originally suggested by Hales and colleagues.

In populations at high risk of diabetes, U-shaped or positive monotonic relationships of diabetes risk to size at birth have been found, in contrast to the inverse relationships identified in European populations. The most likely explanation for this is that gestational

From: *Contemporary Endocrinology: Insulin Resistance*
Edited by: G. Reaven and A. Laws © Humana Press Inc., Totowa, NJ

diabetes is associated both with increased birth weight and with increased risk of diabetes in the offspring. Failure to stratify by gestational age may account for the finding that in some studies glucose intolerance and insulin resistance are related more strongly to thinness at birth, measured by low ponderal index, than to birth weight.

Suggestions that the inverse association between diabetes and size at birth could be accounted for by selective survival of low birth weight infants genetically predisposed to diabetes are not compatible with historical data on infant mortality rates. Because insulin regulates fetal growth, the association of reduced size at birth with insulin resistance in adult life could result from a primary genetic defect in insulin action. Both human and animal models for such an association exist. However, the results of a twin study, and the follow-up of a Dutch cohort exposed to famine *in utero* support the view that impairment of growth in fetal life causes insulin resistance and increased risk of diabetes in adult life. This effect appears to depend upon interaction with adiposity in adult life. It has been suggested that the high rates of non-insulin-dependent diabetes in populations such as Native Americans result from undernutrition in early life: this "thrifty phenotype" hypothesis has been proposed as an alternative to the usual "thrifty genotype" explanation. However, there is compelling evidence from studies of migrants and admixed populations that these ethnic differences in diabetes prevalence are at least partly attributable to genetic factors.

The association of insulin resistance with reduced size at birth is not accounted for by obesity or body fat pattern. Although reduced size at birth predicts insulin resistance, glucose intolerance, and raised blood pressure, it does not predict the lipid disturbances—raised plasma triglyceride and low high-density-lipoprotein (HDL) cholesterol that are associated with insulin resistance and central obesity in the general population. The "small baby syndrome" is thus not the same as "syndrome X." Preliminary evidence suggests that insulin resistance in those who were small at birth is associated with alterations in muscle fuel utilization that resemble those found in obesity. Experimental studies have not clearly demonstrated that insulin resistance in adult life can be produced by undernutrition in fetal life, but have shown that exposure to maternal glucocorticoid hormone in fetal life leads to both raised blood pressure and glucose intolerance in adult life.

As the effects of reduced size at birth on insulin resistance appear to depend upon interaction with obesity in adult life, control of obesity in adult life is likely to be the most effective measure to reduce the risk of diabetes in those who were thin at birth.

INTRODUCTION

The first suggestions that early malnutrition could predispose to diabetes were based on clinical descriptions of malnutrition-associated diabetes, and on animal experiments in which undernutrition in early life produced lasting impairment of the insulin response to glucose *(1)*. To investigate the relation of size at birth to Type 2 diabetes in adult life, it is necessary to study populations where records of size at birth are available from at least 50 yr before, unless the risk of diabetes in the population under study is so high that the disease is common before this age.

DIABETES AND IMPAIRED GLUCOSE TOLERANCE IN RELATION TO SIZE AT BIRTH

Five studies have examined the relation of size at birth to impaired glucose tolerance or non-insulin-dependent diabetes in later life (Table 1).

Table 1
Studies Relating Diabetes or Impaired Glucose Tolerance to Size at Birth

Population	N	Age	Outcome	Measurement of size at birth	Form of relation	Odds ratio highest/lowest categories
Hertfordshire men (2)	468	64	IGT/new NIDDM	Birthweight	Inverse	6.6[a]
Preston adults (3)	266	46–54	IGT/new NIDDM	Birthweight	Inverse	6.4[a]
Pima-American adults (6)	1179	20-39	NIDDM	Birthweight	U-shaped	3.8[a]
US male health professionals (5)	22693	61	Diagnosed NIDDM	Birthweight (recalled)	Inverse	1.9
Uppsala men (25)	1093	60	NIDDM	(i) Birthweight (ii) Ponderal index	Stepwise Stepwise	1.9, 2.3[a] 4.4
Mysore adults	506	39–60	NIDDM	Birthweight	Positive[a]	

[a]Adjusted for body mass index.

Hertfordshire

Of 1157 men born in Hertfordshire between 1920 and 1930 and traced from their birth records, 408 underwent glucose tolerance tests at a mean age of 64 yr (2). Glucose intolerance was defined by 2-h plasma glucose of 7.8 mmol/L or more. There was a linear inverse relationship between prevalence of glucose intolerance and birth weight, from 14% prevalence in the highest two birth weight categories to 36% in the lowest two birth weight categories. Adjustment for body mass index (BMI) strengthened the relationship: the adjusted odds ratios for prevalence in the highest birth weight category compared with the lowest was 6.6. There was an equally strong relationship between glucose intolerance and weight at one year.

Preston

The 266 men and women born in a hospital in Preston between 1935 and 1943 underwent oral glucose tolerance tests at a mean age of 50 years (3). Prevalence of glucose intolerance showed a linear inverse relationship to birth weight. There was a similar relationship with ponderal index. Gestational age at birth (estimated from the date of last menstrual period) was similar in those with and without glucose intolerance. In a further analysis with 2-h glucose as the dependent variable in a regression analysis, both shortness at birth (defined by a high ratio of head circumference to birth length), and thinness at birth (defined by low ponderal index) independently predicted diabetes.

Uppsala

Birth records were traced on 1093 men who were born between 1920 and 1924, resident in Uppsala and examined at age 60 yr. Oral glucose tolerance tests were performed on all those whose fasting glucose was 5.7 mmol/L or higher. When prevalence of diabetes at age 60 yr was compared across the birth weight groups, there was a stepwise increase in diabetes prevalence in the lowest birth weight category (less than 3.25 kg). This association was statistically significant only when adjusted for BMI. A stronger effect of size at birth was seen when prevalence of diabetes was compared across quintiles of ponderal index at birth; prevalence was three times higher in the lowest quintile of ponderal index than in the other four quintiles. This association was independent of BMI.

When the 709 men remaining in this cohort were re-examined at age 70 yr, there was an inverse relationship of glucose intolerance to birth weight but an inverted U-shaped relation of glucose intolerance to ponderal index *(4)*. This change in form of the relationship was partly accounted for by selective loss to follow-up between ages 60 and 70 yr.

US Male Health Professionals

The 22,693 men who had participated in the Health Professionals Follow-up Study were surveyed by questionnaire at a mean age of 61 years *(5)*. Five groupings of recalled birth weight were defined. With the middle group (birth weight 7–8.4 lb) as referent category, the odds ratio for diabetes was 1.9 in those in the lowest birth weight group (birth weight less than 5.5 lb) and 1.4 in the next highest birth weight group (5.5–6.9 lb). At higher levels of birth weight there was no trend in diabetes prevalence.

Native Americans

In Pima Native Americans diabetes is common even in young adults, and cohort studies of predictors of diabetes can therefore be undertaken with younger individuals. The 1179 Pimas whose birth weights had been recorded between 1965 and 1972 were examined between ages 20 and 39 yr *(6)*. There was a U-shaped relationship between birth weight and the prevalence of diabetes. Prevalence of diabetes was raised only in those with birth weight less than 2.5 kg or more than 4.5 kg. Although the odds ratio for diabetes in those with low birth weight compared with those with normal birth weight was 3.8, the excess risk associated with low birth weight accounted for only 6% of all cases in the population. When maternal diabetes was included in the model, the excess prevalence in the high birth weight group was no longer significant.

Mysore

From birth records in a hospital in the south Indian city of Mysore, 506 men and women aged 39–60 yr were traced and examined *(7)*. In contrast to the inverse relationships between diabetes and size at birth seen in European and American populations, the prevalence of diabetes was positively related to ponderal index at birth. The authors suggested that the effects of gestational diabetes on size at birth and β-cell function in adult life might account for this association.

GLUCOSE LEVELS IN YOUNG ADULTS AND CHILDREN IN RELATION TO SIZE AT BIRTH

These studies of glucose intolerance in older adults have been supplemented by other studies of fasting or post-load glucose levels in younger adults or children, for whom records of size at birth are more easily found. As we do not know whether raised glucose levels in children predict diabetes in later life, these studies do not provide direct evidence of a relationship between size at birth and the risk of diabetes. In 40 men aged 21 yr who had been born in a Southampton hospital, there was an inverse relationship between birth weight and glucose levels at 30 minutes after an oral glucose load *(8)*. In contrast a study in San Antonio, Texas, found no associations of birth weight with fasting or 2 h glucose in 541 Mexican-Americans and Anglos examined at a mean age of 32 yr, after adjusting for age, sex and ethnicity *(9)*.

Two studies in children have measured glucose levels at 30 min after oral glucose challenge. In Pune, India, 379 four-year old children whose birth weights had been recorded in hospital were studied *(10)*. The 30-minute glucose levels were inversely correlated with birth weight in those who had been on the routine postnatal wards, but not in those who had been admitted to the special care baby unit. In Salisbury, England, 30-minute glucose levels were inversely related to ponderal index but not to birth weight in a sample of 250 seven-year-old children *(11)*. As an alternative to measuring plasma glucose, glycated hemoglobin levels can be used as a measure of average plasma glucose levels. 659 Jamaican children who were born in the University Hospital were examined at ages from 6 to 16 years *(12)*. Children who were shorter at birth had thicker triceps skinfolds and higher glycated hemoglobin levels.

The studies reviewed above suggest that in inverse associations of size at birth with raised glucose levels in children and adults are consistently seen in populations of European descent. In populations at high risk for diabetes, such as Native Americans, Mexican-Americans and urban Indians, the inverse relationship between glucose intolerance and size at birth is less clear, and the relationship may be U-shaped or reversed. This attenuation or reversal of the inverse association between size at birth and glucose intolerance may be attributable to the effects of glucose intolerance during pregnancy. Maternal hyperglycemia causes fetal hyperinsulinemia which in turn promotes fetal growth, especially in subcutaneous fat depots *(13)*. In experimental studies maternal hyperglycemia itself has been shown to affect glucose homeostasis. Induction of hyperglycemia in female rats leads to glucose intolerance, insulin resistance and impaired β-cell function in the adult offspring *(14,15)*. These effects are transmissible from one generation to the next *(16)*. A possible human counterpart to this experimental model is the observation that in Pima Americans, the risk of diabetes is much higher in the offspring of mothers who were diabetic during pregnancy than in the offspring of mothers who developed diabetes subsequently *(17)*.

In populations where gestational diabetes is common, we would therefore expect to observe a positive association between size at birth and risk of diabetes in adult life. Infants of mothers who are hyperglycemic will be large at birth because of fetal hyperinsulinemia, and will also be at higher than average risk of developing diabetes. This increased risk may be attributable both to genetic effects and to the effects of hyperglycemia in fetal life on glucose homeostasis. One way to test this hypothesis would be to examine the relation of diabetes in adult life to size at birth after excluding births to older mothers and births to mothers who were later diagnosed diabetic.

INSULIN RESISTANCE AND INSULIN SECRETION IN RELATION TO SIZE AT BIRTH

To explain the association between reduced fetal growth and glucose intolerance, Hales and colleagues initially suggested that inadequate fetal nutrition might impair the development of the endocrine pancreas *(2)*. More recent work has led the Southampton-Cambridge group to suggest instead that the association between glucose intolerance and reduced size at birth may be mediated through insulin resistance *(18,19)*. This is consistent with other evidence that insulin resistance has a primary role in the pathogenesis of Type 2 diabetes *(20)*. Defects in β-cell function, such as loss of the acute insulin response to glucose challenge, are seen in people with impaired glucose tolerance and non-insulin-dependent diabetes, but may be a consequence of hyperglycemia rather than a primary cause of it *(20)*.

Hales' hypothesis that malnutrition in early life impairs the development of the endocrine pancreas is compatible with the known timing of differentiation and growth of this tissue *(21)*, and with experimental evidence. Protein-restricted diets administered to rats from weaning until six weeks of age cause impairment of the insulin secretory response to glucose and glucose intolerance, which persists after refeeding *(1,22)*. Similar effects have been reported when rats are exposed to protein restriction *in utero*, followed by a normal diet from birth to adult life *(23)*.

Epidemiological studies however have failed to demonstrate that reduced size at birth predicts impairment of β-cell function. Although inverse associations of weight at one year of age with raised levels of proinsulin and 32–33 split proinsulin in Hertfordshire men aged 64 yr were originally interpreted as evidence of that reduced growth in early life was associated with β-cell dysfunction, subsequent studies from the same group have shown that raised proinsulin levels correlate well with insulin resistance. The most generally accepted measure of β-cell function in humans is the acute insulin response to intravenous glucose challenge, which has been validated in baboons against measurements of β-cell mass at autopsy *(24)*. Reduced size at birth did not predict impairment of the acute insulin response in Preston adults *(18)* or in Uppsala men *(25)*. In Uppsala the measurements of insulin response were recorded at age 50 yr, ten years before the participants were tested for diabetes at age 60 yr. The relationship between size at birth and diabetes could thus be analyzed with insulin response as an intervening variable. In such analyses, adjusting for acute insulin response at age 50 yr strengthened the relationship between reduced size at birth and diabetes at age 60 yr, which is not consistent with the hypothesis that the effect of reduced size at birth is mediated through impairment of β-cell function.

The first direct evidence for an inverse relationship of insulin resistance to size at birth was in a study of Preston adults, in whom insulin resistance was measured by the short insulin tolerance test *(19)*. An inverse relation was found with ponderal index but not with birth weight, head circumference or gestational age. The relationship was present within each stratum of BMI. In a study of 331 Danish subjects aged 18–32 yr studied by the frequently-sampled glucose tolerance test, an inverse relationship of insulin resistance to birth weight was detected in women but not in men *(26)*. In the cohort of Uppsala men examined at age 70 yr, insulin resistance was measured by the euglycemic clamp technique *(4)*. In men born at 38 wk of gestation or later, insulin resistance was inversely related to birth weight. This relationship was reversed in men born before 38 wk of gestation, in whom there was a positive relationship of insulin resistance to birth weight.

In other studies inverse associations have been demonstrated for size at birth with insulin levels either in the fasting state or 1–2 h after an oral glucose load in nondiabetic individuals. In Mexican-Americans aged 32 yr, both fasting and 2 h insulin levels were inversely related to birth weight *(9)*. In Uppsala men at age 60 years, fasting and 60-minute insulin levels in the intravenous glucose tolerance test were inversely correlated with birth weight and with ponderal index *(25)*. These associations were strongest in men who were the highest tertile for BMI. Inverse association between insulin levels and size at birth have also been found in children, although the validity of insulin levels as proxy measures of insulin resistance in children is unknown. In four-year-old children in Pune, India, there was a significant inverse relationship between insulin levels at 30 min after a glucose load and birth weight *(10)*, and in seven-year old children in Salisbury, England an inverse relationship was found between fasting insulin levels and ponderal index at birth *(11)*.

These results are consistent with the hypothesis that the association of reduced size at birth with Type 2 diabetes is mediated through insulin resistance. Because the inverse association between ponderal index and raised post-load insulin level is strongest in overweight individuals, who account for most new cases of diabetes, a weak overall association between reduced size at birth and insulin resistance is compatible with a strong association between reduced size at birth and diabetes. The explanation for the reversal of this relationship among preterm births may be that a high proportion of preterm infants who are heavier than expected for their gestational age are macrosomic infants of mothers with gestational diabetes. Failure to stratify by gestational age may account for inconsistencies in the relationships of insulin resistance and glucose intolerance to size at birth, and for the detection of stronger associations with ponderal index than with birth weight. Because gestational age has less effect on ponderal index than on birth weight, using ponderal index as a measure of size at birth has the effect of partially adjusting size at birth for gestational age.

EXPERIMENTAL STUDIES OF MALNUTRITION IN EARLY LIFE

As yet no experimental model has been clearly established in which malnutrition in fetal life causes impairment of insulin-mediated glucose uptake in adult life. There is some evidence that malnutrition after weaning affects insulin resistance. In comparison with controls, rats fed energy restricted diets from weaning until six weeks of age have a delayed and exaggerated insulin secretory response to glucose as adults, suggesting that they are insulin resistant *(22)*. In contrast, adult rats exposed *in utero* to restriction of protein in the diets of their mothers clear an intravenous glucose load more rapidly than controls *(27,28)*. The basis of this effect appears to be that production of glucose from glycogen by the liver is reduced in rats exposed to protein restriction *in utero*. This effect has been demonstrated under basal conditions *(28)* and when the liver is perfused with glucagon which stimulates glucose production *(29)*. In one of these studies, insulin action was measured directly by the euglycemic clamp *(28)*. Basal glucose uptake was slower in rats exposed to protein restriction *in utero* than in controls, but there was no difference in insulin-stimulated glucose uptake between the two groups.

More recently it has been suggested that impairment of the placental barrier to maternal cortisol may represent a common pathway for the effects of maternal environment, including the effects of intrauterine malnutrition, on blood pressure and glucose tolerance in adult life *(30–32)*. Exposure of the fetus to maternal cortisol is normally prevented by the action of the enzyme 11β-hydroxysteroid dehydrogenase 2 (11β-HSD2) which converts cortisol to inactive cortisone *(33)*. Maternal dietary protein restriction reduces placental 11β-HSD activity by one-third *(34)*, which could impair the placental barrier to maternal cortisol. Exposure to glucocorticoids in fetal life leads to impaired glucose tolerance *(35,36)* in the offspring. Rats exposed *in utero* to maternal protein restriction or glucocorticoids have increased glucocorticoid receptors in peripheral tissues *(37)* and increased activity of glucocorticoid-inducible enzymes *(38)* as adults. However, central glucocorticoid receptor expression is reduced *(39)* so that negative feedback is impaired and plasma corticosterone (the glucocorticoid hormone in rats) is raised. There is some preliminary evidence that reduced fetal growth is associated with alterations in glucocorticoid action in humans. Low birth weight has been shown to predict increased excretion of glucocorticoid metabolites in children *(40)* and raised plasma cortisol levels in adults *(41)*. Insulin resistance in those whose growth was impaired *in utero* could thus result either from increased glucocorticoid production or from increased tissue sensitivity to cortisol.

IS THE ASSOCIATION OF REDUCED SIZE AT BIRTH WITH INSULIN RESISTANCE CAUSAL?

One criticism of the fetal origins hypothesis has been that the association between glucose intolerance and birth weight depends to some extent on adjustment for adult body mass index *(42)*. BMI is strongly related to prevalence of diabetes, and also has a weak positive correlation ($r = 0.1$) with birth weight *(25)*. Associations adjusted for BMI are difficult to interpret because of uncertainties about what underlying physiological variables are adjusted for. Weight for height indexes a combination of factors including fat mass, lean tissue mass and skeletal proportions. This criticism does not apply to associations of insulin resistance and glucose intolerance with ponderal index, as ponderal index at birth is uncorrelated with adult BMI.

Others have suggested that the inverse association between fetal growth and diabetes could be accounted for by an inverse association between genetic susceptibility to diabetes and mortality among low birth weight infants *(6,43)*: in other words, that low birth weight infants are more likely to survive if they are genetically predisposed to diabetes. The Uppsala results are not consistent with this explanation: when the men in this cohort were born in 1920–24, the infant mortality rate in Uppsala County was around 60 per 1000 live births, similar to the national rate for Sweden *(44)*. Even if we make the extreme assumption that all these deaths occurred in the lowest quintile of ponderal index among infants who were not susceptible to diabetes, such selection at birth could account only for a prevalence ratio for diabetes in adults of 1.3 in the lowest quintile compared to the other four quintiles. This contrasts with the observed prevalence ratio of 3.0.

Associations of reduced size at birth with insulin resistance and diabetes could have a genetic explanation. Estimates of heritability based on studying half-sibs (or the offspring of female monozygotic (mz) twins, who are genetically half-sibs) indicate that about 40% of variance in human birth weight is accounted for by genetic effects *(45,46)*. Thus, genetic effects on birth weight are large enough for genetic explanations of associations with birth weight to be plausible. Insulin regulates fetal growth, so that a primary defect in insulin action would reduce growth *in utero* and also predispose to glucose intolerance in later life. Such a mechanism would be consistent with clinical observations that human infants with genetic defects causing severe insulin resistance are small at birth *(47)*. An experimental model is provided by mice in which the gene for insulin receptor substrate-1 has been destroyed: in comparison with their normal littermates, these mice are 30% lighter at birth and more resistant to insulin-stimulated glucose uptake as adults *(48)*.

Recent epidemiological evidence, however, is not compatible with a genetic explanation for the association. A recent study based on the Danish Twin Registry has demonstrated that in 18 monozygotic pairs discordant for Type 2 diabetes whose birth records were traced, the mean birth weight of the diabetic twins was 195 g less than the mean birth weight of their nondiabetic co-twins *(49)*. This difference was statistically significant. A quasi-experimental test of the hypothesis that impaired nutrition in fetal life causes increased risk of diabetes in adult life may be provided by follow-up of groups exposed to famine during fetal life. One study compared 174 Russian adults exposed *in utero* to malnutrition during the 1941–42 siege of Leningrad with controls born before the siege or outside Leningrad *(50)*. Fasting and 2-h glucose levels were not significantly higher in the group exposed to malnutrition *in utero* than in controls. It is uncertain, however, whether malnutrition in this population would have been restricted to those classified as exposed. A more sharply delimited famine occurred in the western part of the Netherlands during 1944–45. A recent follow-up study of 702 people born between 1943 and 1947 in Amsterdam found that mean 2 h glucose levels were 0.4–0.5 mmol/L higher among those exposed to famine during mid gestation or late gestation than in those not exposed *(51)*. Although exposure to famine was associated with increased obesity in adult life, the effect of famine exposure on 2-h glucose levels was independent of BMI. These results, combined with those of the Danish twin study, imply a causal relationship between impaired fetal growth and increased risk of diabetes in adult life.

CAN IMPAIRED FETAL GROWTH ACCOUNT FOR ETHNIC DIFFERENCES IN PREVALENCE OF DIABETES?

The high prevalence of diabetes in many non-European populations where there has been a rapid transition from a rural subsistence economy to urban living has been interpreted in terms of a "thrifty genotype" *(52)*. This term was coined by Neel, who suggested that evolutionary selection for traits that confer the ability to survive when food supplies are unreliable might select also for genes that increase the risk of diabetes when food is abundant. Hales and Barker have suggested as an alternative explanation that the high rates of diabetes in these populations result from undernutrition in fetal and infant life, followed by relative overnutrition later *(53)*. They cite the high rates of diabetes recorded in the Pacific island of Nauru *(54)*, where there has been a recent transition from undernutrition to relative affluence, as an example. Evidence from migrant and admixture studies, however, suggests that differences in diabetes risk between high-risk ethnic groups such as Pacific islanders and low-risk ethnic groups such as Europeans are attributable to genetic factors. Prevalence of diabetes is uniformly high (around 20% in those aged over 35 yr) in urban populations of Indian descent even where migration occurred during the mid-nineteenth century *(55)*. While it is plausible that an effect of maternal environment could persist over one or two generations after migration, it is unlikely that such an effect would persist five or six generations after migration as an exposure specific to Indians. In Singapore, for instance, a rapid transition to affluence has been shared by all three of the main ethnic groups (Chinese, Malays, and Indians) but prevalence of diabetes is much higher in Indians than in Chinese *(56)*. In Nauruans and Pima Native Americans, inverse associations of diabetes with genetic markers of European admixture have been reported *(57,58)*. Admixture in Nauru resulted mainly from unions between Nauruan women and European men; thus the effect was to introduce European genes but not European maternal environment. It is of course possible that ethnic differences in the risk of diabetes could be a consequence of ethnic differences in fetal growth which have a genetic basis: average ponderal index at birth has been reported to be lower in the infants of Indian than European mothers in England. Such an explanation, however would still assign a primary role to genetic influences.

Although reduced fetal growth may be part of the explanation for high prevalence of diabetes in these high-risk populations, the evidence that genetic factors underlie the differences in risk of diabetes between high-risk groups such as Native Australians and low-risk groups such as Europeans remains compelling. This point is of some practical importance, as if ethnic differences in disease risk have a genetic basis it is in principle possible to map the genes underlying these differences by studying populations where there has been recent admixture *(59)*.

SMALL BABY SYNDROME OR INSULIN RESISTANCE SYNDROME?

The clustering in the population of physiological disturbances associated with insulin resistance—hyperinsulinemia, glucose intolerance, hypertension, elevated plasma triglyceride and low HDL cholesterol—is now considered as a distinct syndrome *(60,61)*. In the cohort of Hertfordshire men studied by the Southampton group, Barker and colleagues combined the measurements of glucose intolerance, hypertension and lipid disturbances at age 64 yr are combined to define a single binary trait corresponding to "Syndrome X" as defined by Reaven *(60)*. They found a strong inverse relationship between birth weight and the prevalence of this trait in middle age, with an odds ratio of 18 between the highest and the lowest categories of birth weight *(62)*. They suggested that impaired fetal growth could account for the clustering of glucose intolerance, hypertension and lipid disturbances in the population, and that the insulin resistance syndrome (IRS) should therefore be renamed as "small baby syndrome" *(62)*. In other studies which have examined the associations of size at birth with glucose intolerance, hypertension and disturbances of plasma lipid levels separately, with diabetic individuals excluded *(9,25,63)*, reduced fetal growth has been found to predict hyperinsulinemia, glucose intolerance and hypertension but not to predict the lipid abnormalities characteristic of the IRS—elevated triglyceride and low HDL cholesterol levels. It is thus possible to distinguish two patterns of clustering: a "small baby syndrome" characterized by hypertension, insulin resistance and glucose intolerance, and the "Syndrome X" cluster of raised triglyceride levels, low HDL cholesterol, insulin resistance, glucose intolerance. The lipid disturbances of "Syndrome X" are strongly associated with central obesity, measured by the waist-hip girth ratio (WHR). In two cohort studies—Hertfordshire men *(64)* and Preston adults *(3)*—inverse relations of WHR to birth weight were found. In a subsequent study of 93 Preston adults aged 50 there was no relation between size at birth and WHR *(63)*. Waist-hip ratio is not a pure measure of body fat distribution, and depends also on skeletal proportions. Thus, a higher WHR in those who were small at birth could be a consequence of small pelvic diameter rather than a consequence of intra-abdominal obesity. Further studies with direct measurements using computed tomography or magnetic resonance imaging to measure intra-abdominal fat directly are required to establish whether there is any relationship between body fat distribution and size at birth.

PHYSIOLOGICAL BASIS OF INSULIN RESISTANCE
IN ADULTS WHO WERE SMALL AT BIRTH

As skeletal muscle accounts for most insulin-mediated glucose disposal, some structural or functional defect in skeletal muscle must be present in individuals who were small at birth to account for the resistance to insulin-mediated glucose uptake in this group. In adults born in Preston, muscle mass was correlated with birth weight but not with ponderal index: thus the association with insulin resistance is not explained by alterations in muscle mass *(65)*. Lower capillary density in muscle has been suggested as a possible mechanism which could impair insulin-mediated glucose disposal. However, no relation of thinness at birth with the density of capillaries in the gastrocnemius muscle, or with the percentage of Type I (slow-twitch) muscle fibers was found when biopsy specimens were examined *(66)*. In the general population insulin sensitivity is correlated with post-prandial glycogen synthase activity *(67)*. Glycogen synthase activity in muscle biopsies was found to correlate with insulin sensitivity measured by the short insulin tolerance test and with central obesity, but not with size at birth *(68)*.

The Southampton group and their collaborators have studied the relation of size at birth to fuel utilization in skeletal muscle using phosphorus-31 magnetic resonance spec-troscopy (MRS) in a group of 25 women selected to cover a wide range of birth weight and ponderal index at birth *(69)*. A constant heavy workload was applied to a forearm muscle (flexor digitorum superficialis) to test anerobic glycolysis, and to a calf muscle (gastrocnemius) to test oxidative metabolism. In response to forearm exercise, fatigue was more rapid and the rise in adenosine diphosphate (ADP) levels in the forearm was greater in women who were thin at birth. The halftime of muscle reoxygenation was measured by near-infra-red spectroscopy of hemoglobin during metabolic recovery from ischemic finger exercise *(66)*. Women who had been thin at birth showed higher reoxygenation rates. Reoxygenation rates correlated strongly ($r = 0.6$) with rates of phosphocreatinine depletion and ADP accumulation in the magnetic resonance study. The authors suggested that reduced size at birth might be associated with a reduced ability to generate adenosine triphosphate (ATP) by anerobic glycolysis, and that the increased oxygenation in women could be a compensatory response to this impairment. Reduced generation of ATP by anaerobic glycolysis has been described in obese Zucker rats also *(70)*. Both in women who were small at birth, and in obese rats there appears to be an increased reliance on oxidative metabolism.

In response to oral glucose challenge, individuals who were small at birth suppress plasma NEFA *(63)* to the same extent as those who were large at birth, but fail to suppress total lipid oxidation *(71)*. This suggests that individuals who were small at birth may be oxidizing lipid stored in skeletal muscle cells. Lipolysis of triglyceride stored in muscle cells maintains a supply of nonesterified fatty acids (NEFA) in muscle even when lipoly-sis in adipocytes (the main source of NEFA in plasma) is suppressed by insulin *(72)*. Excess triglyceride stores in muscle cells, or increased lipolysis of these stores, could cause resistance to insulin-mediated glucose uptake through substrate competition between NEFA and glucose *(73)*. Substrate competition from intracellular lipid can be demonstrated in obese insulin-resistant individuals, in whom hyperinsulinemia sup-presses oxidation of lipid derived from plasma NEFA but fails to suppress oxidation of intracellular lipid *(74)*. Triglyceride stores in muscle cells are increased in obese indi-viduals but not in those who were small at birth *(75)*; thus the association of reduced fetal growth with failure of glucose to suppress lipid oxidation cannot be explained simply by increased levels of intracellular triglyceride.

CONCLUSIONS

In populations of European descent, size at birth is inversely related to the risk of Type 2 diabetes in adult life. This relationship appears to be mediated through insulin resistance. Studies of twins and adults exposed *in utero* to famine support the view that this association is causal: in other words, that impairment of growth in fetal life causes insulin resistance and diabetes, rather than that a primary defect in insulin action predisposes to both reduced growth *in utero* and to diabetes in adult life. The association of maternal glucose intolerance with increased size at birth and increased risk of diabetes in later life may account for the U-shaped or inverse associations seen in populations at high risk for Type 2 diabetes. The inverse association of birth weight with insulin resistance is seen only in those born at term. Failure to stratify by gestational age may account for why some studies have found stronger relationships of insulin resistance and diabetes with ponderal index than with birth weight. The effect of reduced fetal growth on insulin resistance appears to depend upon interaction with obesity in adult life. This suggests that whatever the mechanism of the effect, control of obesity is likely to be effective in alleviating insulin resistance and reducing the risk of diabetes in individuals who were thin at birth.

REFERENCES

1. Swenne I, Crace CJ, Milner RD, Milner RDG. Persistent impairment of insulin secretory response to glucose in adult rats after limited period of protein-calorie malnutrition early in life. Diabetes 1987;36:454–458.
2. Hales CN, Barker DJP, Clark PMS, Cox LJ, Fall C, Osmond C, Winter PD. Fetal and infant growth and impaired glucose tolerance at age 64. BMJ 1991;303:1019–1022.
3. Phipps K, Barker DJP, Hales CN, Fall CHD, Osmond C, Clark PMS. Fetal growth and impaired glucose tolerance in men and women. Diabetologia 1993;36:225–228.
4. McKeigue PM, Lithell HO, Leon DA. Glucose tolerance and resistance to insulin-stimulated glucose uptake in men aged 70 years in relation to size at birth. Diabetologia 1998;41;1133–1138.
5. Curhan GC, Willett WC, Rimm EB, Spiegelmann D, Ascherio AL, Stampfer MJ. Birth weight and adult hypertension and diabetes mellitus in US men. Circulation 1996;94:3246–3250.
6. McCance DR, Pettitt DJ, Hanson RL, Jacobson LTH, Knowler WC, Bennett PH. Birthweight and non-insulin-dependent diabetes: thrifty genotype, thrifty phenotype or surviving small baby genotype? BMJ 1994;308:942–945.
7. Fall CHD, Stein CE, Kumaran K, Cox V, Osmond C, Barker DJP, Hales CN. Size at birth, maternal weight, and type 2 diabetes in south India. Diabetic Med 1998;15:220–227.
8. Robinson S, Walton RJ, Clark PM, Barker DJP, Hales CN, Osmond C. The relation of fetal growth to plasma glucose in young men. Diabetologia 1992;35:444–446.
9. Valdez R, Athens MA, Thompson GH, Bradshaw BS, Stern MP. Birth weight and adult health outcomes in a biethnic population in the USA. Diabetologia 1994;37:624–631.
10. Yajnik CS, Fall CH, Vaidya U, et al. Fetal growth and glucose and insulin metabolism in four-year-old Indian children. Diabetic Med 1995;12:330–336.
11. Law CM, Gordon CM, Shiell AW, Barker DJP, Hales CN. Thinness at birth and glucose tolerance in seven-year-old children. Diabetic Med 1995;12:24–249.
12. Forrester TE, Wilks RJ, Bennett FI, et al. Fetal growth and cardiovascular risk factors in Jamaican schoolchildren. BMJ 1996;312:156–160.
13. Freinkel N. Of pregnancy and progeny. Diabetes 1980;29:1023–1035.
14. Aerts L, Sodoyez Goffaux F, Sodoyez JC, Malaisse WJ, Van Assche FA. The diabetic intrauterine milieu has a long-lasting effect on insulin secretion by β-cells and on insulin uptake by target tissues. Am J Obstet Gynecol 1988;159:1287–92.
15. Grill V, Johansson B, Jalkanen P, Eriksson UJ. Influence of severe diabetes mellitus early in pregnancy in the rat: effects on insulin sensitivity and insulin secretion in the offspring. Diabetologia 1991;34:373–378.
16. Gauguier D, Bihoreau MT, Ktorza A, Berthault MF, Picon L. Inheritance of diabetes mellitus as consequence of gestational hyperglycemia in rats. Diabetes 1990;39:734–739.
17. Pettitt DJ, Aleck KA, Baird HR, Carraher MJ, Bennett PH, Knowler WC. Congenital susceptibility to NIDDM: role of intrauterine environment. Diabetes 1988;37:622–628.

18. Phillips DIW, Hirst S, Clark PMS, Hales CN, Osmond C. Fetal growth and insulin secretion in adult life. Diabetologia 1994;37:592–596.
19. Phillips DIW, Barker DJP, Hales CN, Hirst S, Osmond C. Thinness at birth and insulin resistance in adult life. Diabetologia 1994;37:150–154.
20. Yki-Jarvinen H. Evidence for a primary role of insulin resistance in the pathogenesis of Type 2 diabetes. Ann Med 1990;22:197–200.
21. Rahier J, Wallon J, Henquin JC. Cell populations in the endocrine pancreas of human neonates and infants. Diabetologia 1981;20:540–546.
22. Crace CJ, Swenne I, Milner RDG. Long-term effects on glucose-tolerance and insulin secretory response to glucose following a limited period of severe protein or energy malnutrition in young-rats. Uppsala J Med Sci 1991;96:177–183.
23. Dahri S, Snoeck A, Reusensbillen B, Remacle C, Hoet JJ. Islet function in offspring of mothers on low-protein diet during gestation. Diabetes 1991;40:115–120.
24. McCulloch DK, Koerker DJ, Kahn SE, Bonner-Weir S, Palmer JP. Correlations of in vivo beta-cell function tests with beta cell mass and pancreatic insulin content in streptozotocin-treated baboons. Diabetes 1991;40:673–679.
25. Lithell HO, McKeigue PM, Berglund L, Mohsen R, Lithell U, Leon DA. Relationship of size at birth to non-insulin-dependent diabetes and insulin levels in men aged 50–60 years. BMJ 1996;312:406–410.
26. Clausen JO, Borch-Johnsen K, Pedersen O. Relation between birth weight and the insulin sensitivity index in a population sample of 331 young, healthy Caucasians. Am J Epidemiol 1997;146:23–31.
27. Langley SC, Browne RF, Jackson AA. Altered glucose tolerance in rats exposed to maternal low-protein diets in utero. Comp Biochem Physiol 1994;109:223–229.
28. Holness MJ. Impact of early growth-retardation on glucoregulatory control and insulin action in mature rats. Am J Physiol 1996;33:E 946–E954.
29. Ozanne SE, Smith GD, Tikerpae J, Hales CN. Altered regulation of hepatic glucose output in the male offspring of protein-malnourished rat dams. Am J Physiol 1996;33:E 559–E564.
30. Benediktsson R, Lindsay RS, Noble J, Seckl JR, Edwards CR. Glucocorticoid exposure in utero: new model for adult hypertension. Lancet 1993;341:339–341.
31. Seckl JR, Benediktsson R, Lindsay RS, Brown RW. Placental 11-beta-hydroxysteroid dehydrogenase and the programming of hypertension. J Steroid Biochem Mol Biol 1995;55:447–455.
32. Seckl JR. Glucocorticoids, feto-placental 11 beta-hydroxysteroid dehydrogenase Type 2, and the early life origins of adult disease. Steroids 1997;62:89–94.
33. Benediktsson R, Calder AA, Edwards CR, Seckl JR. Placental 11 beta-hydroxysteroid dehydrogenase: a key regulator of fetal glucocorticoid exposure. Clin Endocrinol 1997;46:161–166.
34. Langley-Evans SC, Phillips GJ, Benediktsson R, Gardner DS, Edwards CRW, Jackson AA, Seckl JR. Protein-intake in pregnancy, placental glucocorticoid metabolism and the programming of hypertension in the rat. Placenta 1996;17:169–172.
35. Hales CN, Desai M, Ozanne SE, Crowther NJ. Fishing in the stream of diabetes—from measuring insulin to the control of fetal organogenesis. Biochem Soc Trans 1996;24:341–350.
36. Lindsay RS, Lindsay RM, Waddell BJ, Seckl JR. Prenatal glucocorticoid exposure leads to offspring hyperglycemia in the rat: studies with the 11 beta-hydroxysteroid dehydrogenase inhibitor carbenoxolone. Diabetologia 1996;39:1299–1305.
37. Langley-Evans SC, Gardner DS, Jackson AA. Maternal protein restriction influences the programming of the rat hypothalamic-pituitary-adrenal axis. J Nutr 1996;126:1578–1585.
38. Langley-Evans SC, Welham SJM, Sherman RC, Jackson AA. Weanling rats exposed to maternal low-protein diets during discrete periods of gestation exhibit differing severity of hypertension. Clin Sci 1996;91:607–615.
39. Levitt NS, Lindsay RS, Holmes MC, Seckl JR. Dexamethasone in the last week of pregnancy attenuates hippocampal glucocorticoid receptor gene expression and elevates blood pressure in the adult offspring in the rat. Neuroendocrinology 1996;64:412–418.
40. Clark PM, Hindmarsh PC, Shiell AW, Law CM, Honour JW, Barker DJ. Size at birth and adrenocortical function in childhood. Clin Endocrinol 1996;45:721–726.
41. Phillips DIW, Barker DJ, Fall CHD, Whorwood CB, Walker BR, Wood PJ. Low birthweight and raised plasma cortisol concentrations in adult life. J Endocrinol 1997;152 suppl: P2(abstract).
42. Paneth N, Susser M. Early origin of coronary heart disease: the "Barker hypothesis." BMJ 1995; 310:411–412.

43. Zimmet PZ. The pathogenesis and prevention of diabetes in adults—genes, autoimmunity, and demography. Diabetes Care 1995;18:1050–1064.

44. Sjolin S. Infant mortality in Sweden. In: Wallace HM, ed. Health care of mothers and children in national health services: implications for the United States. Ballinger, Cambridge, MA, 1975, pp. 229–240.

45. Morton NE. The inheritance of human birth weight. Ann Hum Genet 1955;20:125.

46. Magnus P. Further evidence for a significant effect of fetal genes on variation in birth weight. Clin Genet 1984;26:289–296.

47. Gluckman PD. The role of pituitary hormones, growth factors and insulin in the regulation of fetal growth. Oxford Rev Reproductive Biol 1986;8:1–60.

48. Tamemoto H, Kadowaki T, Tobe K, et al. Insulin resistance and growth retardation in mice lacking insulin receptor substrate-1. Nature 1994;372:182–186.

49. Poulsen P, Vaag AA, Kyvik KO, Jensen DM, Beck-Nielsen H. Low birth weight is associated with NIDDM in discordant monozygotic and dizygotic twin pairs. Diabetologia 1997;40:439–446.

50. Yudkin JS, Stanner S, Bulmer K, et al. Is cardiovascular risk related to intrauterine starvation—the Leningrad Siege Study. Diabetes 1996;45 suppl 2:193A(abstract).

51. Ravelli ACJ, van der Meulen JHP, Michels RPJ, Osmond C, Barker DJP, Hales CN, Bleker OP. Glucose intolerance in adults after prenatal exposure to famine. Lancet 1998;351:173–177.

52. Neel JV. Diabetes mellitus: a 'thrifty' genotype rendered detrimental by 'progress.' Am J Hum Genet 1962;14:353–62.

53. Hales CN, Barker DJP. Type 2 (non-insulin-dependent) diabetes mellitus—the thrifty phenotype hypothesis. Diabetologia 1992;35:595–601.

54. Dowse GK, Zimmet PZ, Finch CF, Collins VR. Decline in incidence of epidemic glucose intolerance in Nauruans—implications for the thrifty genotype. Am J Epidemiol 1991;133:1093–1104.

55. McKeigue PM, Miller GJ, Marmot MG. Coronary heart disease in South Asians overseas: a review. J Clin Epidemiol 1989;42:597–609.

56. Hughes K, Yeo PPB, Lun KC, et al. Cardiovascular diseases in Chinese,Malays and Indians in Singapore. II. Differences in risk factor levels. J Epidemiol Commun Health 1990;44:29–35.

57. Serjeantson SW, Owerbach D, Zimmet P, Nerup J, Thoma K. Genetics of diabetes in Nauru: effects of foreign admixture, HLA antigens and the insulin-gene-linked polymorphism. Diabetologia 1983;25:13–17.

58. Knowler WC, Williams RC, Pettitt DJ, Steinberg AG. Gm3;5,13,14 and Type 2 diabetes mellitus: an association in American Indians with genetic admixture. Am J Hum Genet 1988;43:520–526.

59. McKeigue PM. Mapping genes that underlie ethnic differences in disease risk: methods for detecting linkage in admixed populations by conditioning on parental admixture. Am J Hum Genet 1998;63:241–251.

60. Reaven GM. Role of insulin resistance in human disease. Diabetes 1988;37:1595–1607.

61. DeFronzo RA, Ferrannini E. Insulin resistance: a multifaceted syndrome responsible for NIDDM, obesity, hypertension, dyslipidemia, and atherosclerotic cardiovascular disease. Diabetes Care 1991;14:173–194.

62. Barker DJP, Hales CN, Fall CHD, Osmond C, Phipps K, Clark PMS. Type 2 (non-insulin-dependent) diabetes mellitus, hypertension and hyperlipidemia (syndrome X): relation to reduced fetal growth. Diabetologia 1993;36:62–67.

63. Phillips DIW, McLeish R, Osmond C, Hales CN. Fetal growth and insulin resistance in adult life: role of plasma triglyceride and nonesterified fatty acids. Diabetic Med 1995;12:796–801.

64. Law CM, Barker DJP, Osmond C, Fall CHD, Simmonds SJ. Early growth and abdominal fatness in adult life. J Epidemiol Commun Health 1992;46:184–186.

65. Phillips DIW. Relation of fetal growth to adult muscle mass and glucose-tolerance. Diabetic Med 1995;12:686–690.

66. Thompson CH, Stein C, Caddy S, et al. Fetal growth and insulin resistance in adult life: role of skeletal muscle microcirculation and oxygenation. Diabetologia 1995;38:A 136(abstract).

67. Kida Y, Esposito Del Puente A, Bogardus C, Mott DM. Insulin resistance is associated with reduced fasting and insulin-stimulated glycogen synthase phosphatase activity in human skeletal muscle. J Clin Invest 1990;85:476–481.

68. Phillips DIW, Borthwick AC, Stein C, Taylor R. Fetal growth and insulin resistance in adult life: relationship between glycogen synthase activity in adult skeletal muscle and birth weight. Diabetic Med 1996;13:325–329.

69. Taylor DJ, Thompson CH, Kemp GJ, Barnes PRJ, Sanderson AL, Radda GK, Phillips DIW. A relationship between impaired fetal growth and reduced muscle glycolysis revealed by P-31 magnetic resonance spectroscopy. Diabetologia 1995;38:1205–1212.

70. Sanderson AL, Kemp GJ, Thompson CH, Radda GK. Increased oxidative and delayed glycogenolytic ATP synthesis in exercising skeletal muscle of obese (insulin resistant) Zucker rats. Clin Sci 1996;91:691–702.

71. Wootton SA, Murphy JL, Wilson F, Phillips D. Energy expenditure and substrate metabolism after carbohydrate ingestion in relation to fetal growth in women born in Preston. Proc Nutr Soc 1994;53:174A(abstract).

72. Yki-Jarvinen H, Puhakainen I, Saloranta C, Groop L, Taskinen MR. Demonstration of a novel feedback mechanism between FFA oxidation from intracellular and intravascular sources. Am J Physiol 1991;260:E680–E689.

73. Randle PJ, Garland PB, Hales CN, Newsholme EA. The glucose-fatty acid cycle. Its role in insulin sensitivity and the metabolic disturbances of diabetes mellitus. Lancet 1963;1:785–789.

74. Groop LC, Bonadonna RC, Simonson DC, Petrides AS, Shank M, DeFronzo RA. Effect of insulin on oxidative and nonoxidative pathways of free fatty-acid metabolism in human obesity. Am J Physiol 1992;263:79–84.

75. Phillips DIW, Caddy S, Ilic V, Fielding BA, Frayn KN, Borthwick AC, Taylor R. Intramuscular triglyceride and muscle insulin sensitivity: evidence for a relationship in nondiabetic subjects. Metabolism 1996;45:947–950.

4

Obesity and Insulin Resistance

Epidemiologic, Metabolic, and Molecular Aspects

Jean-Pierre Després, PhD
and André Marette, PhD

CONTENTS

INTRODUCTION
OBESITY AND METABOLIC COMPLICATIONS: *IMPORTANCE OF BODY FAT
    DISTRIBUTION AND OF VISCERAL ADIPOSE TISSUE ACCUMULATION*
THE INSULIN RESISTANT-DYSLIPIDEMIC SYNDROME OF VISCERAL
    OBESITY: *BEYOND THE PREVENTION OF NON-INSULIN DEPENDENT
    DIABETES MELLITUS*
POTENTIAL MECHANISMS OF INSULIN RESISTANCE IN OBESITY
MOLECULAR DEFECTS OF INSULIN ACTION IN OBESITY-LINKED
    INSULIN RESISTANCE
THE ATHEROGENIC DYSLIPIDEMIA OF INSULIN RESISTANCE
    IN ABDOMINAL OBESITY: *IMPACT ON THE RISK
    OF ISCHEMIC HEART DISEASE*
SIMPLE TOOLS FOR THE ASSESSMENT OF THE INSULIN RESISTANCE
    SYNDROME IN ABDOMINAL OBESITY
SIMPLE ANTHROPOMETRIC MARKERS OF REGIONAL BODY FAT
    DISTRIBUTION AND OF VISCERAL ADIPOSE TISSUE ACCUMULATION
ARE THERE CRITICAL VALUES OF VISCERAL ADIPOSE TISSUE
    ACCUMULATION AND OF WAIST CIRCUMFERENCE?
ARE THERE SIMPLE CLINICAL MARKERS OF THE INSULIN-RESISTANCE
    DYSLIPIDEMIC SYNDROME?
REFERENCES

INTRODUCTION

It is commonly accepted that obesity is a health hazard associated with complications such as non-insulin-dependent diabetes mellitus (Type 2 diabetes), dyslipidemias, hypertension and cardiovascular diseases *(1–5)*. On the basis of its increasing prevalence in affluent countries *(6–8)*, obesity is considered as a major cause of morbidity and mortality

From: *Contemporary Endocrinology: Insulin Resistance*
Edited by: G. Reaven and A. Laws © Humana Press Inc., Totowa, NJ

which makes a major contribution to our health care expenditures *(9)*. Overall, excess weight is related to an increased mortality rate both from cardiovascular diseases and other causes *(2–5,10,11)*.

Despite the general acceptance of its deleterious impact on health, obesity has long been a puzzling condition for many clinicians as it is characterized by a remarkable heterogeneity *(3,4,11)*. Indeed, a substantial excess of body fat in some individuals is not always associated with severe complications whereas some patients who are only moderately overweight may develop Type 2 diabetes, hypertension and premature cardiovascular diseases *(3,4)*. Whether or not obesity is an "independent" risk factor for cardiovascular diseases and related mortality remains an epidemiological question which has not been fully answered *(12–14)*. However, evidence published over the last 15 years has emphasized that there is a subgroup of obese patients who are characterized by an excess accumulation of "bad," upper body, abdominal fat and who are at very high risk for the development of Type 2 diabetes, dyslipidemias, hypertension and cardiovascular diseases (for reviews see refs. *3,4,15–22*). Thus, although the question of the "independence" of the obesity-cardiovascular disease relationship is interesting from an epidemiologic perspective, it may not be that critical and could even be misleading in the clinical practice. Indeed, from the lack of randomized weight loss-mortality study available, some clinicians may not be tempted to target abdominal obesity as a legitimate therapeutic objective and may rather treat the related insulin resistance, the Type 2 diabetes or the atherogenic dyslipidemic state, which may lead to the "suboptimal" management of risk in these patients. Indeed, such an approach would only deal with the consequences of obesity rather than target the primary factor leading to the metabolic complications. On the other hand, some clinicians may question the relevance of weight loss for reducing mortality risk in an obese patient without insulin resistance or related complications and this issue has also not been satisfactorily addressed in the literature. However, we suggest that the relevance of weight loss should be further emphasized for the abdominal obese patient showing the complications of insulin resistance. Despite this recommendation based on the overall favorable effects of weight loss on the metabolic complications of obesity, it has to be recognized that no randomized weight loss trial has so far been conducted to clearly document the impact of voluntary weight loss on both morbidity and mortality. Such trials, currently under consideration, are urgently needed.

In this chapter, the objectives of the authors are the following:

1. To review the link between adipose tissue distribution, insulin resistance, and metabolic complications, with an emphasis over visceral adipose tissue.
2. To discuss some potential mechanisms of insulin resistance in obesity.
3. To provide further epidemiologic evidence that even in the absence of Type 2 diabetes or of impaired glucose tolerance, the cluster of metabolic abnormalities found in the insulin resistance dyslipidemic syndrome of visceral obesity is a very atherogenic condition requiring careful attention.
4. To provide clinicians with simple tools (anthropometric and metabolic markers) for the assessment of the insulin resistance syndrome (IRS) in abdominal obesity.

This chapter is by no means a bibliographic review. The paper is rather an attempt to discuss some of the issues relevant to obesity and insulin resistance which are related to the interests and expertise of the authors. Several review articles that may address additional aspects of the IRS in obesity are available in the literature *(3,4,15–22)*.

OBESITY AND METABOLIC COMPLICATIONS:
IMPORTANCE OF BODY FAT DISTRIBUTION
AND OF VISCERAL ADIPOSE TISSUE ACCUMULATION

It is more and more widely recognized that body fat distribution, especially abdominal fat deposition, is an important factor to consider in the clinical evaluation of the obese patient. Abdominal obesity is now considered as a powerful risk factor for the development of Type 2 diabetes and cardiovascular disease *(23–26)*. Over the last ten years, we have used computed tomography, an imaging technique which had been reported to be a relevant tool to study regional adipose tissue accumulation *(27–30)* and we found significant associations between abdominal visceral adipose tissue deposition and metabolic complications known to increase the risk of Type 2 diabetes and cardiovascular diseases *(31–36)*. This technique was especially helpful to distinguish intra-abdominal (visceral) adipose tissue from subcutaneous abdominal fat. As several review articles from our laboratory have been published to describe the contribution of our group to the understanding of some pathophysiologic aspects of visceral obesity, we will not provide the reader with an extensive description of our previously published results. In the present section, our main observations will be summarized with discussion of additional material recently published by our group. The reader is once again referred to our previous literature for further details regarding our descriptive studies of the visceral obesity syndrome *(15–18,31–38)*. In brief, we found that excess visceral adipose tissue accumulation, in the presence or absence of obesity, is associated with insulin resistance, hyperinsulinemia, glucose intolerance, these metabolic abnormalities being predictive of an increased risk of Type 2 diabetes *(15–18,31–38)*. Furthermore, we also reported that excess visceral adipose tissue accumulation was associated with a potentially atherogenic lipoprotein profile which includes hypertriglyceridemia, elevated apoB levels, an increased proportion of small, dense low-density lipoprotein (LDL) particles, and low high-density lipoprotein (HDL)-cholesterol concentrations *(15–18,31–38)*. Furthermore, evidence has accumulated that the insulin resistance-dyslipidemic syndrome of visceral obesity is also associated with alterations in hemostatic variables which contribute to increase the risk of atherothrombotic events in these patients *(39,40)*.

From a public health standpoint, it is critically important to emphasize that these features of the IRS of visceral obesity are not only observed in the diabetic and prediabetic patients, but also in a large proportion of insulin resistant individuals who are relatively euglycemic and who may never develop Type 2 diabetes *(41)*. Thus, although insulin resistance is a major risk factor for the development of glucose intolerance and Type 2 diabetes *(42–44)*, the majority of insulin resistant individuals will never develop Type 2 diabetes, but they are at very high risk for atherothrombotic events. We propose "preventive endocrinology" to describe an approach where early markers of risk could be used for the identification of patients with the features of the IRS.

THE INSULIN RESISTANT-DYSLIPIDEMIC SYNDROME
OF VISCERAL OBESITY: *BEYOND THE PREVENTION*
OF NON-INSULIN-DEPENDENT DIABETES MELLITUS

The "Preventive Endocrinology" Concept

Cardiovascular disease (CVD) is a major cause of mortality among patients with non-insulin dependent diabetes mellitus (Type 2 diabetes) *(45–47)*. Indeed, prospective studies have shown that the risk of CVD is increased by several folds among Type 2 diabetes patients in comparison with nondiabetic controls *(45–47)*. It has been previously reported that this increased CVD risk is already observed among newly diagnosed Type 2 diabetes patients *(48,49)* probably due to the fact that the condition of several Type 2 diabetes patients had remained undiagnosed for several years. In addition, it is more and more recognized that metabolic alterations already present in the prediabetic state may increase the risk of CVD several years before the condition evolves to glucose intolerance and eventually to Type 2 diabetes *(41,50)*. Indeed, it is well accepted that Type 2 diabetes is associated with in vivo insulin resistance and with an impaired insulin secretion and prospective studies have shown that these two metabolic abnormalities are good predictors of the risk of Type 2 diabetes *(42–44,51–55)*. Although the identification of the primary abnormality(ies) leading to Type 2 diabetes remains a matter of considerable ongoing work and debate, especially regarding the genetic factors involved, a reduced insulin secretion appears to be an important triggering factor which may lead to relative insulin deficiency and Type 2 diabetes among insulin resistant individuals *(42,44,53,54)*.

This notion has important implications regarding the etiology of macrovascular disease. Type 2 diabetes is commonly accompanied by a typical dyslipidemic state which includes hypertriglyceridemia, low HDL-cholesterol levels, normal to marginally elevated LDL-cholesterol concentrations and an increased proportion of small, dense LDL particles *(55–60)*. Furthermore, hemostatic alterations and an impaired fibrinolytic potential, an impaired endothelial reactivity as well as alterations in growth factors could exacerbate CVD risk in Type 2 diabetes patients *(57)*. Prospective studies in diabetic and nondiabetic individuals have all suggested that these metabolic abnormalities could contribute to CVD risk, especially as they tend to cluster in Type 2 diabetes patients *(55–57)*.

However, it is now more and more recognized that these metabolic alterations precede Type 2 diabetes as long as insulin resistance and hyperinsulinemia are present *(50,55–57)*. Insulin resistant individuals with no defect in pancreatic insulin secretion potential have marked hyperinsulinemia but may display normal fasting glycemia and even a normal glucose tolerance *(50)*. As only a portion of insulin resistant or glucose intolerant individuals will convert to Type 2 diabetes *(42–44,51–55)*, the majority of these insulin resistant-hyperinsulinemic individuals will not develop Type 2 diabetes. However, the price associated with this hyperinsulinemic state may be a substantial increase in the risk of macrovascular atherosclerotic disease *(41,50)*.

In a landmark article introducing his insulin resistance syndrome (Syndrome X) concept *(50)*, Reaven emphasized that about 25% of sedentary individuals with normal glucose tolerance (because of an adequate compensatory increase in insulin secretion) are characterized by an insulin resistant state which is almost as severe as in glucose intolerant and in Type 2 diabetes patients. Insulin resistance in nondiabetic individuals has been associated with a dyslipidemia which was later described as including the main alterations in plasma lipoprotein lipid levels found in Type 2 diabetes patients, i.e., hypertriglyceridemia and low HDL-cholesterol levels but plasma cholesterol and LDL-cholesterol levels in the normal range or only marginally elevated *(37,41,50,58,59)*. More recent studies have indicated that one should not be misled by these apparently normal plasma LDL-cholesterol concentrations as additional analytical techniques such as gradient polyacrylamide gel electrophoresis have shown that insulin resistant-dyslipidemic subjects are characterized by an increased proportion of small, dense LDL particles *(60,61)*. The presence of an increased proportion of these dense LDL particles has been recently reported in prospective studies to increase the risk of coronary heart disease *(62–64)*.

Due to the presence of insulin resistance in non-obese individuals, Reaven did not initially include obesity among the original features of the syndrome *(50)*. However, it is now recognized that abdominal obesity associated with an excess accumulation of visceral adipose tissue (which can even been found in non-obese individuals) is an important correlate of the insulin resistance-dyslipidemic syndrome *(3,15–22)*. The insulin resistance syndrome concept has important implications from a prevention standpoint. Indeed, although it is recognized that the hyperglycemic state of Type 2 diabetes increases CVD risk and that even a slight "dysglycemia" may also contribute to an increased risk of macrovascular disease *(65)*, it is emphasized that insulin resistant individuals who may never develop Type 2 diabetes due to an adequate pancreatic insulin secretion potential may develop CVD in the absence of any dysglycemia *(41,50)*.

POTENTIAL MECHANISMS OF INSULIN RESISTANCE IN OBESITY

The Pathogenesis of Obesity-Linked Insulin Resistance

One of the most challenging tasks for scientists working on insulin action and insulin resistance has been to unravel the molecular basis of this cellular defect. Insulin resistance is defined as a diminished response of a target cell or organ to a physiological concentration of insulin. Whereas this definition can be applied to all insulin-responsive tissues (skeletal and cardiac muscle, adipose tissue, and liver), the mechanisms behind this cellular resistance to insulin action are not necessarily the same. Indeed, whereas the binding and early signaling events involved in insulin action are for the most part identical between all the above tissues, there are notable differences in downstream effectors and intracellular metabolic pathways between muscle, fat and liver cells. Thus, insulin resistance is heterogeneous and can take different forms depending on its site of occurrence. In the following section, we will first briefly review the pathogenesis of obesity-linked insulin resistance. We will then survey the molecular defects that have been reported in cells from obese insulin-resistant subjects. A particular attention will be given to the peripheral targets of insulin (muscle and adipose cells) since our understanding of the molecular mechanisms of insulin action on glucose transport in these cells, and their dysregulation in the obese insulin-resistant state, has greatly improved in recent years.

Obesity-Related Insulin Resistance in Different Tissues

Insulin resistance develops in both the liver and peripheral tissues (fat and muscle) in obesity-linked diabetes. However, important tissue-specific differences exist in both its development over time and in its primary causes. Thus, insulin resistance can be detected very early in skeletal muscle and liver, even in non-obese nondiabetic relatives of Type 2 diabetes subjects *(see* Molecular Defects of Insulin Action in Obesity-Linked Insulin Resistance*)*. In contrast, insulin resistance develops much later in adipose tissue when there is a marked lipid accretion in adipocytes. The temporal distinction in the development of insulin resistance between skeletal muscle and adipose tissue has been elegantly demonstrated by the classical work of Pénicaud and colleagues *(66)* using the genetically obese Zucker rat as a model of insulin resistance. In that model, insulin-mediated glucose uptake in skeletal muscle was already impaired in young (4-weeks) obese Zucker rats. In marked contrast, (white) adipose tissue from the same animal was not resistant to insulin for glucose utilization. Isolated adipocytes from young obese Zucker rats showed a greater insulin responsiveness for glucose transport and a greater capacity for lipogenesis than cells from lean littermates *(67,68)*. In older animals, insulin-induced glucose uptake is also impaired in adipocytes and may be linked to the overexpression of TNF-α (or leptin) by the enlarged fat cells *(see next section)*. The accumulation of fat, particularly in the visceral region, further exacerbates the insulin resistance syndrome (both hepatic and peripheral). Thus, whereas obesity *per se* may be an essential condition for the development of insulin resistance in fat cells of obese insulin-resistant individuals, it only exacerbates a primary defect that is already present in skeletal muscle and liver.

CANDIDATE MEDIATORS OF OBESITY-RELATED INSULIN RESISTANCE IN SKELETAL MUSCLE AND FAT

Several factors have been postulated to be responsible for the development of peripheral insulin resistance in obesity. The reader is referred to previous reviews and book chapters on the subject *(37,69)*. One molecule that has received considerable attention in the last five years is the cytokine TNF-α *(see Fig. 1)*.

There are now several pieces of evidence implicating TNF-α as a candidate mediator of obesity-associated insulin resistance (70,71). TNF-α is expressed at high levels in the enlarged adipose tissue from virtually all rodent models of genetic obesity as well as in obese humans *(72–74)*. The cytokine is also overexpressed in muscle cells isolated from Type 2 diabetes subjects *(74)*. Moreover, TNF-α was shown to reduce insulin-stimulated glucose uptake both in vivo and in adipose cells in vitro *(75,76)*. Importantly, both experimental neutralization and genetic ablation of TNF-α or TNF-α function were reported to improve insulin sensitivity in various animal models of insulin resistance. Thus, neutralization of TNF-α action in vivo was found to improve the insulin-resistant glucose utilization of obese Zucker rats *(71)*. However, neutralization experiments failed to improve insulin sensitivity in obese Type 2 diabetes subjects *(77)*. Two recent studies in mice lacking TNF-α expression or function have further confirmed the role of TNF-α in obesity-linked insulin resistance in animals. Uysal et al. *(78)* and Ventre et al. *(79)* generated obese mice with a targeted null mutation in the gene encoding TNF-α or those encoding the two receptors (p55 and p75) for TNF-α. The lack of TNF-α (or TNF-α action) significantly (but not completely) restored insulin sensitivity in rodent models of either diet-induced (high-fat), experimental (gold-thioglucose-injected) or genetic (*ob/ob* mouse) obesity. In the high-fat fed animals, mice lacking TNF-α showed an improved signaling capacity of the insulin receptor in both muscle and fat as compared with TNF-α+/+ mice *(78)*. Two conclusions can be drawn from these studies: 1) TNF-α is a mediator of insulin resistance in obesity, 2) the absence of TNF-α or of its action is not sufficient to protect completely against insulin resistance and therefore other candidate mediators must be considered.

Interestingly, TNF-α may also explain the well recognized negative relationship between plasma free fatty acids (FFA) and insulin resistance. Indeed, Hotamisligil et al. *(80)* reported that a targeted mutation of aP2, an adipocyte fatty acid binding protein, uncoupled obesity from insulin resistance in mice. The aP2-deficient mice failed to express TNF-α in adipose tissue, thus suggesting that binding of FFA and their transport to intracellular compartments by aP2 could regulate the expression of TNF-α (and perhaps other genes) in that tissue. On the other hand, these studies cannot rule out the classical but still updated hypothesis that FFA can reduce insulin-stimulated glucose utilization in muscle through substrate competition (the glucose-fatty acid cycle) (Randle), as reviewed elsewhere *(81)*.

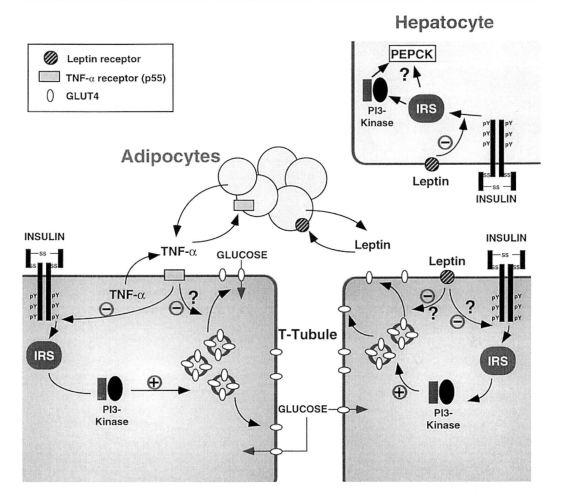

Fig. 1. Mechanisms postulated to be implicated in the development of insulin resistance in obesity. The enlarged fat cells oversecrete TNF-α and leptin in the local circulation. TNF-α impairs insulin action by inhibiting insulin receptor signaling, possibly by increasing IRS-1 serine phosphorylation *(see text)*. Other effects of TNF-α on GLUT4 expression and translocation to the cell surface may also be implicated. Leptin released from visceral adipocytes may inhibit insulin action in the liver by impairing insulin receptor signaling, leading to reduced down-regulation of PEPCK, the rate-limiting enzyme in gluconeogenesis. Possible long-term effects of leptin on insulin action in skeletal muscle remain to be demonstrated. Both TNF-α and leptin have been shown to have autocrine effects and to impair insulin action also in adipocytes.

Taken together, these data strongly support a role for TNF-α (acting either locally or systemically) in obesity-related insulin resistance, although more definitive evidence for such a role in humans is still lacking. One important question that remains to be answered is how TNF-α causes insulin resistance. Whereas direct inhibitory effects of TNF-α on insulin action has been demonstrated in adipocytes *(76)*, most studies failed to observe such an effect of the cytokine on skeletal muscle or cultured muscle cells *(82,83)*. One possible reason for these discrepant findings is that longer time (days) of exposure to the cytokine is necessary to observe the impairment of insulin action in skeletal muscle. Alternatively, TNF-α may be acting in concert with other cytokines in vivo. Indeed, TNF-α acts in synergy with other cytokines during activation of inflammatory processes and this may also be the case in the obese insulin-resistant state. Interestingly, exposure of L6 myotubes to a combination of cytokines was recently reported to inhibit insulin-stimulated glucose transport whereas TNF-α alone had no effect *(84)*. Whether the action of cytokines other than TNF-α is contributing to the insulin-resistant effects of TNF-α in vivo remains to be explored.

Another molecule that has lately received a great deal of attention is leptin, the protein product of the ob gene. With the exception of the *ob/ob* mice (which have a point mutation in the leptin gene that encodes a nonfunctional protein), all animal models of obesity and the vast majority of obese humans have increased adipose tissue leptin expression and circulating leptin levels *(85,86)*. Thus, it has been proposed that hyperleptinemia may contribute to the development of peripheral insulin resistance in obesity (Fig. 1). Recent studies have shown that leptin have direct effects on isolated rat adipocytes. Long-term exposure of adipose cells to leptin was shown to impair insulin's ability to induce glucose transport, glycogen synthase, lipogenesis, antilipolysis, and protein synthesis *(87)*. On the other hand, the implication of leptin in obesity-linked insulin resistance is complicated by the lack of direct action of leptin on skeletal muscle, the main site of peripheral insulin resistance in obesity. Whereas previous studies showed that leptin could exert acute insulin-like effects in C2C12 myotubes in culture *(88)*, other studies failed to confirm these findings in isolated skeletal muscles *(89)*. However, longer exposure to leptin may be necessary to affect insulin action in muscle, or leptin is possibly acting together with other factors in vivo. Further studies are warranted to verify these possibilities.

MECHANISMS OF INSULIN RESISTANCE IN LIVER

Among the factors believed to play a potential role in causing liver insulin resistance, elevated FFA levels have received considerable attention. Intra-abdominal obesity is believed to be associated with increased portal FFA flux which may lead to a reduced hepatic insulin extraction, enhanced lipoprotein synthesis and increased gluconeogenesis, all features of insulin resistance *(22,90–92)*. Among the various hormones which regulate adipose tissue lipolysis, catecholamines and insulin play primary roles *(90,91,93)*. Adrenaline modulates lipolysis through its antilipolytic α2-AR and lipolytic β-AR components *(94,95)*, whereas insulin is a potent inhibitor of lipolysis at low physiological concentrations *(96–98)*. Previous studies have established that visceral adipocytes are more lipolytic than subcutaneous fat cells, probably because of an increased β-AR (and more particularly, β3-AR component *(99–102)* as well as of both reduced α2-AR (125,126)) and insulin antilipolytic components *(94,96,98)*.

The molecular mechanisms behind this FFA-mediated liver insulin resistance are still not fully unraveled. Previous studies reported that elevated ambient FFA levels were associated with impaired insulin cell surface binding to isolated hepatocytes, possibly through an effect of lipid oxidation on the internalization/recycling of the insulin-receptor complex, and lower receptor-mediated insulin degradation *(103,104)*. No defect in receptor tyrosine kinase (TK) activity was detected in FFA-treated cells. It is unlikely that FFA impairs insulin action in hepatocytes by increasing TNF-α expression like in fat and muscle cells. Indeed, TNF-α-induced insulin resistance has been shown to occur in fat and muscle but not in liver *(71)*.

Leptin could also be an additional potential mediator of hepatic insulin resistance in obesity. It has been previously reported that concentrations of leptin similar to those measured in obese individuals attenuated insulin signaling in human hepatic cells *(105)*. Thus, insulin-mediated down-regulation of the mRNA encoding phosphoenolpyruvate carboxykinase (PEPCK), the rate-limiting enzyme for gluconeogenesis, was found to be reduced by leptin. This suggests that hyperleptinemia in obesity-related insulin resistance may be responsible for increased hepatic gluconeogenesis.

MOLECULAR DEFECTS OF INSULIN ACTION IN OBESITY-LINKED INSULIN RESISTANCE

It is conceivable that an impaired expression or regulation of insulin signaling molecules or metabolic effectors could be a primary defect in the insulin resistance of obesity and Type 2 diabetes. Whereas mutations in genes encoding several of these proteins have been previously reported, none of them could explain the common form of insulin resistance associated with the development of obesity in the population. Insulin resistance is a heterogeneous syndrome that likely arises from the combination of subtle genetic defects in key molecules involved in insulin action and susceptibility to environmental risk factors. Consumption of high amounts of dietary fat and a sedentary life style represent conditions that favor the development of the syndrome in genetically susceptible individuals *(37)*.

In the next section, we will first briefly discuss the molecular mechanisms of insulin action in normal cells and then review the molecular defects that have been identified in obesity and Type 2 diabetes.

Mechanisms of Insulin Action in Intact Cells

The diversity of signals that are initiated by insulin have been discussed in recent reviews *(106,107)*. The known key events in the stimulation of glucose transport by insulin are summarized in Fig. 2.

Upon binding to its receptor, insulin induces the autophosphorylation of the β-subunits and the intrinsic activation of the receptor tyrosine kinase activity. The activated receptor increases tyrosine phosphorylation of several docking proteins but it is generally accepted that the acute metabolic actions of insulin on glucose transport are principally mediated by the insulin receptor substrates-1 and -2 (IRS-1, IRS-2) *(108,109)*, and also in adipocytes by a recently identified 60 kDa protein named IRS-3 *(110,111)*.

There is now strong evidence that activation of PI 3-kinase by insulin plays an essential role in mediating the hormone's metabolic actions. Through its lipid kinase activity, PI 3-kinase phosphorylates the lipid PI on the 3' position of the myoinositol ring, yielding PI-3-phosphate. The enzyme can also use other forms of PI in vivo to yield PI(3,4)P2 and PI(3,4,5)P3. PI 3-kinase is a heterodimer consisting of a regulatory subunit of 85 kDa (p85) that contains two SH2 domains, as well as a catalytic subunit of 100 kDa (p110). To date, several isoforms of the regulatory subunits (p85α, p85β, p55α/AS53 and p55γ/p55PIK) and the catalytic subunits (p110α, p110β, p110γ and p170) of PI 3-kinases have been identified in mammalian cells *(112–117)*. However, insulin treatment activates p110α and p110β but not p170 or p110γ. Binding of tyrosine phosphorylated IRS proteins to p85 induces a conformation change leading to activation of the p110 catalytic activity. It is believed that PI 3-kinase activation by insulin is essential for stimulation of glucose transporter (GLUT4) translocation and glucose transport. Indeed, several studies

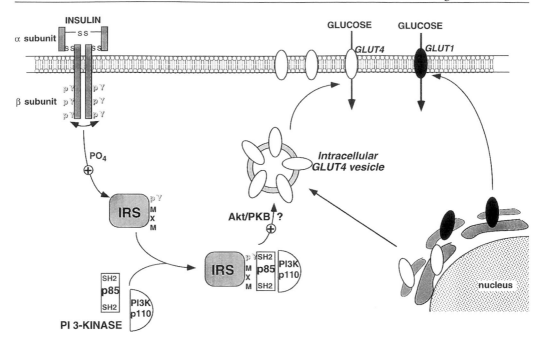

Fig. 2. Insulin stimulation of glucose transport in skeletal muscle. Upon binding to the insulin receptor alpha subunits, insulin activates the tyrosine kinase activity of the beta subunits and receptor autophosphorylation. The activated receptor kinase phosphorylates IRS proteins (IRS-1, IRS-2 in muscle and fat cells, and IRS-3 in adipocytes) on tyrosines which then bind to the p85 regulatory subunit of the PI 3-kinase. Binding of tyrosyl phosphorylated IRS proteins to p85 induces a conformation change leading to activation of the p110 subunit catalytic activity. Insulin appears to redistribute PI 3-kinase to the intracellular GLUT4-containing vesicles suggesting that this enzyme participates in the traffic, docking and/or fusion of these vesicles with the cell surface. One potential targets of the PI products that may be involved in glucose transport stimulation by insulin is c-Akt or PKB (see text for detail). Both GLUT4 and the ubiquitous GLUT1 glucose transporters are expressed in muscle cells but only GLUT4 is stored in specialized vesicles and translocated by insulin. GLUT1 is only present at the plasma membrane in skeletal muscle.

have shown that relatively specific inhibitors of PI 3-kinase (wortmannin and LY294002), or overexpression of a mutated p85 regulatory subunit lacking the ability to bind and activate the p110 catalytic subunit, inhibit insulin-mediated GLUT4 translocation and glucose transport in adipocytes and skeletal muscle cells *(69)*. However, activation of PI 3-kinase by insulin is not sufficient to stimulate glucose transport since other receptors that activate the enzyme such as the platelet-derived growth factor (PDGF) and interleukin-4 receptors do not increase glucose transport in adipose or muscle cells *(118–120)*. This may be related to the finding that in contrast to PDGF, insulin directs the association of PI 3-kinase with the GLUT4-containing vesicles in adipocytes *(118,121)*. These recent studies suggest that activation of PI 3-kinase activity in the unique intracellular GLUT4-enriched vesicles (or membranes closely associated with these vesicles) is a key event involved in insulin action to stimulate GLUT4 translocation to the cell surface. Importantly, activation of PI 3-kinase is essential not only for the stimulation of glucose transport, but also for other metabolic actions of insulin such as stimulation of amino acid uptake *(122)* glycogen synthesis *(123,124)* and antilipolysis *(125)*.

The downstream targets of the PI products remain to be identified. The fact that insulin appears to redistribute PI 3-kinase to the GLUT4-containing vesicles suggests that this enzyme participates in vesicle traffic, docking and/or fusion with the cell surface. It is tempting to think that some of the substrate PI's of PI 3-kinase may be found on the GLUT4-containing vesicles, but this remains to be shown. One potential target of the PI products that may be involved in glucose transport stimulation by insulin is c-Akt or PKB (Protein Kinase B). c-Akt was identified as a serine/threonine protein kinase that is activated by insulin *(126,127)*. Importantly, its activation is prevented by prior inhibition of PI 3-kinase with wortmannin *(126,128)*. The potential importance of Akt as a downstream effector of insulin-stimulated glucose transport was recently suggested by the observation that expression of constitutively activated Akt in adipocytes increased glucose uptake and augmented the presence of GLUT4 transporters at the cell surface *(129,130)*. It will be important to prove that activation of the endogenous Akt by insulin is indeed an essential event in the hormone's effect to induce glucose transport.

When muscle and fat cells are activated by insulin, GLUT4-enriched vesicles are translocated from intracellular storage site(s) to the cell surface by a mechanism that is still not fully understood but appears to depend on an intact cytoskeleton *(131)*. It is currently believed that insulin largely stimulates the exocytic rate of this process and produces a small reduction in the endocytic rate *(132–135)*. The nature of the intracellular GLUT4 storage compartment(s) remains obscure. Whereas the majority of GLUT4 proteins is found in unique vesicular structures clustered in the cytoplasm, a significant proportion can also be observed in several elements of the endocytic pathway (clathrin-coated vesicles, endosomes, and trans-Golgi network) *(136)*. However, recent studies suggest that the bulk of GLUT4 molecules appearing at the cell surface upon insulin stimulation are recruited from storage vesicles that are segregated from the endosomal system *(137)*. On the other hand, a minor proportion of the translocated GLUT4 proteins may be originating from the endocytic compartment, as for GLUT1 in adipose cells and several other recycling proteins (ex. transferrin receptor, mannose-6-phosphate/IGF-II receptor, etc.) known to be recruited to the plasma membrane during insulin stimulation *(137)*.

Molecular Defects in Insulin Action in Obesity

It is likely that insulin resistance in obesity develops as a consequence of more than one cellular defect. Insulin resistance may result from an altered expression and/or activity of key proteins involved in both insulin signaling as well as in effector molecules mediating the different metabolic pathways activated by the hormone (glucose metabolism, antilipolysis, LPL activation, etc.). Among the known metabolic actions of insulin, the stimulation of glucose transport and metabolism in fat and muscle, and their dysregulation in insulin-resistant tissues have been extensively studied and will therefore be the focus here.

INSULIN SIGNALING MOLECULES

Insulin Receptor. Abnormalities in either insulin receptor content or function have been frequently described in obese insulin-resistant subjects. Insulin receptor number has been reported to be reduced in isolated adipose cells from obese Type 2 diabetes patients (138). However, insulin receptor content has been shown to be normal or only slightly decreased in skeletal muscles from such patients (139,140). On the other hand, a decreased tyrosine kinase (TK) activity of the insulin receptor has been reported in both muscle and fat cells of obese rodents and Type 2 diabetes individuals (138–141).

Impaired insulin receptor TK function in muscle and fat cells of insulin-resistant subjects is not related to genetic alterations in the insulin receptor gene. Indeed, whereas several mutations in the insulin receptor gene have been previously reported in markedly insulin-resistant patients with acanthosis nigricans or ovarian hyperandrogenism, there is no evidence of such a genetic defect for the common form of insulin resistance in obesity. Hence, the altered insulin receptor function is not intrinsic but rather thought to be caused by the presence of other cellular or circulating factors (proteins, metabolites, etc.) in obese insulin-resistant individuals. One likely candidate factor is again TNF-α, whose expression is greatly increased in adipose tissue of obese individuals *(70)*. Accordingly, the cytokine impairs insulin receptor TK activity in adipocytes *(75,76)* and this defect is significantly reversed in mice lacking TNF-α expression *(78)*. On the other hand, a reduced TK function of the insulin receptor has also been observed in muscle of first-degree relatives of Type 2 diabetes subjects as well as in poorly-insulin-sensitive individuals without any genetic background of Type 2 diabetes *(142,143)*. Thus, it is likely that obesity-related TNF-α expression is not the only factor involved in the development of an impaired insulin receptor TK activity in skeletal muscle of obese insulin-resistant subjects.

IRS Proteins and PI 3-Kinase. A potential role for a defective expression or function of IRS proteins and PI 3-kinase in the pathogenesis of insulin resistance has been the subject of intense investigation in recent years. It has been reported that IRS-1 phosphorylation and PI 3-kinase activation by insulin are reduced in adipocytes, skeletal muscles, and liver of animal models of obesity and insulin resistance *(144–146)*. A reduced IRS-1 phosphorylation and associated PI 3-kinase activity upon insulin stimulation has also been demonstrated in skeletal muscle from Type 2 diabetes subjects *(147,148)*. In morbidly obese diabetic subjects, a further decrease in IRS-1 protein content was also observed *(148)*. Interestingly, IRS-1 protein content and tyrosine phosphorylation as well as IRS-1-associated PI 3-kinase activity are markedly reduced in adipocytes from Type 2 diabetes subjects but IRS-2 protein levels and phosphorylation, and associated PI 3-kinase activity are intact in the same cells *(149)*. This suggests that IRS-2 becomes an important docking protein for PI 3-kinase in muscle of Type 2 diabetes subjects, a finding that is in good agreement with the observations made in mice deficient for IRS-1 *(150,151)*. However, since insulin-induced IRS-2 tyrosine phosphorylation and PI 3-kinase activation is about half that obtained for a similar concentration of insulin, the former docking protein cannot fully compensate for the lack of insulin action in adipose cells from Type 2 diabetes subjects *(149)*. On the other hand, it is still unknown whether the specific action of insulin to increase PI 3-kinase in the GLUT4-containing intracellular pool is impaired in skeletal muscle and adipose cells from obese insulin-resistant subjects.

In addition to their numerous (>20) putative tyrosine (ser/thr) phosphorylation sites, IRS-1 and IRS-2 also contains over 30 potential serine/threonine phosphorylation sites in motifs recognized by numerous kinases. Recent studies suggest that an increased ser/thr phosphorylation of IRS-1 may be implicated in the development of insulin resistance in obesity-linked diabetes. Thus, ser/thr phosphorylation of IRS-1 is markedly increased by TNF-α *(152)*. Moreover, IRS-1 ser/thr phosphorylation is increased in cardiomyocytes from obese Zucker rats *(153)*. In the latter study, insulin-mediated IRS-1 tyrosine phosphorylation was not decreased but IRS-1-associated PI 3-kinase activity was reduced in parallel with increased ser/thr phosphorylation. Ser/thr phosphorylated IRS-1 has been shown to act as an inhibitor of the insulin receptor tyrosine kinase activity *(152)*. Moreover, Paz et al. *(154)* recently showed that increased ser/thr phosphorylation of IRS-1 and IRS-2 inhibits their binding to the juxtamembrane region of the insulin receptor in vitro and thus impairs their ability to undergo insulin-induced tyrosine phosphorylation. These studies strongly support the hypothesis that elevated ser/thr phosphorylation of IRS-1 (and perhaps IRS-2) in muscle and fat cells is an important molecular defect causing insulin resistance in obesity and diabetes. Additional studies will be necessary to confirm the existence of this defect in humans and whether it is a primary defect in the pathogenesis of the metabolic syndrome.

Over the past few years, several studies have reported various IRS-1 gene polymorphisms in patients with Type 2 diabetes *(155–162)*. Whether these mutations in IRS-1 gene contribute to the occurrence of insulin resistance in Type 2 diabetes remains unclear as most of these polymorphisms were also found in nondiabetic subjects. Almind et al. *(163)* and Yoshimura et al. (164) showed that one of those natural mutations present in both normal and diabetic individuals (G971R, missense mutation of Gly971 to Arg) results in impaired insulin signaling when expressed in the 32D cell line overexpressing the insulin receptor, particularly at the level of PI 3-kinase activation. On the other hand, the ability of insulin to induce G971R binding to the insulin receptor and G971R tyrosine phosphorylation were not altered. These studies suggest that the G971R mutation reduces IRS-1 association with the p85 subunit of PI 3-kinase and that this defect may be important for the pathogenesis of insulin resistance and also contribute to explain the presence of low-insulin-sensitive subjects in the normal population.

GLUCOSE TRANSPORTERS

The potential role of glucose transporters in the insulin-resistant glucose transport of muscle and adipose cells has been reviewed extensively in the past few years *(69,165,166)*. Insulin resistance for cellular glucose transport could be explained by a variety of defects in GLUT4 regulation including its level of expression, its translocation to and insertion in the cell surface membrane, or its intrinsic activity. In the present chapter, we have briefly summarized the knowledge gained from previous studies and we focus more on recent studies that have suggested potential mechanisms for GLUT4 dysregulation in insulin resistance.

GLUT4 Expression. As discussed above, GLUT4 is by far the predominant transporter protein used by insulin to increase glucose transport in muscle and fat cells. Thus, it appears possible that a reduced GLUT4 expression may explain the insulin-resistant glucose transport that typifies insulin-resistant subjects. GLUT4 expression is markedly altered in adipose tissue of animals with obesity and Type 2 diabetes. During the dynamic phase of obesity in young Zucker *fa/fa* rats, GLUT4 levels rise in adipocytes in conjunction with an hyper-responsiveness of these cells for insulin-induced glucose transport and fatty acid synthesis (165). Subsequently, GLUT4 expression drops as insulin resistance develops in adipose tissue of older Zucker rats as well as in other models of Type 2 diabetes like the viable yellow Avy/a and the KKAy mice *(165)*. In humans with Type 2 diabetes there is also a marked reduction in GLUT4 expression in isolated adipocytes *(159,167–169)*. Whether the reduced GLUT4 expression in fat cells from Type 2 diabetes patients is in part related to obesity has been difficult to sort out. GLUT4 protein levels in subcutaneous fat were negatively correlated with the BMI in control subjects and moderately obese patients *(170)*. Importantly, a similar decrease in GLUT4 protein content was found in the adipose tissue of obese subjects with or without diabetes but with similar body mass indices (BMI) *(170)*. Furthermore, GLUT4 protein content is strongly and negatively correlated with accumulation of abdominal fat in severely obese premenopausal women without Type 2 diabetes *(98)*. In the latter study, adipose tissue GLUT4 expression (protein and mRNA) was also found to vary in function of the anatomical location of the fat depot. This regional variation in adipose tissue GLUT4 has been recently confirmed at the level of the mRNA in non-obese subjects *(171)*, indicating that it is misleading to extrapolate GLUT4 expression data from one fat depot to the total adipose mass. Importantly, these studies strongly suggest that obesity *per se* may be responsible for the reduced GLUT4 expression in adipose tissue of insulin-resistant Type 2 diabetes subjects. In agreement with this proposal, subcutaneous adipose tissue GLUT4 expression is not different between poorly insulin-sensitive (but healthy) and highly insulin sensitive subjects *(170)*. It is therefore unlikely that a decreased GLUT4 expression in adipose tissue is involved in the early development of insulin resistance.

Unlike the reported data in adipose tissue, insulin resistance in Type 2 diabetes subjects is not related to a decrease GLUT4 expression in skeletal muscle, the main site of glucose disposal in the post-absorptive state. Indeed, several groups found no net reduction in the total cellular content of GLUT4 proteins or GLUT4 mRNA in muscles of these subjects *(172–174)*. A small reduction in muscle cell GLUT4 protein content was reported in only one study, in which Type 2 diabetes was associated with morbid obesity *(175)*. Similar results were obtained in animal models of Type 2 diabetes such as the obese (*db/db*) mouse and Zucker (*fa/fa*) rats *(165)*. Moderate (20 to 25%) to significant (40%) reductions in GLUT4 protein levels in muscle were reported in obese Zucker diabetic and obese SHR/N-*cp* rats *(165,176)*, whose diabetes is much more severe. In contrast to these mild or insignificant changes in GLUT4 in genetically determined diabetes, the insulin resistance of rats fed high-fat diets is associated with a reduced GLUT4 expression in muscle *(177,178)*. This may be due to the lower insulin levels that the fat-fed rats display in the fed state *(177,178)*. Thus, the impaired action of insulin to increase glucose uptake in muscles of Type 2 diabetes individuals is unlikely to be mainly related to a decreased expression of GLUT4 but may be caused by an impaired translocation or insertion of the transporter protein to the plasma membrane or by a malfunction of the GLUT4 protein.

GLUT4 Translocation. Several groups have evaluated the effect of insulin on GLUT4 translocation in skeletal muscle of the obese Zucker rat. Using subcellular fractionation techniques, GLUT4 translocation to a plasma membrane-enriched fraction was found to be either impaired *(179,180)* or unaffected *(181)*. Furthermore, it has been suggested that the intrinsic activity of the translocated transporters is reduced in muscle of obese Zucker rats *(179,181)* although this latter conclusion is not unanimously recognized *(182)*. Furthermore, normal translocation of GLUT4 but reduced intrinsic activity of the transporter was reported in muscle of obese high-fat fed rats *(183)*. We have recently proposed that these inconsistent findings may in part be explained by the presence of variable amounts of T-tubule membranes in the isolated plasma membranes *(184)*. Since the tubular extensions of the plasma membrane contain GLUT4 and cover most (>60%) of the muscle cell surface area, even a small contamination with these structures may greatly influence the amount of GLUT4 proteins in plasma membrane preparations. Few studies have looked at the effect of insulin on GLUT4 distribution in normal and obese insulin-resistant human subjects. This is mainly related to the fact that significant amount of muscle fibers must be removed by open biopsies. Zierath and colleagues recently reported that in response to insulin, GLUT4 protein increased in the plasma membranes derived from muscle of control individuals but not of Type 2 diabetes patients *(185)*. The small magnitude of change observed in the control samples and the relatively high amount of GLUT4 transporters seen in the plasma membranes of the Type 2 diabetes patients before insulin stimulation, does not allow to establish the quantitative nature of this defect in GLUT4 translocation in Type 2 diabetes.

In summary, the available data suggest that an impaired GLUT4 translocation is the principal defect responsible for reduced insulin-stimulated glucose transport in obese and diabetic animals and perhaps in humans, but more studies are needed to clarify the aforementioned discrepancies. It will be important to develop procedures to more precisely quantitate GLUT4 translocation to both the plasma membrane and the T-tubules in human muscle in order to assess the true extent of the translocation defect.

One of the most challenging tasks for the coming years is to unravel the molecular defects responsible for the defective insulin-mediated GLUT4 translocation in insulin-resistant muscle and adipose cells. As discussed, under Insulin Signaling Molecules, PI 3-kinase activation by insulin is reduced in adipocytes and skeletal muscles of obese insulin-resistant subjects. It is still unknown whether the PI 3-kinase activity that associates with GLUT4-containing vesicles is impaired in insulin-resistant skeletal muscle and adipose cells. A better understanding of the molecular events downstream PI 3-kinase activation by insulin may lead to the identification of the defects responsible for impaired GLUT4 translocation in insulin-resistant tissues of obese Type 2 diabetes patients in the near future.

One area in which significant progress has been made over the last couple of years is in how GLUT4 vesicles are recognized and inserted at the cell surface. It is now realized that the processes of docking and fusion of these vesicles with the plasma membrane resembles to a significant degree the traffic or small synaptic vesicles in neurosecretory cells. This process is orchestrated by membrane proteins known as the SNAREs *(69,137)*. This process is mediated by a triad of SNARE proteins—one in the incoming vesicle (v-SNARE) and two in the target membrane (t-SNAREs)—that form a strong complex allowing membrane recognition and docking. The v-SNAREs of the incoming vesicles belong to the VAMP/synaptobrevin family, of which three members have been identified: VAMP1, VAMP2 and cellubrevin/VAMP3. The t-SNAREs of the target membranes are members of the syntaxin and SNAP-25 families. Additional soluble regulators of this complex are proteins belonging to the munc18 family that may be negative regulators of vesicle docking *(69,137)*. It will be important to test the possibility that an altered expression and/or insulin-dependent regulation of the SNARE proteins may result in an impaired docking or fusion of GLUT4 vesicles with the cell surface in adipose and muscle cells of obese insulin-resistant subjects.

THE ATHEROGENIC DYSLIPIDEMIA
OF INSULIN RESISTANCE IN ABDOMINAL OBESITY:
IMPACT ON THE RISK OF ISCHEMIC HEART DISEASE

Our previously published reports on the metabolic complications of visceral obesity and our recently published findings on the Québec Cardiovascular Study cohort of men emphasize the early identification of high risk individuals long before they develop impaired glucose tolerance (IGT) or Type 2 diabetes. Several papers from our laboratory have highlighted the metabolic complications found in obese men and women with an excess accumulation of visceral adipose tissue (15,18,31-37). In nondiabetic subjects, we found visceral obesity to be associated with a cluster of metabolic abnormalities that included hyperinsulinemia resulting from an insulin resistant state, a greater glycemic response to an oral glucose load, hypertriglyceridemia, normal or marginally elevated plasma LDL-cholesterol levels and reduced HDL-cholesterol concentrations *(15–18,31–38)*. Furthermore, despite the apparently normal or close to normal plasma LDL-cholesterol concentrations, smaller LDL particles *(38)* and a 15–20% increase in plasma apoB and LDL-apoB concentrations *(36)* were noted in visceral obesity, indicating a greater concentration of denser, cholesterol-ester depleted LDL particles. This cluster of metabolic abnormalities is also found in Type 2 diabetes patients but is common in nondiabetic individuals with the insulin resistance syndrome. On the basis of the similarities between the metabolic alterations of visceral obesity and the features of the insulin resistance syndrome and considering the fact that visceral adipose tissue has been found to be a stronger correlate of these metabolic abnormalities than obesity *per se*, we have proposed that excess visceral adipose tissue accumulation is also a component of the insulin resistance syndrome. We have therefore described this condition as the insulin resistance-dyslipidemic syndrome of visceral obesity *(15,36)*.

Recent publications of analyses conducted on the cohort of the Québec Cardiovascular Study have emphasized the atherogenic nature of the dyslipidemia of the insulin resistance syndrome even in the absence of diabetes mellitus. Indeed, when a cohort of more than 2000 men free from clinical signs of ischemic heart disease (IHD) were followed for a period of 5 yr for incidence of IHD events (angina pectoris, myocardial infarction, CHD-related death), multivariate analyses revealed that diabetes mellitus and apolipoprotein B concentrations were the two best predictors of IHD risk *(186)*. After inclusion of these two variables, plasma triglycerides and HDL-cholesterol failed to remain independent predictors of IHD in this cohort *(186)*.

We have also examined the IHD risk associated with hyperinsulinemia among nondiabetic men of the Québec Cardiovascular Study cohort by matching each man who developed IHD for age, BMI, smoking and alcohol consumption with an individual who remained free from IHD over the follow-up period *(187)*. After exclusion of men with diabetes, we were able to match 91 IHD cases with 105 men who had remained healthy. Fasting plasma insulin concentrations were initially 18% higher in men who developed IHD compared to those who remained IHD-free. Hyperinsulinemia was found to be an independent predictor of IHD in this cohort and a remarkable synergy was found with apoB concentration: indeed, men in the top tertile of fasting insulin levels and above the 50th percentile of the apoB distribution were characterized by a more than 11-fold increase in IHD risk compared to men with low apoB levels (<50th percentile) who were also in the first tertile of fasting insulin levels *(187)*. We have also recently reported that men of the Québec Cardiovascular Study with small, dense LDL particles and with apoB concentrations above the 50th percentile were characterized by more than a sixfold increase in IHD risk *(63)*. All these metabolic abnormalities (hyperinsulinemia, elevated apoB, small dense LDL phenotype) are found in the insulin resistance syndrome of visceral obesity, even in the absence of Type 2 diabetes *(15–18,38)*. Unpublished observations from the Québec Cardiovascular Study have suggested that this triad of "unconventional" metabolic risk factors (hyperinsulinemia, elevated apoB levels, small dense LDL particles) was associated with an 18-fold increase in IHD risk, even after adjustment for conventional risk factors such as plasma triglyceride, LDL-cholesterol and HDL-cholesterol concentrations (Lamarche et al., unpublished observations).

Although it is more and more accepted that the cluster of metabolic alterations of insulin resistance increases IHD risk, to what extent the IRS is as atherogenic as a marked elevation in plasma LDL-cholesterol concentration (such as in hypercholesterolemia) is unclear. We have used a simple experimental design as an attempt to address this question when we examined the relationship of abdominal obesity, fasting hyperinsulinemia and of familial hypercholesterolemia (FH) (a monogenic dyslipidemia associated with a marked increase in plasma LDL-cholesterol levels and with premature coronary artery disease (CAD) among affected patients) to angiographically assessed CAD in a sample of 120 nondiabetic heterozygous FH male patients and in 280 nonFH, nondiabetic controls matched for age and smoking *(188)*. An oral glucose tolerance test was performed in all patients to exclude Type 2 diabetes patients or individuals with impaired glucose tolerance. Using nonFH subjects with low waist circumference values and low plasma insulin concentrations as the reference group (odds ratio of finding CAD by angiography established at a value of 1.0 in this "control" group for comparison purposes), we then quantified the risk of finding significant CAD as assessed by a greater than 50% stenosis in one of the main coronary vessels *(188)*. Among nonFH patients, abdominal obesity (as crudely assessed by an increased waist circumference) combined with hyperinsulinemia was associated with a CAD odds ratio of about 2.5, a finding essentially similar to our previous observations in the prospective Québec Cardiovascular Study, where hyperinsulinemia *per se* was associated with a 3-fold increase in IHD risk *(187)*. Familial hypercholesterolemic patients without abdominal obesity and hyperinsulinemia had about a 2-fold increase in their risk of CAD, which was also an expected finding consistent with the premature CAD found among patients with this monogenic dyslipidemia *(189–190)*. However, FH patients with abdominal obesity and hyperinsulinemia displayed an almost 13-fold increase in the risk of finding significant CAD (188). These results emphasize two complementary notions. First, a raised plasma LDL-cholesterol concentration is indeed a major CAD risk factor and the premature CAD of FH supports this notion. However, even within a group of homogeneous patients with the same molecular defect in the LDL receptor gene leading to hypercholesterolemia and with markedly elevated plasma LDL-cholesterol concentration, hyperinsulinemia and abdominal obesity are potent markers of CAD risk. These results add fuel to the current debate on the contribution of the IRS as a risk factor for CAD and on therapeutic options. Indeed, reducing plasma LDL-cholesterol concentration is a legitimate objective in the prevention (primary or secondary) of CAD, even in Type 2 diabetes patients and in nondiabetic insulin resistant individuals. However, considering the high prevalence of the IRS and of obesity in our affluent societies, it is proposed that more emphasis should be placed on the management of insulin resistance through proper lifestyle modification programs (management of abdominal obesity through proper diet and physical activity) *(191)*. Otherwise, it is proposed that pharmacological therapies aimed at the management of the consequences of the insulin resistance syndrome (hyperglycemia, hypertension, dyslipidemia) may only lead to the suboptimal reduction of risk in the insulin resistant patient. Further work in this area is clearly warranted and it is hoped that the development of safe weight loss drugs will allow the testing of this hypothesis.

SIMPLE TOOLS FOR THE ASSESSMENT OF THE INSULIN RESISTANCE SYNDROME IN ABDOMINAL OBESITY

Although the health burden of the insulin resistance syndrome is more and more widely recognized, there is also the need to provide clinicians with simple methods in order to assess the critical features of this syndrome. Such tools would allow clinicians and health professionals to better evaluate risk and help them to assess success of therapy.

Anthropometric Variables

More than a century ago, Quetelet *(192)* reported that body weight was proportional to height squared. Later on, Keys *(193)* proposed the body mass index (BMI) defined as the body weight in kg divided by height squared (m^2) as an index of obesity, this ratio being independent of height and strongly correlated with weight. Several studies have shown that the BMI is related to Type 2 diabetes, cardiovascular disease and to related mortality *(1–5,10,22)*. Although there is no consensus in the literature, BMI values between 20 and 25 kg/m^2 appear to be associated with little variation in mortality risk *(10)*. There appears to be an increase in risk for BMI values above 27 kg/m^2 and a more substantial increase among patients with BMI values above 30 kg/m^2 *(11)*. On the basis of these observations, the term "overweight" is often used for individuals with BMI values between 27 kg/m^2 and 30 kg/m^2 whereas men and women with BMI values above 30 kg/m^2 are generally considered as obese *(11)*. These values have been reported to approximately correspond to the 85th and 95th percentiles of the population of the United States *(6)*. In Europe, average BMI values of 30,9 kg/m^2 in men and of 33 kg/m^2 in women correspond to the 90th percentiles of the European MONICA populations studied *(7)*. This classification is essentially in accordance with the definition of obesity (BMI > 30 kg/m^2) initially put forward by Garrow *(194)*.

When the relationship of anthropometric correlates of obesity to insulin resistance and Type 2 diabetes is examined, two issues need to be raised:

1. The critical threshold above which an individual may develop insulin resistance or may be at increased risk of Type 2 diabetes varies among ethnic groups. Indeed, it appears that some ethnic populations may develop Type 2 diabetes at lower BMI values than Caucasians *(195)*. It is therefore quite important to examine the relationship of BMI to Type 2 diabetes risk in all populations in order to develop public health recommendations that are appropriate for each population of interest.
2. Within a given ethnic group, there is considerable individual variation in the risk associated with a given BMI or with a given excess of total body fat. In this regard, prospective epidemiologic studies and numerous metabolic studies conducted in the 1980s have re-emphasized clinical observations made by Jean Vague (196) in the forties: The distribution of body fat is an important correlate of the metabolic complications that have been associated with excess fatness per se *(3,4,15–26,197)*.

Is There a Critical BMI Value or Amount of Total Body Fat?

The BMI as an index of body fatness has limitations, especially in lean to moderately overweight people. Obese patients with very high BMI values are clearly characterized by an excess mass of adipose tissue. However, some moderately overweight individuals may be misclassified or their amount of total body fat be overestimated due to a high muscle mass *(198)*. Thus, these subjects may be poorly assessed in terms of health risk. A simple approach to deal with this problem is to assess subcutaneous skinfold thicknesses *(198,199)*. It is indeed possible to measure the thickness of several subcutaneous fat depots by using calipers, the most frequently assessed skinfolds being triceps, biceps, subscapular, suprailiac, abdomen (lateral to the umbilicus), mid-thigh, and mid-calf. The sum of these skinfolds would provide a satisfactory estimate of the amount of subcutaneous body fat.

However, the relation of the BMI to body composition may be different among ethnic groups *(200)* and this point has not been completely addressed in the current literature. Furthermore, the relationship of the BMI or of subcutaneous fat (as assessed by skinfolds) to metabolic complications may vary from one ethnic group to the other and some groups (for example: the Asian population) may be more susceptible to Type 2 diabetes for a given BMI or amount of subcutaneous fat *(195)*.

SIMPLE ANTHROPOMETRIC MARKERS OF REGIONAL BODY FAT DISTRIBUTION AND OF VISCERAL ADIPOSE TISSUE ACCUMULATION

Metabolic and prospective studies have shown that the amount of abdominal fat, which has been crudely assessed by the ratio of waist-to-hip circumferences (WHR) was a much closer correlate of the metabolic complications found in obese individuals (including Type 2 diabetes) than excess fatness *per se (3,4,197)*. As discussed in the previous sections of this chapter, more recent studies which have used imaging techniques to assess abdominal fat accumulation have indicated that it is the amount of fat located in the abdominal cavity, the so-called intra-abdominal or visceral adipose tissue, which is the critical correlate of a cluster of metabolic abnormalities that not only increase the risk of Type 2 diabetes *(3,4,196)* but also of coronary heart disease (insulin resistance, hyperinsulinemia, glucose intolerance, hypertriglyceridemia, hyperapoB, increased proportion of small, dense LDL particles and reduced HDL-cholesterol levels *(3–4,15–22)*. As these alterations are reminiscent of the features of the IRS, it has been proposed that excess visceral fat accumulation (visceral obesity) is a common component of the insulin resistance syndrome *(15,17)*. Thus, the measurement of visceral adipose tissue accumulation is relevant but to recommend the use of a costly radiological technique such as CT to assess visceral adipose tissue would be unrealistic from a public health standpoint. There is therefore a need to develop simple anthropometric methods to estimate visceral adipose tissue accumulation for the clinical practice. The first anthropometric candidate for the prediction of visceral adipose tissue accumulation has been the ratio of WHR which had been used in many epidemiologic and metabolic studies.

Unfortunately, if not used in combination with the BMI in a complicated algorithm *(11)*, we found that the WHR alone had a limited ability to predict visceral fat deposition *(201–203)*. In this regard, it has been suggested that the waist circumference and the sagittal diameter could represent two useful predictors of visceral adipose tissue accumulation *(201–203)* (Table 1). However, the shared variance between waist circumference, the sagittal diameter and visceral adipose tissue accumulation barely reaches 70–75% *(201)*. Thus, some individuals with high waist circumference values may be misclassified as having too much visceral fat whereas they have too much subcutaneous abdominal fat.

ARE THERE CRITICAL VALUES OF VISCERAL ADIPOSE TISSUE ACCUMULATION AND OF WAIST CIRCUMFERENCE?

It has been suggested that a visceral accumulation above 130 cm^2 was associated, in both men and women, with an increased likelihood of finding metabolic abnormalities predictive of an increased risk of Type 2 diabetes, this value corresponding to a waist circumference of about one meter *(191,201,203)*. However, it is important to point out

Table 1
**Useful Anthropometric Variables for the Assessment of Total Fatness
and for the Estimation of Visceral Adipose Tissue Deposition**

1. BMI	Weight in kg divided by height in m^2
2. Skinfolds	Commonly assessed skinfolds are triceps, biceps, subscapular, abdomen, suprailiac, mid-thigh and mid-calf
3. Waist	Measured at the level of the mid-distance between the bottom of the rib cage to the top of the iliac crest
4. Sagittal diameter	Measured at the level of the umbilicus

that no large prospective study has examined the relationship of visceral fat to the risk of Type 2 diabetes and CVD. Furthermore, results have been mostly obtained from the study of Caucasians and it will be critically important to verify the threshold of visceral fat above which complications are found in all ethnic groups. Finally, visceral fat increases with age and a given waist circumference has been associated with a higher deposition of visceral fat in middle-aged men and women than in young adults *(203)*. Thus, age-specific waist circumference or sagittal diameter values will have to be generated (Table 2).

Although it is clear that obesity combined with an excess of abdominal visceral adipose tissue increases the risk of Type 2 diabetes, several important issues remain to be addressed before making recommendations on anthropometric procedures relevant to public health. First, there is a need to examine the relationship of BMI to the incidence of Type 2 diabetes in all ethnic populations as BMI cut-points specific to ethnicity are likely to be found. Secondly, the relationship of BMI to body composition may also be affected by ethnicity. In addition, subcutaneous fat can be crudely but adequately estimated by skinfolds which can be assessed with the use of simple calipers. However, only a few skinfolds have been simultaneously assessed in most epidemiologic studies, which often failed to consider individual differences in subcutaneous fat distribution. Furthermore, even with the use of several skinfolds to assess subcutaneous fat, a multiple skinfold procedure cannot assess intra-abdominal fat accumulation, this latter variable being the critical correlate of complications predictive of an increased risk of Type 2 diabetes. Imaging techniques such as computed tomography and magnetic resonance imaging (MRI) are considered as gold standard methods to assess visceral fat accumulation. Unfortunately, these methods are costly and not practical for field work and the development of anthropometric indices should be a priority. Finally, although the waist circumference and the sagittal diameter have been suggested as useful predictors, albeit imperfect, of visceral adipose tissue accumulation, additional issues will have to be addressed before critical values can be identified for these variables. Indeed, the relationship of these anthropometric variables to visceral adipose tissue accumulation may differ among ethnic groups and may also be affected by age. Thus, older adults have more visceral fat for a given waist circumference than young adults.

On the basis of these observations, prospective studies should be conducted in every ethnic population in order to examine the relationships of anthropometric correlates of obesity and of abdominal (visceral) adipose tissue accumulation to the incidence of Type 2 diabetes. Such studies would allow the implementation of population specific public health programs aiming at identifying patients at risk for the development of Type 2 diabetes. At the present time, the optimal BMI range has been largely estimated from the

Table 2
Proposed Values of Waist Girth That are Either Desirable
(Less than 100 cm^2 of Visceral Adipose Tissue) or Associated
with an Increased Risk (More Than 130 cm^2
of Visceral Adipose Tissue) in Caucasian Men and Women[a]

	Visceral at accumulation	
Waist values per age groups[b]	*100 cm^2*	*130 cm^2*
<40 yr	90 cm	100 cm
40 yr < age < 60 yr	80 cm	90 cm

[a]Adapted from ref. *(83)*.
[b]For post-menopausal women, a desirable waist girth should be below 75 cm, whereas a girth > 85 cm is associated with an increased likelihood of finding an altered metabolic risk profile.

study of Caucasian populations. Furthermore, some individuals with moderate increases in their BMI are misclassified for their body composition due to a high muscle mass. In addition, the BMI does not provide information on the distribution of body fat. Thus, some non-obese individuals by current BMI standards may have too much visceral adipose tissue. It has been proposed that the waist circumference and the sagittal diameter are useful, although not perfect, correlates of visceral adipose tissue accumulation. However, the critical values identified so far have been generated from the study of Caucasians. It will be of great importance, from a public health standpoint, to establish the relationship of anthropometric variables to visceral fat accumulation and to metabolic complications in all ethnic groups in order to generate useful critical values.

ARE THERE SIMPLE CLINICAL MARKERS
OF THE INSULIN-RESISTANCE DYSLIPIDEMIC SYNDROME?

The insulin resistance concept has important clinical and public health implications. Thus, the identification of simple markers of its most critical features is also of considerable importance. The consequences of Type 2 diabetes on CVD are manifest and it is important to improve the metabolic control of the Type 2 diabetes patient. However, results of the Québec Cardiovascular Study are consistent with the notion that "the clock for macrovascular disease starts ticking long before the one for diabetes mellitus" *(41)*. Endocrinologists are legitimately focusing on the complications of Type 2 diabetes and on its treatment. However, the question must be raised about the cost-benefit of an approach where prediabetic or nondiabetic patients with the features of the IRS would be optimally identified and primary prevention measures implemented. Would fasting dysglycemia *(65)* represent an adequate early marker of insulin resistance? We believe that this approach is an improvement over current screening procedures but even moderate dysglycemia may not be the first manifestation of the insulin resistance dyslipidemic syndrome. As some insulin resistant individuals may have an excellent β-cell capacity for insulin secretion, insulin resistance could therefore develop in some subjects even in the absence of any sign of disturbed plasma glucose homeostasis. We therefore propose that fasting hyperinsulinemia may be, as previously suggested *(204,205)* the simplest and best marker (although not perfect) of early insulin resistance in nondiabetic individuals (Table 3).

Table 3
Working Model for Simple Markers
of the Insulin-Resistant Dyslipidemic Syndrome of Abdominal Obesity

Variable	Justification
Waist	Simple, inexpensive correlate of abdominal obesity.
Triglyceride	Good correlate of small, dense LDL particles currently assessed in clinical biochemistry laboratories
Apo B	Best marker of the concentration of atherogenic lipoproteins (the cholesterol/HDL-cholesterol ratio could be used if an apo B measurement is not available)
Insulin	Crude but useful correlate of insulin resistance in nondiabetic individuals

As this condition is often associated with normal or only marginally elevated LDL-cholesterol levels (which provides the clinician with misleading information on the concentration of LDL particles), the measurement of apoB is also recommended to screen for elevated plasma LDL concentrations. Regarding the dense LDL phenotype, the methodology currently available is labor intensive and rather tedious *(38,62,63)*. However, numerous studies have shown that most individuals with hypertriglyceridemia and low HDL-cholesterol levels have dense LDL particles *(206,207)*. Thus, it is very likely that the patients with hyperinsulinemia, elevated apoB levels, hypertriglyceridemia and low HDL-cholesterol levels have the small, dense LDL phenotype. Finally, abdominal visceral obesity can be crudely identified on the basis of an increased waist circumference, as we have shown this variable to be the simplest and best correlate of visceral adipose tissue accumulation in men and women *(201–203)*. Values above 1 meter in men and women below 40 yr of age and above 90 cm in individuals between 40 and 60 yr of age have been suggested to be the best predictive of an excess accumulation of visceral adipose tissue among Caucasian subjects *(203)*.

Current cutoff points for hypertriglyceridemia (above 2.3 mmol) and low HDL-cholesterol (below 0.9 mmol) are based on the consensus of experts and not on a sound physiological rationale *(206)*. We are further remote from universally accepted values for hyperinsulinemia and hyperapoB although it is our common clinical practice to use the 75th percentile of the distribution found in a group of healthy men and women. However, irrespective of these considerations that will have to receive more attention, it is suggested that we need to go far beyond the screening and treatment of Type 2 diabetes. How our proposed screening modalities should be implemented is an issue of considerable public health implications which will require further attention. However, we are convinced that this new metabolic triad of risk factors (hyperinsulinemia, hyperapoB, dense LDL phenotype) represents the most prevalent cause of macrovascular disease in our affluent, sedentary societies. It is therefore important that further work is conducted to examine epidemiologic, metabolic, molecular, genetic and therapeutic aspects of this atherogenic IRS with careful consideration for the contribution of abdominal obesity in its etiology and its treatment.

REFERENCES

1. Turner RC. The role of obesity in diabetes. Int J Obes 1992;16(Suppl.2):S43–S46.
2. Pi-Sunyer FX. Medical hazards of obesity. Ann Intern Med 1993;119:655–660.
3. Kissebah AH, Freedman DS, Peiris AN. Health risks of obesity. Med Clin North Am 1989;73:111–138.

4. Bjorntorp P. Abdominal obesity and the development of noninsulin dependent diabetes mellitus. Diabetes Metab Rev 1988;4:615–622.
5. Barrett-Connor E. Epidemiology, obesity, and non-insulin dependent diabetes mellitus. Epidemiol Rev 1989;11:172–181.
6. Kuczmarski RJ. Prevalence of overweight and weight gain in the United States. Am J Clin Nutr 1992;55:495S–502S.
7. Seidell JC. Obesity in Europe: scaling an epidemic. Int J Obes 1995;19(Suppl3):S1-S4.
8. Stamler J. Epidemic obesity in the United States. Arch In Med 1993;153:1040–1044.
9. Wolf AM, Colditz GA. Social and economic effects of body weight in the United States. Am J Clin Nutr 1996;63(Suppl)466S–469S.
10. National Institutes of Health Consensus Development Panel on the Health implications of Obesity: Health implications of obesity: National Institutes of Health consensus development conference statement. Ann Intern Med 1985;103:1073–1077.
11. Bray, GA. Pathophysiology of obesity. Ann J Clin Nutr 1992;55:488S–494S.
12. Barrett-Connor E. Obesity, atherosclerosis, and coronary artery disease. Ann Intern Med 1985; 103:1010–1019.
13. Manson JE, Willett WC, Stampfer MJ, Colditz GA, Hunter DJ, Hankinson SE, Hennekens CH, Speizer FE. Body weight and mortality among women. N Engl J Med 1995;333:677–685.
14. Bouchard C, Després JP. Variation in fat distribution with age and health implications. In: Eckert HM, Spirduso W, eds. Physical activity and aging. American Academy of Physical Education, 1989;78–106.
15. Després JP. Visceral obesity: A component of the insulin resistance-dyslipidemic syndrome. Can J Cardiol 1994;10:17B–22B.
16. Després JP. Obesity and lipid metabolism: Relevance of body fat distribution. Curr Opin Lipidol 1991;2:5–15.
17. Després JP. Dyslipidemia and obesity. Ballière's Clinical Endocrinology and Metabolism. 1994; 8:629–60.
18. Després JP, Moorjani S, Lupien PJ, Tremblay A, Nadeau A, Bouchard C. Regional distribution of body fat, plasma lipoproteins, and cardiovascular disease. Arteriosclerosis 1990;10:497–511.
19. Kissebah AH, Peiris AN. Biology of regional body fat distribution: Relationship to non- insulin-dependent diabetes mellitus. Diabetes Metab Rev 1989; 5:83–109.
20. Björntorp P. "Portal" adipose tissue as a generator of risk factors for cardiovascular disease and diabetes. Arteriosclerosis 1990;10:493–496.
21. Kissebah AH, Evans DJ, Peiris A, Wilson CR. Endocrine characteristics in regional obesities: Role of sex steroids. In: Metabolic complications of human obesities, Vague J, Björntorp P, Guy-Grand B, et al, eds. Amsterdam: Elsevier Science Publ 1985;115–130.
22. Kissebah AH, Krakower GR. Regional adiposity and morbidity. Physiol Rev 1984;74:761-811.
23. Lapidus L, Bengtsson C, Larsson B, Pennert K, Rybo E, Sjöström L. Distribution of adipose tissue and risk of cardiovascular disease and death: A 12 year follow-up of participants in the population study of women in Gothenburg, Sweden. BMJ 1984;289:1261–1263.
24. Larsson B, Svardsudd K, Welin L, Wilhemsen L, Björntorp P, Tibblin G. Abdominal adipose tissue distribution, obesity and risk of cardiovascular disease and death: 13 year follow-up of participants in the study of men born in 1913. BMJ 1984;288:1401-1404.
25. Ducimetière P, Richard J, Cambien F. The pattern of subcutaneous fat distribution in middle-aged men and the risk of coronary heart disease: The Paris Prospective study. Int J Obes 1986;10:229–240.
26. Ohlson LO, Larsson B, Svärdsudd K, Welin L, Eriksson H, Wilhelmsen L, Björntorp P, Tibblin G. The influence of body fat distribution on the incidence of diabetes mellitus—13.5 years of follow-up of the participants in the study of men born in 1913. Diabetes 1985;34:1055–1058.
27. Borkan GA, Gerzof SG, Robbins AH, Hults DE, Silbert CK, Silbert JE. Assessment of abdominal fat content by computed tomography. Am J Clin Nutr 1982;36:172–177.
28. Tokunaga K, Matsuzawa Y, Ishikawa K, Tarui S. A novel technique for the determination of body fat by computed tomogrphy. Int J Obes 1983;7:437–445.
29. Sjöström L, Kvist H, Cederblad A, Tylen U. Determination of total adipose tissue and body fat in women by computed tomography, 40K, and tritium. Am J Physiol (Endocrinol Metab) 1986;250:E736–E745.
30. Kvist H, Chowdhury B, Grangard U, Tylén U, Sjöström L. Total and visceral adipose tissue volumes derived from measurements with computed tomography in adult men and women: Predictive equations. Am J Clin Nutr 1988;48:1351–1361.

31. Després JP, Nadeau A, Tremblay A, Ferland M, Lupien PJ. Role of deep abdominal fat in the association between regional adipose tissue distribution and glucose tolerance in obese women. Diabetes 1989;38:304–309.

32. Pouliot MC, Després JP, Nadeau A, Moorjani S, Prud'homme D, Lupien PJ, Tremblay A, Bouchard C. Visceral obesity in men. Associations with glucose tolerance, plasma insulin, and lipoprotein levels. Diabetes 1992;41:826–834.

33. Després JP, Moorjani S, Ferland M, Tremblay A, Lupien PJ, Nadeau A, Pinault S, Thériault G, Bouchard C. Adipose tissue distribution and plasma lipoprotein levels in obese women: Importance of intra-abdominal fat. Arteriosclerosis 1989;9:203–210.

34. Després JP, Ferland M, Moorjani S, Tremblay A, Lupien PJ, Thériault G, Bouchard C. Role of hepatic-triglyceride lipase activity in the association between intra-abdominal fat and plasma HDL-cholesterol in obese women. Arteriosclerosis 1989;9:485–492.

35. Després JP, Moorjani S, Tremblay A, Ferland M, Lupien PJ, Nadeau A, Bouchard C. Relation of high plasma triglyceride levels associated with obesity and regional adipose tissue distribution to plasma lipoprotein-lipid composition in premenopausal women. Clin Invest Med 1989;12:374–380.

36. Després JP, Lemieux S, Lamarche B, Prud'homme D, Moorjani S, Brun LD, Gagné C, Lupien PJ. The insulin-resistance syndrome: Contribution of visceral obesity and therapeutic implications. Int J Obes 1995;19(suppl):S76-S86.

37. Després JP, Marette A. Relation of components of insulin resistance syndrome to coronary disease risk. Curr Opin Lipidol 1994;5:274–289.

38. Tchernof A, Lamarche B, Prud'homme D et al. The dense LDL phenotype: association with plasma lipoprotein levels, visceral obesity, and hyperinsulinemia in men. Diabetes Care 1996;19(6):629–637.

39. Juhan-Vague I, Pyke SDM, Alessi ML, et al. Fibrinolytic factors and the risk of myocardial infarction or sudden death in patients with angina pectoris. Circulation 1996;94:2057–2063.

40. Alessi MC, Peiretti F, Morange P, Henry M, Nalbone G, Juhan-Vague I. Production of plasminogen activator inhibitor 1 by human adipose tissue: possible link between visceral fat accumulation and vascular disease. Diabetes 1997;46:860–867.

41. Haffner SM, Stern MP, Hazuda HP, Mitchell BD, Patterson JK. Cardiovascular risk factors in confirmed prediabetic individuals. Does the clock for coronary heart disease start ticking before the onset of clinical diabetes? JAMA 1990;263:2893–2898.

42. Lillioja S, Mott DM, Spraul M et al. Insulin resistance and insulin secretory dysfunction as precursors of non-insulin dependent diabetes mellitus: prospective studies of Pima Indians. N Engl J Med 1993;329:1988–1992.

43. Warram JH, Martin BC, Krolewski AS, Soeldner JS, Kahn CR. Slow glucose removal rate and hyperinsulinemia precede the development of type II diabetes in the offspring of diabetic patients. Ann Intern Med 1990;113:909–915.

44. Martin BC, Warram JH, Krolewski AS, Bergman RN, Soeldner JS, Kahn CR. Role of glucose and insulin resistance in development of type 2 diabetes mellitus: results from a 25-year follow-up study. Lancet 1992;340:925–929.

45. Stamler J, Vaccaro O, Neaton JD, Wentworth D. Diabetes, other risk factors, and 12-yr cardiovascular mortality for men screened in the Multiple Risk Factor Intervention Trial. Diabetes Care 1993;16:434–444.

46. Damsgaard EM, Froland A, Jorgensen OD, Mogensen CE. Eight to nine year mortality in known non-insulin dependent diabetes and controls. Kidney Int 1992;42:731–735.

47. Donahue RP, Orchard TJ. Diabetes Mellitus and macrovascular complications: an epidemiological perspective. Diabetes Care 1992;15:1141–1155.

48. Jarrett RJ, Shipley MJ. Type 2 (non-insulin dependent) diabetes mellitus and cardiovascular disease-putative association via common antecedents; further evidence from the Whitehall study. Diabetologia 1988;31:737–740.

49. Herman JB, Medalie JH, Goldbourt U. Differences in cardiovascular morbidity and mortality between previously known and newly diagnosed adult diabetics. Diabetologia 1977;13:229–234.

50. Reaven GM. Role of insulin resistance in human disease. Diabetes 1988;37:1595–1606.

51. Sicree RA, Zimmet PZ, King HOM, Coventry JS. Plasma insulin response among Nauruans: prediction of deterioration in glucose tolerance over 6 yrs. Diabetes 1987;36:179–186.

52. Bergstrom RW, Newell-Morris LL, Leonetti DL, Shuman WP, Wahl PW, Fujimoto WY. Association of elevated fasting C-peptide level and increased intra-abdominal fat distribution with development of NIDDM in Japanese American men. Diabetes 1990;39:104–111.

53. Saad MF, Knowler WC, Pettitt DJ, Nelson RG, Mott DM, Bennett PH. The natural history of impaired glucose tolerance in the Pima Indians. N Engl J Med 1988;319:1500–1506.

54. Haffner SM, Miettinen H, Gaskill SP, Stern MP. Decreased insulin secretion and increased insulin resistance are independently related to the seven year risk of non-insulin dependent diabetes mellitus in Mexican Americans. Diabetes 1995;44:1386–1391.

55. Pyorala K, Laakso M, Vusitupa M. Diabetes and atherosclerosis: an epidemiologic view. Diabetes Metab Rev 1987;3:463–524.

56. Lewis GF, Steiner G. Hypertriglyceridemia and its metabolic consequences as a risk factor for atherosclerotic cardiovascular disease in non-insulin-dependent diabetes mellitus. Diabetes Metab Rev 1996;12:37–56.

57. Bierman EL. Atherogenesis in diabetes. Arterioscler Thromb 1992;12:647–656.

58. Frayn KN. Insulin resistance and lipid metabolism. Curr Opin Lipidolol 1993;4:197–204.

59. Laws A. Free fatty acids, insulin resistance and lipoprotein metabolism. Curr Opin Lipidolol 1996;7:172–177.

60. Reaven GM, Chen IYD, Jeppesen J, Krauss RM. Insulin resistance and hyperinsulinemia in individuals with small, dense, low density lipoprotein particles. J Clin Invest 1993;92:141–146.

61. Selby JB, Austin MA, Newman B et al. LDL subclass phenotypes and the insulin resistance syndrome in women. Circulation 1993;88:381–387.

62. Gardner CD, Fortmann SP, Krauss RM. Association of small low-density lipoprotein particles with the incidence of coronary artery disease in men and women. JAMA 1996;276:875–881.

63. Lamarche B, Tchernof A, Moorjani S. Small, dense low-density lipoprotein particles as predictors of the risk of ischemic heart disease in men: prospective results from the Québec Cardiovascular Study. Circulation 1997;95:69–75.

64. Stampfer MJ, Krauss RM, Ma J, et al. A prospective study of triglyceride level, low-density lipoprotein particle diameter, and risk of myocardial infarction. JAMA 1996;276:882–888.

65. Gerstein HC, Yusuf S. Dysglycemia and the risk of cardiovascular disease. Lancet 1996;347:949–950.

66. Pénicaud L, Ferré P, Terretaz J, Kinebanyan MF, Leturque A, Doré E, Girard J, Jeanrenaud B, Picon L. Development of obesity in Zucker rats. Early insulin resistance in muscles but normal sensitivity in white adipose tissue. Diabetes 1987;36:626–631.

67. Lavau M, Bazin R, Guerre-Millo M. Increased capacity for fatty acid synthesis in white and brown adipose tissues from 7-day-old obese Zucker pups. Int J Obes 1985;9:61–66.

68. Pénicaud L, Ferré P, Assimacopoulos-Jeannet F, Perdereau D, Leturque A, Jeanrenaud B, Picon L, Girard J. Increased gene expression of lipogenic enzymes and glucose transporter in white adipose tissue of suckling and weaned obese Zucker rats. Biochem J 1991;279:303–308.

69. Klip A, Marette A. Regulation of glucose transporters by insulin and exercise: cellular effects and implications for diabetes In: Rowell LB, ed. Handbook of Physiology, J.T.S. Oxford University Press, 1998, 2 (part II) Target tissues for metabolic regulatory hormones; in press.

70. Hotamisligil GS, Spiegelman BM. Tumor necrosis factor alpha: a key component of the obesity-diabetes link. Diabetes 1994;43:1271–1278.

71. Hotamisligil, G S, Spiegelman BM. Adipose expression of tumor necrosis factor-alpha: direct role in obesity-linked insulin resistance. Science 1993;259:87–91.

72. Kern PA, Saghizadeh M, Ong JM, Bosch RJ, Deem R, Simsolo RB. The expression of tumor necrosis factor in human adipose tissue. Regulation by obesity, weight loss, and relationship to lipoprotein lipase. J Clin Invest 1995;95:2111–2119.

73. Hotamisligil GS, Arner P, Caro JF, Atkinson RL, Spiegelman BM. Increased adipose tissue expression of tumor necrosis factor-alpha in human obesity and insulin resistance. J Clin Invest 1995;95: 2409–2415.

74. Saghizadeh M, Ong JM, Garvey WT, Henry RR, Kern PA. The expression of TNF-α by human muscle. Relationship to insulin resistance. J Clin Invest 1996;97:1111–1116.

75. Hotamisligil GS, Budavari A, Murray D, Spiegelman BM. Reduced tyrosine kinase activity of the insulin receptor in obesity-diabetes—central role of tumor necrosis factor-alpha. J Clin Invest 1994;94:1543–1549.

76. Hotamisligil GS, Murray DL, Choy LN, Spiegelman BM. Tumor necrosis factor a inhibits signaling from the insulin receptor. Proc Natl Acad Sci USA 1994;91:4854–4858.

77. Ofei F, Hurel S, Newkirk J, Sopwith M, Taylor R. Effects of an engineered human anti-TNF-alpha antibody (CDP571) on insulin sensitivity and glycemic control in patients with NIDDM. Diabetes 1996;45:881–885.

78. Uysal KT, Wiesbrock SM, Marino MW, Hotamisligil GS. Protection from obesity-induced insulin resistance in mice lacking TNF-alpha function. Nature 1997;389: 610–614.

79. Ventre J, Doebber T, Wu M, MacNaul K, Stevens K, Pasparakis M, Kollias G, Moller DE. Targeted disruption of the tumor necrosis actor-alpha gene: metabolic consequences in obese and nonobese mice. Diabetes 1997;46:1526–1531.

80. Hotamisligil GS, Johnson RS, Distel RJ, Ellis R, Papaioannou VE, Spiegelman BM. Uncoupling of obesity from insulin resistance through a targeted mutation in aP2, the adipocyte fatty acid binding protein. Science 1996;274(5291):1377–1379.

81. Randle PJ, Priestman DA, Mistry SC, Halsall A. Glucose fatty acid interactions and the regulation of glucose disposal. J Cell Biochem 1994;55:1–11.

82. Ranganathan S, Davidson MB. Effect of tumor-necrosis-factor-alpha on basal and insulin-stimulated glucose-transport in cultured muscle and fat-cells. Metabolism-clinical and experimental 1996; 45:1089–1094.

83. Furnsinn C, Neschen S, Wagner O, Roden M, Bisschop M, Waldhausl W. Acute and chronic exposure to tumor necrosis factor-alpha fails to affect insulin-stimulated glucose metabolism of isolated rat soleus muscle. Endocrinology 1997;138(7):2674–2679.

84. Bédard S, Marcotte B, Marette A. Cytokines modulate glucose transport in skeletal muscle by inducing the expression of inducible nitric oxide synthase. Biochem J 1997;325:487–493.

85. Girard J. Is leptin the link between obesity and insulin resistance? Diabetes Metab 1997;23:16–24.

86. Spiegelman BM, Flier JS. Adipogenesis and obesity: rounding out the big picture. Cell 1996;87:377–389.

87. Muller, G., J. Ertl, M. Gerl, and G. Preibisch. Leptin impairs metabolic actions of insulin in isolated rat adipocytes. J Biol Chem 272:10585–93, 1997.

88. Berti L, Kellerer M, Capp E, Haring HU. Leptin stimulates glucose transport and glycogen synthesis in C2C12 myotubes: evidence for a PI3-kinase mediated effect. Diabetologia 1997;40:606–609.

89. Zierath JR, Frevert EU, Ryder JW, Berggren PO, Kahn BB. Evidence against a direct effect of leptin on glucose transport in skeletal muscle and adipocytes. Diabetes 1998;47:1–4.

90. Björntorp P. Visceral obesity: A "Civilization Syndrome." Obesity Res 1993;1:206–222.

91. Arner P. Regulation of adipose tissue lipolysis, importance for the metabolic syndrome. Adv Exp Med Biol 1993;334:259–267.

92. Frayn KN, Williams CM, Arner P. Are increased plasma non-esterified fatty acid concentrations a risk marker for coronary heart disease and other chronic diseases? [editorial]. Clin Sci 1996;90:243–253.

93. Bouchard C, Després JP, Mauriège P. Genetic and nongenetic determinants of regional fat distribution. Endocr Rev 1993;14:72–93.

94. Mauriège P, Galitzky J, Berlan M, Lafontan M. Heterogeneous distribution of beta and alpha–2 adrenoceptor binding sites in human fat cells from various fat deposits: functional consequences. Eur J Clin Invest 1987;17:156–165.

95. Mauriège P, Després JP, Prud'homme D, Pouliot MC, Marcotte M, Tremblay A, Bouchard C. Regional variation in adipose tissue lipolysis in lean and obese men. J Lipid Res 1991;32:1625–1633.

96. Mauriège P, Marette A, Atgie C, Bouchard C, Theriault G, Bukowiecki LK, Marceau P, Biron S, Nadeau A, Després JP. Regional variation in adipose tissue metabolism of severely obese premeno-pausal women. J Lipid Res 1995;36:672–684.

97. Mauriège P, Prud'homme D, Lemieux S, Tremblay A, Després JP. Regional differences in adipose tissue lipolysis from lean and obese women: existence of postreceptor alterations. Am J Physiol 1995;269:E341-E350.

98. Marette A, Mauriège P, Atgié C, Bouchard C, Thériault G, Bukowiecki L, Marceau P, Biron S, Nadeau A, Després JP. Regional variation in adipose tissue insulin action and GLUT4 glucose transporter expression in severely obese premenauposal women. Diabetologia 1997;40:590–598.

99. Lönnqvist F, Thorne A, Nilsell K, Hoffstedt J, Arner P. A pathogenic role of visceral fat beta3-adrenoceptors in obesity. J Clin Invest 1995;95:1109–1116.

100. Lönnqvist F, Krief S, Strosberg AD, Nyberg B, Emorine LJ, Arner P. Evidence for a Functional beta(3)-Adrenoceptor in Man. Br J Pharmacol 1993;110:929–936.

101. Hoffstedt J, Wahrenberg H, Thorne A, Lonnqvist F. The metabolic syndrome is related to beta 3-adrenoceptor sensitivity in visceral adipose tissue. Diabetologia 1996;39:838–844.

102. Hoffstedt J, Arner P, Hellers G, Lonnqvist F. Variation in adrenergic regulation of lipolysis between omental and subcutaneous adipocytes from obese and non-obese men. J Lipid Res 1997;38:795–804.

103. Hennes MM, Shrago E, Kissebah AH. Receptor and postreceptor effects of free fatty acids (FFA) on hepatocyte insulin dynamics. Int J Obes 1990;14:831–841.

104. Svedberg J, Bjorntorp P, Smith U, Lonnroth P. Effect of free fatty acids on insulin receptor binding and tyrosine kinase activity in hepatocytes isolated from lean and obese rats. Diabetes 1992;41:294–298.

105. Cohen B, Novick D, Rubinstein M. Modulation of insulin activities by leptin. Science 1996;274:1185–1188.

106. Myers MG, White MF. Insulin signal-transduction and the IRS proteins. Annual review of pharmacology and toxicology. 1996;36:615–658.

107. White MF. The insulin signalling system and the IRS proteins. Diabetologia 1997;40:S2–S17.

108. Quon MJ, Butte AJ, Zarnowski MJ, Sesti G, Cushman SW, Taylor SI. Insulin receptor substrate 1 mediates the stimulatory effect of insulin on GLUT4 translocation in transfected rat adipose cells. J Biol Chem 1994;269:27920–27924.

109. Zhou L, Chen H, Lin CH, Cong LN, McGibbon MA, Sciacchitano S, Lesniak MA, Quon MJ, Taylor SI. Insulin receptor substrate–2 (IRS–2) can mediate the action of insulin to stimulate translocation of GLUT4 to the cell surface in rat adipose cells. J Biol Chem 1997;272: 29829–29833.

110. Lavan BE, Lane WS, Lienhard GE. The 60-kDa phosphotyrosine protein in insulin-treated adipocytes is a new member of the insulin receptor substrate family. J Biol Chem 1997;272:11439–11443.

111. Kaburagi Y, Satoh S, Tamemoto H, Yamamoto-Honda R, Tobe K, Veki K, Yamauchi T, Kono-Sugita E, Sekihara H, Aizawa S, Cushman SW, Akanuma Y, Yazaki Y, Kadowaki T. Role of insulin receptor substrate-1 and pp60 in the regulation of insulin-induced glucose transport and GLUT4 translocation in primary adipocytes. J Biol Chem 1997;272:25839–25844.

112. Virbasius JV, Guilherme A, Czech MP. Mouse p170 is a novel phosphatidylinositol 3-kinase containing a C2 domain. J. Biol. Chem. 1996;271:13304–13307.

113. Stoyanov B, Volinia S, Hanck T, Rubio I, Loubtchenkov M, Malek D, Stoyanova S, Vanhaesebroeck B, Dhand R, Nurnberg B, Gierschik P, Seedorf K, Justin Hsuan J, Waterfield MD, Wetzker R. Cloning and characterization of a G protein-activated human phosphoinositide–3 kinase. Science 1995; 269:690–693.

114. Thomason PA, James SR, Casey PJ, Downes CP. A G-protein bg-subunits-responsive phosphoinositide 3-kinase activity in human platelet cytosol. J Biol Chem 1994;269:16525–16528.

115. Stephens L, Smrcka A, Cooke FT, Jackson TR, Sternweis PC, Hawkins PT. A novel phosphoinositide 3-kinase activity in myeloid-derived cells is activated by G Protein bg subunits. Cell 1994;77:83–93.

116. Antonetti DA, Algenstaedt P, Kahn RC. Insulin receptor substrate-1 binds two novel splice variants of the regulatory subunit of phosphatidylinositol 3-kinase in muscle and brain. Mol Cell Biol 1996;16:2195–2203.

117. Fry MJ. Structure, regulation and function of phosphoinositide 3-kinases. Biochim. Biophys Acta 1994;1226:237–268.

118. Ricort JM, Tanti JF, Van Obberghen E, Le Marchand-Brustel Y. Different effects of insulin and platelet-derived growth factor on phosphatidylinositol 3-kinase at the subcellular level in 3T3-L1 adipocytes. A possible explanation for their specific effects on glucose transport. Eur J Biochem 1996;239:17–22.

119. Nave BT, Haigh RJ, Hayward AC, Siddle K, Shepherd PR. Compartment-specific regulation of phosphoinositide 3-kinase by platlet-derived growth factor and insulin in 3T3-L1 adipocytes. Biochem J 1996;318:55–60.

120. Isakoff SJ, Taha C, Rose E, Marcusohn J, Klip A, Skolnik EY. The inability of phosphatidylinositol 3-kinase activation to stimulate GLUT4 translocation indicates additional signaling pathways are required for insulin-stimulated glucose uptake. Proc Natl Acad Sci USA 1995;92:10247–10251.

121. Heller-Harrison RA, Morin M, Guilherme A, Czech MP. Insulin-mediated targeting of phosphatidylinositol 3-kinase to GLUT4-containing vesicles. J Biol Chem 1996;271:10200–10204.

122. Tsakiridis T, McDowell HE, Walker T, Downes CP, Hundal HS, Vranic M, Klip A. Multiple roles of phosphatidylinositol 3-kinase in regulation of glucose transport, amino acid transport, and glucose transporters in L6 skeletal muscle cells. Endocrinology 1995;136:4315–4322.

123. Yamamoto-Honda R, Tobe K, Kaburagi Y, Ueki K, Asai S, Yachi M, Shirouzu M, Yodoi J, Akanuma Y, Yokoyama S, Yazaki Y, Kadowaki T. Upstream mechanisms of glycogen synthase activation by insulin and inulin-like growth factor–1: Glycogen synthase activation is antagonized by wortmannin or LY294002 but not by rapamycin or by inhibiting p21ras. J Biol Chem 1995;270:2729–2734.

124. Shepherd PR, Nave BT, Siddle K. Insulin Stimulation of Glycogen Synthesis and Glycogen Synthase Activity is Blocked by Wortmannin and Rapamycin in 3T3-L1 Adipocytes: Evidence for the Involvement of Phosphoinositide 3-Kinase and P70 Ribosomal protein-S6 Kinase. Biochem J 1995;305:25–28.

125. Okada T, Kawano Y, Sakakibara T, Hazeki O, Ui M. Essential role of phosphatidylinositol 3-kinase in insulin-induced glucose transport and antilipolysis in rat adipocytes. J Biol Chem 1994;269:3568–3573.

126. Burgering BMT, Coffer PJ. Protein kinase B (c-Akt) in phosphatidylinositol–3-OH kinase signal transduction. Nature 1995;376:599–602.

127. Franke TF, Yang SI, Chan TO, Datta K, Kazlauskas A, Morrison DK, Kaplan DR, Tsichlis PN. The protein kinase encoded by the Akt proto-oncogene is a target of the PDGF-activated phosphatidylinositol 3-kinase. Cell 1995;81:727–736.

128. Alessi DR, Andjelkovic M, Caudwell B, Cron P, Morrice N, Cohen P, Hemmings BA. Mechanism of activation of protein kinase B by insulin and IGF-1. EMBO J 1996;15:6541–6551.

129. Kohn AD, Summers SA, Birnbaum MJ, Roth RA. Expression of a constitutively active akt Ser/Thr kinase in 3T3-L1 adipocytes stimulates glucose uptake and glucose transporter 4 translocation. J Biol Chem 1996;271:31372–31378.

130. Tanti JF, Grillo S, Gremeaux T, Coffer PJ, Van Obberghen E, Le Marchand-Brustel Y. Potential role of protein kinase B in glucose transporter 4 translocation in adipocytes. Endocrinology 1997;138:2005–2010.

131. Tsakiridis T, Vranic M, Klip A. Disassembly of the actin network inhibits insulin-dependent stimulation of glucose transport and prevents recruitment of glucose transporters to the plasma membrane. J Biol Chem 1994;269:29934–29942.

132. Satoh S, Nishimura H, Clark AE, Kozka IJ, Vannucci SJ, Simpson IA, Quon MJ, Cushman SW, Holman GD. Use of bimannose photolabel to elucidate insulin-regulated GLUT4 subcellular trafficking kinetics in rat adipose cells. Evidence that exocytosis is a critical site of hormone action. J Biol Chem 1993;268:17820–17829.

133. Jhun BH, Rampal AL, Liu H, Lachaal M, Jung CY. Effects of insulin on steady state kinetics of GLUT4 subcellular distribution in rat adipocytes. Evidence of constitutive GLUT4 recycling. J Biol Chem 1992;267:17710–17715.

134. Czech MP, Buxton JM. Insulin action on the internalization of the GLUT4 glucose transporter in isolated rat adipocytes. J Biol Chem 1993;268:9187–9190.

135. Yang J, Holman GD. Comparison of GLUT4 and GLUT1 subcellular trafficking in basal and insulin-stimulated 3T3-L1 cells. J Biol Chem 1993;268:4600–4603.

136. Slot JW, Geuze HJ, Gigendack S, James DE, Lienhard GE. Translocation of the glucose transporter GLUT4 in cardiac myocytes of the rat. Proc Natl Acad Sci USA 1991;88:7815–7819.

137. Rea S, James DE. Moving GLUT4: the biogenesis and trafficking of GLUT4 storage vesicles. Diabetes 1997;46:1667–1677.

138. Sinha MK, Pories WJ, Flickinger EG, Meelheim D, Caro JF. Insulin-receptor kinase activity of adipose tissue from morbidly obese humans with and without NIDDM. Diabetes 1987;36:620–625.

139. Arner P, Pollare T, Lithell H, Livingston JN. Defective insulin receptor tyrosine kinase in human skeletal muscle in obesity and type 2 (non-insulin-dependent) diabetes mellitus. Diabetologia 1987;30:437–440.

140. Caro JF, Sinha MK, Raju SM, Ittoop O, Pories WJ, Flickinger EG, Meelheim D, Dohm GL. Insulin receptor kinase in human skeletal muscle from obese subjects with and without noninsulin dependent diabetes. J Clin Invest 1987;79:1330–1337.

141. Le Marchand-Brustel Y, Grémeaux T, Ballotti R, Van Obberghen E. Insulin receptor tyrosine kinase is defective in skeletal muscle of insulin-resistant obese mice. Nature 1985;315:676–679.

142. Grasso G, Frittitta L, Anello M, Russo P, Sesti G, Trischitta V. Insulin receptor tyrosine-kinase activity is altered in both muscle and adipose tissue from non-obese normoglycaemic insulin-resistant subjects. Diabetologia 1995;38:55–61.

143. Handberg A, Vaag A, Vinten J, Beck-Nielsen H. Decreased tyrosine kinase activity in partially purified insulin receptors from muscle of young, non-obese first degree relatives of patients with type 2 (non-insulin-dependent) diabetes mellitus. Diabetologia 1993;36:668–674.

144. Folli F, Saad MJA, Backer JM, Kahn CR. Regulation of phosphatidylinositol 3-kinase activity in liver and muscle of animal models of insulin-resistant and insulin-deficient diabetes-mellitus. J Clin Invest 1993;92:1787–1794.

145. Heydrick SJ, Jullien D, Gautier N, Tanti JF, Giorgetti S, Van Obberghen E, Le Marchand Brustel Y. Defect in skeletal muscle phosphatidylinositol–3-kinase in obese insulin-resistant mice. J Clin Invest 1993;91:1358–1366.

146. Heydrick SJ, Gautier N, Olichon Berthe C, Van Obberghen E, Le Marchand Brustel Y. Early alteration of insulin stimulation of PI 3-kinase in muscle and adipocyte from gold thioglucose obese mice. Am J Physiol 1995;268:E604–E612.

147. Bjornholm M, Kawano Y, Lehtihet M, Zierath JR. Insulin receptor substrate-1 phosphorylation and phosphatidylinositol 3- kinase activity in skeletal muscle from NIDDM subjects after in vivo insulin stimulation. Diabetes 1997;46:524–527.

148. Goodyear LJ, Giorgino F, Sherman LA, Carey J, Smith RJ, Dohm GL. Insulin receptor phosphorylation, insulin receptor substrate-1 phosphorylation, and phosphatidylinositol 3-kinase activity are decreased in intact skeletal muscle strips from obese subjects. J Clin Invest 1995;95:2195–2204.

149. Rondinone CM, Wang LM, Lonnroth P, Wesslau C, Pierce JH, Smith U. Insulin receptor substrate (IRS) 1 is reduced and IRS-2 is the main docking protein for phosphatidylinositol 3-kinase in adipocytes from subjects with non-insulin-dependent diabetes mellitus. Proc Natl Acad Sci USA 1997;94:4171–4175.

150. Tamemoto H, Kadowaki T, Tobe K, Yagi T, Sakura H, Hayakawa T, Terauchi Y, Ueki K, Kaburagi Y, Satoh S, et al. Insulin resistance and growth retardation in mice lacking insulin receptor substrate-1 [see comments]. Nature 1994;372:182–186.

151. Araki E, Lipes MA, Patti ME, Bruning JC, Haag BR, Johnson RS, Kahn CR. Alternative pathway of insulin signalling in mice with targeted disruption of the IRS-1 gene [see comments]. Nature 1994;372:186–190.

152. Hotamisligil GS, Peraldi P, Budavari A, Ellis R, White MF, Spiegelman BM. IRS-1-mediated inhibition of insulin receptor tyrosine kinase activity in TNF-α- and obesity-induced insulin resistance. Science 1996;271:665–668.

153. Kolter T, Uphues I, Eckel J. Molecular analysis of insulin resistance in isolated ventricular cardiomyocytes of obese Zucker rats. Am J Physiol 1997;273:E59–E67.

154. Paz K, Hemi R, LeRoith D, Karasik A, Elhanany E, Kanety H, Zick Y. A molecular basis for insulin resistance. Elevated serine/threonine phosphorylation of IRS-1 and IRS–2 inhibits their binding to the juxtamembrane region of the insulin receptor and impairs their ability to undergo insulin-induced tyrosine phosphorylation. J Biol Chem 1997;272:29911–29918.

155. Stoffel M, Espinosa RD, Keller SR, Lienhard GE, Le Beau MM, Bell GI. Human insulin receptor substrate-1 gene (IRS1): chromosomal localization to 2q35-q36.1 and identification of a simple tandem repeat DNA polymorphism. Diabetologia 1993;36:335–337.

156. Hager J, Zouali H, Velho G, Froguel P. Insulin receptor substrate (IRS-1) gene polymorphisms in French NIDDM families [letter]. Lancet 1993;342:1430.

157. Laakso M, Malkki M, Kekalainen P, Kuusisto J, Deeb SS. Insulin receptor substrate-1 variants in non-insulin-dependent diabetes. J Clin Invest 1994;94:1141–1146.

158. Imai Y, Fusco A, Suzuki Y, Lesniak MA, D'Alfonso R, Sesti G, Bertoli A, Lauro R, Accili D, Taylor SI. Variant sequences of insulin receptor substrate-1 in patients with noninsulin-dependent diabetes mellitus. J Clin Endocrinol Metab 1994;79:1655–1658.

159. Clausen JO, Hansen T, Bjorbaek C, Echwald SM, Urhammer SA, Rasmussen S, Andersen CB, Hansen L, Almind K, Winther K et al. Insulin resistance: interactions between obesity and a common variant of insulin receptor substrate-1. Lancet 1995;346:397–402.

160. Almind K, Bjorbaek C, Vestergaard H, Hansen T, Echwald S, Pedersen O. Aminoacid polymorphisms of insulin receptor substrate-1 in non-insulin- dependent diabetes mellitus. Lancet 1993;342:828–832.

161. Ura S, Araki E, Kishikawa H, Shirotani T, Todaka M, Isami S, Shimoda S, Yoshimura R, Matsuda K, Motoyoshi S, Miyamura N, Kahn CR, Shichiri M. Molecular scanning of the insulin receptor substrate-1 (IRS-1) gene in Japanese patients with NIDDM: identification of five novel polymorphisms. Diabetologia 1996;39:600–608.

162. Zhang Y, Wat N, Stratton IM, Warren-Perry MG, Orho M, Groop L, Turner RC. UKPDS 19: heterogeneity in NIDDM: separate contributions of IRS-1 and beta 3-adrenergic-receptor mutations to insulin resistance and obesity respectively with no evidence for glycogen synthase gene mutations. UK Prospective Diabetes Study. Diabetologia 1996;39:1505–1511.

163. Almind K, Inoue G, Pedersen O, Kahn CR. A common amino acid polymorphism in insulin receptor substrate-1 causes impaired insulin signaling. Evidence from transfection studies. J Clin Invest 1996;97:2569–2575.

164. Yoshimura R, Araki E, Ura S, Todaka M, Tsuruzoe K, Furukawa N, Motoshima H, Yoshizato K, Kaneko K, Matsuda K, Kishikawa H, Shichiri M. Impact of natural IRS-1 mutations on insulin signals: mutations of IRS-1 in the PTB domain and near SH2 protein binding sites result in impaired function at different steps of IRS-1 signaling. Diabetes 1997;46:929–936.

165. Tsakiridis T, Marette A, Klip A. Glucose transporters in skeletal muscle of animal models of diabetes In: Shafrir E, ed. Lessons from Animal Models of Diabetes V. 1994;141–159.

166. James DE, Piper RC. Insulin resistance, diabetes, and the insulin-regulated trafficking of GLUT-4. J Cell Biol 1994;126:1123–1126.

167. Chisholm DJ, Campbell LV, Kraegen EW. Pathogenesis of the insulin resistance syndrome (syndrome X). Clin Exp Pharmacol Physiol 1997;24:782–784.

168. Garvey WT. Glucose transport and NIDDM. Diabetes Care 1992;15: 396–417.

169. Sinha MK, Raineri-Maldonado C, Buchanan C, Pories WJ, Carter-Su C, Pilch PF, Caro JF. Adipose tissue glucose transporters in NIDDM. Decreased levels of muscle/fat isoform. Diabetes 1991;40:472–477.

170. Trischitta V, Frittitta L, Vigneri R. Early molecular defects in human insulin resistance: studies in healthy subjects with low insulin sensitivity. Diabetes Metab Rev 1997;13:147–162.

171. Lefebvre AM, Laville M, Vega N, Riou JP, van Gaal L, Auwerx J, Vidal H. Depot-specific differences in adipose tissue gene expression in lean and obese subjects. Diabetes 1998;47:98–103.

172. Handberg A, Vaag A, Damsbo P, Beck-Nielsen H, Vinten J. Expression of insulin regulatable glucose transporters in skeletal muscle from Type II (non-insulin-dependent) diabetic patients. Diabetologia 1990;33:625–627.

173. Eriksson J, Koranyi L, Bourey R, Schalin-Jantti C, Widen E, Mueckler M, Permutt AM, Groop LC. Insulin resistance in Type 2 (non-insulin-dependent) diabetic patients and their relatives is not associated with a defect in the expression of the insulin-responsive glucose transporter (GLUT4) gene in human skeletal muscle. Diabetologia 1992;35:143–147.

174. Pedersen O, Bak JF, Andersen PH, Lund S, Moller DE, Flier JS, Kahn BB. Evidence against altered expression of GLUT1 or GLUT4 in skeletal muscle of patients with obesity or NIDDM. Diabetes 1990;39:865–870.

175. Dohm LG, Elton CW, Friedman JE, Pilch PF, Pories WJ, Atkinson SM, Caro JF. Decreased expression of glucose transporter in muscle from insulin-resistant patients. Am J Physiol 1991;260:E459-E463.

176. Marette A, Atgié C, Liu Z, Bukowiecki LJ, Klip A. Differential regulation of GLUT1 and GLUT4 glucose transporters in skeletal muscle of a new model of type II diabetes. The obese SHR/N-cp rat. Diabetes 1993;42:1195–1201.

177. Kahn BB, Pedersen O. Suppression of GLUT4 expression in skeletal muscle of rats that are obese from high fat feeding but not from high carbohydrate feeding or genetic obesity. Endocrinology 1993;132:13–22.

178. Kim Y, Tamura T, Iwashita S, Tokuyama K, Suzuki M. Effect of high-fat diet on gene expression of GLUT4 and insulin receptor in soleus muscle. Biochem Biophys Res Commun 1994;202:519–526.

179. King PA, Horton ED, Hirshman MF, Horton ES. Insulin resistance in obese Zucker rat (fa/fa) skeletal muscle is associated with a failure of glucose transporter translocation. J Clin Invest 1992;90:1568–1575.

180. Brozinick JTJ, Etgen GJ, Yaspelkis III BB, Ivy JL. Glucose uptake and GLUT–4 protein distribution in skeletal muscle of the obese Zucker rat. Am J Physiol 1994;267:R236–R243.

181. Galante P, Maerker E, Scholz R, Rett K, Herberg L, Mosthaf L, Haring HU. Insulin-induced translocation of GLUT 4 in skeletal muscle of insulin-resistant Zucker rats. Diabetologia 1994;37:3–9.

182. Etgen GJ, Wilson CM, Jensen J, Cushman SW, Ivy JL. Glucose-transport and cell-surface glut-4 protein in skeletal-muscle of the obese zucker rat. Am J Physiol 1996;34:E294–E301.

183. Rosholt MN, King PA, Horton ES. High-fat diet reduces glucose transporter responses to both insulin and exercise. Am J Physiol 1994;266:R95.

184. Dombrowski L, Roy D, Marette A. Selective impairment in GLUT4 translocation to transverse tubules in skeletal muscle of streptozotocin-induced diabetic rats. Diabetes 1998;47:5–12.

185. Zierath JR, He L, Guma A, Wahlstrom EO, Klip A, Wallberg-Henriksson H. Insulin action on glucose transport and plasma membrane glut4 content in skeletal muscle from patients with NIDDM. Diabetologia 1996;39:1180–1189.

186. Lamarche B, Moorjani S, Lupien PJ et al. Apolipoprotein A-I and B levels and the risk of ischemic heart disease during a five-year follow-up of men in the Québec Cardiovascular Study. Circulation 1996;94:273–278.

187. Després JP, Lamarche B, Mauriège P et al. Hyperinsulinemia as an independent risk factor for ischemic heart disease. N Engl J Med 1996;334:952–957.

188. Gaudet D, Vohl MC, Perron P, Tremblay G, Gagné C, Lesiège D, Bergeron J, Moorjani S, Després JP. Relationships of abdominal obesity and hyperinsulinemia to angiographically assessed coronary artery disease in men with known mutations in the LDL-receptor gene. Circulation 1998;97:871–877.

189. Brown MS, Goldstein J.L. A receptor-mediated pathway for cholesterol homeostasis. Science 1986;232:34–47.

190. Gagné C, Moorjani S, Brun D, Toussaint M, Lupien PJ. Heterozygous familial hypercholesterolemia. Relationship between plasma lipids, lipoproteins, clinical manifestations and ischemic heart disease in men and women. Atherosclerosis 1979;34:13–24.

191. Després JP, Lamarche B. Effects of diet and physical activity on adiposity and body fat distribution: Implications for the prevention of cardiovascular disease. Nutr Res Rev 1993;6:137–159.

192. Quetelet LAJ. Physique sociale 2. Muquardt C, Brussels 1869:92.

193. Keys A, Fidanza F, Karvonen MJ, et al. Indices of relative weight and obesity. J Chron Dis 1972;25:329–343.

194. Garrow J. Energy balance and obesity in man. Elsevier, London, 1974.

195. McKeigue PM, Shah B, Marmot MG. Relation of central obesity and insulin resistance with high diabetes prevalence and cardiovascular risk in South Asians. Lancet 1991;337:382–386.

196. Vague, J. La différenciation sexuelle : facteur déterminant des formes de l'obésité. Presse Med 1947;30:339–340.

197. Lemieux S, Després JP. Metabolic complications of visceral obesity: contribution to the aetiology of type II diabetes and implications for prevention and treatment. Diabète & Métab 1994;20:375–393.

198. Baumgartner RN, Heymsfield SB, Roche AF. Human body composition and the epidemiology of chronic disease. Obes Res 1995;3:73–95.

199. Lohman TG. Skinfolds and body density and their relation to body fatness: a review. Hum Biol 1981;53:181–225.

200. Wang J, Thornton JC, Russell M, et al. Asians have lower body mass index (BMI) but higher percent body fat than do whites: comparisons of anthropometric measurements. Am J Clin Nutr 1994;60:23–28.

201. Pouliot MC, Després JP, Lemieux S, et al. Waist circumference and abdominal sagittal diameter: best simple anthropometric indexes of abdominal visceral adipose tissue accumulation and related cardiovascular risk in men and women. Am J Cardiol 1994;73:460–468.

202. Lemieux S, Prud'homme D, Tremblay A, Bouchard C, Després JP. Anthropometric correlates to changes in visceral adipose tissue over 7 years in women. Int J Obes 1996;20:618–624.

203. Lemieux S, Prud'homme D, Bouchard C, Tremblay A, Després JP. A single threshold value of waist girth identifies normal-weight and overweight subjects with excess visceral adipose tissue. Am J Clin Nutr 1996;64:685–693.

204. Laakso M. How good a marker is insulin level for insulin resistance? Am J Epidemiol 1993;137:959–965.

205. Ferrannini E, Haffner SM, Mitchell BD, Stern MP. Hyperinsulinemia: The key feature of a cardiovascular and metabolic syndrome. Diabetologia 1991;34:416–422.

206. Austin MA, King MC, Vranizan KM, Krauss RM. Atherogenic lipoprotein phenotype: A proposed genetic marker for coronary heart disease. Circulation 1990;82:495–506.

207. Grundy SM. Small LDL, atherogenic dyslipidemia, and the metabolic syndrome. Circulation 1997;95:1–4.

5

The Role of Body Fat Distribution in Insulin Resistance

Abhimanyu Garg, MD

Contents

Introduction
Metabolic Heterogeneity of Adipose Tissue
Regional Distribution of Adipose Tissue
(Anatomic Considerations)
Regional Adiposity and Insulin Resistance
(Clinical Studies)
Summary and Conclusions
References

INTRODUCTION

The association of generalized obesity with insulin resistance has been well-described. However, it is becoming increasingly apparent that beyond the effects of overall adiposity, the location of fat in different adipose tissue compartments may have additional impact in causing insulin resistance and other metabolic complications of obesity such as atherosclerotic vascular disease, Type 2 diabetes mellitus, dyslipidemia and hypertension.

The concept of unique contribution of body fat distribution or regional adiposity to the metabolic complications was initiated by Vague *(1)* who in 1947 described two patterns of body fat distribution based on somatotypes, i.e., "android" or male pattern and "gynoid" or female pattern. He later proposed that different patterns of body fat distribution in obese patients are associated with different risk of metabolic complications *(2)*. In his original study *(1)*, android obesity was found to be more frequently associated with diabetes mellitus, coronary artery disease, gout and uric acid renal stones than was gynoid obesity. Subsequently, various terms have been used to identify different patterns of body fat distribution and the "android" pattern is usually synonymous with upper body, truncal, central, abdominal or visceral obesity; the "gynoid" pattern being synonymous with lower body, gluteofemoral or peripheral obesity.

In subsequent years, many different anthropometric indices have been used to characterize body fat distribution (Table 1). Some investigators have used indices such as

From: *Contemporary Endocrinology: Insulin Resistance*
Edited by: G. Reaven and A. Laws © Humana Press Inc., Totowa, NJ

Table 1
Methods to Determine Body Fat Distribution

Body circumference ratios
    Waist-to-hip circumference ratio (WHR)
    Iliac-to-thigh circumference ratio
Skinfold ratios
    Subscapular-to-triceps skinfold ratio
    Femoral-to-subscapular skinfold ratio
Ultrasonography of abdomen
    Distance from anterior abdominal wall to vertebral body
Dual energy Photon X-ray absorptiometry
Computerized tomography scan
    Visceral/sc abdominal fat area ratio
Nuclear magnetic resonance imaging
    Visceral/sc abdominal fat area ratio
    Intraperitoneal/sc abdominal fat mass ratio

waist-to-hip circumference ratio (WHR) and skinfold thickness ratios which involve simple and easy body measurements using tape measures and calipers, respectively. An increasing WHR has been shown to be more frequently associated with insulin resistance, impaired glucose tolerance, hypertriglyceridemia, hypercholesterolemia, and hyperuricemia in several cross-sectional studies (3–9). Recent longitudinal studies have further shown that upper body obesity is associated with increased incidence of coronary artery disease, Type 2 diabetes mellitus and stroke (10–15). The predisposition of individuals with upper body obesity to metabolic complications is mainly attributed to the excess of "visceral" or intra-abdominal fat.

Recently, therefore, in order to assess "visceral" adipose tissue directly, many investigators have utilized computed tomography (CT) or magnetic resonance imaging (MRI) techniques (9,16–18). These studies have identified two subsets of individuals with increased WHR: 1. those with increased subcutaneous (sc) abdominal fat, and 2. those with increased intra-abdominal or visceral fat. Some investigators have also proposed using a visceral fat-to-sc abdominal fat area ratio to identify subsets of individuals with increased intra-abdominal fat (9). A further refinement of the concept of adverse metabolic consequences of intra-abdominal adiposity has also been put forward which suggests that accumulation of fat in the intraperitoneal region ("portal" fat) has a unique influence on insulin sensitivity (19).

Two theoretical reasons are put forth to explain the deleterious effects of intraperitoneal fat on insulin sensitivity. The first reasoning is based upon the peculiar anatomic location of the intraperitoneal adipose tissue and its venous drainage into the portal system. Consequently, excessively high concentration of free fatty acids (FFA) and glycerol released from this depot directly affect hepatic metabolism. The high FFA flux to the liver may decrease hepatic insulin sensitivity (20) and can increase hepatic glucose output (21). Increased FFA flux in the portal circulation is also hypothesized to reduce hepatic insulin clearance, resulting in hyperinsulinemia in the systemic circulation. Excess FFAs also provide substrate for hepatic triglyceride synthesis and thus may contribute to hypertriglyceridemia. The other reason put forth is that intraperitoneal adipose tissue may be metabolically more active than adipose tissue located in other sites and thus may

Table 2
Classification of Adipose Tissue

Metabolically active	Mechanical
A. Subcutaneous sites other than mechanical	A. Subcutaneous sites Scalp, temporal, buccal, palm, sole, vulvar
B. Intra-abdominal Omental, mesenteric, retroperitoneal	B. Orbit
C. Intrathoracic Mediastinal, epidardial, retrosternal	C. Periarticular
D. Bone marrow	D. Epidural
E. Intraparenchymal parathyroids	E. Crista galli
	F. Perineal
	G. Pericalyceal (kidneys)

contribute more to the overall flux of FFAs and glycerol in the systemic circulation. According to the Randle's hypothesis *(22)*, excessive FFA release may induce peripheral insulin resistance by inhibiting skeletal muscle glucose uptake. In the following discussion, the evidence for and against the "portal" fat hypothesis is reviewed. First, the metabolic properties of adipose tissue from various different compartments of the body, particularly with respect to lipolytic activity, will be reviewed, followed by a review of anatomic considerations and recent clinical studies assessing the relationships of regional adiposity to insulin sensitivity.

METABOLIC HETEROGENEITY OF ADIPOSE TISSUE

Adipose tissue performs several important functions in the human body including, energy storage and release, conservation of body heat, protection to vital structures, storage of fat soluble vitamins and aromatization of sex steroids. Our recent studies of body fat distribution in patients with congenital generalized lipodystrophy (CGL), a rare autosomal-recessive disorder characterized by almost complete absence of adipose tissue since birth, have led us to propose that two distinct types of white adipose tissue may be present in humans; "metabolically-active" adipose tissue which participates in storage and release of energy, and "mechanical" adipose tissue, which is metabolically inert and may only serve supportive or protective functions *(23,24)*. Patients with CGL have provided a unique opportunity to identify various anatomic sites where mechanical adipose tissue is present in the human body (Table 2). Although the ultrastructure of mechanical adipose tissue may be similar to that of metabolically-active adipose tissue, it may have a unique embryological origin, lipid and membrane composition, as well as distinct vascular and nerve supply, which needs further studies.

Beyond the distinction between the "metabolically-active" and "mechanical" adipose tissues, whether "metabolically-active" adipose tissue from various anatomic sites have differences in metabolic activity will be reviewed in the following section. Most of the information is derived from the in vitro studies related to energy storage and release, however, recently some investigators have studied the metabolic heterogeneity of adipose tissue in vivo using microdialysis technique. Energy storage involves the enzyme lipoprotein lipase which is present in capillary endothelium and hydrolyzes triglycerides in lipoproteins to FFAs and glycerol. FFAs are taken up by the adipocytes and are reesterified to store energy as triglycerides. Release of energy from adipocytes involves the enzyme hormone sensitive lipase (HSL) which hydrolyzes stored triglycerides into FFA and glycerol.

Lipolytic Activity

Hormones such as insulin and catecholamines (epinephrine [E], and norepinephrine [NE]) regulate HSL activity mainly *(25,26)*. Nonhormonal factors such as diet, trauma and physical activity may affect HSL activity through changes in hormone levels or hormone sensitivity. Lipolytic activity of adipose tissue from various anatomic sites has been mainly studied in vitro using isolated adipocytes or adipose tissue. In addition, recently, using microdialysis technique, investigators have been able to assess in vivo rates of lipolysis.

BASAL LIPOLYSIS

Early investigation by Carlson et al. *(27)* noted higher basal lipolytic rate in sc adipose tissue compared to omental adipose tissue (0.43 ± 0.05 and 0.31 ± 0.03 µmol of glycerol/g/h, respectively). In a subsequent study by the same investigators *(28)*, however, no differences in basal lipolysis were observed among the two types of adipose tissue (0.61 ± 0.08 and 0.62 ± 0.06 µmol of glycerol/g/h, respectively). Subsequently, several investigators have reported an increased basal glycerol release from sc adipose tissue than from omental tissue *(29–31)*. The difference in basal lipolysis may possibly be due to increased size of sc adipocytes compared to those from omental area, however, other factors may also play a role.

Differences in lipolytic activity of adipocytes from various sc sites have also been reported. For example, Smith et al. *(32)* noted higher basal rate of lipolysis in sc adipose tissue from femoral area than that from abdominal area. The same group of investigators *(33)*, however, recently reported no differences in basal lipolysis in adipose tissue from abdominal and gluteofemoral region from obese and nonobese women. Rebuffe-Scrive et al. *(34)* using adipocyte suspensions also noted no difference in basal rate of lipolysis in femoral and abdominal sc adipose tissue.

Recently Jansson et al. *(35)* studied regional differences in adipose tissue lipolysis in vivo using a microdialysis technique. Although interstitial glycerol concentration was reported to be significantly higher in sc abdominal adipose tissue compared to femoral adipose tissue in obese men, overall glycerol release was the same. Obese men, however, had an increased release of glycerol compared to lean men, irrespective of adipose tissue distribution. Studies of Martin and Jensen *(36)* on the other hand suggest that regional distribution of fat may affect in vivo whole body lipolysis. They noted an increased [1-^{14}C] palmitate release in women with upper-body obesity than those with lower body obesity or nonobese women (161 ± 16, 111 ± 9, 92 ± 9 µmol/min, respectively). Upper-body obese women also had higher lipolysis from upper body compared to lower body obese women *(36)*.

CATECHOLAMINE-INDUCED LIPOLYSIS

The results of in vitro studies of regional adipose tissue metabolism pertaining to effects of hormones on lipolysis are somewhat variable. Several workers have studied lipolytic response to catecholamines in adipose tissue from different regions. Wertheimer et al. *(37)* were the first to study lipolytic response to E in rat adipose tissue and noted that sc adipose tissue released less fatty acids than mesenteric, epididymal and perirenal adipose tissue. Mosinger et al. *(38)* showed that human sc tissue responded less to E than omental tissue. On the contrary, Hamosh et al. *(39)* did not observe any difference in lipolytic response of human sc and omental adipose tissue to E.

Carlson et al. *(28)* reported higher glycerol release from omental adipose tissue after NE than that from sc adipose tissue (1.94 ± 0.20 and 1.09 ± 0.09 µmol of glycerol/g/h, respectively). Goldrich et al. *(29)* also observed an increase in E- stimulated lipolysis in omental tissue compared to sc adipose tissue. Efendic *(31)* noted an increased maximum NE-induced lipolysis in omental adipose tissue compared to sc adipose tissue. Ostman et al. *(30)*, however, did not show any differences in NE sensitivity of sc and omental adipocytes.

Recent studies further suggest that various types of sc adipose tissue may also have different lipolytic activity. Smith et al. *(32)* noted that the response of sc abdominal tissue to NE and isoproterenol was much greater than that of femoral adipose tissue. Increased sensitivity to isoproterenol-induced lipolysis in sc abdominal adipose tissue was observed only in obese women with increased WHR. Rebuffe-Scrive et al. *(34)* also reported an increased lipolytic response to NE in sc abdominal adipocytes compared to femoral adipocytes.

A recent study by Rebuffe-Scrive et al. *(40)* compared lipolytic responses of three intra-abdominal depots (mesenteric, omental and retroperitoneal) to sc abdominal adipose tissue in men and women. Interestingly, retroperitoneal adipose tissue responded like sc tissue (nonportal adipose tissue) and both responded differently than the omental and mesenteric adipose tissues (portal adipose tissues). Compared to nonportal adipose tissue, NE- and isoproterenol-stimulated lipolysis in portal adipose tissue was higher in men but lower in premenopausal women, whereas postmenopausal women showed no differences.

Since the lipolytic effect of catecholamines in human adipose tissue is mediated by β-adrenoreceptors, Arner et al. *(41)* studied β-adrenoreceptor (BAR) expression in abdominal and gluteal fat cells. Abdominal fat cells had twice the number of BAR binding sites and mRNA levels of BAR 1 and BAR 2 compared to gluteal cells in both men and women. This variation in gene expression may underly the regional differences in catecholamine-induced lipolysis in various types of adipose tissue.

Insulin-Mediated Inhibition of Lipolysis

Effect of insulin on suppression of lipolysis has not been well studied. Recently, Bolinder et al. *(42)* noted an increased sensitivity to the antilipolytic effect of insulin in sc adipose tissue than in the omental adipose tissue which was probably due to differences in receptor affinity or due to differences in insulin action at the post-receptor level. However, Goldrich et al. *(29)* reported no differences in insulin inhibition of E-stimulated lipolysis in the sc abdominal and omental adipose tissue. Smith et al. *(32)* reported higher antilipolytic effect of insulin in sc abdominal adipose tissue than that in femoral adipose tissue. Further no difference was observed in inhibition of isoproterenol-induced lipolysis by insulin in abdominal and gluteofemoral adipose tissues. In contrast to these observations, total insulin receptor mRNA levels were reported to be higher in omental than in sc abdominal adipose tissue *(43)*. Interestingly, the mRNA levels of insulin receptor variant with exon 11: the form considered to transmit insulin signal more efficiently, were essentially the same in the two types of adipose tissue.

Effects of Other Hormones

Other hormones such as estrogens and prolactin also may have significant effects on adipose tissue lipolysis. Rebuffe-Scrive et al. *(34)* have elegantly demonstrated differences in regional lipolytic activity of sc femoral and abdominal adipose tissues in women during normal menstrual cycle, during pregnancy and during lactation. Taking into account the cell size (femoral adipocytes are larger than abdominal adipocytes), no differences were observed in basal lipolysis. During lactation, however, lipolysis in femoral adipocytes was significantly higher.

Hormone Sensitive Lipase Expression

Consistent with the higher basal lipolytic rate in sc adipose tissue compared to the omental adipose tissue, Reynisdottir et al. *(44)*, recently found higher HSL activity (mean 27.5 vs 14.4 mU/10^7 cells, respectively, an increase of 80%) and mRNA levels (mean 2.4 vs 1.8 pg/pg γ-actin, respectively) in sc adipocytes than in omental adipocytes. However, recent studies of Lefebvre et al. *(43)* failed to notice any differences in HSL mRNA levels from omental and sc abdominal adipose tissue (mean 468 vs 465 amol/μg total RNA, respectively). Therefore, increased catecholamine-induced lipolysis may be due to differences in hormonal control of this pathway rather than to absolute differences in the expression of the enzymes involved.

Lipoprotein Lipase (LPL) Activity and Triglyceride Synthesis

Hamosh et al. *(39)* reported that de-novo fatty acid synthesis was much more active in omental adipose tissue than in sc adipose tissue. Arner et al. *(45)* studied 25 obese women and noted that LPL activity of femoral adipose tissue was 20% higher than that of sc abdominal adipose tissue. In recent studies, Arner et al. *(46)* confirmed their previous observation in women, however, men were found to have increased LPL activity in abdominal region than in gluteal region. Rebuffe-Scrive et al. *(40)* also did not find an increase in femoral LPL activity in men. Arner et al. *(46)* further reported that in both sexes LPL mRNA levels were threefold higher in the abdominal as compared to the gluteal site. These findings suggest that regional variation in LPL activity in adipose tissue may be due to both gene expression and posttranslational modification of LPL enzyme activity.

Rebuffe-Scrive et al. *(34)* noted higher LPL activity in femoral adipose tissue of premenopausal women as well as pregnant women compared to abdominal sc tissue. In lactating women, however, LPL activity in the femoral region was markedly decreased. No major differences in LPL activity were observed when sc abdominal, retroperitoneal, mesenteric and omental adipose tissue were studied from men, premenopausal and postmenopausal women *(40,47)*. Omental adipose tissue in premenopausal women had low LPL activity compared to other sites. In further studies, no differences in LPL activity was noted in various intra-abdominal depots and sc abdominal adipose tissue in severely obese men and women *(47)*.

In a recent study, Marin et al. *(48)* observed an increased LPL activity in omental tissue as compared to sc abdominal tissue (9.6 ± 0.9, 7.2 ± 0.8 mU/cell surface area, $p < 0.05$, mean [SEM]), while not different from the activity in the retroperitoneal tissue (8.4 ± 1.0 mU/cell surface area). Lipid uptake was determined by oral administration of 9,10-^{3}H oleic acid before surgery and counting radioactivity in various adipose tissue samples. Interestingly, lipid uptake was higher in omental and retroperitoneal adipose tissue compared to sc abdominal tissue. Lefebvre et al. *(43)* however noted no differences in LPL mRNA levels from omental and sc abdominal adipose tissue.

To summarize, adipose tissue from various sites show metabolic heterogeneity; however, only modest differences can be documented (Table 3). Further studies are needed to elucidate the underlying basic mechanisms for such regional changes.

Table 3
Metabolic Heterogeneity of Adipose Tissue

	Adipose Tissue Site		
		Subcutaneous	
	Omental	Abdominal	Gluteofemoral
In Vitro Studies			
Adipocyte size	↓	↑	↑↑
Basal lipolysis	~ or ↓	~ or ↑	↑↑
E- or NE-stimulated lipolysis	~ or ↑	~ or ↓	↓
Lipolysis-inhibition by insulin	↓	↑	↓
In Vivo Studies			
Interstitial glycerol concentration	↓	↑	—
Glycerol release	~	~	—

~ = No change.

REGIONAL DISTRIBUTION OF ADIPOSE TISSUE (ANATOMIC CONSIDERATIONS)

Total amount of FFA and glycerol released in the circulation from an adipose tissue site are dependent not only upon its metabolic properties but also upon its total mass. Therefore consideration needs to be given to the relative mass of adipose tissue located in various anatomic sites.

It is known for several decades that adult women have increased amount of body fat than men, usually by about 10% (49–51). The sex difference in overall adiposity may be present even before the onset of puberty. Beyond the overall difference in adiposity, the pattern of distribution of body fat is also distinctly different among men and women (50,51). Figure 1 shows the anthropometric data on skinfold thickness among men and women (50,51). It is clear that men have more sc truncal fat but less sc fat in the peripheral sites than women. Recent studies using CT and MRI also support these findings. These studies further reveal that women have much less intra-abdominal, both intraperitoneal and retroperitoneal adipose tissue mass, compared to men but have more total sc fat, particularly in the extremities (Table 4; Fig. 2 [52–57]). The intraperitoneal fat mass accounts for only ~10–11% and ~5% of the total body fat mass in men and women, respectively (52–56). The intraperitoneal fat therefore should be at least 10X more active than the sc fat to contribute more FFA and glycerol to the systemic circulation and thus to have a unique influence in inducing peripheral insulin resistance. Certainly, data reviewed in the previous section do not support such an increase in lipolytic activity of the intraperitoneal fat.

REGIONAL ADIPOSITY AND INSULIN RESISTANCE (CLINICAL STUDIES)

To address the question of the specific contribution of regional abdominal adiposity, especially intraperitoneal, retroperitoneal and sc abdominal fat, to the metabolic consequences of excess fat, we have recently developed an MRI technique to estimate the total mass of each region (18). The MRI technique has several potential advantages over CT

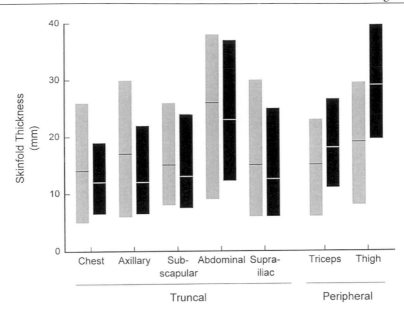

Fig. 1. Comparison of skinfold thickness at various body sites in adult men and women. The grey and black bars represent median, 10th and 90th percentile values of skinfold thickness for normal adult men and women, respectively. (Data from Jackson et al., refs. *50* and *51.*)

scan for the estimation of adipose tissue mass. The main advantage is that it does not entail any radiation exposure. It also provides a better definition of adipose tissue mass than that provided by CT scan. This is because of a short T1 and a long T2 proton relaxation time of fat, which differs markedly from those of the other tissues. Therefore, adipose tissue is distinctly visualized as bright areas with high signal intensity that contrast with other tissues on T1-weighted images. Visual mapping of the anatomical areas on the computer screen using a track ball further prevents possible overestimation due to the nonadipose tissue on T1-weighted images. The disadvantages of MRI include the high cost and the complexity of the measurements involved. Therefore, its applicability, at this time, is confined to studies involving small number of subjects.

The MRI method involves scanning the entire abdominal region using contiguous axial 10-mm slices (Fig. 3). Intra-abdominal adipose tissue is distinguished and separated into intraperitoneal and retroperitoneal adipose tissue compartments using anatomical points, such as ascending and descending colon, aorta and inferior vena cava. The number of pixels counted in each compartment, i.e., sc abdominal, intraperitoneal and retroperitoneal, are converted into a volume by multiplying the number of pixels by 0.04 cm^3. Assuming the density of adipose tissue to be 0.9196 kg/L *(58)*, adipose tissue mass in each compartment can be calculated.

We recently documented the accuracy and precision of the MRI method in the estimation of adipose tissue mass in the abdominal region of human cadavers *(18)*. The masses of the three abdominal compartments estimated by this method were compared to those obtained by direct weighing of adipose tissue after dissection. The difference between MRI estimate and direct measurement by dissection was less than 5%. The intra-observer coefficient of variation for various adipose tissue compartments was found to be below 14% *(18)*.

Table 4
Sex Differences in Intra-Abdominal Fat Distribution Based on MRI Studies

| Sex | n | % of total body fat | | | Reference |
		Total intra-abdominal fat	Intraperitoneal fat	Retroperitoneal fat	
M	17	15.0	10.4	2.9	Ross et al. *(53)*
M	39	17.6	10.9	6.7	Abate et al. *(55)*
M	31	17.9	11.2	7.2	Abate et al. *(56)*
F	15	7.3	NA	NA	Ross et al. *(52)*
F	24	7.6	5.0	1.3	Ross et al. *(54)*
F	40	7.0	4.6	1.2	Ross et al. *(53)*

M = male; F = female; NA = not available.

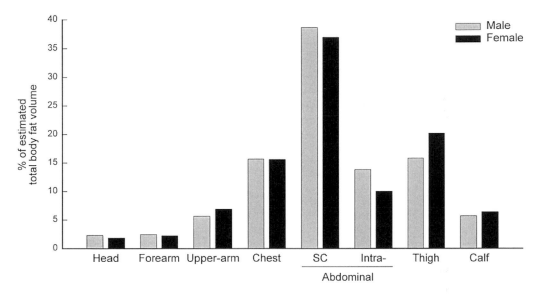

Fig. 2. Comparison of body composition differences among adult (20–50-year-old) men and women based on estimation of fat volume using CT scanning *(57)*. The grey and black bars indicate mean % total body fat in each compartment for men and women, respectively.

Subsequently, this method was applied to study the relationships between regional adiposity and insulin sensitivity in a group of nondiabetic, middle-aged men with varying degrees of obesity *(55)*. In this study *(55)*, increased amounts of total body fat were correlated with decreases in insulin-mediated glucose disposal (Rd value). Variation in intraperitoneal fat mass, however, failed to provide additional prediction of insulin sensitivity beyond that noted with total body fat. In contrast, sc abdominal fat mass and the sum of truncal skinfolds thickness gave significant incremental prediction of insulin sensitivity (Fig. 4). The data suggested that sc truncal fat was a better predictor of insulin resistance than intraperitoneal, retroperitoneal or peripheral sc fat. SC truncal obesity also showed a relationship to hepatic insulin sensitivity. Further analysis of the data revealed that posterior sc abdominal fat mass was ~1.6 times more than that of the anterior compartment *(58)*. The posterior sc abdominal fat mass was a better predictor of insulin sensitivity than the anterior sc abdominal fat mass *(59)*.

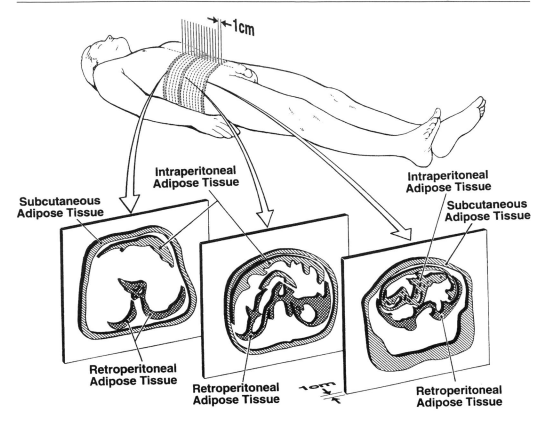

Fig. 3. Schematic illustration of the MRI technique to measure masses of various abdominal fat compartments. A series of contiguous 10-mm thick slices are obtained to scan the entire abdomen. Intra-abdominal adipose tissue is distinguished as intraperitoneal or retroperitoneal adipose tissue using anatomical landmarks. The number of pixels are counted in each slice for the three compartments. (Reprinted with permission from Journal of Lipid Research, ref. *18*.)

Our studies of men with non-insulin-dependent diabetes mellitus (NIDDM or Type 2 diabetes) further showed a strong relationship between amounts of sc truncal fat and the Rd values *(56)*. However, Type 2 diabetes patients were more insulin resistant at every level of total or regional adiposity compared to nondiabetic men (Fig. 4). Our results, therefore, suggest that intraperitoneal fat plays only a minor role in the causation of insulin resistance in men. Although others have proposed a ratio of visceral-to-sc abdominal fat areas or volumes as a sensitive predictor of insulin sensitivity *(9,60–62)*, our previous data in nondiabetic and Type 2 diabetes men did not support the ratio as a major determinant of insulin sensitivity *(55,56)*.

Although the precise mechanisms for our observations are not entirely clear, a simple explanation may arise from anatomic considerations. Our MRI data revealed that sc abdominal fat mass in men was ~2 times compared to the intraperitoneal fat mass. Although the total sc truncal fat mass was not quantified, it could be ~4 to 5 times larger than the intraperitoneal fat mass. It is possible that sc truncal fat releases more FFA and glycerol in the systemic circulation than the intraperitoneal fat mass and thus may have a unique influence in determining peripheral insulin sensitivity. Further studies are needed to investigate if excess of intraperitoneal fat has any other effects on hepatic

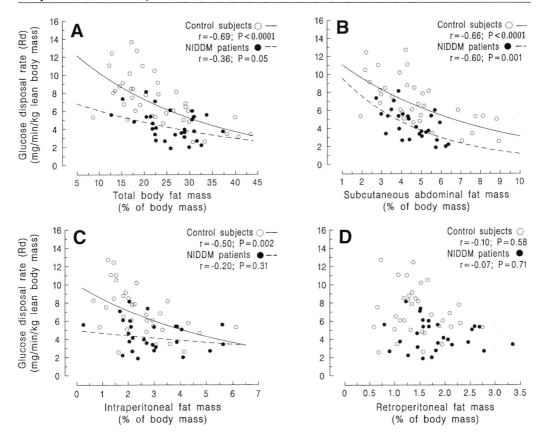

Fig. 4. The relationship of insulin-mediated glucose disposal rate (Rd value, during euglycemic, hyperinsulinemic glucose clamp study at 40mUm^{-2}min^{-1} insulin infusion rate) and total body (**A**), sc abdominal (**B**), intraperitoneal (**C**), and retroperitoneal (**D**) fat masses in control subjects (○) and patients with Type 2 diabetes (●). Pearson product moment analysis was used for computing the correlation coefficients after log$_e$ transformation of Rd value, the independent variable. The best fit regression curves for control subjects and patients with Type 2 diabetes are represented by solid and interrupted lines, respectively. (From Abate et al., ref. *56*. Reprinted with permission from The American Diabetes Association.)

metabolism, particularly hepatic triglyceride synthesis and release of very-low density lipoprotein particles.

SUMMARY AND CONCLUSIONS

It is well recognized that overall obesity causes insulin resistance. However, whether regional adiposity, particularly excess of intraperitoneal fat contributes additionally to the causation of insulin resistance remains debatable. Although the results of in vivo and in vitro studies of metabolic heterogeneity of adipose tissue are variable, omental adipose tissue appears to be more responsive to E- or NE-stimulated lipolysis and less responsive to insulin-induced inhibition of lipolysis. However, release of FFA in the circulation is dependent both upon the metabolic activity and total mass of adipose tissue compartment. Recent advances in methodology to study adipose tissue distribution reveal that intraperitoneal fat mass accounts for only 10% or 5% of the total fat mass in men and women, respectively. Further, our studies in men with and without Type 2 diabetes, investigating the relationship of insulin sensitivity with MRI-based determination of the masses of abdominal adipose tissue compartments do not reveal a unique influence of excess of intraperitoneal fat in causing insulin resistance. On the other hand, sc truncal fat was found to be a better predictor of insulin sensitivity. Thus, our findings change the focus of fat distribution-insulin resistance relationship from intraperitoneal or "portal" fat to sc truncal fat. Further studies are needed to elucidate the mechanisms by which sc truncal adiposity influences whole body insulin sensitivity.

REFERENCES

1. Vague J. La differenciation sexuelle: facteur determinant des formes: de l'obesite. La Presse Medicale 1947;55:39–340.
2. Vague J. The degree of masculine differentiation of obesities: a factor determining predisposition to diabetes, atherosclerosis, gout, and uric calculous disease. Am J Clin Nutr 1956;4:20–34.
3. Pouliot MC, Despres JP, Moorjani S, et al. Regional variation in adipose tissue lipoprotein lipase activity: association with plasma high density lipoprotein levels. Eur J Clin Invest 1991;21:398–405.
4. Kissebah AH, Vydelingum N, Murray R, et al. Relation of body fat distribution to metabolic complications of obesity. J Clin Endocrinol Metab 1982;54:254–260.
5. Peiris AN, Mueller RA, Smith GA, Struve MF, Kissebah AH. Splanchnic insulin metabolism in obesity: influence of body fat distribution. J Clin Invest 1986;78:1648–1657.
6. Peiris AN, Struve MF, Mueller RA, Lee MB Kissebah AH. Glucose metabolism in obesity: influence of body fat distribution. J Clin Endocrinol Metab 1988;67:760–767.
7. Peiris AN, Sothmann MS, Hennes MI., et al. Relative contribution of obesity and body fat distribution to alterations in glucose insulin homeostasis: predictive values of selected indices in premenopausal women. Am J Clin Nutr 1989;49:758–764.
8. Peiris AN, Sothmann MS, Hoffmann RG, et al. Adiposity, fat distribution, and cardiovascular risk. Ann Intern Med 1989;110:867–872.
9. Fujioka S, Matsuzawa Y, Tokunaga K, Tarui S. Contribution of intra-abdominal fat accumulation to the impairment of glucose and lipid metabolism in human obesity. Metabolism 1987;36:54–59.
10. Lapidus L, Bengtsson C, Larsson B, Pennert K, Rybo E, Sjostrom L. Distribution of adipose tissue and risk of cardiovascular disease and death: A 12-year follow-up of participants in the population study of women in Gothenburg. BMJ 1984;289:1257–1261.
11. Ohlson LO, Larsson B, Svardsudd K, Welin L, Eriksson H, Wilhelmsen L, Bjorntorp P, Tibblin G. The influence of body fat distribution on the incidence of diabetes mellitus: 13.5 years of follow-up on the participants in the study of men born in 1913. Diabetes 1985;34:1055–1058.
12. Ducimetiere P, Richard J, Cambien F. The pattern of subcutaneous fat distribution in middle-aged men and the risk of coronary heart disease: the Paris Prospective Study. Int J Obes 1986;10:229–240.
13. Casassus P, Fontbonne A, Thibult N, Ducimetiere P, Richard JL, Claude JR, Warnet JM, Rosselin G, Eschwege E. Upper-body fat distribution: a hyperinsulinemia-independent predictor of coronary heart disease mortality. The Paris Prospective Study. Arterioscler Thromb 1992;12:1387–1392.
14. Donahue RP, Bloom E, Abbott RD, Reed DM, Yano K. Central obesity and coronary heart disease in men. Lancet 1:1987;821–823.
15. Welin L, Svardsudd K, Wilhelmsen L, Larsson B, Tibblin G. Analysis of risk factors for stroke in a cohort of men born in 1913. N Engl J Med 1987;317:521–526.
16. Weingand KW, Hartke GT, Noordsy TW, Ledeboer DA. A minipig model of body adipose tissue distribution. Int J Obes 1989;13:347–355.
17. Rossner S, Bo WJ, Hiltbrandt E, Hinson W, Karstaedt N, Santago P, Sobol WT, Crouse JR. Adipose tissue determinations in cadavers—a comparison between cross-sectional planimetry and computed tomography. Int J Obes 1990;14:893–902.
18. Abate N, Burns D, Peshock R, Garg A, Grundy SM. Estimation of adipose tissue mass by magnetic resonance imaging: validation against dissection in human cadavers. J Lipid Res 1994;35:1490–1496.
19. Bjorntorp P. "Portal" adipose tissue as a generator of risk factors for cardiovascular disease and diabetes. Arteriosclerosis 1990;10:493–498.
20. Ferrannini E, Barrett EJ, Bevilacqua S, DeFronzo RA. Effect of fatty acids on glucose production and utilization in man. J Clin Invest 1983;72:1737–1747.

21. Bevilacqua S, Bonadonna R, Buzzigoli G, Boni C, Ciociaro D, Maccari F, Giorico MA, Ferrannini E. Acute elevation of free fatty acid levels leads to hepatic insulin resistance in obese subjects. Metabolism 1987;36:502–506.

22. Randle PJ, Garland PB, Hales CN, Newsholme, EA. The glucose-fatty acid cycle. Its role in insulin sensitivity and the metabolic disturbances of diabetes mellitus. Lancet 1963;I, 785–789.

23. Garg A, Fleckenstein JL, Peshock RM, Grundy SM. Peculiar distribution of adipose tissue in patients with congenital generalized lipodystrophy. J Clin Endocrinol Metab 1992;75:358–361.

24. Chandalia M, Garg A, Vuitch F, Nizzi F. Postmortem findings in congenital generalized lipodystrophy. J Clin Endocrinol Metab 1995;80:3077–3081.

25. Hales CN, Luzio JP, Siddle K. Hormonal control of adipose-tissue lipolysis. Biochem Soc Symp 1978;43:97–135.

26. Bjorntorp P, Ostman J. Human adipose tissue dynamics and regulation. Adv Metab Disord 1971; 5:277–327.

27. Carlson LA, Hallberg D. Basal lipolysis and effects of norepinephrine and prostaglandin E1 on lipolysis in human subcutaneous and omental adipose tissue. J Lab Clin Med 1968;71:368–377.

28. Carlson LA, Hallberg D, Micheli H. Quantitative studies on the lipolytic response of human subcutaneous and omental adipose tissue to noradrenaline and theophylline. Acta Med Scand 1969;185:465–469.

29. Goldrick RB, McLaughlin GM. Lipolysis and lipogenesis from glucose in human fat cells of different sizes. J Clin Invest 1970;49:1213–1223.

30. Ostman J, Arner P, Engfeldt P, Kager L. Regional differences in the control of lipolysis in human adipose tissue. Metabolism 1979;28:1198–1205.

31. Efendic, S. Catecholamines and metabolism of human adipose tissue. III. Comparison between the regulation of lipolysis in omental and subcutaneous adipose tissue. Acta Med Scand 1970;187:477–483.

32. Smith U, Hammerstein J, Bjorntorp P, Kral JG. Regional differences and effect of weight reduction on human fat cell metabolism. Eur J Clin Invest 1979;9:327–332.

33. Landin K, Lonnroth P, Krotkiewski M, Holm G, Smith U. Increased insulin resistance and fat cell lipolysis in obese but not lean women with a high waist/hip ratio. Eur J Clin Invest 1990;20:530–535.

34. Rebuffe-Scrive M, Enk L, Crona N, et al. Fat cell metabolism in different regions in women: effect of menstrual cycle, pregnancy, and lactation. J Clin Invest 1985;75:1973–1976.

35. Jansson PA, Larsson A, Smith U, Lonnroth P. Glycerol production in subcutaneous adipose tissue in lean and obese humans. J Clin Invest 1992;89:1610–1617.

36. Martin ML, Jensen MD. Effects of body fat distribution on regional lipolysis in obesity. J Clin Invest 1991;88:609–613.

37. Wertheimer HE, Hamosh M, Shafrir E. Factors affecting fat mobilization from adipose tissue. Am J Clin Nutr 1960;8:705.

38. Mosinger B, Kuhn E, Kujalova, V. Action of adipokinetic hormones on human adipose tissue in vitro. J Lab Clin Med 1965;66:380.

39. Hamosh M, Hamosh P, Bar-Maor JA, Cohen H. Fatty acid metabolism by human adipose tissues. J Clin Invest 1963;42:1648.

40. Scrive-Rebuffe M, Andersson B, Olbe L, Bjorntorp P. Metabolism of adipose tissue in intraabdominal depots of nonobese men and women. Metabolism 1989;38:453–458.

41. Arner P, Hellstrom L, Wahrenberg H, Bronnegard M. Beta-adrenoceptor expression in human fat cells from different regions. J Clin Invest 1990;86:1595–1600.

42. Bolinder J, Kager L, Ostman J, Arner P. Differences at the receptor and post-receptor levels between human omental and subcutaneous adipose tissue in the action of insulin on lipolysis. Diabetes 1983;32:117–123.

43. Lefebvre A-M, Laville M, Vega N, Riou JP, van Gaal L, Auwerx J. Vidal H. Depot-specific differences in adipose tissue gene expression in lean and obese subjects. Diabetes 1998;47:98–103.

44. Reynisdottir S, Dauzats M, Thorne A, Langin D. Comparison of hormone-sensitive lipase activity in visceral and subcutaneous human adipose tissue. J Clin Endocrinol Metab 1997;82:4162–4166.

45. Arner P, Engfeldt P, Lithell H. Site differences in the basal metabolism of subcutaneous fat in obese women. J Clin Endocrinol Metab 1981;53:948–952.

46. Arner P, Lithell H, Wahrenberg H, Bronnegard M. Expression of lipoprotein lipase in different human subcutaneous adipose tissue regions. J Lipid Res 1991;32:423–429.

47. Scrive-Rebuffe M, Anderson B, Olbe L, Bjorntorp P. Metabolism of adipose tissue in intraabdominal depots in severely obese men and women. Metabolism 1990;39:1021–1025.

48. Marin P, Andersson B, Ottosson M, et al. The morphology and metabolism of intraabdominal adipose tissue in men. Metabolism 1992;41:1242–1248.
49. Behnke, AR. New concepts of height-weight relationships. In: Wilson NL, ed. Obesity. Davis, Philadelphia, PA, 1969, pp. 25–53.
50. Jackson AS, Pollock ML, Ward A. Generalized equations for predicting body density of women. Med Sci Sports Ex 1980;12:175–182.
51. Jackson AS, Pollock ML. Generalized equations for predicting body density of men. Br J Nutr 1978;40:497.
52. Ross R, Shaw KD, Martel Y, De Guise J, Avruch L. Adipose tissue distribution measured by magnetic resonance imaging in obese women. Am J Clin Nutr 1993;57:470–475.
53. Ross R, Shaw KD, Rissanen J, Martel Y, De Guise J, Avruch L. Sex differences in lean and adipose tissue distribution by magnetic resonance imaging: anthropometric relationships. Am J Clin Nutr 1994;59:1277–1285.
54. Ross R, Rissanen J. Mobilization of visceral and subcutaneous adipose tissue in response to energy restriction and exercise. Am J Clin Nutr 1994;60:695–703.
55. Abate N, Garg A, Peshock RM, Stray-Gundersen J, Grundy SM. Relationship of generalized and regional adiposity to insulin sensitivity in men. J Clin Invest 1995;96:88–98.
56. Abate N, Garg A, Peshock RM, Stray-Gundersen J, Adams-Huet B, Grundy SM. Relationship of generalized and regional adiposity to insulin sensitivity in men with NIDDM. Diabetes 1996;45:1684–1693.
57. Kotani K, Tokunaga K, Fujioka S, Kobatake T, Keno Y, Yoshida S, Shimomura I, Tarui S, Matsuzawa Y. Sexual dimorphism of age-related changes in whole-body fat distribution in the obese. Int J Obes Related Metabolic Disorders 1994;18(4):207–212.
58. Thomas LW. The chemical composition of adipose tissue of man and mice. Q J Exp Physiol 1962; 47:179–188.
59. Misra A, Garg A, Abate N, Peshock RM, Stray-Gundersen J, Grundy SM. Relationship of anterior and posterior subcutaneous abdominal fat to insulin sensitivity in nondiabetic men. Obes Res 1997;5:93–99.
60. Zamboni M, Armellini F, Turcato E, De Pergola G, Todesco T, Bissoli L, Bergamo IA, Bosello O. Relationship between visceral fat, steroid hormanes and insulin sensitivity in premenopausal obese women. J Intern Med 1994;236:521–527.
61. Bonora E, Prato S, Bonadonna R, Gulli G, Solini A, Shank M, Ghiatas A, Lancaster J, Kilcoyne R, Alyassin A, DeFronzo R. Total body fat content and fat topography are associated differently with in vivo glucose metabolism in nonobese and obese nondiabetic women. Diabetes 1992;41:1151–1159.
62. Caprio S, Hyman L, Limb C, McCarthy S, Lange R, Sherwin R, Shulman G, Tamborlane W. Central adiposity and its metabolic correlates in obese adolescent girls. Am J Physiol 1995;269:E118–E126.

6

Physical Activity and Insulin Resistance in Man

Flemming Dela, MD, DMSC,
Kári Mikines, MD, DMSC,
and Henrik Galbo, MD, DMSC

CONTENTS

ADAPTATIONS OF INSULIN ACTION AND SECRETION TO PHYSICAL
ACTIVITY IN HEALTHY SUBJECTS
ADAPTATIONS OF INSULIN ACTION AND SECRETION TO PHYSICAL
ACTIVITY IN VARIOUS INSULIN RESISTANT GROUPS
GENERAL CONCLUSION
REFERENCES

ADAPTATIONS OF INSULIN ACTION AND SECRETION TO PHYSICAL ACTIVITY IN HEALTHY SUBJECTS

An Overall View

After both acute exercise and physical training, i.e., regularly performed exercise, increased glucose tolerance or unchanged glucose tolerance in the face of lower plasma insulin concentrations may be seen during oral (OGTT) and intravenous (IVGTT) glucose loading *(85,89,116,148)*. Conversely, physical inactivity during bed rest or resulting from spinal cord injury decreases glucose tolerance in the face of increased insulin concentrations *(39,88,107)*. The deterioration in glucose tolerance during bed rest can be diminished by exercise *(39,88)*. These findings indicate a direct relationship between physical activity and insulin action and also suggest an inverse relationship between physical activity and glucose induced insulin secretion.

The view that the effect of insulin increases over the full range of activity levels from inactivity to daily endurance training has been confirmed by studies using the hyperinsulinemic euglycemic clamp technique (Fig. 1) *(74,98–101)*. The influence of physical activity on pancreatic β-cell secretion has been studied in detail by the hyperglycemic clamp technique *(96,97,102)*. No effect on insulin secretion was found after 1 h of ergometer cycling *(97)*. However, in trained subjects the capacity to secrete insulin was reduced (Fig. 2) *(102)* as also evidenced by studies using arginine infusion *(33)*.

From: *Contemporary Endocrinology: Insulin Resistance*
Edited by: G. Reaven and A. Laws © Humana Press Inc., Totowa, NJ

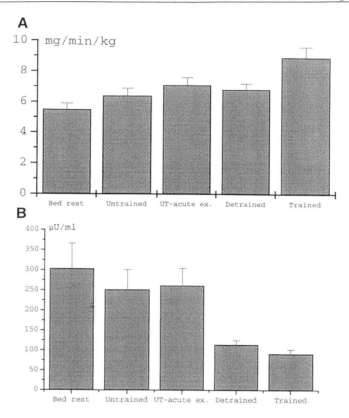

Fig. 1. Steady state glucose disposal rate during insulin infusion of 0.7 μU · min^{-1} · kg^{-1} (plasma insulin approximately 40–50 μU · mL^{-1}) (**A**) and plasma insulin concentration in the 90th min of a 20 m*M* glucose stimulation (**B**). Note inverse relationship between insulin action and secretion. Values are mean ± SE. (Data from refs. *96–102.*)

Conversely, both detraining (Fig. 2) and bed rest increased glucose stimulated insulin secretion *(96,102)*. In these studies the training-induced decrease in β-cell secretory capacity was very accurately matched to the increase in insulin action because during clamping of plasma glucose from 7–20 m*M* glucose disposal was identical in trained, detrained, and untrained subjects despite widely differing plasma insulin concentrations *(102)*.

Interestingly, however, in athletes who trained even harder and had higher maximal oxygen uptake rates than the trained subjects in the aforementioned studies, oral glucose tolerance was better than seen in untrained subjects indicating that upon extreme training enhancement of insulin action is not fully compensated by reduced β-cell function *(28)*. Conversely, the inactivity induced insulin resistance seen in bedridden sedentary subjects is not fully overcome by the accompanying enhancement of glucose-stimulated insulin secretion *(96)*. Apparently, in terms of influence on glucose homeostasis the adaptive effect of physical activity on β-cell function is at most as high as that on insulin action and may, accordingly, be considered a compensatory phenomenon. The described findings over the entire spectrum of physical activity levels strongly add to the view from studies of obesity *(115)* fasting *(10)* and dexamethazone treatment *(8)* that the insulin secretory capacity of the healthy pancreas is inversely related to the sensitivity of target tissues to insulin (Fig. 1).

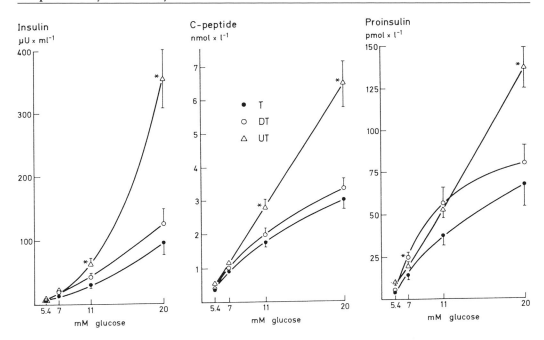

Fig. 2. Dose response relation for glucose stimulated β-cell secretion. Plasma concentrations of insulin (left), C-peptide (middle), and proinsulin (right) at basal and in the 90th min of each of 3 sequential hyperglycemic (7, 11, and 20 m*M* glucose) clamps. Subjects were 7 untrained (UT) and 7 trained men studied 12–16 h after last training session (T) and after 5 days of detraining (DT). Values are mean ± SE. * significantly different from T (*p* < 0.05). (Adapted from ref. *102*.)

The training-induced increase in insulin sensitivity and decrease in glucose-stimulated β-cell secretion revealed by the described laboratory experiments would suggest that training may be beneficial to health by diminishing glucose and/or insulin concentrations in plasma and decreasing the load on the β-cells. Such changes imply reduced risk of developing Type 2 diabetes, atherosclerosis and hypertension *(9,133,134,141)*. However, the reasoning does not allow for the fact that training necessitates an increased food intake that tends to increase glucose levels as well as secretion and plasma concentrations of insulin. In fact, daily intake of carbohydrate and overall energy have been found to be 2.3 and 1.5 times higher, respectively, in athletes compared to sedentary young men *(28)*. Thus, the sparing effect of training on insulin secretion and/or glucose levels, at given glucose loads might under ordinary living conditions be offset by a higher food intake in trained compared with untrained subjects.

In order to test this possibility heavily trained and untrained subjects had both identical absolute oral glucose loads and, in order to mimic daily living conditions, oral glucose loads making up identical fractions of daily carbohydrate intake, i.e., identical relative glucose loads *(28)*. In the athletes glucose, C-peptide and insulin responses were all markedly reduced in response to conventional identical absolute glucose loads, whereas in response to identical relative glucose loads, glucose and C-peptide responses were identical in the two groups while athletes had lower insulin responses *(28)* (Table 1). Evidently this laboratory experiment did not exactly imitate real life. For instance, glucose is not a major component of usual meals, and acute effects of exercise bouts were not considered. However, when the same subjects were studied during ordinary living conditions similar results were found *(29)*. Thus, 24 h integrated plasma concentrations of glucose and C-peptide, 24 h urinary C-peptide excretion and blood HbA_1C concentrations did not differ between athletes and sedentary subjects whereas 24 h integrated insulin concentrations tended to be 30% diminished in the athletes (Table 2) *(29)*.

The conclusion from these studies is that the adaptations induced by physical training in secretion and action of insulin seem accurately matched to the increase in fuel turnover that accompanies the training regimen. Trained subjects have, compared with untrained subjects, the same overall insulin secretion and average plasma glucose concentration despite a higher food intake. This means that during training, adaptations in pancreas and insulin-sensitive tissues allow the necessary increase in food intake without potentially harmful hyperglycemia and overloading of β-cells. However, being only relative to food intake, the training-induced sparing of insulin secretion and reduction in plasma glucose concentrations have been overrated in the past and do not indicate a health benefit compared with the untrained state. In contrast, the lowering of arterial insulin levels, which probably reflects a training-induced increase in hepatic insulin extraction *(33,148,149)*, may be wholesome.

The ratio between on the one hand daily carbohydrate intake and, in turn, disposal and on the other hand 24 h integrated C-peptide concentration, which is a measure of daily insulin secretion, is an index of physiological insulin sensitivity. It is interesting to note that judged from this ratio applied during ordinary living conditions *(29)* the insulin-saving effect of training is at least as big as suggested by laboratory studies using the hyperinsulinemic, euglycemic clamp technique *(100)*. The fact that during ordinary living conditions, in contrast to findings during intravenous glucose infusion, integrated C-peptide levels were not reduced relative to glucose levels in athletes compared to sedentary subjects probably reflects that the overall β-cell stimulus was higher in the athletes due to a higher incretin secretion from the gut resulting from their higher food intake *(29)*.

Effects of Training vs Acute Exercise on Insulin Action

Trained subjects are most appropriately characterized in their "habitual" state, i.e., between two regular training sessions. However, this state may be influenced by the last exercise bout per se as well as by more long-lived adaptations to training. Several lines of evidence indicate that the enhanced insulin action seen in trained subjects does not merely reflect residual effects of the last exercise. Thus, insulin responsiveness has been found to be higher in trained subjects in the habitual state than in untrained subjects studied either at rest or 3 h after one hour of exhausting bicycle exercise *(100)*. Furthermore, in untrained subjects one hour of moderate ergometer cycling may enhance whole-body insulin responsiveness for two but not for five days *(99)*, whereas the effect of training is not lost during five days of abstinence from exercise *(101)*. Similarly, in untrained subjects whole-body insulin responsiveness is not diminished during seven days of bedrest *(98)*. In contrast, the training-induced enhancement of whole-body insulin sensitivity is not more marked than the enhancement seen by a single exercise bout *(100)*, and sensitivity decreases rapidly with detraining and bedrest *(98,101)*.

The enhancing effect of acute exercise on insulin-mediated glucose disposal to a large extent reflects muscle glycogen depletion and accompanying glycogen synthase activation *(99,101)*. This explains that an enhanced insulin effect on muscle may be hard to find when a main meal has been taken between acute exercise and measurement *(14,31)*. The

Table 1

Integrated Glucose, C-Peptide, and Insulin Responses to Oral Glucose
in Seven Trained and Eight Untrained Subjects[a]

		Glucose ($mmol \cdot L^{-1} \cdot 180\ min$)	C-Peptide ($pmol \cdot mL^{-1} \cdot 180\ min$)	Insulin ($pmol \cdot mL^{-1} \cdot 180\ min$)
Low relative glucose load	UT ($0.4\ g \cdot kg^{-1}$)	1066 ± 29	181 ± 23	32 ± 3^b
	T ($1.0\ g \cdot kg^{-1}$)	1040 ± 29	158 ± 17	24 ± 4
High relative glucose load	UT ($1.0\ g \cdot kg^{-1}$)	1277 ± 47^c	285 ± 27^c	58 ± 4^c
	T ($2.3\ g \cdot kg^{-1}$)	1173 ± 47	270 ± 25	44 ± 6

[a]Trained (T) and untrained (UT) healthy, young subjects were compared at the same absolute glucose loads ($1.0\ g \cdot kg^{-1}$) and oral glucose loads that made out identical fractions of daily carbohydrate intake, $11.8 \pm 0.5\%$ (same low relative glucose load) or $27.7 \pm 1.1\%$ (same high relative glucose load). Glucose loads are given in parentheses. Total areas under concentration vs time curves were calculated. Values are mean $\pm$ SE.
[b]$p < 0.05$ for comparison at same relative glucose load.
[c]$p < 0.05$ for comparisons at same absolute glucose load.

Table 2

HbA$_1$C and 24-h Integrated Concentrations in Plasma and Urine[a]

	HbA$_1$C (%)	P-Glucose ($mol \cdot L^{-1} \cdot 1440\ min$)	P-C-peptide ($pmol \cdot mL^{-1} \cdot 1440\ min$)	P-Insulin ($pmol \cdot mL^{-1} \cdot 1440\ min$)	U-C-peptide ($nmol \cdot 1440\ min^{-1}$)
Untrained	4.6 ± 0.2	7.3 ± 0.6	1047 ± 175	175 ± 38	22 ± 2
Trained	5.2 ± 0.2	7.4 ± 0.2	923 ± 99	124 ± 13	20 ± 4

[a]Seven trained and eight untrained healthy, young subjects had blood drawn frequently and urine sampled during 24 h of ordinary living conditions. Measurements were made in plasma (P) and urine (U). Total areas under concentration vs time (1440 min) curves were calculated. Values are mean $\pm$ SE.

adaptations explaining the long-lived effects of training on insulin action are probably initiated during a single exercise bout *(110)*. However, exercise has to be regularly repeated to obtain a measurable cumulated effect, and it is of note that the effect of a change in physical activity level will be lost within less than 2 wk *(19,31,101)*.

Site of Exercise-Induced Increase in Insulin Effect

Studies using arterial and femoral venous catheterizations have indicated that both acute leg exercise *(119)* and leg training *(31)* increase sensitivity and responsiveness of glucose uptake to insulin in the involved muscle whereas these variables decrease during inactivity *(98)*. The effects seen in muscle are more marked than those measured at the whole-body level. However, exercise may enhance insulin action also in extramuscular tissues. In trained subjects the suppressive action of insulin on hepatic glucose production seems to be increased probably reflecting an effect of the last exercise bout *(33,100,101)*. The suppressive action of insulin on pancreatic secretion of insulin and glucagon may also be enhanced by exercise *(99–101)* making it difficult to tell whether exercise-induced changes in hepatic sensitivity to insulin are direct or secondary to changes in glucagon secretion. Anyhow, in line with the view that the insulin sparing effect of training is more pronounced in peripheral tissues than in liver, studies carried out during ordinary living conditions have shown that a relatively smaller fraction of secreted insulin is delivered to "posthepatic" tissues in athletes compared to sedentary subjects *(29)*.

Microdialysis studies of subcutaneous abdominal fat tissue have revealed a small effect of training on insulin-mediated glucose uptake in human adipose tissue (B. Stallknecht, personal communication). Interestingly, with similar techniques training has also recently been shown to enhance insulin-mediated glucose disposal in several intra-abdominal adipose tissues in rats (B. Stallknecht, personal communication). In support of an influence of exercise on insulin action in human adipose tissues, the insulin-mediated suppression of plasma glycerol and free fatty acid (FFA) levels may be enhanced after acute exercise and in trained compared to untrained subjects *(28,33,99,100)*. It appears that exercise enhances insulin action on both carbohydrate and fat metabolism. In addition, evidence has been provided in rats that a few resistance exercise sessions may enhance the effect of insulin on protein synthesis in muscle *(50)*. In line with this resistance exercise has recently been shown to enhance the protein anabolic action of insulin in human muscle (RR Wolfe, personal communication). Furthermore, during insulin infusion net protein breakdown, as reflected by tyrosine release, is lower in control compared with immobilized legs *(118)*.

Mechanisms of Exercise-Induced Adaptations in Insulin Action and Secretion

The exercise-induced enhancement of insulin action in muscle is predominantly due to local contraction dependent mechanisms, because it can be demonstrated in comparisons between an acutely exercised or trained leg and the contralateral resting and untrained leg *(31,119)*. Insulin increases muscle blood flow *(31,119)* and this effect tends to be enhanced by training *(31)*, whereas muscle blood flow may be reduced by inactivity *(98)*. These differences in flow as well as the training-induced increase in muscle capillarization *(1)* will directly influence glucose delivery to available glucose transporters in the muscle cell membrane and, in turn, glucose uptake during insulin stimulation. The importance of glucose delivery is illustrated by the fact that superimposed exercise can add markedly to the effect of maximal insulin concentrations on muscle glucose uptake in the face of a marked increase in blood flow while glucose extraction decreases *(32)*.

On the other hand, activity associated variations in insulin delivery do probably not explain accompanying variations in insulin action, because muscle insulin clearance is not influenced by inactivity *(118)*, acute exercise *(119)* and training *(31)*. The fact that local insulin clearance is not changed agrees with the finding that insulin receptor binding is also not altered by training *(25)*. Apparently the activity related enhancement of insulin action on muscle cells is exerted at the postreceptor level. Studies of rat muscle have shown that acute exercise increases sensitivity but not responsiveness of insulin-mediated glucose transport *(120)*. In contrast, training may increase responsiveness, which agrees with an increase in GLUT4 transporters *(114)*. The number of these transporters is also increased by ordinary training in normal human muscle *(25)* as well as in atrophied human muscle subjected to functional electrical stimulation *(107)*. Conversely, the muscle GLUT4 content is diminished by bedrest *(135)*.

The increase in GLUT4 content and capillarization of muscle with increase in level of physical activity may to some extent reflect conversion of muscle fibers from type II B to II A and perhaps further on to type I *(1,106,132)*. In line with this skeletal muscle fiber type composition is a determinant for insulin sensitivity, the latter being positively associated with type I fibers and negatively associated with type II B fibers *(140)*. Higher surface membrane content of GLUT4, due to higher total content or higher fractional recruitment of the transporter, as well as higher diffusion capacity and longer mean transit time resulting from higher capillary density will tend to increase the arteriovenous concentration difference for glucose. Correspondingly, glucose extraction during insulin stimulation may be increased by acute exercise *(119)* and training *(31)* and decreased by inactivity *(98)*.

As regards the fate of glucose taken up from plasma during insulin stimulation the non-oxidative glucose disposal measured on the whole-body level is increased by acute exercise and training and decreased by inactivity *(99,101)*. At least partly this reflects activity related variations in non-oxidative glucose storage as glycogen in muscle *(31,98,101,119)*. These variations are favored by the fact that acute exercise increases the active fraction of the glycogen synthase enzyme and the insulin-mediated increase in this fraction *(99,119)* while training increases the total glycogen synthase activity *(101,144)*. After acute exercise the enhancement of insulin-mediated muscle glycogen storage takes place at the expense of a diminished glycolysis *(119)*, whereas after training and inactivity changes in glycogen storage and glycolysis, respectively, essentially vary in parallel *(31,98)*.

Extramuscular effects of physical activity on insulin action have been less studied than muscular effects. However, studies in rats have shown that the responsiveness of glucose transport in adipocytes is increased by training but not by acute exercise *(145)*. This reflects increased concentrations of GLUT4 mRNA and protein *(130,146)*. In the liver training increases glucose storage capacity by increasing the glycogen synthase concentration *(56)*. In addition to enhancing glucose disposal acute exercise may, like insulin, enhance plasma triglyceride clearance after a meal *(124,125)*. The mechanism probably includes exercise-induced increases in lipoprotein lipase activity in plasma *(125)* and recruited muscle *(73)*, whereas lipoprotein lipase activity in adipose tissue has not been studied. In states of insulin resistance the adipocyte lipoprotein lipase sensitivity to insulin may be reduced while the postprandial lipidemia is increased *(16)*, a fact which may contribute to enhanced development of atherosclerosis *(71,125)*. Postprandial lipidemia is reduced by training. This potentially beneficial effect probably reflects increased lipoprotein lipase activity in muscle rather than in adipose tissue *(71,72)*. Still, the interplay between physical activity, insulin, and muscle and adipocyte lipoprotein lipase activity in plasma triglyceride metabolism needs further study. Regarding the mechanisms responsible for the development of the extramuscular metabolic adaptations to exercise little is known. However, studies on rats have shown that neither local sympathetic nerve activity nor circulating catecholamines are important for the training-induced decrease in size and increase in insulin-mediated glucose transport of adipocytes *(131)*.

In vitro studies have indicated that the training-induced decrease in insulin secretion capacity *(33,102)* is at least partially due to adaptations within the pancreatic β-cells *(45,54)*. These adaptations, surprisingly, include increased glucose metabolism *(131)*. It might be speculated that a diminished average glucose level during the day in consequence of an increased tissue sensitivity to insulin is responsible for the development of reduced β-cell responsiveness to glucose during training. However, this idea is not in line with the finding of identical HbA$_1$C levels and 24 h integrated plasma glucose profiles in athletes compared to untrained subjects during ordinary living conditions (Table 2) *(29)*. On the other hand, average plasma catecholamine concentrations are twice as high in athletes compared to untrained subjects which is compatible with the hypothesis that increased sympathoadrenomedullary activity may elicit the β-cell adaptation *(30)*. If so, sympathetic nervous norepinephrine release within the pancreas, rather than circulating catecholamines, is responsible *(131)*.

In addition to producing adaptations within the β-cells training may also cause adaptations in stimuli influencing β-cell secretion. Thus, the glucose induced secretion from the gut of glucose-dependent insulin-stimulating polypeptide (gastric inhibitory peptide, GIP) is diminished in the trained state *(82)* as well as after a single bout of exercise *(12)*. These findings, and possible analogous changes in secretion of other gut incretins, may explain that the training-induced reduction in insulin and C-peptide responses may be more pronounced during oral compared with intravenous glucose tolerance testing *(11)*, and that the last exercise bout may account for a major part of the difference between trained and untrained subjects in response to oral glucose testing *(59)*. Despite the downregulation of secretion in response to given stimulations the overall incretin secretion during the day seems to be higher in trained compared to untrained subjects. This view is based on the finding of identical daily insulin secretion rates in the two groups even though the former group would be expected to show less insulin secretion as judged from reduced β-cell sensitivity to plasma glucose concentrations and comparable average glucose concentrations during the day *(29)*.

A higher incretin secretion in trained compared to untrained subjects should be provoked by their higher food intake *(28)*. A higher food intake may also explain that trained subjects have a higher average hepatic insulin extraction than untrained subjects during normal living *(28,29)*. However, also in the postabsorptive state trained subjects may have a higher clearance of both endogenous *(33)* and exogenous *(100)* insulin, a fact which probably reflects a hepatic adaptation *(149)*. In contrast training does not influence insulin clearance in muscle *(25,31)*.

Role of Exercise Modality

When not otherwise specifically stated the exposition presented so far has been based on studies of non-exhausting endurance type exercises including predominantly concentric muscle contractions, e.g., bicycle or swimming exercise. Apparently, physical activity of this kind tends to increase insulin action and reduce insulin secretion. However, reverse responses to exercise may be seen during special conditions. Thus, in both untrained and trained subjects insulin action is in fact reduced in the early recovery period after short term maximal exercise *(78,79)*, and insulin action is also reduced after marathon running *(139)*. These findings have been ascribed to elevated levels of counterregulatory hormones as well as metabolic inhibition of glucose uptake in muscle by accumulated glycolytic intermediates and fat metabolism, respectively *(78,79,139)*. After a marathon the reduced insulin action is accompanied by impaired muscle glycogen resynthesis in the face of unaltered GLUT4 content and increased glycogen synthase activity *(6,139)*.

Unaccustomed, severe exercise that causes muscle damage also seems to impair insulin action, an effect accompanied by enhanced glucose-stimulated insulin secretion. This has appeared from studies of untrained subjects carried out 12 h after heavy running to exhaustion *(76)* or 1–2 d after eccentric exercise *(3,75)*. The reduced insulin action after eccentric exercise includes diminished insulin action on glucose uptake and glycogen synthesis in the recruited muscle *(3)*. This is seen in the face of diminished total GLUT4 content but unaltered glycogen synthase activity in the exercised muscle *(3,4)*. In accordance with these findings insulin-mediated glucose transport has been shown to be decreased in rat muscle after eccentric contractions, while glycogen synthase responded normally *(5)*. In rats also heavy resistance exercise repeated for a few days has been found to diminish insulin effect on muscle glucose transport and uptake while enhancing glucose-induced insulin secretion *(48,49)*. The described responses to unaccustomed and eccentric severe exercise are probably reversed if the exercise is regularly repeated. In accordance with this view insulin action is clearly enhanced and secretion spared in athletes studied during ordinary living conditions during which their activities include both eccentric and exhausting exercise *(29)*. Furthermore, regular strength training has been shown to enhance insulin action *(104,151)*. It has been claimed that this reflects an increase in muscle mass rather than a change in muscle character *(151)*. However, because strength training usually includes also concentric contractions and increases maximal oxygen uptake it appears unlikely that the ability of muscle to respond to insulin was unaltered. In fact, even heavy isometric resistance training carried out for 20 days has been shown to increase the GLUT4 content in human muscle *(135)*.

ADAPTATIONS OF INSULIN ACTION
AND SECRETION TO PHYSICAL ACTIVITY
IN VARIOUS INSULIN RESISTANT GROUPS

Aging People

Glucose tolerance and whole-body insulin action decline with advancing age although the variability among the elderly is substantial *(22,46,66,122)*. The decrease in insulin action with aging has tentatively been ascribed to reduced insulin action in skeletal muscle *(22,46)*. However, whole-body insulin-stimulated glucose clearance does not differ between aged and young subjects when expressed per unit fat free body mass *(26)*. Also indicating that the age-induced impairment of whole-body insulin action is rather due to accumulation of poorly responding adipose tissue, insulin action in muscle is not reduced by aging (Fig. 3) *(26)*. Aerobic performance is reduced in aged muscle and is, accordingly, dissociated from local insulin action *(26)*. Similarly, in comparisons

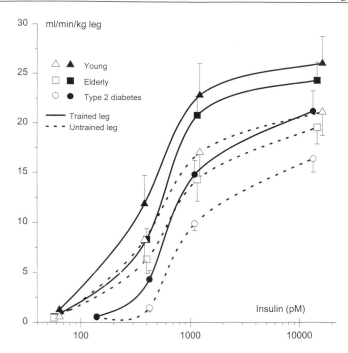

Fig. 3. Insulin mediated glucose clearance rates in trained and untrained legs in healthy young (23 ± 1 yr, n = 7) or elderly (59 ± 1 yr, n = 8) subjects and in patients with NIDDM (58 ± 2 yr, n = 7). All subjects endurance trained one leg 30 min/day, 6 days/week for ten weeks. Measurements of glucose clearance rates were performed during hyperinsulinemic, isoglycemic clamps combined with arterio-venous catheterization of both legs. During insulin infusion, glucose clearance rates are always higher in the trained compared with the untrained leg (*p* < 0.05). (Adapted from ref. *24*.)

between young and elderly subjects VO$_2$ max and insulin-stimulated whole-body glucose disposal do not vary in parallel *(15)*.

Insulin-mediated whole-body glucose disposal is higher in elderly athletes and lower in elderly bedridden patients compared with elderly controls *(150)*. In response to endurance training insulin-mediated muscle glucose clearance increases similarly in aged compared with young subjects, the effect reflecting local genuine adaptations to regularly repeated exercise *(26,27,63)*. Insulin-mediated increase in muscle blood flow is always enhanced by training but, both before and after training, at high insulin concentrations blood flow is lower and glucose extraction higher in aged compared with young subjects *(26)*. Muscle GLUT4 concentrations increase similarly in the two groups and also in the aged subjects an increase in glycogen synthase mRNA is seen while hexokinase activity is unaltered *(27,34)*. In the aged as in young subjects the training-induced increase in insulin-mediated glucose uptake in muscle is accompanied by an enhanced glycogenesis as well as an enhanced lactate release *(27,31)*. In aged subjects the increase in insulin-mediated glucose clearance in trained muscle cannot fully account for the training-induced increase in whole-body glucose clearance, a fact which points at improvement of insulin action also in other tissues. Agreeing with the fact that training induces marked adaptations in muscle, whole-body insulin sensitivity may in the elderly be improved independent of changes in weight and body composition *(26,69,77,136)*. The enhancement of insulin action by aerobic endurance training is accompanied by a diminished glucose-stimulated insulin secretion *(69,77)*. Finally, also in the elderly strength training may improve insulin action *(21,103)*.

Obese People

Heredity is undoubtedly important for development of excessive obesity and probably also directly involved in the accompanying impaired insulin action in muscle *(16)*. The latter has been demonstrated in vivo as well as in vitro and includes impairment of glucose transport as well as non-oxidative and oxidative glucose disposal *(16)*. As would be expected from knowledge of effects of exercise on normal muscle, in obese subjects both acute exercise and training may improve insulin action measured on the whole-body level *(18,23,38)*. Improved insulin action has been found in response to both endurance and strength type exercises *(47)*. The effect of training includes an increased hepatic sensitivity to insulin *(23)* and the effect vanishes within a week *(128)*.

While acknowledging a role of heredity the predominant lifestyle with little exercise and high energy intake is probably the major determinant of the rapidly increasing prevalence of excessive obesity. The latter in itself causes insulin resistance in particular when the adiposity is intra-abdominal *(70,111)*. Accordingly, the insulin resistance may be alleviated by weight loss. Exercise may enhance a weight loss induced by restricted energy intake and may serve to preserve the weight loss *(16,43)*. Exercise-mediated weight loss depends on genetic factors *(60,137)* and seems to occur in particular in males and at the expense of intra-abdominal fat *(16,36,43,81,127)*. Thus, in obese subjects exercise may enhance insulin action both by reducing adiposity and by mechanisms independent of fat loss *(27,35,64)*. A combination of aerobic endurance and resistance exercise seems ideal by allowing both a noticeable increase in energy expenditure and maintenance of muscle mass *(43)*.

Patients with Type 2 Diabetes Mellitus

The general view is that typically Type 2 diabetes develops in obese people whose pancreas fails in continuously maintaining the hypersecretion of insulin necessary for compensating their insulin resistance. Accordingly, the genetic predisposition involved in both obesity and accompanying decrease in insulin action in target tissues and also a genetic predisposition to β-cell exhaustion are determinants of Type 2 diabetes, but the modern western lifestyle with little exercise and high energy intake is the cause of the rapid increase in prevalence of the disease (*see* Obese People). In agreement with this, strong epidemiological evidence indicates that a physically active lifestyle reduces the risk of developing impaired glucose tolerance and Type 2 diabetes *(44,61,67,92–94,112,153)*. The protective effect of regular exercise is only partly due to less body weight gain. The fact that exercise reduces the occurrence of Type 2 diabetes indicates that physical activity does reduce the overall load on the pancreas in subjects at risk. The reason that such an effect has not appeared from comparisons between healthy athletes and controls (*see* An Overall View) may be that after all the activity level of the studied controls was higher than the average for sedentary diabetes prone subjects and sufficient to elicit the maximally achievable effect. In line with this explanation first degree relatives of patients with Type 2 diabetes have a low physical fitness *(108)*. Alternatively, however, a β-cell relieving effect of exercise depends on a genetic predisposition. In support of this, the diabetes preventing effect of regular exercise seems to be strongest for those individuals at highest risk of Type 2 diabetes *(61)*.

In the postabsorptive state patients who have developed Type 2 diabetes may show a marked decrease in plasma glucose concentration during prolonged submaximal dynamic exercise (80,95,105). After this type of exercise (37,80) as well as after a bout of resistance exercise (47) their insulin sensitivity may be improved. In contrast, in response to brief intense dynamic exercise the plasma glucose concentration increases and insulin sensitivity shows a biphasic response being reduced for the first 1–2 h but increased 24 h after such exercise (79). However, during daily life physical exercise is mostly taken in the postprandial rather than in the postabsorptive state. When prolonged dynamic exercise is performed after breakfast glycemia and insulin secretion are reduced (84). However, glucose and insulin responses to a subsequent meal are not affected (84). Furthermore, in terms of reducing insulin secretion and glucose levels acute postprandial exercise apparently has no effect beyond that of increasing energy expenditure because the overall effects of exercise on these variables can be mimicked by a reduction in energy intake equivalent to the exercise-induced energy expenditure (84). In line with this conclusion, in the postprandial state moderate and high intensity, respectively, isocaloric acute exercise protocols have similar overall effects on glucose and insulin levels (JJ Larsen, personal communication).

It is reasonable to suppose that regularly repeated exercise may improve glucose homeostasis more in Type 2 diabetes patients than can be inferred from the effect of a single bout of exercise, because training may elicit more profound tissue adaptations. Training *per se* can increase whole-body insulin action in Type 2 diabetes patients (Table 3) (80,121). Studies in which Type 2 diabetes patients performed regular one-legged dynamic exercise have shown that this effect is in part due to the fact that training increases the glucose clearance in muscle by local contraction dependent mechanisms (Fig. 3) (27). This reflects training-induced enhancement of the insulin-mediated increase in muscle blood flow as well as of the ability of muscle to extract glucose from the blood (27). The latter effect may partly be due to an increase in muscle GLUT4 content (34). The training-induced increase in muscle glucose clearance is accompanied by increases in both non-oxidative glycolysis and glucose storage (27). The total activities of hexokinase and glycogen synthase in muscle are unaltered whereas the fractional velocity of glycogen synthase and the mRNA for this enzyme are increased by training in Type 2 diabetes patients (27). Interestingly, in Type 2 diabetes patients training may increase insulin-mediated muscle glucose clearance to values seen in healthy, untrained control subjects (Fig. 3) (27). It is of note, however, that training does not exactly revert the muscle defect in Type 2 diabetes, because training, at least partly, exerts its effect by enhancing blood flow and GLUT4 concentrations, variables that are not subnormal in the untrained state (27,34).

The effect of training on muscle glucose clearance in Type 2 diabetes patients represents a genuine adaptation to repeated exercise but it is gone within a week, if training is stopped (27). Because the increase in glucose clearance in the trained diabetic muscle cannot fully account for the increase in whole-body glucose clearance, training must also increase insulin action in other tissues (27). In addition to the described effects which may be seen in weight stable patients, training may increase diet-induced weight loss, and this occurrence may, in itself, increase insulin sensitivity (51,62,86,123).

A training induced reduction in glucose stimulated β-cell secretion as seen in healthy subjects (*see* An Overall View) would appear less expedient in Type 2 diabetes patients. However, it has been proposed that β-cells in diabetics and healthy subjects, respectively,

Table 3
Prospective Studies on the Effect of Training on Whole Body Insulin Action
(Hyperinsulinemic Clamp) in Patients with Type 2 Diabetes Mellitus[a]

Study	n =	Duration (wk)	Bouts/wk	Duration of bouts (min)	Type of training	% VO_2max	Time since last training	Change in VO_2max	Effect on insulin action
Reitman et al. (117)	6	8	5–6	20–40	Intermittent	Rest → 60–90[e]	1.5 day	+17%	No
Bogadus et al. (13)	10[b]	12	Minimum 3	20–30	?	75 % of HR_{max}	6 days	+13%	Yes (+27%)[c]
Trovati et al. (138)	5	6	7	60	Continuous	50–60	2 days	+15%	Yes (+28%)
Krotkiewski et al. (83)	10	12	3	50	Intermittent	"light" → 80–90	4 days	+14%	Yes (+20%)
Segal et al. (128)	6	12	4	60	Continuous	70	4–5 days	+27%	No
Dela et al. (27)	7	10	6	30	Continuous	70	16 hours	+11%[d]	Yes (+23%)[d]

[a]Adapted from ref. 24.
[b]Only five subjects met criteria for Type 2 diabetes. Five others had impaired glucose tolerance.
[c]Including effects of diet intervention. However, no weight loss.
[d]Training was performed with one leg only. Average of increases in whole body effect during the two highest insulin infusion rates is given.
[e]HR_{max} denotes maximal heart rate.

respond in opposite directions to training: In Type 2 diabetes patients a diminished glucose stress resulting from an increase in target tissue insulin sensitivity might improve the secretory capacity of overloaded β-cells *(55)*. In favor of this hypothesis in some studies enhanced insulin responses to oral or intravenous glucose tolerance testing have been found in diabetics following training *(13,117)*.

In one study correlation analysis indicated that patients with the lowest pre-training C-peptide response to OGTT had the largest increase in C-peptide response during training *(83)*. This might just reflect a regression towards the mean, low values tending to increase and high values to decrease if measurements are repeated. However, different responses of subgroups within the heterogenous group of Type 2 diabetes patients would explain why not all studies using glucose tolerance tests have indicated that training alters β-cell function *(80,126,138)*. For clarification we applied the sequential hyperglycemic clamp technique with an arginine bolus at the end in Type 2 diabetes patients who prior to training were allocated to high and low insulin secreting groups, respectively, by an independent stimulation test (iv glucagon). Overall C-peptide and insulin responses were enhanced by training in high secretors (Table 4) but unaltered in low secretors (M. v Linstow et al., unpublished). Thus, training may improve diabetic β-cell function when residual secretory capacity is not minimal.

It appears from the above that various laboratory examinations have disclosed training-induced adaptations in both secretion and effect of insulin in Type 2 diabetes patients. However, what really matters is the influence of training on overall glucose homeostasis during normal living conditions. Accordingly, we sampled venous blood regularly for 24 h from 14 Type 2 diabetes patients, 9 high and 5 low insulin secretors, who carried out their usual activities (M. v Linstow et al., unpublished). This was done before and at the end of 12 wk ergometer cycle training which increased VO_2 max 20% ($p < 0.05$) and reduced heart rate at 100 Watt 8% ($p < 0.05$). We found that areas under plasma concentration versus time curves were identical for glucose, but significantly lower for insulin and C-peptide after compared to before training (Fig. 4). Energy intake was not restricted and was probably at least as high after as before training. Thus, 3 day's diet recordings showed unaltered energy intake during training. Furthermore, the patients maintained bodyweight despite a training associated energy expenditure of about 1200 kJ per bout (equivalent to approximately 12–15% of daily metabolic rate), and total number of heart beats during the 24 h was unchanged. One may conclude that during physiological conditions insulin action is enhanced by training in Type 2 diabetes patients, because overall disposal of glucose and other nutrients is increased relative to both average peripheral insulin concentrations and overall insulin secretion.

After training daily insulin secretion, as judged from integrated C-peptide levels, was reduced despite unchanged average plasma glucose levels and possibly enhanced glucose stimulated secretion in the high secretors. This implies that net non-glucose stimulation was diminished, a fact which at least partly could be ascribed to increased β-cell suppressing sympathetic nervous activity during exercise and to diminished food-induced gut incretin secretion as seen in non-diabetics after exercise and training (*see* Mechanisms of Exercise-Induced Adaptations in Insulin Action and Secretion). In agreement with unchanged integrated plasma glucose concentrations also HbA_1C levels were identical before and after training (M. v Linstow et al., unpublished) as generally found in Type 2 diabetes-patients *(27,52)*. In the clinic such findings would be taken to indicate no improvement of overall metabolic control in response to training. This is, however,

Table 4
Insulin and C-Peptide Areas Under Concentration Curves During Hyperglycemic Clamps
in Patients with NIDDM (High Secretors)[a]

Glucose concentration	18 mM	25 mM	25 mM + 5 mg Arginine bolus
Insulin	$(nmol \cdot L^{-1} \cdot 90\ min)$	$(nmol \cdot L^{-1} \cdot 90\ min)$	$(nmol \cdot L^{-1} \cdot 35\ min)$
Study start	18 ± 3	24 ± 4	24 ± 4
After 3 mo	22 ± 5	33 ± 8^{b}	32 ± 8
C-peptide	$(nmol \cdot L^{-1} \cdot 90\ min)$	$(nmol \cdot L^{-1} \cdot 90\ min)$	$(nmol \cdot L^{-1} \cdot 35\ min)$
Study start	122 ± 16	168 ± 23	109 ± 13
After 3 mo	138 ± 20^{b}	188 ± 29^{b}	126 ± 19^{b}

[a]Nine patients with Type 2 diabetes (6 min C-peptide response to 1 mg glucagon iv > 1.1 nmol·L^{-1} [high secretors]) were studied before and after 3 months of bicycle ergometer training. Sequential hyperglycemic clamps with superimposed arginine bolus were performed. Values are mean ± SE.
[b]$p < 0.05$.

wrong because insulin secretion is spared and peripheral insulin levels diminished indicating delayed progression of β-cell failure and atherosclerosis (*see* An Overall View). It is not impossible for ambulatory Type 2 diabetes patients to achieve an improvement in diural glycemia by training, but it seems to require restricted energy intake and a considerable weight loss *(2,90,129,147)*. In contrast, in line with findings in healthy subjects (*see* An Overall View) it is a common clinical experience that mobilization of bedridden Type 2 diabetes-patients improves glycemia.

It can be concluded that regular exercise reduces the occurrence of Type 2 diabetes and may improve glucose homeostasis in those who have developed the disease. The latter effect may be more marked in younger patients and patients with short duration of disease *(65,123,143,152)* and may vary directly with volume of training and weight loss. The fundamental training-induced adaptations in muscle compensate for rather than correct the basal diabetic defect. The beneficial effects on insulin action and secretion are due to a combination of acute effects of exercise and of short lived genuine adaptations Consequently, the Type 2 diabetes patient has to keep up a physically active lifestyle in order to preserve acquired health benefits. Unfortunately, it is a well-known fact that in this regard compliance of Type 2 diabetes patients is poor *(129)*. Another obstacle to gaining benefits from exercise is presence of long-term diabetic complications *(52,53,152)*.

Women with Gestational Diabetes Mellitus

Women who develop gestational diabetes mellitus in response to the hormonal changes and increase in body mass seen during pregnancy have a predisposition to an insulin resistance closely resembling that of Type 2 diabetes *(20)*. So, it is no wonder that also the risk of developing gestational diabetes can be reduced by a physically active lifestyle *(40)*. Also in women who have contracted gestational diabetes effects of exercise are similar to those seen in Type 2 diabetes (*see* Patients with Type 2 Diabetes Mellitus). Thus, a single 30 min bout of moderate exercise is not sufficient to blunt the glycemic response to a mixed meal taken 14 h later and after an intervening meal *(87)*. Furthermore, supervised physical training programs of moderate intensity may decrease the insulin response to an oral glucose load and may even normalize fasting plasma glucose

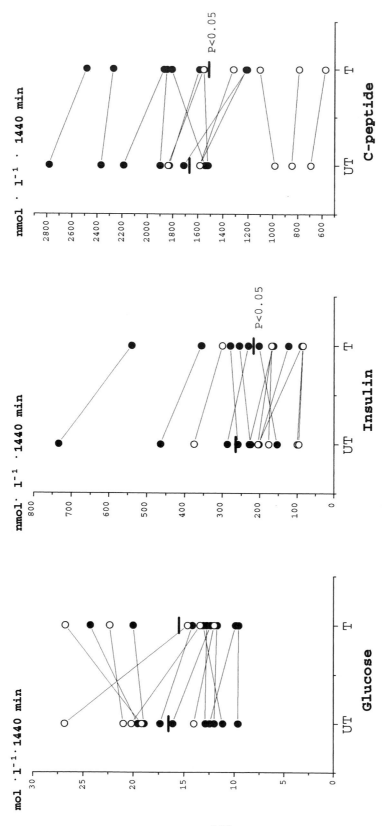

Fig. 4. Fourteen Type 2 diabetes patients had blood sampled frequently during 24-h of ordinary living conditions. This was done before and at the end of 12 wk ergometer cycle training. The figure shows individual 24-h integrated plasma concentrations. Horizontal bar indicates group mean. Open symbols denote low secretors, closed symbols denote high secretors.

concentrations *(17,68)*. Partially supervised training programs may be less efficient *(7)*. It is a general experience that pregnancy itself puts the necessary limitations on exercise performance so that physical activity can be recommended as a therapeutic option in the treatment of gestational diabetes *(17)*.

First-Degree Relatives of Patients with Type 2 Diabetes

Compared to subjects with no family record of diabetes first-degree relatives of Type 2 diabetes patients have a lower physical fitness and a higher fraction of II B muscle fibers *(108,109)*. They are also insulin resistant and show reduced insulin mediated glucose extraction, phosphorylation and storage as glycogen in muscle *(42,108,113,142)*. The extent to which the latter defects reflect genetic predisposition or physical inactivity is not known. Whatever the cause may be, exercise may improve the condition. Thus, in the diabetic relatives insulin-mediated whole-body glucose uptake is increased 20% the day after a single exercise bout and 40% after six weeks of moderate endurance training *(113)*. In the diabetic relatives the training-induced enhancement of insulin action is associated with a reversal of the defect in glucose phosphorylation and storage in muscle *(113)*. However, the improvement in insulin action may not be accompanied by altered glucose stimulated insulin secretion *(113)*.

Patients with Chronic Renal Failure

Chronic renal failure is accompanied by impairment of insulin action the primary site of which is muscle *(91)*. Insulin resistance develops in direct consequence of reduced kidney function, which causes endocrine and metabolic derangement, including diminished renal insulin clearance. However, the patients are also relatively physically inactive as reflected in low VO_2 max, and their insulin resistance is inversely related to VO_2 max *(41,58)*. In patients with end stage renal failure a one year training program, which increases VO_2 max by 21%, increases insulin sensitivity, reduces basal plasma insulin levels and improves plasma lipoprotein pattern *(57)*. However, in patients with only mild to moderate chronic renal failure no changes in these variables have been found during one year of training despite a similar increase in VO_2 max (I Eidemark, personal communication).

GENERAL CONCLUSION

Physical activity increases insulin action on glucose disposal. This effect is predominantly but not only located in the recruited muscles. When changes in level of physical activity are moderate the effect of insulin action is outbalanced by adaptations in insulin secretion. Accordingly, glucose tolerance is well preserved but in the face of changes in plasma insulin levels inversely related to the level of physical activity. However, if training or inactivity are more extreme, glucose tolerance may be improved or deteriorate, respectively. The β-cell relieving and plasma insulin depressing effects of exercise are potentially wholesome but may be overestimated from standard glucose tolerance tests if increase in level of physical activity is accompanied by an increase in energy intake. Regular exercise may facilitate weight loss, an effect which will further improve glucose homeostasis. Finally, insulin action and secretion reflect the habitual level of physical activity and will change rapidly if this level is changed.

REFERENCES

1. Andersen P, Henriksson J. Capillary supply of the quadriceps femoris muscle of man: adaptive response to exercise. J Physiol 1977;270:677–690.

2. Anonymous. Consensus Development Conference on Diet and Exercise in non-insulin-dependent diabetes mellitus. National Institutes of Health. Diabetes Care 1987;10:639–644.

3. Asp S, Daugaard JR, Kristiansen S, Kiens B, Richter EA. Eccentric exercise decreases maximal insulin action in humans: muscle and systemic effects. J Physiol 1996;494:891–898.

4. Asp S, Daugaard JR, Richter EA. Eccentric exercise decreases GLUT4 protein in human skeletal muscle. J Physiol 1995;482:705–712.

5. Asp S, Richter EA. Decreased insulin action on muscle glucose transport after eccentric contractions in rats. J Appl Physiol 1996;81:1924–1928.

6. Asp S, Rohde T, Richter EA. Impaired muscle glycogen resynthesis after a marathon is not caused by decreased muscle GLUT4 content. J Appl Physiol 1997;83:1482–1485.

7. Avery MD, Leon AS, Kopher RA. Effects of a partially home-based exercise program for women with gestational diabetes. Obst Gynecol 1997;89:10–15.

8. Beard JC, Halter JB, Best JD, Pfeifer MA, Porte D Jr. Dexamethasone-induced insulin resistance enhances β-cell responsiveness to glucose level in normal men. Am J Physiol 1984;247:E592–E596.

9. Berger M, Kemmer FW. Discussion: Exercise, fitness, and diabetes. In: Bouchard C, Shephard RL, Stephens T, Sutton JR, McPherson BD, ed. Exercise, Fitness, and Health. Human Kinetics, Champaign IL, 1990, pp. 491–495.

10. Björkman O, Eriksson LS. Influence of a 60-hour fast on insulin-mediated splanchnic and peripheral glucose metabolism in humans. J Clin Invest 1985;76:87–92.

11. Björntorp P Effects of exercise on plasma insulin and glucose tolerance. In: Enzi G, Crepaldi G, Pozza G, Renold AE, ed. Serano Symposium No. 28. Obesity: Pathogenesis and Treatment. Academic, London and New York, 1981, pp. 197–205.

12. Blom PC, Hostmark AT, Flaten O, Hermansen L. Modification by exercise of the plasma gastric inhibitory polypeptide response to glucose ingestion in young men. Acta Physiol Scand 1985; 123:367–368.

13. Bogardus C, Ravussin E, Robbins DC, Wolfe RR, Horton ES, Sims EAH. Effects of physical training and diet theraphy on carbohydrate metabolism in patients with glucose intolerance and non-insulin-dependent diabetes mellitus. Diabetes 1984;33:311–318.

14. Bogardus C, Thuillez P, Ravussin E, Vasquez B, Narimiga M, Azhar S. Effect of muscle glycogen depletion on in vivo insulin action in man. J Clin Invest 1983;72:1605–1610.

15. Broughton DL, James OWF, Alberti KGMM, Taylor R. Peripheral and hepatic insulin sensitivity in healthy elderly human subjects. Eur J Clin Invest 1991;21:13–21.

16. Buemann B, Tremblay A. Effects of exercise training on abdominal obesity and related metabolic complications. Sports Med 1996;21:191–212.

17. Bung P, Artal R. Gestational diabetes and exercise: a survey. Seminars in Perinatology 1996; 20:328–333.

18. Burstein R, Epstein Y, Shapiro Y, Charuzi I, Karneili E. Effect of an acute bout of exercise on glucose disposal in human obesity. J Appl Physiol 1990;69(1):299–304.

19. Burstein R, Polychronakos C, Toews CJ, MacDougall JD, Guyda HJ, Posner BI. Acute reversal of the enhanced insulin action in trained athletes. Association with insulin receptor changes. Diabetes 1985;34:756–760.

20. Catalano PM, Tyzbir ED, Wolfe RR, Calles J, Roman NM, Amini SB, Sims EA Carbohydrate metabolism during pregnancy in control subjects and women with gestational diabetes. Am J Physiol 1993;264:E60–E67.

21. Craig BW, Everhart J, Brown R. The influence of high-resistance training on glucose tolerance in young and elderly subjects. Mech Ageing Develop 1989;49:147–157.

22. DeFronzo RA. Glucose tolerance and ageing. Evidence for tissue insensitivity to insulin. Diabetes 1979;28:1095–1101.

23. DeFronzo RA, Sherwin RS, Kraemer N. Effect of physical training on insulin action in obesity. Diabetes 1987;36:1379–1385.

24. Dela F. On the influence of physical training on glucose homeostasis. Acta Physiol Scand 1996; 158:5–41.

25. Dela F, Handberg A, Mikines KJ, Vinten J, Galbo H. GLUT4 and insulin receptor binding and kinase activity in trained human muscle. J Physiol 1993;469:615–624.

26. Dela F, Mikines KJ, Larsen JJ, Galbo H. Training-induced enhancement of insulin action in human skeletal muscle: The influence of aging. J Gerontol 1996;51A:B247–B252.

27. Dela F, Mikines KJ, Larsen JJ, Ploug T, Petersen LN, Galbo H. Insulin stimulated muscle glucose clearance in patients with Type 2 diabetes mellitus. Effects of one-legged physical training. Diabetes 1995;44:1010–1020.

28. Dela F, Mikines KJ, Linstow vM, Galbo H. Effect of training on response to a glucose load adjusted for daily carbohydrate intake. Am J Physiol 1991;260(23):E14–E20.
29. Dela F, Mikines KJ, Linstow vM, Galbo H. Twenty-four-hour profile of plasma glucose and glucoregulatory hormones during normal living conditions in trained and untrained men. J Clin Endocrinol Metab 1991;73:982–989.
30. Dela F, Mikines KJ, Linstow vM, Galbo H. Heart rate and plasma catecholamines during 24 h of everyday life in trained and untrained men. J Appl Physiol 1992;73(6): 2389–2395.
31. Dela F, Mikines KJ, Linstow vM, Secher NH, Galbo H. Effect of training on insulin mediated glucose uptake in human skeletal muscle. Am J Physiol 1992;263:E1134–E1143.
32. Dela F, Mikines KJ, Sonne B, Galbo H. Effect of training on the interaction between insulin and exercise in human muscle. J Appl Physiol 1994;76:2386–2396.
33. Dela F, Mikines KJ, Tronier B, Galbo H. Diminished arginine-stimulated insulin secretion in trained men. J Appl Physiol 1990;69(1):261–267.
34. Dela F, Ploug T, Handberg A, Petersen LN, Larsen JJ, Mikines KJ, Galbo H. Physical training increases muscle GLUT4 protein and mRNA in patients with NIDDM Diabetes 1994;43:862–865.
35. Dengel DR, Pratley RE, Hagberg JM, Rogus EM, Goldberg AP. Distinct effects of aerobic exercise training and weight loss on glucose homeostasis in obese sedentary men. J Appl Physiol 1996;81: 318–325.
36. Despres JP. Visceral obesity, insulin resistance, and dyslipidemia: contribution of endurance exercise training to the treatment of the plurimetabolic syndrome. Exerc Sport Sci Rev 1997;25:271–300.
37. Devlin JT, Hirshman M, Horton ED, Horton ES. Enhanced peripheral and splanchnic insulin sensitivity in NIDDM men after a single bout of exercise. Diabetes 1987;36:434–439.
38. Devlin JT, Horton ES. Effects of prior high-intensity exercise on glucose metabolism in normal and insulin-resistent man. Diabetes 1985;34:973–979.
39. Dolkas CB, Greenleaf JE. Insulin and glucose responses during bed rest with isotonic and isometric exercise. J Appl Physiol 1977;43:1033–1038.
40. Dye TD, Knox KL, Artal R, Aubry RH, Wojtowycz MA. Physical activity, obesity, and diabetes in pregnancy. Am J Epidemiol 1997;146:961–965.
41. Eidemak I, Feldt-Rasmussen B, Kanstrup IL, Nielsen SL, Schmitz O, Strandgaard S. Insulin resistance and hyperinsulinemia in mild to moderate progressive chronic renal failure and its association with aerobic work capacity. Diabetologia 1995;38:565–572.
42. Eriksson J, Franssila-Kallunki A, Ekstrand A, Saloranta C, Widen E, Schalin C, Groop L. Early metabolic defects in persons at increased risk for non-insulin-dependent diabetes mellitus. N Engl J Med 1989;321:337–343.
43. Eriksson J, Taimela S, Koivisto VA. Exercise and the metabolic syndrome. Diabetologia 1997;40:125–135.
44. Eriksson K-F, Lindgärde F. Prevention of Type 2 (non-insulin-dependent) diabetes mellitus by diet and physical exercise. Diabetologia 1991;34:891–898.
45. Farrell PA, Caston AL, Rodd D, Engdahl J. Effect of training on insulin secretion from single pancreatic beta cells. Med Sci Sports Exerc 1992;24:426–433.
46. Fink RI, Kolterman OG, Griffin J, Olefsky JM. Mechanisms of insulin resistance in aging. J Clin Invest 1983;71:1523–1535.
47. Fluckey JD, Hickey MS, Brambrink JK, Hart KK, Alexander K, Craig BW. Effects of resistance exercise on glucose tolerance in normal and glucose-intolerant subjects. J Appl Physiol 1994;77: 1087–1092.
48. Fluckey JD, Kraemer WJ, Farrell PA. Pancreatic islet insulin secretion is increased after resistance exercise in rats. J Appl Physiol 1995;79:1100–1105.
49. Fluckey JD, Ploug T, Galbo H. Attenuated insulin action on glucose uptake and transport in muscle following resistance exercise in rats, 1998, submitted for publication.
50. Fluckey JD, Vary TC, Jefferson LS, Farrell PA. Augmented insulin action on rates of protein synthesis after resistance exercise in rats. Am J Physiol 1996;270:E313–E319.
51. Fujii S, Okuno Y, Okada K, Tanaka S, Seki J, Wada M, Iseki T. Effects of physical training on glucose tolerance and insulin response in diabetics. Osaka City Med J 1982;28:1–8.
52. Galbo H. Exercise and diabetes. Scand J Sports Sci 1988;10:89–95.
53. Galbo H Exercise protocols in diabetes. In: Mogensen CE, Standl E, eds. Research Methodologies in Human Diabetes. Walter de Gruyter, Berlin, 1995, pp. 191–206.
54. Galbo H, Hedeskov CJ, Capito K, Vinten J. The effect of physical training on insulin secretion of rat pancreatic islets. Acta Physiol Scand 1981;111:75–79.

55. Galbo H, Kjær M. Endocrinology and metabolism in exercise: future research directions. Can J Spt Sci 1987;12(Suppl 1):102S–107S.

56. Galbo H, Saugmann P, Richter EA. Increased hepatic glycogen synthetase and decreased phosphory-lase in trained rats. Acta Physiol Scand 1979;107:269–272.

57. Goldberg AP, Geltman EM, Gavin JR, Carney RM, Hagberg JM, Delmez JA, Naumovich A, Oldfield MH, Harter HR. Exercise training reduces coronary risk and effectively rehabilitates hemodialysis patients. Nephron 1986;42:311–316.

58. Goldberg AP, Hagberg JM, Delmez JA, Haynes ME, Harter HR. Metabolic effects of exercise training in hemodialysis patients. Kidney Int 1980;18:754–761.

59. Heath GW, Gavin JRI, Hinderliter JM, Hagberg JM, Bloomfield SA, Holloszy JO. Effects of exercise and lack of exercise on glucose tolerance and insulin sensitivity. J Appl Physiol 1983;55(2):512–517.

60. Heitmann BL, Kaprio J, Harris JR, Rissanen A, Korkeila M, Koskenvuo M. Are genetic determinants of weight gain modified by leisure-time physical activity? A prospective study of Finnish twins. Am J Clin Nutr 1997;66:672–678.

61. Helmrich SP, Ragland DR, Leung RW, Paffenbarger RS. Physical activity and reduced occurrence of non-insulin-dependent diabetes-mellitus. N Engl J Med 1991;325:147–152.

62. Holloszy JO, Schultz J, Kusnierkiewicz J, Hagberg JM, Ehsani AA. Effects of exercise on glucose tolerance and insulin resistance. Brief review and some preliminary results. Acta Medica Scandinavica—Supplementum 1986;711:55–65.

63. Houmard JA, Tyndall GL, Midyette JB, Hickey MS, Dolan PL, Gavigan KE, Weidner ML, Dohm GL. Effect of reduced training and training cessation on insulin action and muscle GLUT4. J Appl Physiol 1996;81:1162–1168.

64. Hughes VA, Fiatarone MA, Fielding RA, Kahn BB, Ferrara CM, Shepherd P, Fisher EC, Wolfe RR, Elahi D, Evans WJ. Exercise increases muscle GLUT4 levels and insulin action in subjects with impaired glucose tolerance. Am J Physiol 1993;264:E855–E862.

65. Ivy JL. Role of exercise training in the prevention and treatment of insulin resistance and non-insulin-dependent diabetes mellitus. Sports Med 1997;24:321–336.

66. Jackson RA. Mechanisms of age-related glucose intolerance. Diabetes Care 1990;13(suppl. 2):9–19.

67. Jarrett RJ. Epidemiology and public health aspects of non-insulin-dependent diabetes mellitus. Epide-miol Rev 1989;11:151–171.

68. Jovanovic-Peterson L, Durak EP, Peterson CM. Randomized trial of diet versus diet plus cardiovas-cular conditioning on glucose levels in gestational diabetes. Am J Obstet Gynecol 1989;161:415–419.

69. Kahn SE, Larson VG, Beard JE, Cain KC, Fellingham GW, Schwartz RS, Veith RC, Stratton JR, Cerqueira MD, Abrass IB. Effect of exercise on insulin action, glucose tolerance, and insulin secretion in ageing. Am J Physiol 1990;258(21):E937–E943.

70. Karter AJ, Mayer-Davis EJ, Selby JV, D'Agostino RBJ, Haffner SM, Sholinsky P, Bergman R, Saad MF, Hamman RF. Insulin sensitivity and abdominal obesity in African-American Hispanic, and non-Hispanic caucasion men and women. The Insulin Resistance and Atherosclerosis Study. Diabetes 1996;45:1547–1555.

71. Katzel LI, Busby-Whitehead MJ, Rogus EM, Krauss RM, Goldberg AP. Reduced adipose tissue lipoprotein lipase responses, postprandial lipemia, and low high-density lipoprotein-2 subspecies levels in older athletes with silent myocardial ischemia. Metabolism: Clin Exper 1994;43:190–198.

72. Kiens B, Lithell H. Lipoprotein metabolism influenced by training-induced changes in human skeletal muscle. J Clin Invest 1989;83:558–564.

73. Kiens B, Lithell H, Mikines KJ, Richter EA. Effects of insulin and exercise on muscle lipoprotein lipase activity in man and its relation to insulin action. J Clin Invest 1989;84:1124–1129.

74. King DS, Dalsky GP, Staten MA, Clutter WE, Van Houten DR, Holloszy JO. Insulin action and secretion in endurance-trained and untrained humans. J Appl Physiol 1987;63:2247–2252.

75. King DS, Feltmeyer TL, Baldus PJ, Sharp RL, Nespor J. Effects of eccentric exercise on insulin secretion and action in humans. J Appl Physiol 1993;75:2151–2156.

76. Kirwan JP, Bourey RE, Kohrt WM, Staten MA, Holloszy JO. Effects of treadmill exercise to exhaus-tion on the insulin response to hyperglycemia in untrained men. J Appl Physiol 1991;70:246–250.

77. Kirwan JP, Kohrt WM, Wojta DM, Bourey RE, Holloszy JO. Endurance exercise training reduces glucose-stimulated insulin levels in 60- to 70-year-old men and women. J Gerontol 1993; 48: M84–M90.

78. Kjær M, Farrell PA, Christensen NJ, Galbo H. Increased epinephrine response and inaccurate glucoregulation in exercising athletes. J Appl Physiol 1986;61(5):1693–1700.

79. Kjær M, Hollenbeck CB, Frey-Hewitt B, Galbo H, Haskell W, Reaven GM. Glucoregulation and hormonal responses to maximal exercise in non-insulin-dependent diabetics. J Appl Physiol 1990;68(5):2067–2074.

80. Koivisto VA, Yki-Järvinen H, DeFronzo RA. Physical training and insulin sensitivity. Diabetes-Metabolism Rev 1986;1:445–481.

81. Krotkiewski M, Björntorp P. Muscle tissue in obesity with different distribution of adipose tissue. Effects of physical training. Int J Obes 1986;10:331–341.

82. Krotkiewski M, Björntorp P, Holm G, Marks V, Morgan L, Smith U, Feurle GE. Effects of physical training on insulin, connecting peptide (C-peptide), gastric inhibitory polypeptide (GIP) and pancreatic polypeptide (PP) levels in obese subjects. Int J Obes 1984;8:193–199.

83. Krotkiewski M, Lönnroth P, Mandroukas K, Wroblewski Z, Rebuffé-Scrive M. The effects of physical training on insulin secretion and effectiveness and on glucose metabolism in obesity and Type 2 (non-insulin-dependent) diabetes mellitus. Diabetologia 1985;28:881–890.

84. Larsen JJ, Dela F, Kjær M, Galbo H. The effect of moderate exercise on postprandial glucose homeostasis in NIDDM patients. Diabetologia 1997;40:447–453.

85. LeBlanc J, Nadeau A, Richard D, Tremblay A. Studies on the sparing effect of exercise on insulin requirements in human subjects. Metabolism 1981;30:1119–1124.

86. Lehmann R, Vokac A, Niedermann K, Agosti K, Spinas GA. Loss of abdominal fat and improvement of the cardiovascular risk profile by regular moderate exercise training in patients with NIDDM Diabetologia 1995;38:1313–1319.

87. Lesser KB, Gruppuso PA, Terry RB, Carpenter MW. Exercise fails to improve postprandial glycemic excursion in women with gestational diabetes. J Maternal-Fetal Med 1996;5:211–217.

88. Lipman RL, Schnure JJ, Bradley EM, Lecocq FR. Impairment of peripheral glucose utilization in normal subjects by prolonged bed rest. J Lab Clin Med 1970;76:221–230.

89. Lohmann D, Liebold F, Heilmann W, Senger H, Pohl A. Diminished insulin response in highly trained athletes. Metabolism 1978;27:521–524.

90. Lucas CP, Patton S, Stepke T, Kinhal V, Darga LL, Carroll-Michals L, Spafford TR, Kasim S. Achieving therapeutic goals in insulin-using diabetic patients with non-insulin-dependent diabetes mellitus. Am J Med 1987;83(Suppl 3A):3–9.

91. Mak RHK, DeFronzo RA. Glucose and insulin metabolism in uremia. Nephron 1992;61:377–382.

92. Manson JE, Nathan DM, Krolewski AS, Stampfer MJ, Willett WC, Hennekens CH. A prospective study of exercise and incidence of diabetes among United States male physicians. JAMA 1992;268:63–67.

93. Manson JE, Rimm EB, Stampfer MJ, Colditz GA, Willett WC, Krolewski AS, Rosner B, Hennekens CH, Speizer FE. Physical activity and incidence of non-insulin-dependent diabetes-mellitus in women. Lancet 1991;338:774–778.

94. Manson JE, Spelsberg A. Primary prevention of non-insulin-dependent diabetes mellitus. Am J Prev Med 1994;10:172–184.

95. Martin IK, Katz A, Wahren J. Splanchnic and muscle metabolism during exercise in NIDDM patients. Am J Physiol 1995;269:E583-E590.

96. Mikines KJ, Dela F, Tronier B, Galbo H. Effect of 7 days of bedrest on dose-response relation between glucose and insulin secretion. Am J Physiol 1989;257:E43–E48.

97. Mikines KJ, Farrell PA, Sonne B, Tronier B, Galbo H. Postexercise dose-response relationship between plasma glucose and insulin secretion. J Appl Physiol 1988;64(3):988–999.

98. Mikines KJ, Richter EA, Dela F, Galbo H. Seven days of bedrest decrease insulin action on glucose uptake in leg and whole body. J Appl Physiol 1991;70(3):1245–1254.

99. Mikines KJ, Sonne B, Farrell PA, Tronier B, Galbo H. Effect of physical exercise on sensitivity and responsiveness to insulin in humans. Am J Physiol 1988;254:E248–E259.

100. Mikines KJ, Sonne B, Farrell PA, Tronier B, Galbo H. Effect of training on the dose-response relationship for insulin action in men. J Appl Physiol 1989;66(2):695–703.

101. Mikines KJ, Sonne B, Tronier B, Galbo H. Effects of acute exercise and detraining on insulin action in trained men. J Appl Physiol 1989;66(2):704–711.

102. Mikines KJ, Sonne B, Tronier B, Galbo H. Effects of training and detraining on dose-response relationship between glucose and insulin secretion. Am J Physiol 1989;256:E588–E596.

103. Miller JP, Pratley RE, Goldberg AP, Gordon P, Rubin M, Treuth MS, Ryan AS, Hurley BF. Strength training increases insulin action in healthy 50- to 65-yr-old men. J Appl Physiol 1994;77:1122–1127.

104. Miller WJ, Sherman WM, Ivy JL. Effect of strength training on glucose tolerance and post-glucose insulin response. Med Sci Sports Exer 1984;16:539–543.

105. Minuk HL, Vranic M, Marliss EB, Hanna AK, Albisser AM, Zinman B. Glucoregulatory and metabolic response to exercise in obese non-insulin-dependent diabetes. Am J Physiol 1981;240:E458–E464.

106. Mohr T, Andersen JL, Biering-Sørensen F, Galbo H, Bangsbo J, Wagner Aa, and Kjaer M. Long term adaptation to electrically induced cycle training in severe spinal cord injured individuals. Spinal Cord 1997;35:1–16.

107. Mohr T, Dela F, Handberg A, Galbo H, Biering-Sørensen F, Kjær M. Insulin action and long-term electrically induced cycle training in spinal cord injured individuals. Med Sci Sports Exer 1998, submitted.

108. Nyholm B, Mengel A, Nielsen S, Skjærbaek C, Møller N, Alberti KG, Schmitz O. Insulin resistance in relatives of NIDDM patients: the role of physical fitness and muscle metabolism. Diabetologia 1996;39:813–822.

109. Nyholm B, Qu Z, Kaal A, Pedersen SB, Gravholt CH, Andersen JL, Saltin B, Schmitz O. Evidence of an increased number of type IIb muscle fibers in insulin-resistant first-degree relatives of patients with NIDDM Diabetes 1997;46:1822–1828.

110. O'Doherty RM, Bracy DP, Osawa H, Wasserman DH, Granner DK. Rat skeletal muscle hexokinase II mRNA and activity are increased by a single bout of acute exercise. Am J Physiol 1994; 266:E171–E178.

111. Pedersen SB, Borglum JD, Schmitz O, Bak JF, Sørensen NS, Richelsen B. Abdominal obesity is associated with insulin resistance and reduced glycogen synthase activity in skeletal muscle. Metabolism 1993;42:998–1005.

112. Perry IJ, Wannamethee SG, Walker MK, Thomson AG, Whincup PH, Shaper AG. Prospective study of risk factors for development of non-insulin dependent diabetes in middle aged British men. BMJ 1995;310:560–564.

113. Perseghin G, Price TB, Petersen KF, Roden M, Cline GW, Gerow K, Rothman DL, Shulman GI. Increased glucose transport-phosphorylation and muscle glycogen synthesis after exercise training in insulin-resistant subjects. N Engl J Med 1996;335:1357–1362.

114. Ploug T, Stallknecht BM, Pedersen O, Kahn BB, Ohkuwa T, Vinten J, Galbo H. Effect of endurance training on glucose transport capacity and glucose transporter expression in rat skeletal muscle. Am J Physiol 1990;259(22): E778–E786.

115. Polonsky KS, Given BD, Hirsch L, Shapiro ET, Tillil H, Beebe C, Galloway JA, Frank BH, Karrison T, and Van CE. Quantitative study of insulin secretion and clearance in normal and obese subjects. J Clin Invest 1988;81:435–441.

116. Pruett ED, Oseid S. Effect of exercise on glucose and insulin response to glucose infusion. Scand J Clin Lab Invest 1970;26:277–285.

117. Reitman JS, Vasquez B, Klimes I, Nagulesparan M. Improvement of glucose homeostasis after exercise training in non-insulin-dependent diabetes. Diabetes Care 1984;7:434–441.

118. Richter EA, Kiens B, Mizuno M, Strange S. Insulin action in human thighs after one-legged immobilization. J Appl Physiol 1989;67(1):19–23.

119. Richter EA, Mikines KJ, Galbo H, Kiens B. Effect of exercise on insulin action in human skeletal muscle. J Appl Physiol 1989;66(2):876–885.

120. Richter EA, Ploug T, Galbo H. Increased muscle glucose uptake after exercise. No need for insulin during exercise. Diabetes 1985;34:1041–1048.

121. Rogers MA, Yamamoto C, King DS, Hagberg JM, Ehsani AA, Holloszy JO. Improvement in glucose tolerance after 1 wk of exercise in patients with mild NIDDM. Diabetes Care 1988;11:613–618.

122. Rosenthal M, Doberne L, Greenfield M, Widstrom A, Reaven GM. Effect of age on glucose tolerance, insulin secretion, and in vivo insulin action. J Am Geriatr Soc 1982;30:562–567.

123. Rönnemaa T, Mattila K, Lehtonen A, Kallio V. A controlled randomized study on the effect of long-term physical exercise on the metabolic control in Type 2 diabetic patients. Acta Med Scand 1986;220:219–224.

124. Sady SP, Thompson PD, Cullinane EM, Kantor MA, Domagala E, Herbert PN. Prolonged exercise augments plasma triglyceride clearance. JAMA 1986;256:2552–2555.

125. Schlierf G, Dinsenbacher A, Kather H, Kohlmeier M, Haberbosch W. Mitigation of alimentary lipemia by postprandial exercise—phenomena and mechanisms. Metabolism: Clin Exp 1987; 36:726–730.

126. Schneider SH, Amorosa LF, Khachadurian AK, Ruderman NB. Studies on the mechanism of improved glucose control during regular exercise in Type 2 (non-insulin-dependent) diabetes. Diabetologia 1984;26:355–360.

127. Schwartz RS, Shuman WP, Larson V, Cain KC, Fellingham GW, Beard JC, Kahn SE, Stratton JR, Cerqueira MD, Abrass IB. The effect of intensive endurance exercise training on body fat distribution in young and older men. Metabolism: Clin Exp 1991;40:545–551.

128. Segal KR, Edano A, Abalos A, Albu J, Blando L, Tomas MB, Pi-Sunyer FX. Effect of exercise training on insulin sensitivity and glucose metabolism in lean, obese, and diabetic men. J Appl Physiol 1991;71(6):2402–2411.

129. Skarfors ET, Wegener TA, Lithell H, Selinus I. Physical training as treatment for Type 2 (non-insulin-dependent) diabetes in elderly men. A feasibility study over 2 years. Diabetologia 1987;30:930–933.

130. Stallknecht B, Andersen PH, Vinten J, Bendtsen LL, Sibbersen J, Pedersen O, Galbo H. Effect of physical training on glucose transporter protein and mRNA levels in rat adipocytes. Am J Physiol 1993;265:E128–E134.

131. Stallknecht B, Roesdahl M, Vinten J, Capito K, Galbo H. The effect of lesions of the sympathoadrenal system on training induced adaptations in adipocytes and pancreatic islets in rats. Acta Physiol Scand 1996;156:465–473.

132. Staron RS, Johnson P. Myosin polymorphism and differential expression in adult human skeletal muscle. Comp Biochem 106B(3):463–475.

133. Stout RW. Insulin and atheroma. Diabetes Care 1990;13:631–654.

134. Stout RW. The Impact of Insulin upon Atherosclerosis. Horm Metab Res 1994;26:125–128.

135. Tabata I, Suzuki Y, Fukunaga T, Yokozeki T, Akima H, Funato K. Effect of resistance training on GLUT4 content in skeletal muscle of humans subjected to 20 days of –6 degrees head-down bed rest. J Appl Physiol 1998.

136. Torino RP. Effect of physical training on the insulin resistance of aging. Am J Physiol 1989; 256:E352–E356.

137. Tremblay A ET Poehlman JP Despres G Theriault E Danforth, and C Bouchard. Endurance training with constant energy intake in identical twins: changes over time in energy expenditure and related hormones. Metabolism: Clinical & Experimental 1997;46:499–503.

138. Trovati M, Carta Q, Cavalot F, Vitali S, Banaudi C, Lucchina PG, Fiocchi F, Emanuelli G, Lenti G. Influence of physical training on blood glucose control, glucose tolerance, insulin secretion, and insulin action in non-insulin-dependent diabetic patients. Diabetes Care 1984;7:416–420.

139. Tuominen JA, Ebeling P, Bourey R, Koranyi L, Lamminen A, Rapola J, Sane T, Vuorinen-Markkola H, Koivisto VA. Postmarathon paradox: insulin resistance in the face of glycogen depletion. Am J Physiol 1996;270:E336–E343.

140. Utriainen T, Holmäng A, Björntorp P, Makimattila S, Sovijarvi A, Lindholm H, Yki-Järvinen H. Physical fitness, muscle morphology, and insulin-stimulated limb blood flow in normal subjects. Am J Physiol 1996;270:E905–E911.

141. Uusitupa MIJ, Niskanen LK, Siitonen O, Voutilainen E, Pyörälä K. 5-year incidence of atherosclerotic vascular disease in relation to general risk factors, insulin level, and abnormalities in lipoprotein composition in non-insulin-dependent diabetic and nondiabetic subjects. Circulation 1990;82:27–36.

142. Vaag A, Henriksen JE, Beck-Nielsen H. Decreased insulin activation of glycogen synthase in skeletal muscles in young nonobese caucasian 1st-degree relatives of patients with non-insulin-dependent diabetes mellitus. J Clin Invest 1992;89:782–788.

143. Vanninen E, Uusitupa M, Siitonen O, Laitinen J, Lansimies E. Habitual physical activity, aerobic capacity and metabolic control in patients with newly-diagnosed Type 2 (non-insulin-dependent) diabetes mellitus: effect of 1-yr diet and exercise intervention. Diabetologia 1992;35:340–346.

144. Vestergaard H, Andersen PH, Lund S, Schmitz O, Junker S, Pedersen O. Pre- and posttranslational upregulation of muscle-specific glycogen synthase in athletes. Am J Physiol 1994;266:E92–E101.

145. Vinten J, Galbo H. Effect of physical training on transport and metabolism of glucose in adipocytes. Am J Physiol 1983;244(7):E129–E1341983.

146. Vinten J, Petersen LN, Sonne B, Galbo H. Effect of physical training on glucose transporters in fat cell fractions. Biochim Biophys Acta 1985;841:223–227.

147. Wing RR, Epstein LH, Paternostro-Bayles M, Kriska A, Nowalk MP, Gooding W. Exercise in a behavioural weight control programme for obese patients with Type 2 (non-insulin-dependent) diabetes. Diabetologia 1988;31:902–909.

148. Wirth A, Diehm C, Mayer H, Mörl H, Vogel I, Björntorp P, Schlierf G. Plasma C-peptide and insulin in trained and untrained subjects. J Appl Physiol 1981;50:71–77.

149. Wirth A, Holm G, Björntorp P. Effect of physical training on insulin uptake by the perfused rat liver. Metabolism 1982;31:457–462.

150. Yamanouchi K, Nakajima H, Shinozaki T, Chikada K, Kato K, Oshida Y, Osawa I, Sato J, Sato Y, Higuchi M. Effects of daily physical activity on insulin action in the elderly. J Appl Physiol 1992;73:2241–2245.
151. Yki-Järvinen H, Koivisto VA. Effects of body composition on insulin sensitivity. Diabetes 1983;32:965–969.
152. Zierath JR, Wallberg-Henriksson H. Exercise training in obese diabetic patients. Special considerations. Sports Med 1992;14:171–189.
153. Zimmet P, Dowse G, Finch C, Serjeantson S, King H. The epidemiology and natural history of NIDDM—lessons from the South Pacific. Diabetes-Metabolism Rev 1990;6:91–124.

7

Insulin Resistance in Smokers and Other Long-Term Users of Nicotine

Björn Eliasson, MD *and Ulf Smith,* MD

CONTENTS

INTRODUCTION
PREVALENCE OF CIGARET SMOKING
ROLE AS A RISK FACTOR
METABOLIC RISK PROFILE IN SMOKERS
POTENTIAL MECHANISMS OF ACTION
SMOKING VS CONFOUNDING FACTORS
IMPLICATIONS
REFERENCES

INTRODUCTION

Smoking has long been considered a major health hazard, leading to both malignant disorders and cardiovascular disease (CVD). However, smoke contains many potentially harmful substances and it is currently unclear which agents can play a major role. Recent developments have implicated smoking as an important environmental factor in eliciting insulin resistance and the insulin resistance syndrome (IRS). IRS is the clustering of several important risk factors for CVD where insulin resistance appears to play a pivotal role. These risk factors include dyslipidemia, dysfibrinolysis and impaired glucose tolerance including Type 2 diabetes mellitus.

In this chapter, we review the current understanding of the role and mechanisms whereby smoking can lead to insulin resistance, IRS and risk for CVD.

PREVALENCE OF CIGARET SMOKING

The estimated prevalence of smoking in men in different countries of the world ranges from 68% (Republic of Korea) to 19% (Bahamas) *(1)*. In women, the prevalence is lower, ranging from 37% (Denmark) to less than 1% (Sri Lanka, Turkmenistan). The tobacco consumption is higher in men in the developing countries than in the developed countries (48 and 42%, respectively), while women in the industrialized part of the world smoke

From: *Contemporary Endocrinology: Insulin Resistance*
Edited by: G. Reaven and A. Laws © Humana Press Inc., Totowa, NJ

more than their sisters in the developing countries (24 and 7%, respectively) *(1)*. WHO estimates that there are 1,100 million smokers in the world, which is equal to one-third of the global population aged 15 years or older. There are, however, large variations in smoking habits in different areas of the world, due to both the effects of restrictive legislation as well as the influence of religion and regional tradition. Throughout the world there are also several other tobacco products as well as smokeless tobacco, although manufactured cigarets constitute 65–85% of all tobacco consumed annually *(1)*.

In Göteborg, Sweden, the prevalence of cigaret smoking in 50-yr-old men has decreased during the last 30 years, from 56% (1963) to 30% (1993) (A. Rosengren 1998, personal communication). This decrease agrees with the trend in the developed countries after 1975, when the cigaret consumption in adults started to decrease *(1)*. In contrast, smoking is slowly increasing in the rest of the world.

ROLE AS A RISK FACTOR

Cigaret smoking is a major cause of disease and death in the Western world *(2)*. Unfortunately, the habit of smoking tobacco is becoming increasingly widespread throughout the world as discussed above. This will, in all likelihood, cause the incidence of cardiovascular and pulmonary diseases as well as smoking-related cancer to increase in years to come.

Smoking is a strong risk factor for several forms of cancer, chronic obstructive pulmonary disease as well as other respiratory disorders, cardiovascular morbidity and, consequently, premature death *(1)*. Doll et al. have, in fact, stated that "half of all regular cigaret smokers will eventually be killed by their habit", but also demonstrated that smoking cessation (SC) increases life expectancy radically *(3)*.

Blood pressure increases after acute smoking *(4)*. Resting blood pressure in healthy, smoking subjects is, however, lower than in nonsmokers *(5)* and, consequently, the prevalence of hypertension is reduced in smokers compared with smoke-free consumers of tobacco and nonsmokers *(6)*. This discrepancy between the acute and chronic effects of smoking on arterial blood pressure is still unexplained.

Smoking also influences several other cardiovascular risk factors. Smokers exhibit a more atherogenic lipoprotein profile with elevated triglyceride levels, low HDL-cholesterol and possibly elevated total, VLDL-, and LDL-cholesterol *(7)*. They also have elevated levels of fibrinogen *(8)*, which also is considered to be a cardiovascular risk factor *(9)*.

Smoking has been shown to have profound effects on blood vessel function *(10)* and is a major risk factor for atherosclerotic lesions as demonstrated with noninvasive ultrasound techniques *(11–13)*.

METABOLIC RISK PROFILE IN SMOKERS

Anthropometry

Smokers have lower body weight than nonsmokers but have a greater proportion of abdominal fat *(14,15)*. This is manifested as a higher waist/hip circumference ratio (WHR) which also has been shown to be a cardiovascular risk factor *(16)*. WHR increases in spite of weight loss in subjects beginning to smoke, but it does not increase proportionally with the weight increase after SC. Furthermore, there is a positive correlation between smoking habits and WHR in both women and men *(14,15)*.

Although smokers have different lifestyles than nonsmokers which, in turn, can influence body composition, it has been suggested that cigaret smoking has a direct effect on body fat distribution also after adjustment for the effects of age, body mass index (BMI), dietary intake and physical activity *(17)*.

Effects on Glucose Metabolism

Fasting blood glucose levels are usually not elevated in smokers, but a recent survey demonstrated a relative glucose intolerance and hyperinsulinemia following an oral glucose tolerance test (OGTT) *(18)*. Fasting insulin levels are elevated in smokers compared with nonsmokers as demonstrated by surveys in Finland and Sweden *(19,20)*. Acute smoking in both smokers and nonsmokers was recently shown to significantly impair glucose tolerance. This was also accompanied by higher insulin levels in the smokers *(21)*.

These recent data support and extend the results by Attvall et al. *(22)* and Facchini et al. *(23)*, showing that insulin sensitivity is reduced in smokers. In addition, Attvall et al. showed that insulin sensitivity, measured with the euglycemic hyperinsulinemic clamp technique, decreased in young smokers after smoking one cigaret per hour for six hours *(22)*. Similar results were found in habitually smoking Type 2 diabetic patients using a similar protocol, demonstrating decreased glucose utilization and glucose storage after smoking one cigaret per hour for six hours *(24)*.

Facchini et al. performed a cross-sectional study of 20 smokers and 20 well-matched nonsmoking control subjects and found that the smokers were hyperinsulinemic during an OGTT *(23)*. In the same study, using a modified insulin suppression test which measures insulin sensitivity, smokers were insulin resistant compared with nonsmoking controls.

In a recent cross-sectional study we compared insulin sensitivity in 36 healthy but smoking men and 25 age- and BMI-matched nonsmoking control subjects *(25)*. In spite of matching for BMI the smokers were again found to have higher WHR. The smokers were also insulin resistant as determined with the euglycemic hyperinsulinemic clamp technique *(25)*, the "golden standard" for measuring insulin sensitivity in vivo *(26)*.

We also studied the relations between smoking habits and metabolic variables in 57 healthy male smokers (Fig. 1) *(27)*. Smoking habits, i.e., average nicotine consumption, correlated positively with degree of insulin resistance as well as with various manifestations of IRS, including fasting insulin levels. Stepwise regression analyses, considering the effects of age, lean body mass, body fat mass (BF), BMI, WHR and alcohol consumption, showed that only smoking habits and percent BF were independently related to degree of insulin resistance *(27)*.

In contrast, Godsland et al. were not able to demonstrate similar abnormalities in glucose metabolism in a study in women, using mathematical modeling of an iv glucose tolerance test (IVGTT) and measuring glucose, insulin and C-peptide concentrations *(28)*. In this report, which was a subanalysis of previously published data *(29)*, no differences were found between smokers and nonsmokers. However, the subjects in that study smoked less than the subjects participating in the other studies and, furthermore, the study was not designed to evaluate the metabolic effects of smoking.

In Type 2 diabetic patients, Targher et al. *(30)*, recently showed that glucose disposal was reduced about 40% in smokers compared with well-matched nonsmokers. The smokers also had higher insulin and C-peptide levels and degree of insulin resistance was a function of smoking habits.

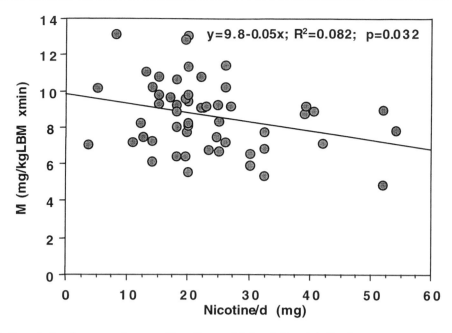

Fig. 1. Correlation between degree of insulin sensitivity (M) and daily cigaret consumption. (Data from ref. *27.*)

In Type 1 diabetic subjects, Helve et al. found no differences in insulin sensitivity between smoking and nonsmoking individuals or any acute effects of smoking on insulin sensitivity, in spite of increased adrenaline, cortisol, GH and glucagon levels *(31).* The reason for this is unclear. However, it is possible that when the smoking and nonsmoking Type 1 diabetes subjects were compared, fluctuations in blood glucose and metabolic control disguised the influence of smoking habits.

In a study by Nilsson et al., normo- and hypertensive smokers and nonsmoking control subjects did not exhibit impairments in glucose metabolism measured by IVGTT and the euglycemic hyperinsulinemic clamp *(32).* The effects of cigaret smoking *per se*, as opposed to the metabolic consequences of hypertension, also an insulin resistant state *(33),* are difficult to define from the results of that study, since only a small number of subjects were normotensive nonsmokers. Furthermore, the HbA1c levels were elevated in the smokers. This suggests that the smokers had higher blood glucose levels as seen in glucose intolerance and in insulin resistant states.

Effects on Lipoproteins and Lipoprotein Metabolism

Smokers are characterized by several abnormalities in lipoprotein levels and activity of enzymes regulating lipoprotein metabolism.

Cigaret smoking and nicotine administration have been shown to increase plasma glycerol and free fatty acid (FFA) levels, indicating an increased lipolysis via adrenergic mechanisms *(34–38).* In addition, the ability of insulin to suppress plasma FFA levels is impaired in smokers *(27,39).*

Smokers are characterized by elevated postabsorptive levels of triglyceride-rich lipoproteins (TRL), low HDL-cholesterol *(7,23)* as well as an increased prevalence of small dense LDL-particles *(25),* which are readily oxidized and considered particularly atherogenic. It is likely that the higher TRL are, at least in part, caused by the elevated FFA levels, leading to an increased hepatic production of these lipoproteins. It has been clearly shown by Hellerstein et al. that hepatic esterification of FFA increases after cigaret smoking *(36)*.

Adipose tissue lipoprotein lipase activity (LPL), which is the rate-limiting enzyme for uptake and storage of triglyceride fatty acids by the adipocytes, seems to be differently regulated by insulin in smokers compared with nonsmoking subjects *(40–42)*. Both adipose and muscle LPL activity are positively correlated to degree of insulin sensitivity *(43)*. We recently found that plasma postheparin LPL activity was positively correlated with degree of insulin sensitivity among the nonsmokers *(25)*. However, smokers do not appear to have low postheparin LPL activity although, as discussed above, the adipose tissue response after an OGTT seems to be abnormal *(42)*. In contrast, hepatic-lipase (HL) levels seem to be increased *(25)*, producing a low LPL/HL ratio which is compatible with IRS *(44)*.

Lecithin:cholesteryl acyl transferase (LCAT) is an important enzyme for the reverse cholesterol transport and converts circulating small HDL particles into larger, cholesteryl ester-rich HDL. Cholesteryl ester transfer protein (CETP) is instrumental in the distribution of cholesteryl ester between lipoproteins. Several studies have found impairments in the activity of these enzymes, which may contribute to the abnormalities in the lipoprotein profile in smokers *(45–49)*.

A novel finding in smokers is the marked postprandial lipid intolerance and that this is seen even in the absence of elevated fasting triglyceride levels (Fig. 2) *(25,50)*. Postprandial lipid metabolism has attracted growing interest in the last years. Zilversmit, already in 1979, suggested that the large triglyceride-rich lipoproteins (TRL), i.e., chylomicrons, chylomicron remnants and VLDL-lipoproteins, are atherogenic and since these lipoproteins predominantly occur in the postprandial state, the importance of postprandial lipid handling should be evaluated and related to the occurrence of CVD *(51)*. Several recent studies have also shown an association between postprandial lipemia and CVD *(52,53)* and Type 2 diabetes *(54,55)*, also in subjects with fasting normotriglyceridemia, although the fasting triglyceride level is the major determinant for the degree of postprandial hypertriglyceridemia *(56)*. The close correlation between postprandial lipemia and insulin sensitivity in healthy subjects, demonstrated recently by Jeppesen et al. *(44)*, was recently verified in nonsmoking subjects *(25)*.

The mechanisms for the postprandial lipid intolerance are currently unclear. However, in a recent study using ApoB48, ApoB100 and retinyl palmitate determinations after a fat load, we found that smokers had markedly elevated chylomicrons, chylomicron remnants and VLDL1- and VLDL2-lipoprotein levels compared with nonsmoking control subjects *(57)*. These results show that smokers have an impairment in the clearance of TRL after a fat load, either caused by deficient LPL activity and/or impaired hepatic clearance via the LDL-receptor (small VLDL remnants and intermediate-density lipoproteins (IDL) particles) or LRP (LDL-receptor related protein; large VLDL-particles) pathways. There are no reports, however, demonstrating a decreased plasma LPL activity in smokers, although the LPL-lipoprotein interaction could possibly be altered in smokers because of abnormal lipoprotein composition. Furthermore, adipose tissue LPL activity, which has been shown to be high in smokers but with an abnormal response to glucose/insulin *(40,42)*, could possibly contribute to an impaired postprandial TRL removal.

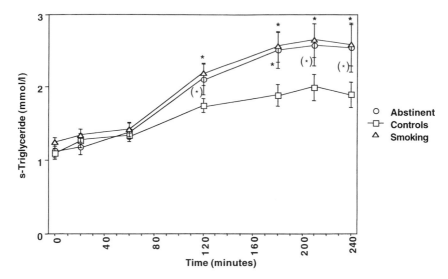

Fig. 2. Postprandial triglyceride levels in nonsmokers and smokers. The smokers were examined while smoking and after two days of smoking abstinence. (From ref. *50.* With permission from *Journal of Internal Medicine.*)

Recent data suggest that hepatic insulin resistance, leading to a decreased ability of insulin to suppress endogenous VLDL-lipoprotein production, can be an important reason for the increased TRL levels in IRS *(58–60)*. A similar mechanism could also exist in the smokers, since the VLDL1- and VLDL2-lipoprotein levels are clearly higher than in a matched group of nonsmoking control subjects *(57)*.

Effects of Nicotine Replacement Therapy

Nicotine replacement therapy (NRT) is an effective aid for smoking cessation (61). Long-term use of smoke-free tobacco (e.g., moist snuff) is associated with a lower risk for cardiovascular disease than smoking, although the relative risk in snuff users is higher than in nonsmokers (62), and the risk for hypertension is markedly elevated compared with both smokers and nonsmokers (6). However, the metabolic effects of NRT and smoke-free tobacco use are not well studied, although there is reason to believe that they are not metabolically neutral since intravenously administered nicotine elicits several responses, including similar neuroendocrine effects as smoking (63).

In a recent study, 20 long-term nicotine gum chewers (NGC; nicotine gum use >11 months) were compared with 20 nonsmoking control subjects, who were carefully selected to have similar ranges of age, BMI and BF, and who had not regularly smoked or consumed nicotine in any form for >20 yr *(39)*.

NGCs had significantly higher WHR than the nonsmokers. The NGC had higher plasminogen activator inhibitor 1 (PAI-1) activity, fasting insulin, and C-peptide levels but lower degree of insulin sensitivity as measured with the euglycemic hyperinsulinemic clamp. During the clamp, the NGC suppressed the FFA and C-peptide levels less than the nonsmoking control subjects and the steady-state levels of insulin were also higher in NGC.

Plasma cotinine levels, a measure of the extent of long-term nicotine use, were significantly and negatively correlated to degree of insulin sensitivity (Fig. 3). BF, alcohol and

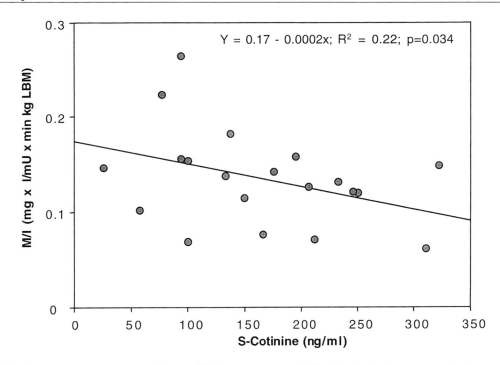

Fig. 3. Regression plot: Insulin sensitivity vs serum cotinine levels in long-term nicotine gum chewers. (From ref. *39.*)

nicotine consumption were analyzed in a multiple linear regression analysis where the insulin sensitivity index was used as the dependent variable. The regression model was statistically significant and showed that nicotine use and percent BF were negatively related to insulin sensitivity while alcohol use was positively correlated *(39).*

Only two studies have appeared on the acute effects of NRT or smoke-free tobacco on glucose metabolism. Epifano et al. examined the effects of nicotine patches in Type 2 diabetic patients with the euglycemic hyperinsulinemic clamp technique and found similar results as after smoking, i.e., impaired glucose utilization and storage, although to a lesser degree *(24).*

However, Attvall et al. did not find the same impairment in insulin sensitivity after one portion of bag-packed moist snuff per hour as after smoking one cigaret per hour for six hours *(22).* A possible cause for this discrepancy may be the differences in pharmacokinetics. Inhaled cigaret smoke and nicotine reach the brain at high peak concentrations and exert an effect within seconds, while nicotine absorbed via the oral mucosa is transported via the venous blood to the liver and, thereafter, reaches the brain at a lower concentration *(64).*

Effects of Smoking Cessation

Smoking cessation has dramatic effects on risk for mortality from all causes in men and women *(3,65).* The risk for Type 2 diabetes is also lower in previous compared with current smokers *(66,67).*

Ex-smokers have normal HDL-cholesterol levels *(68)* and a rapid improvement in HDL-cholesterol after SC has been verified in several studies *(69,70),* although changes in diet after SC may also contribute *(71)*. Reports on positive effects of SC on LDL-cholesterol levels are scarce *(72)*. Fibrinogen and other rheologic factors normalize after SC *(73)* and resting arterial blood pressure increases *(72,74)*.

Studies on the effects of SC on glucose, insulin, C-peptide levels or insulin sensitivity are also scarce, but a recent study in healthy middle-aged men and women did not report any significant changes in these variables four months after SC *(69)*. However, no direct measurement of insulin sensitivity was performed. The absence of consistent beneficial changes may be related to divergent effects on insulin sensitivity, i.e., potential divergent effects of an increased body weight vs SC *per se*. Furthermore, the results may be influenced by the use of NRT following SC.

In a recent study from our laboratory we examined the effects of SC *(75)*. Seventeen smokers were examined before and after SC for eight weeks, while 23 smokers were unable to stop smoking and served as control (smoking) subjects in the calculations.

SC was associated with increased insulin sensitivity and increased levels of HDL-cholesterol as well as Apoproteins A-I and A-II in spite of a concomitant modest 2.7 kg increase in body weight. The initial cotinine levels, reflecting smoking habits, were positively correlated to increases in HDL-cholesterol and BMI following SC. The increase in BF was positively correlated to increases in Glucose infusion rate (GIR) and HDL-cholesterol. Thus, the greater the initial nicotine consumption, the greater the increases in BMI and percent BF as well as in HDL-cholesterol, Apoproteins A-I, A-II, and insulin sensitivity after SC *(75)*. These results clearly document that SC leads to divergent effects but the repercussions of a modest increase in body weight is more than compensated for by the beneficial effects of stopping smoking.

In a large prospective study, the weight gain after SC for more than one year was 2.8 kg in men and 3.8 kg in women, after adjustment for environmental factors *(76)*. In that study, initial body weight was related to the extent of weight gain. Although the smokers initially weighed less than the nonsmokers, their weights after SC were approximately the same as for the subjects who had never smoked *(76)*.

The increase in body weight after SC has been attributed to an increased body fat due to a reduced resting metabolic rate and an increased caloric intake *(77,78)*. The weight increase correlates to initial weight, physical activity and smoking habits *(79)*. Dietary changes also occur after SC and studies have documented both increased or unchanged caloric intake *(79–81)*.

POTENTIAL MECHANISMS OF ACTION

Several neuroendocrine and circulatory effects can be registered after cigaret smoking. Acute smoking activates several neurohumoral pathways and increases circulating levels of adrenaline, noradrenaline, cortisol and growth hormone (GH), as well as β-endorphin, acetylcholine, dopamine, serotonin, vasopressin and ACTH *(35,63)*.

There are several studies emphasizing the importance of the increased catecholamine levels after smoking. In one study, the energy expenditure was increased by approximately 10% in smokers compared with nonsmokers when examined under standardized conditions in a metabolic chamber *(82)*. In that study, the urinary excretion rate of noradrenaline was notably elevated during smoking compared with nonsmoking conditions. These findings may contribute to the lower body weight in smokers, although the role of total body energy expenditure for the long-term control of body weight is not well defined.

In an interesting study by Cryer et al. *(35)* some of the acute effects of cigaret smoking, i.e., increased pulse rate and blood pressure, blood glycerol and lactate/pyruvate ratio, were prevented by adrenergic blockade. The effects on pulse rate and blood pressure by smoking actually preceded the increases in plasma levels of catecholamines, suggestive of an immediate action on peripheral nerve terminals as a mechanism of action *(35)*. The increments in cortisol and GH levels were not prevented by adrenergic blockade.

Further support for the concept that smoking alters the activity of the sympathetic nervous system was supplied by Grassi et al. who recently showed that smoking-induced increases in heart rate, arterial blood pressure, calf vascular resistance and catecholamine levels are accompanied by a marked reduction in muscle sympathetic nerve activity *(4)*. These data suggest that there are regional differences in the activation of the sympathetic nervous system. Alternatively, the effect of smoking is due to an increased release and/ or impaired clearance of catecholamines in the peripheral nerve junctions, while the central sympathetic activity is decreased, presumably due to baroreceptor stimulation following the pressor effect of smoking.

Several other effects of smoking on vascular and hemostatic function have been demonstrated, most of which indicate a pro-atherothrombotic state in smoking individuals. These perturbations include activated platelets *(83)*, increased levels of von Willebrand factor *(84)*, increased white blood cell count and levels of PAI-1 activity *(69,83,85)*.

From the data discussed it is clear that cigaret smoking and long-term nicotine consumption are associated with insulin resistance, hyperinsulinemia and a relative glucose intolerance *(18,21–23,25,27,39)*. This may be caused by direct or indirect effects on intracellular insulin-signaling and action.

Nicotine may have direct or indirect effects via interactions with the insulin receptor and/or postreceptor events. Such effects could, for instance, be mediated via the neuroendocrine cascade elicited by smoking, i.e., increased release of catecholamines, cortisol, GH, somatostatin, vasopressin and possibly other substances *(63)*. Chronically elevated catecholamine levels may be particularly relevant in this context. It is well known that catecholamines, via increased levels of cyclic AMP (cAMP) *(57)* reduce the number of binding sites for insulin as well as influence the normal intracellular sequence of events following insulin receptor tyrosine kinase activation. Furthermore, the translocation of functional intracellular glucose transporters (GLUT4) to the plasma membrane as well as the synthesis of GLUT4 are impaired by chronically elevated catecholamine levels (Reviewed in *[86]*). There may also be other indirect effects of smoking/nicotine via, for instance, elevated levels of FFA which impair insulin-mediated glucose uptake *(87)*.

SMOKING VS CONFOUNDING FACTORS

In agreement with the concept that smoking/nicotine elicits insulin resistance, large surveys have demonstrated two- to fourfold increased risk for Type 2 diabetes mellitus in smoking men and women *(66,67,88)*. Furthermore, for the patients with Type 1 or Type 2 diabetes mellitus, cigaret smoking dramatically increases the risk for the diabetes-related complications, i.e., nephropathy, neuropathy and retinopathy as well as for macrovascular disease *(89)*.

Insulin sensitivity is modulated by a number of other life-style factors like physical activity, fitness *(90)* and obesity in addition to a genetic predisposition *(91)*.

The effects on the cardiovascular risk factors by a sedentary lifestyle are well-known; increased risk for obesity, dyslipidemia and glucose intolerance. The beneficial effects

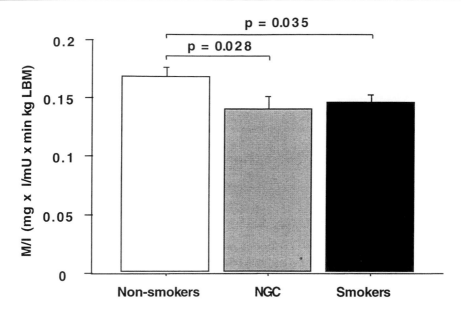

Fig. 4. Insulin sensitivity in smokers and long-term users of nicotine gum (NGC). (Data from refs. *25* and *39*.)

of a physically active lifestyle on cardiovascular risk factors have also been documented including the recent large survey by Blair et al. *(92)*. Physical fitness was actually shown to override the adverse effects of smoking or other risk factors such as cholesterol levels, blood pressure and health status. In the same study, the age-adjusted relative risk, compared with a low-risk group, for mortality from all causes was 1.89 and 2.12 in smoking men and women, respectively, while the same risk score was 1.33 and 1.18, respectively, in individuals with BMI > 27.

Dietary habits seem to be different in smokers compared with nonsmokers *(93,94)*. Smokers consume more saturated fat and short-chain carbohydrates. After SC some temporary dietary changes occur *(81)*, possibly increasing the energy intake *(78)*. Several studies have shown that individuals who quit smoking have an increased urge for sweets and snacks *(81)*. However, the extent to which modest changes in the diet *per se* can influence insulin sensitivity is unclear *(95–97)*.

Alcohol consumption, on the other hand, has very clear effects on cardiovascular risk factors and moderate consumers of alcohol have a lower cardiovascular risk *(98,99)*, higher HDL-cholesterol levels *(100)* as well as insulin sensitivity than individuals who do not drink alcohol at all *(101)*. Also other environmental factors could conceivably play a role for degree of insulin sensitivity. These include psychological stress, unemployment and socio-economic class but their direct effects on metabolic variables have not been evaluated.

IMPLICATIONS

As discussed above and shown in Fig. 4, cigaret smoking and long-term nicotine consumption are associated with insulin resistance and IRS *(23,25,39)*, the degree of which is positively correlated to smoking habits and nicotine consumption *(27,39)*. SC for eight weeks significantly improves degree of insulin resistance and lipoprotein levels in spite of a concomitant 2.7 kg weight gain *(75)*. This weight gain is positively correlated to initial smoking habits as well as the degree of improvement in the metabolic variables. These findings are consistent with our estimate that a comparable impairment in insulin sensitivity as that elicited by smoking requires a body weight gain of at least 6.5 kg. Thus, a lesser gain in body weight following SC is also expected to lead to an improved insulin sensitivity.

The various components of IRS, i.e., hyperinsulinemia, hypertriglyceridemia, low HDL-cholesterol and elevated PAI-1 activity levels, are all established risk factors for CVD *(102–106)*. Since cigaret smoking is related to IRS it would be important to establish to which extent the smoking-associated insulin resistance and IRS can account for the increased cardiovascular risk. This risk, in turn, is two- to threefold higher in moderately smoking men and women compared with nonsmokers *(8,107,108)*.

No study has addressed this question and such calculations are also difficult to perform because of the close interrelationships between the metabolic variables. However, recent studies have shown that a 20% or 1 S.D. increase in fasting insulin levels are associated with odds ratios of 1.2 and 1.7, respectively, for ischemic heart disease in nondiabetic middle-aged men *(103,104)*. Data from the Framingham study demonstrate that the risk for CVD increases with 3–4% for every percent lower HDL-cholesterol value in men and women *(106)*. It has also recently been reported from the Helsinki Heart Study that the relative risk for cardiac events during five years follow-up, after correction for age and smoking, is 2.7 in individuals with triglyceride levels >2.3 mmol/L and HDL-cholesterol <1.12 mmol/L *(109)*. In middle-aged men, PAI-1 antigen levels correlate with early atherosclerosis measured by carotid ultrasonography (odds ratios 1.2, 1.5 and 1.6 in second, third and fourth quartiles of PAI-1 antigen levels) *(105)*. Since 1960 the mean BMI in 50–59-yr-old US men has increased from 25.6 to 27.6 kg/m^2 *(110)*. This has caused the prevalence of obesity to increase from 25.6% to 42.1%, if obesity is defined as BMI > 27.8 kg/m^2 *(110)*. The risk for Type 2 diabetes mellitus increases with degree of obesity; the relative risk for diabetes is more than 13-fold higher in men with BMI > 27.0 kg/m^2 than in nonobese subjects (BMI < 23 kg/m^2) *(111)*.

The risk for diabetes in smokers is elevated compared with nonsmokers also after adjustment for age and BMI, as already pointed out *(66,67,88,112,113)*. In middle-aged men, for instance, the age-adjusted relative risk is doubled compared with nonsmokers during six years *(66)*. However, smokers have lower body weight than nonsmokers but after smoking cessation their weight increases by about 2.8 kg discussed above *(75,76)*. This normalizes body weight when compared to individuals who have never smoked *(76)*.

Does the lower body weight in smokers then exert a significant protection from risk of developing diabetes? As expected from the discussion above this does not seem to be the case, since Rimm et al. showed that the risk for diabetes was actually higher (relative risk 3.3; nonobese nonsmokers relative risk 1) in smoking subjects with BMI less than 27.8 kg/m^2 than in nonsmoking obese subjects with BMI > 27.8 kg/m^2 (relative risk 1.7) *(66)*. Furthermore, the authors conclude: "Though the relative risk of diabetes for smokers vs nonsmokers was not as large among the more obese men, the attributable risk was larger because rates of diabetes were much greater in obese men" *(66)*.

Since approximately one-third of the adult population in the world are smokers *(1)*, we conclude that cigaret smoking must be a major global risk factor for Type 2 diabetes.

Thus, taken together, it seems quite likely that insulin resistance and IRS can explain most of the increased risk for CVD and Type 2 diabetes in smokers, as well as the elevated risk for cardiovascular complications in smoking diabetic subjects *(89)*. It has also been shown that smoking diabetic patients have slightly higher HbA1c-levels in spite of higher insulin doses compared with nonsmoking Type 1 diabetes patients *(114,115)*. This finding is in agreement with an enhanced insulin resistance also in diabetic subjects who smoke.

The results of studies reviewed in this paper also provide support for the hypothesis that nicotine is the main responsible agent in smoke for the metabolic aberrations. Nicotine administration has been shown to cause increased FFA and glycerol levels, suggesting increased lipolysis *(34)*, as well as acute cardiovascular effects, including pulse rate and blood pressure increases *(63,116)*. Furthermore, epidemiological studies have demonstrated an increased risk for CVD and hypertension in users of moist snuff *(6,62)*. Studies evaluating the acute and long-term metabolic effects of smoke-free nicotine are scarce. However, the present and other available data show that long-term use of smoke-free nicotine is associated with insulin resistance and IRS. Thus, although nicotine replacement therapy during the nicotine abstinence phase in smoking cessation can be helpful it should both be transient and of limited extent.

REFERENCES

1. Collishaw NE, Lopez AD. The tobacco epidemic: A global public health emergency. In: Geneva, Switzerland: WHO. Available at online URL: http://www.who.ch/programmes/psa/toh/alert. 1996, pp. 1–28.
2. McGinnis JM, Foege WH. Actual causes of death in the United States. JAMA 1993;270:2207–2012.
3. Doll R, Peto R, Wheatley K, Gray R, Sutherland I. Mortality in relation to smoking: 40 years' observations on male British doctors. BMJ 1994;309:901–911.
4. Grassi G, Seravalle G, Calhoun DA, Bolla GB, Giannattasio C, Marabini M, et al. Mechanisms responsible for sympathetic activation by cigarette smoking in humans. Circulation 1994;90:248–253.
5. Green MS, Jucha E, Luz Y. Blood pressure in smokers and nonsmokers: Epidemiologic findings. Am Heart J 1986;111:932–939.
6. Bolinder GM, Ahlborg BO, Lindell JH. Use of smokeless tobacco: blood pressure elevation and other health hazards found in a large-scale population survey. J Intern Med 1992;232:327–334.
7. Craig WY, Palomaki GE, Haddow JE. Cigarette smoking and serum lipid and lipoprotein concentrations: An analysis of published data. BMJ 1989;298:784–788.
8. Kannel WB, D'Agostino RB, Belanger AJ. Fibrinogen, cigarette smoking and risk of cardiovascular disease: Insights from the Framingham study. Am Heart J 1987;113:1006–1010.
9. Ernst E, Resch KL. Fibrinogen as a cardiovascular risk factor: A meta-analysis and review of the literature. Ann Intern Med 1993;118:956–963.
10. Kool MJ, Hoeks AP, Struijker BHA, Reneman RS, Van BLM. Short- and long-term effects of smoking on arterial wall properties in habitual smokers. J Am Coll Cardiol 1993;22:1881–1886.
11. Crouse J, Toole J, McKinney W, Dignan M. Risk factors for extracranial carotid artery atherosclerosis. Stroke 1987;18:990–996.
12. Dempsey RJ, Moore RW. Amount of smoking independently predicts carotid artery atherosclerosis severity. Stroke 1992;23:693–696.
13. Lassila HC, Tyrrell KS, Matthews KA, Wolfson SK, Kuller LH. Prevalence and determinants of carotid atherosclerosis in healthy postmenopausal women. Stroke 1997;28:513–517.
14. Lissner L, Bengtsson C, Lapidus L, Björkelund C. Smoking initiation and cessation in relation to body fat distribution based on data from a study of Swedish women. Am J Public Health, 82:273–275.
15. Shimokata H, Muller DC, Andres R. (1989).Studies in the distribution of fat: Effects of cigarette smoking. JAMA 1992;261:1169–1173.
16. Lapidus L, Bengtsson C, Larsson B, Pennert K, Rybo E, Sjöström L. Distribution of adipose tissue and risk of cardiovascular disease and death: A 12 year follow up of participants in the population study of women in Gothenburg, Sweden. BMJ 1984;289:1257–1261.

17. Troisi RJ, Heinold JW, Vokonas PS, Weiss ST. Cigarette smoking, dietary intake and physical activity: Effects on body fat distribution-the Normative Aging Study. Am J Clin Nutr 1991;53:1104–1111.

18. Zavaroni I, Bonini L, Gasparini P, Dall'Aglio E, Passeri M, Reaven GM. Cigarette smokers are relatively glucose intolerant, hyperinsulinemic and dyslipidemic. Am J Cardiol 1994;73:904–905.

19. Eliasson M, Lundblad D, Hägg E. Cardiovascular risk factors in young snuff-users and cigarette smokers. J Intern Med 1991;230:17–22.

20. Rönnemaa T, Rönnemaa EM, Puukka P, Pyörälä K, Laakso M. Smoking is independently associated with high plasma insulin levels in nondiabetic men. Diabetes Care 1996;19:1229–1132.

21. Frati AC, Iniestra F, Raul Ariza C. Acute effect of cigarette smoking on glucose tolerance and other cardiovascular risk factors. Diabetes Care 1996;19:112–118.

22. Attvall S, Fowelin J, Lager I, von Schenck H, Smith U. Smoking induces insulin resistance—A potential link with the insulin resistance syndrome. J Intern Med 1993;233:327–332.

23. Facchini FS, Hollenbeck CB, Jeppesen J, Chen Y-DI, Reaven GM. Insulin resistance and cigarette smoking. Lancet 1992;339:1128–1130.

24. Epifano L, Di Vincenzo A, Fanelli C, Porcellati F, Perriello G, De Feo P, et al. Effect of cigarette smoking and of a transdermal nicotine delivery system on glucoregulation in type 2 diabetes mellitus. Eur J Clin Pharmacol 1992;43:257–263.

25. Eliasson B, Mero N, Taskinen M-R, Smith U. The insulin resistance syndrome and postprandial lipid intolerance in smokers. Atherosclerosis 1997;129:79–88.

26. DeFronzo RA, Tobin JD, Andres R. Glucose clamp technique: A method for quantifying insulin secretion and resistance. Am J Physiol 1979;237:E214–E223.

27. Eliasson B, Attvall S, Taskinen MR, Smith U. The insulin resistance syndrome in smokers is related to smoking habits. Arterioscl Thromb 1994;14:1946–1950.

28. Godsland IF, Wynn V, Walton C, Stevenson JC. Insulin resistance and cigarette smoking :letter. Lancet 1992;339:1619–1620.

29. Godsland IF, Walton C, Felton C, Proudler A, Patel A, Wynn V. Insulin resistance, secretion and metabolism in users of oral contraceptives. J Clin Endocrinol Metab 1992;74:64–70.

30. Targher G, Alberiche M, Zenere MB, Bonadonna RC, Muggeo M, Bonora E. Cigarette smoking and insulin resistance in patients with noninsulin-dependent diabetes mellitus. J Clin Endocrinol Metab 1997;82:3619–3624.

31. Helve E, Yki-Järvinen H, Koivisto VA. Smoking and insulin sensitivity in type I diabetic patients. Metabolism 1986;35:874–877.

32. Nilsson PM, Lind L, Pollare T, Berne C, Lithell HO. Increased levels of Hemoglobin A1c, but not impaired insulin sensitivity, found in hypertensive and normotensive smokers. Metabolism 1995;44:557–561.

33. Pollare T, Lithell H, Berne C. Insulin resistance is a characteristic feature of primary hypertension independant of obesity. Metabolism 1990;39:167–174.

34. Andersson K, Eneroth P, Arner P. Changes in circulating lipid and carbohydrate metabolites following systemic nicotine treatment in healthy men. Int J Obesity 1993;17:675–680.

35. Cryer PE, Haymond MW, Santiago JV, Shah SD. Norepinephrine and epinephrine release and adrenergic mediation of smoking-associated hemodynamic and metabolic events. N Engl J Med 1976;295:573–577.

36. Hellerstein MK, Benowitz NL, Neese RA, Schwartz J-M, Hoh R, Jacob P, III, et al. Effects of cigarette smoking and its cessation on lipid metabolism and energy expenditure in heavy smokers. J Clin Invest 1994;93:265–272.

37. Kershbaum A, Bellet S, Dickstein ER, Feinberg LJ. Effect of cigarette smoking and nicotine on serum fatty acids. Based on a study in the human subject and the experimental animal. Circ Res 1961;9:631–638.

38. Kershbaum A, Khorsandian R, Caplan RF, Bellet S, Feinberg LJ. The role of catecholamines in the free fatty acid respons to cigarette smoking. Circulation 1963;28:52–57.

39. Eliasson B, Taskinen M-R, Smith U. Long-term use of nicotine gum is associated with hyperinsulinemia and insulin resistance. Circulation 1996;94:878–881.

40. Brunzell JD, Goldberg AP, Schwartz RS. Cigarette smoking and adipose tissue lipoprotein lipase. Int J Obesity 1980;4:101–103.

41. Carney RM, Goldberg AP. Weight gain after cessation of cigarette smoking. A possible role for adipose-tissue lipoprotein lipase. N Engl J Med 1984;310:614–616.

42. Chajek-Shaul, Berry EM, Ziv E, Friedman G, Stein O, Sherer G, et al. Smoking depresses adipose lipoprotein lipase response to oral glucose. Eur J Clin Invest 1990;20:299–304.

43. Pollare T, Vessby B, Lithell H. Lipoprotein lipase activity in skeletal muscle is related to insulin sensitivity. Arterioscl Thromb 1991;11:1192–1203.
44. Jeppesen J, Hollenbeck CB, Zhou M-Y, Coulston AM, Jones C, Chen Y-DI, et al. Relation between insulin resistance, hyperinsulinemia, postheparin plasma lipoprotein lipase activity, and postprandial lipemia. Arterioscl Thromb Vasc Biol 1995;15:320–324.
45. Bielicki JK, McCall MR, van den Berg JJM, Kuypers FA, Forte TM. Copper and gas-phase cigarette smoke inhibit plasma lecithin:cholesterol acyltransferase activity by different mechanisms. J Lipid Res 1995;36:322–331.
46. Dullaart RP, Groener JE, Dikkeschei BD, Erkelens DW, Doorenbos H. Elevated cholesteryl ester transfer protein activity in IDDM men who smoke. Possible factor for unfavorable lipoprotein profile. Diabetes Care 1991;14:338–341.
47. Dullaart RP, Hoogenberg K, Dikkeschei BD, van Tol A. Higher plasma lipid transfer protein activities and unfavorable lipoprotein changes in cigarette-smoking men. Arterioscl Thromb 1994; 14:1581–1585.
48. Hannuksela ML, Liinamaa MJ, Kesäniemi YA, Savolainen MJ. Relation of polymorphisms in the cholesteryl ester transfer protein gene to transfer protein activity and plasma lipoprotein levels in alcohol drinkers. Atherosclerosis 1994;110:35–44.
49. McCall MR, van den Berg JJ, Kuypers FA, Tribble DL, Krauss RM, Knoff LJ, et al. Modification of LCAT activity and HDL structure. New links between cigarette smoke and coronary heart disease risk. Arterioscl Thromb 1994;14:248–253.
50. Axelsen M, Eliasson B, Joheim T, Lenner R, Taskinen M-R, Smith U. Lipid intolerance in smokers. J Intern Med 1995;237:449–455.
51. Zilversmit DB. Atherogenesis: A postprandial phenomenon. Circulation 1979;60:473–485.
52. Karpe F. Alimentary lipemia and coronary atherosclerosis . Stockholm, Sweden: King Gustaf V research institute and Karolinska institute, University of Stockholm; 1992.
53. Patsch W, Sharrett AR, Sorlie PD, Davis CE, Brown SA. The relation of high density lipoprotein cholesterol and its subfractions to apolipoprotein A-I and fasting triglycerides: the role of environmental factors. The Atherosclerosis Risk in Communities (ARIC) Study. Am J Epidemiol 1992;136:546–557.
54. Chen Y-DI, Swami S, Skowronski R, Coulston A, Reaven G. Differences in postprandial lipemia between patients with normal glucose tolerance and noninsulin dependent diabetes mellitus. J Clin Endocrinol Metab 1993;76:172–177.
55. Syvänne M, Hilden H, Taskinen M-R. Abnormal metabolism of postprandial lipoproteins in patients with non-insulin-dependent diabetes mellitus is not related to coronary artery disease. J Lipid Res 1994;35:15–26.
56. Patsch JR, Miesenböck G, Hopferwieser T, Mühlberger V, Knapp E, Dunn JK, et al. Relation of triglyceride metabolism and coronary artery disease. Studies in the postprandial state. Arterioscl Thromb 1992;12:1336–1345.
57. Mero N, Syvänne M, Eliasson B, Smith U, Taskinen M-R. Postprandial elevation of Apo B-48-containing triglyceride rich particles and retinyl palmitate in normolipemic men who smoke. Arterioscl Thromb Vasc Biol 1997;17:2096–2102.
58. Lewis GF, Uffelman KD, Szeto LW, Steiner G. Effects of acute hyperinsulinemia on VLDL triglyceride and VLDL apoB production in normal weight and obese individuals. Diabetes 1993;42:833–842.
59. Malmström R, Packard CJ, Caslake M, Bedford D, Stewart P, Shepard J, et al. Defective suppression of VLDL1 Apo B production by insulin is an inherent feature of dyslipidemia in NIDDM. Diabetologia 1996;39(Suppl 1):A65:238.
60. Naoumova RP, Cummings MH, Watts GF, Rendell NB, Taylor GW, Sönksen PH, et al. Acute hyperinsulinaemia decreases cholesterol synthesis less in subjects with non-insulin-dependent diabetes mellitus than in non-diabetic subjects. Eur J Clin Invest 1996;26:332–340.
61. Silagy C, Mant D, Fowler G, Lodge M. Meta-analysis on efficacy of nicotine replacement therapies in smoking cessation. Lancet 1994;343:139–142.
62. Bolinder G, Alfredsson L, Englund A, de Faire U. Smokeless tobacco use and increased cardiovascular mortality among Swedish construction workers. Am J Public Health 1994;84:399–404.
63. Benowitz NL. Pharmacologic aspects of cigarette smoking and nicotine addiction. N Engl J Med 1988;319:1318–1330.
64. Svensson CK. Clinical pharmacokinetics of nicotine. Clin Pharmacokinetics 1987;12:30–40.

65. Kawachi I, Colditz GA, Stampfer MJ, Willett WC, Manson JE, Rosner B, et al. Smoking cessation in relation to total mortality rates in women. A prospective cohort study. Ann Intern Med 1993;119:992–1000.

66. Rimm EB, Chan J, Stampfer MJ, Colditz GA, Willett WC. Prospective study of cigarette smoking, alcohol use, and the risk of diabetes in men. BMJ 1995;310:555–559.

67. Rimm EB, Manson JE, Stampfer MJ, Colditz GA, Willett WC, Rosner B, et al. Cigarette smoking and the risk of diabetes in women. Am J Public Health 1993;83:211–214.

68. Brischetto CS, Connor WE, Connor SL, Matarazzo JD. Plasma lipid and lipoprotein profiles of cigarette smokers from randomly selected families: enhancement of hyperlipidemia and depression of high-density lipoprotein. Am J Cardiol 1983;52:675–680.

69. Nilsson P, Lundgren H, Söderström M, Fagerström K-O, Nilsson-Ehle P. Effects of smoking cessation on insulin and cardiovascular risk factors—A controlled study of 4 months duration. J Intern Med 1996;240:189–194.

70. Stubbe I, Eskilsson J, Nilsson-Ehle P. High-density lipoprotein concentrations increase after stopping smoking. BMJ 1982;284:1511–1513.

71. Quensel M, Söderström A, Agardh CD, Nilsson-Ehle P. High density lipoprotein concentrations after cessation of smoking: The importance of alterations in diet. Atherosclerosis 1989;75:189–193.

72. Terres W, Becker P, Rosenberg A. Changes in cardiovascular risk profile during the cessation of smoking. Am J Med 1994;97:242–249.

73. Ernst E, Matrai A. Abstention from chronic cigarette smoking normalizes blood rheology. Atherosclerosis 1987;64:75–77.

74. Seltzer CC. Effect of smoking on blood pressure. Am Heart J 1974;87:558–564.

75. Eliasson B, Attvall S, Taskinen M-R, Smith U. Smoking cessation improves insulin sensitivity in healthy middle-aged men. Eur J Clin Invest 1997;27:450–456.

76. Williamson DF, Madans J, Anda RF, Kleinman JC, Giovino GA, Byers T. Smoking cessation and severity of weight gain in a national cohort. N Engl J Med 1991;324:739–745.

77. Dallosso HM, James WPT. The role of smoking in the regulation of energy balance. Int J Obesity 1984;8:365–375.

78. Moffatt RJ, Owens SG. Cessation from cigarette smoking: changes in body weight, body composition, resting metabolism and energy consumption. Metabolism 1991;40:465–470.

79. Gerace TA, Hollis J, Ockene JK, Svendsen K. Smoking cessation and change in diastolic blood pressure, body weight, and plasma lipids. Prev Med 1991;20:602–620.

80. Hall SM, McGee R, Tunstall C, Duffy J, Benowitz N. Changes in food intake and activity after quitting smoking. J Consult Clin Psychol 1989;57:81–86.

81. Rodin J. Weight change following smoking cessation: The role of food intake and exercise. Addict Behav 1987;12:303–317.

82. Hofstetter A, Schutz Y, Jéquier E, Wahren J. Increased 24-hour energy expenditure in cigarette smokers. N Engl J Med 1986;314:79–82.

83. Dotevall A, Rångemark C, Eriksson E, Kutti J, Wadenvik H, Wennmalm Å. Cigarette smoking increases thromboxane A2 formation without affecting platelet survival in healthy young females. Thromb Haemost 1992;68:583–588.

84. Blann AD, McCollum CN. Adverse influence of cigarette smoking on the endothelium. Thromb Hemost 1993;70:707–711.

85. Haire WD, Goldsmith JC, Rasmussen J. Abnormal fibrinolysis in healthy male cigarette smokers: Role of plasminogen activator inhibitors. Am J Hematol 1989;31:36–40.

86. Smith U, Attvall S, Eriksson J, Fowelin J, Lönnroth P, Wesslau C. The insulin-antagonistic effect of the counterregulatory hormones—Clinical and mechanistic aspects. In: Östenson CG, Efendic S, Vranic M, eds. New concepts in the pathogenesis of NIDDM. Plenum, New York, 1992, pp. 169–180.

87. Boden G, Chen X, Ruiz J, White JV, Rossetti L. Mechanisms of fatty acid-induced inhibition of glucose uptake. J Clin Invest 1994;93:2438–2446.

88. Feskens EJM, Kromhout D. Cardiovascular risk factors and the 25-year incidence of diabetes mellitus in middle-aged men. The Zutphen study. Am J Epidemiol 1989;130:1101–1108.

89. Mühlhauser I. Cigarette smoking and diabetes: An update. Diabetic Med 1994;11:336–343.

90. Rosenthal M, Haskell WL, Solomon R, Widstrom A, Reaven GM. Demonstration of a relationship between level of physical training and insulin-stimulated glucose utilization in normal humans. Diabetes 1983;32:408–411.

91. Reaven GM. Pathophysiology of insulin resistance in human disease. Physiol Rev 1995;75:473–486.
92. Blair SN, Kampert JB, Kohl HW, III, Barlow CE, Macera CA, Paffenberger RS, et al. Influences of cardiorespiratory fitness and other precursors on cardiovascular disease and all-cause mortality in men and women. JAMA 1996;276:205–210.
93. Margetts BM, Jackson AA. Interactions between people´s diet and their smoking habits: The dietary and nutritional survey of British adults. BMJ 1993;307:1381–1384.
94. Nuttens MC, Romon M, Ruidavets JB, Arveiler D, Ducimetiere P, Lecerf JM, et al. Relationship between smoking and diet: The MONICA-France project. J Intern Med 1992;231:349–356.
95. Feskens EJM, Virtanen SM, Räsänen L, Tuomilehto J, Stengård J, Pekkanen J, et al. Dietary factors determining diabetes and impaired glucose tolerance. Diabetes Care 1995;18:1104–1112.
96. Storlien LH, Baur LA, Kriketos AD, Pan DA, Cooney GJ, Jenkins AB, et al. Dietary fats and insulin action. Diabetologia 1996;39:621–631.
97. Willett WC. Diet and health: what should we eat? Science 1994;264:532–537.
98. Doll R, Peto R, Hall E, Wheatley K, Gary R. Mortality in relation to consumption of alcohol: 13 years' observations on male British doctors. BMJ 1994;309:911–918.
99. Fuchs CS, Stampfer MJ, Colditz GA, Giovannucci EL, Manson JE, Kawachi I, et al. Alcohol consumption and mortality among women. N Engl J Med 1995;332:1245–1250.
100. Gaziano JM, Buring JE, Breslow JL, Goldhaber SZ, Rosner B, VanDenburgh M, et al. Moderate alcohol intake, increased levels of high-density lipoprotein and its subfractions and decreased risk of myocardial infarction. N Engl J Med 1993;329:1829–1834.
101. Facchini F, Chen Y-DI, Reaven GM. Light-to-moderate alcohol intake is associated with enhanced insulin sensitivity. Diabetes Care 1994;17:115–119.
102. Assmann G, Schulte H. Relation of high-density lipoprotein cholesterol and triglycerides to incidence of atherosclerotic coronary artery disease (the PROCAM experience). Am J Cardiol 1992;70:733–737.
103. Després J-P, Lamarche B, Mauriège P, Cantin B, Dagenais GR, Moorjani S, et al. Hyperinsulinemia as an independent risk factor for ischemic heart disease. N Engl J Med 1996;334:952–957.
104. Katz RJ, R.E R, Cohen RM, Eisenhower E, Verme D. Are insulin and proinsulin independent risk markers for premature coronary artery disease? Diabetes 1996;45:736–741.
105. Salomaa V, Stinson V, Kark JD, Folsom AR, Davis CE, Wu KK. Association of fibrinolytic parameters with early atherosclerosis. The ARIC Study. Circulation 1995;91:284–290.
106. Wilson PWF. High-density lipoprotein, low-density lipoprotein and coronary artery disease. Am J Cardiol 1990;66:7A–10A.
107. Rosengren A, Wilhelmsen L, Wedel H. Coronary heart disease, cancer and mortality in male middle-aged smokers. J Intern Med 1992;231:357–362.
108. Slone D, Shapiro S, Rosenberg L, Kaufman DW, Hartz SC, Rossi AC, et al. Relation of cigarette smoking to myocardial infarction in young women. N Engl J Med 1978;298:1273–1276.
109. Tenkanen L, Pietila K, Manninen V, Manttari M. The triglyceride issue revisited. Findings from the Helsinki Heart Study. Arch Int Med 1994;154:2714–2720.
110. VanItallie TB. Prevalence of obesity. Endocrinol Metab Clin North Am 1996;25:887–905.
111. Chan JM, Rimm EB, Colditz GA, Stampfer MJ, Willett WC. Obesity, fat distribution, and the weight gain as risk factors for clinical diabetes in men. Diabetes Care 1994;17:961–969.
112. Kawakami N, Takatsuka N, Shimizu H, Ishibashi H. Effects of smoking on the incidence of non-insulin-dependent diabetes mellitus. Replication and extension in a Japanese cohort of male employees. Am J Epidemiol 1997;145:103–109.
113. Perry IJ, Wannamethee SG, Walker MK, Thomson AG, Whincup PH, Shaper AG. Prospective study of risk factors for development of non-insulin dependent diabetes in middle aged British men. BMJ 1995;310:560–564.
114. Bott U, Jörgens V, Grüsser M, Bender R, Mühlhauser I, Berger M. Predictors of glycemic control in type 1 diabetic patients after participation in an intensfied treatment and teaching programme. Diabetic Med 1994;11:362–371.
115. Lundman BM, Asplund K, Norberg A. Smoking and metabolic control in patients with insulin-dependent diabetes mellitus. J Intern Med 1990;227:101–106.
116. Roth GM, McDonald JB, Sheard C. The effect of smoking cigarettes and the intravenous administration of nicotine on the electrocardiogram, basal metabolic rate, cutaneous temperature, blood pressure and pulse rate of normal persons. JAMA 1944;125:761–767.

II   PATHOPHYSIOLOGY OF INSULIN RESISTANCE

8

Insulin Resistance and Inhibitors of Insulin Receptor Tyrosine Kinase

Jack F. Youngren, PhD, Ira D. Goldfine, MD, Vincenzo Trischitta, MD, and Betty A. Maddux, BS

Contents

Introduction
Signaling Through The Insulin Receptor
Diminished Insulin Action in Muscle and Adipose Tissues
Potential Sites for Cellular Insulin Resistance
Inhibitors of the Insulin Receptor Tyrosine Kinase
Characteristics of PC-1
Conclusion
References

INTRODUCTION

Noninsulin dependent diabetes mellitus (NIDDM or Type 2 diabetes mellitus) occurs in approximately 5% of the US population *(1)*. The vast majority of these patients display resistance to the biological actions of insulin *(2)*. Insulin resistance both precedes and contributes to the development of the diabetic state *(3,4)*. In addition to Type 2 diabetes patients, insulin resistance occurs in most patients with impaired glucose tolerance and some individuals with normal glucose tolerance *(1,4,5)*. In these people, normoglycemia is maintained by a compensatory hypersecretion of insulin. Progression to frank diabetes generally occurs when insulin secretion by the pancreatic β-cells is no longer sufficient to overcome the peripheral resistance to the hormone *(1)*. There are both genetic and acquired factors which can produce insulin resistance, and thus predispose an individual to Type 2 diabetes *(6)*. Obesity is the most common cause of acquired insulin resistance in Western Society. One-third to one-half of Americans are defined as overweight, and up to 80% of Type 2 diabetes patients are obese. Numerous studies have shown that insulin stimulated glucose disposal declines as a function of increasing obesity (Fig. 1) *(7)*.

Insulin resistance also occurs in a large number of normal weight individuals. Reaven and colleagues have produced compelling evidence that as much as 25% of the general,

From: *Contemporary Endocrinology: Insulin Resistance*
Edited by: G. Reaven and A. Laws © Humana Press Inc., Totowa, NJ

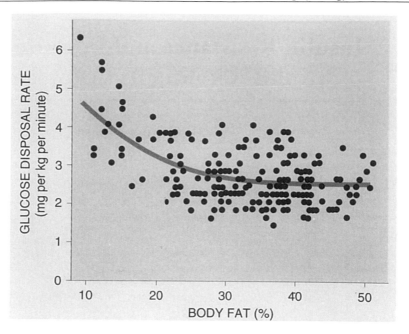

Fig. 1. Relationship between insulin action and obesity. Insulin activity measured as glucose disposal is plotted as % of body fat. Note while there is a correlation between these 2 variables at any degree of obesity. But, at any degree of obesity, there is a range of insulin action values suggesting that other factors are involved. From Science & Medicine 1997;4:18–27. Adapted from C. Bogandus (Diabetes Care 1993; Suppl 1:228–231).

nonobese population are just as insulin resistant as individuals with Type 2 diabetes *(5)*. While in lean subjects it can be difficult to separate the genetic and lifestyle contributions to insulin resistance, the evidence for a genetic component for insulin resistance is very strong. Lean offspring of Type 2 diabetes patients are themselves insulin resistant *(8)*. In families there is clustering of insulin sensitivity *(9,10)* (Fig. 2) and, studies of families and monozygotic (MZ) twins suggest that insulin resistance is an inherited trait *(11)*. Insulin resistance therefore appears to be an intrinsic characteristic of certain individuals.

In any individual, therefore, the degree of insulin sensitivity is determined by numerous factors, both genetic and environmental. It is unclear whether separate determinants of insulin resistance utilize similar mechanisms, or whether the various factors that influence insulin action might act through several distinct avenues. For all but a few genetic cases of severe insulin resistance the causal defects in the cellular insulin signaling pathway remain unknown *(12)*.

SIGNALING THROUGH THE INSULIN RECEPTOR

The cellular response to insulin is mediated through a specific tetrameric $\alpha_2\beta_2$ glycoprotein receptor in the plasma membrane (Fig. 3). The β-subunits contain the insulin binding domains. The β-subunits traverse the plasma membrane, and have tyrosine kinase activity in their intracellular domains *(13)*. When insulin binds to the α-subunit of the receptor, the β-subunit undergoes a conformational change that results in the autophosphorylation of several tyrosine residues on the β-subunit *(14)*. Full receptor

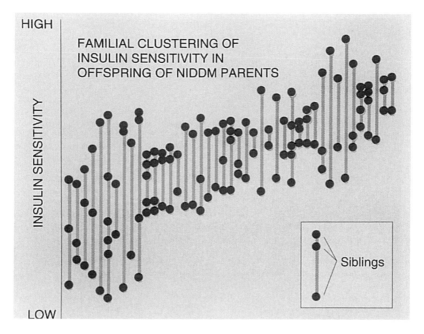

Fig. 2. Familial Clusters of insulin action in offspring of Type 2 diabetes patient. Insulin action measured as glucose disposal, is shown for multiple offspring of Type 2 diabetes patients. Note, while there is famial clustering, there is a range within each family suggesting other factors are involved. From Science & Medicine 1997;4:18–27. Adapted from B. C. Martin, et al. (Diabetes 1992;41:850–854)

autophosphorylation subsequently activates the protein tyrosine kinase activity of the receptor *(15)*. It has been shown that receptor autophosphorylation and tyrosine kinase activity are necessary for the cellular response to insulin *(14)*.

For related receptor tyrosine kinases such as the EGF receptor and the PDGF receptor, it has been demonstrated that intracellular adaptor and effector molecules attach to specific phosphorylated tyrosine residues of the receptors via the protein's Src homology 2 (SH2) domains (Fig. 3). In most intermediate signaling proteins, binding of SH2 domains leads to an activation of the signaling capacity of the protein *(16)*. In contrast, the majority of insulin receptor signaling events are mediated through insulin receptor substrate 1 (IRS-1), a 185 kD protein substrate for the insulin receptor tyrosine kinase activity *(17)*. IRS-1 has 20–22 potential tyrosine phosphorylation sites and has been shown to serve as a docking protein, binding various SH2 containing proteins *(17)* (Fig. 3). One important molecule that associates with phosphorylated IRS-1 is the heterodimeric enzyme, phosphotidylinositol-3-kinase (PI 3-kinase). The active IRS-1/PI 3-kinase complex leads to the phosphorylation of several phosphotidylinositol compounds to produce the signaling molecules PI-3-P, PI-3,4-P_2 and PI-3,4,5-P_3. This branch of the divergent insulin signaling pathway is believed to be critical for the increase in cellular glucose transport that occurs in response to insulin binding *(18,19)*. Treatment of cells with specific inhibitors of PI 3-kinase blocks insulin-stimulated glucose transport, but not insulin's mitogenic effects *(19)*.

The final effector system involved in increasing the rate of glucose uptake into the cell in response to insulin involves the insulin regulatable glucose transporter (GLUT4)

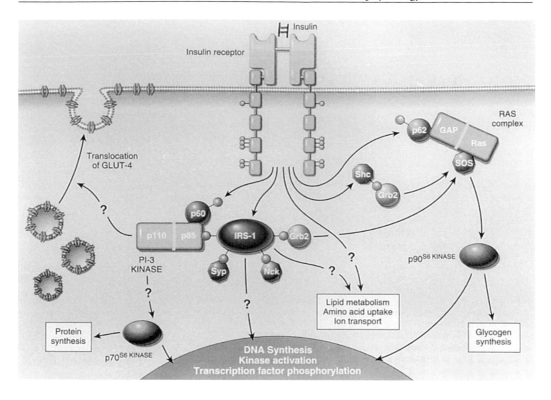

Fig. 3. Pathways of insulin receptor signaling. When insulin activates the receptor, the β-subunit is autophosphorylated at the juxtamembrane domain (tyr 960), the kinase domain (tyrs 1146, 1150, and 1151) and the C-terminal domain (tyr 1316 and 1322). Subsequently, endogenous substrates including IRS-1, IRS-2 and SHC are tyrosine phosphorylated. These phosphorylated substrates act as docking molecules to activate SH2 domain molecules including: GRB-2 which activates the ras pathway; the p85 subunit of PI-3-kinase; protein tyrosine phosphatase PTP2/SYP, PLCγ/NCK, and others. From Science & Medicine 1997;4:18–27.

(Fig. 3). The stimulation of cellular glucose transport by insulin is accomplished by the translocation of GLUT4 proteins from a sequestered intracellular pool to the plasma membrane *(14)*. The large increase in plasma membrane GLUT4 produces the rapid increase in the rate of facilitated diffusion of glucose into the cell in response to insulin. The exact intracellular location and composition of intracellular GLUT4 containing vesicles remains unknown, as does the precise mechanism of insulin-induced translocation. While the cellular signal responsible for translocation has not been discovered, the best evidence suggests that activation of PI 3-kinase is essential for this effect of insulin *(19)*.

DIMINISHED INSULIN ACTION IN MUSCLE AND ADIPOSE TISSUES

Studies on the mechanisms of insulin resistance have focused on the insulin target tissues in which a diminished insulin responsiveness has significant physiological impact. Resistance to insulin has been demonstrated in both skeletal muscle and adipose tissue from insulin resistant subjects, and defects at these sites are responsible for the majority of the altered metabolic profile of the insulin resistant subject *(20,21)*.

Skeletal muscle accounts for approximately 75% of whole body glucose disposal, and in insulin resistant subjects, decreased muscle glucose uptake accounts for nearly the entire decrement in whole body glucose disposal *(20)*. Therefore, while numerous tissues may display resistance to insulin, studies reporting diminished whole body glucose disposal are in fact describing skeletal muscle insulin resistance. Diminished skeletal muscle glucose uptake has also been demonstrated in vitro in incubated muscle strips from insulin resistant subjects *(22,23)*.

Adipocytes isolated from obese and Type 2 diabetes patients also show diminished insulin stimulation of glucose uptake *(24,25)*, and in vivo, the suppression by insulin of plasma free fatty acid (FFA) concentrations and FFA turnover in adipose tissue is impaired in insulin resistant subjects *(26,27)*. Still, the physiological impact of impaired insulin action in this tissue is poorly understood. In contrast to muscle, it is unclear whether the insulin resistance in adipocytes from Type 2 diabetes patients is a precursor to developing the disease. In addition, it is unknown whether insulin resistance in adipose tissue is an intrinsic characteristic of some individuals, or to what degree insulin action in fat and muscle are regulated independently. It has been shown, however, that in morbidly obese subjects, surgically induced weight loss produces enhanced insulin-stimulated glucose disposal well before any improvement in insulin suppression of FFA release is seen *(26)*, suggesting a separate regulation of insulin action in muscle and adipose tissue.

While adipose tissue accounts for a small portion of whole body glucose disposal, insulin resistance in adipose tissue may play a significant role in hyperglycemia. Evidence suggests that, beyond a direct effect of insulin on liver, adipose tissue release of FFA is a main determinant of hepatic glucose output (HGO) *(28)*. Thus, it is likely that impaired insulin suppression of FFA release in adipose tissue of insulin resistant patients is a significant contributor to hyperglycemia via elevations in HGO *(21,28)*. However, in the insulin resistant, nondiabetic state, the prevailing hyperinsulinemia has been shown to be sufficient to inhibit lipolysis *(27)*. It has also been suggested that skeletal muscle insulin resistance accompanying obesity is secondary to elevated FFA which down regulate glucose utilization through the substrate competition model proposed by Randle *(29)*.

POTENTIAL SITES FOR CELLULAR INSULIN RESISTANCE

The potential sites for cellular insulin resistance can be grouped into three major categories: defects in the glucose transport effector system; proximal post-receptor defects; and insulin receptor defects.

The Glucose Transport Effector System

The diminished insulin-stimulated glucose uptake in insulin resistant tissues results from a decreased translocation of GLUT4 to the cell membrane. It is unlikely, however, that defects in the glucose transport effector system represent a primary cause of insulin resistance. While cellular GLUT4 levels are diminished in adipose tissue from Type 2 diabetes patients *(30)*, expression of GLUT4 in adipose tissue is much more labile than in muscle. In contrast to muscle, in adipose tissue, GLUT4 levels are altered by fasting or modulating the dietary fat content *(31,32)*. GLUT4 expression in skeletal muscle appears to be regulated not in a unique manner but in concert with a number of enzymes involved in carbohydrate metabolism and oxidative phosphorylation *(33,34)*. Muscle from insulin resistant human subjects does not show diminished levels of GLUT4 *(35)*.

Proximal Post-Receptor Defects

Defects in in vivo activation of intermediate components of the insulin signal pathway have been demonstrated in models of insulin resistance. Muscle strips from severely insulin resistant, morbidly obese subjects show a dramatic reduction in the IRS-1 immunoprecipitable PI 3-kinase activity following incubation with insulin compared to muscle from lean controls *(36)*. The significance of this finding is unclear, given the dramatic decrease in muscle content of insulin receptors, IRS-1 protein, and IRS-1 phosphorylation in these obese subjects *(36)*. Similarly, reports of reduced activation of glycogen synthetase and S6 kinase in muscle of insulin resistant subjects in response to insulin were not demonstrated in the absence of impaired upstream signaling *(8,37)*. Thus, it is unclear whether defects in intermediate second messenger molecules can by themselves induce insulin resistance. In fact, other cellular signaling pathways utilize these same second messengers yet are apparently not affected in insulin resistance. This argues against a primary role for these molecules in the underlying pathology (e.g., IRS-1 is also a substrate for the activated IGF-1 receptor, though the cellular response to IGF-1 is not impaired in insulin resistant states *[38]*).

Recent findings have demonstrated that intermediate second messenger proteins may be able to actively participate in modulating cellular insulin signaling. IRS-1 is apparently a substrate for cellular serine/threonine kinases *(39)*. Studies have shown that the serine phosphorylated IRS-1 protein is a less effective substrate for insulin receptor tyrosine kinase activity, and may even feed back to inhibit insulin receptor function *(40)*. Thus, mechanisms downstream of the insulin receptor may be involved in insulin resistance, though primary defects in signaling molecules have not been demonstrated in muscle of insulin resistant humans.

Insulin Receptor Defects

Various groups, including our own, have reported that IR tyrosine kinase activity is impaired in muscle, fat, fibroblasts, and other tissues in patients with Type 2 diabetes *(36,41–56)* (Table 1). Decrements in skeletal muscle IR tyrosine kinase activity have been documented in both diabetic *(41,45–49)* and nondiabetic *(41,43,44,48,54,56)* insulin resistant subjects. It appears that these skeletal muscle IR defects are heritable, as lean, prediabetic offspring of Type 2 diabetes patients have impaired muscle insulin receptor function *(44)*. In adipose tissue, while IR tyrosine kinase activity is diminished in Type 2 diabetes *(53)*, in nondiabetic individuals, reports on IR tyrosine kinase activity are controversial. It has been reported that fat cell IR tyrosine kinase activity is unchanged in obesity *(53)*, but studies in lean, insulin resistant subjects *(43)*, and in Pima Indians representing a wide range of body composition *(51)* demonstrate that diminished IR signaling is associated with the insulin resistant state. In the study of Pima Indians, correlations were established between IR autophosphorylation and the ability of insulin to both stimulate glucose uptake and inhibit lipolysis in isolated adipocytes. Thus, impaired IR function in adipose tissue may play a significant role in the dysregulation of adipose FFA release and the subsequent disruption of glucose homeostasis.

Table 1
Studies of Insulin Receptor Tyrosine Kinase Activity in Human Insulin Resistance

Study	Tissue	Patients	IRTK vs Controls	Ref #
Caro, 1987	Muscle	Obese, nondiabetic	Decreased	
		Obese, Type 2 diabetes	Decreased	41
Nyomba, 1990	Muscle	Pima Type 2 diabetes	Decreased	42
Grasso 1994	Muscle	Lean, insulin resistant	Decreased	
	Adipose	Lean, insulin resistant	Decreased	43
Handberg, 1993	Muscle	Type 2 diabetes offspring	Decreased	44
Maegawa, 1991	Muscle	Lean, Type 2 diabetes	Decreased	45
Obermaier-Kusser, 1989	Muscle	Lean, Type 2 diabetes	Decreased	46
Scheck, 1991	Muscle	Type 2 diabetes	Decreased	47
Arner, 1987	Muscle	Obese, nondiabetic	Decreased	48
		Lean, Type 2 diabetes	Decreased	
		Lean, nondiabetic	Decreased	
Nolan, 1994	Muscle	Obese, nondiabetic	Unchanged	49
		Obese, Type 2 diabetes	Decreased	
Goodyear, 1995	Muscle	Obese, nondiabetic	Unchanged	36
Dunaif, 1995	Fibroblasts	Polycystic ovary syndrome (PCOS)	Decreased	
	Muscle	PCOS	Decreased	50
Takayama	Adipose	Obese Pimas	Decreased	51
Klein	Muscle	Lean Type 2 diabetes	Unchanged	52
Freidenberg, 1987	Adipose	Obese, nondiabetic	Unchanged	
		Obese, Type 2 diabetes	Decreased	53
Frittitta, 1996	Muscle	Lean, insulin resistant	Decreased	54
Frittitta, 1997	Adipose	Lean, insulin resistant	Decreased	55
Youngren, 1997	Muscle	Obese, nondiabetic	Decreased	
		Lean, insulin resistant	Decreased	56

While impaired IR function may exist in both fat and muscle of insulin resistant individuals, it is unknown whether the IR tyrosine kinase activity of these very different tissues are related within subjects, or how this relationship is affected by the presence of obesity or Type 2 diabetes. While the hyperglycemia that defines the diabetic state could produce similar impairments in IR signaling in both tissues, it is unclear how the effects of obesity, which might arise through alterations in adipocyte morphology, are then transmitted to muscle. In addition, it is unknown whether the IR defects demonstrated in muscle of individuals with inherited insulin resistance are present in adipose tissue as well.

A recent study investigated insulin receptor function in the Pima Indians of Arizona, a Native American group for whom the high prevalence of obesity and inherited insulin resistance lead to the highest prevalence of Type 2 diabetes for any ethnic group (1). Employing a new, highly sensitive and specific ELISA-based technique to measure insulin receptor autophosphorylation capacity, muscle biopsies were studied from a population of nondiabetic Pima Indians representing a wide range of obesity and insulin sensitivity (56). In these individuals, the tyrosine kinase activity of immunopurified insulin receptors was inversely correlated with percent body fat, clearly demonstrating the negative impact of obesity on insulin receptor function (Fig. 4). In addition, insulin receptor tyrosine kinase activity was positively correlated with insulin-stimulated glucose disposal measured during a hyperinsulinemic glucose clamp (Fig. 4). Together, these findings provide some of the strongest evidence that insulin receptor signaling capacity in skeletal muscle may be one of, if not the major determinant of in vivo insulin action.

Thus, a defect in insulin receptor signaling capacity remains the most promising candidate for the site of insulin resistance. An impaired signaling capacity of the insulin receptor would explain the defects specific to the insulin signal pathway, which is made up of second messenger molecules utilized by other, unaffected pathways. Perhaps the most convincing evidence that defects in insulin receptor function may play a causal role in human insulin resistance comes from transgenic mice that overexpress dominant negative, kinase-deficient insulin receptors exclusively in skeletal and cardiac muscle (57). This targeted expression of mutant receptors produces substantial impairments in insulin stimulated muscle insulin receptor tyrosine kinase activity, as well as diminished activation of downstream signaling intermediates IRS-1 and PI 3-kinase. These transgenic mice develop obesity, hyperinsulinemia, glucose intolerance, and hypertriglyceridemia. These data suggest that impairments in skeletal muscle insulin receptor tyrosine kinase activity are sufficient to produce a physiological state very similar to that of the majority of insulin resistant, nondiabetic humans.

INHIBITORS OF THE INSULIN RECEPTOR TYROSINE KINASE

While insulin receptor gene defects are not present in the vast majority of insulin resistant subjects (12), impairments in insulin receptor tyrosine kinase activity can occur without alterations in the receptor gene. Alterations in insulin receptor function have been reported to result from numerous secondary factors, including serine phosphorylation, phosphatases, and other inhibiting proteins (Fig. 5).

Serine Phosphorylation

Serine phosphorylation has been shown to impair insulin receptor tyrosine kinase activity (58), and excessive serine phosphorylation has been demonstrated in insulin receptors of skeletal muscle and fibroblasts from insulin resistant patients with polycystic ovary syndrome (50), but not routine Type 2 diabetes patients (59). Although protein kinase C has been shown to serine phosphorylate the insulin receptor in cultured cells and down regulate receptor tyrosine kinase activity (58), muscle insulin receptors are not phosphorylated to a greater degree on putative regulatory residues Ser 1327 or Thr 1348 in Type 2 diabetes patients (59). Still, this mechanism may explain the diminished insulin receptor kinase in some hyperglycemic states.

TNFα

Elevations in tumor necrosis factor alpha (TNFα) levels have been proposed to account for the insulin resistance of obesity. Enlarged adipocytes from obese individuals overproduce TNFα and secrete increased levels of this cytokine (60). Signaling through specific TNFα receptors results in increased serine phosphorylation of the insulin receptor substrate IRS-1 (40). The serine phosphorylated protein is a less efficient substrate for the insulin receptor, and, through as yet unknown mechanisms, the serine phosphorylated

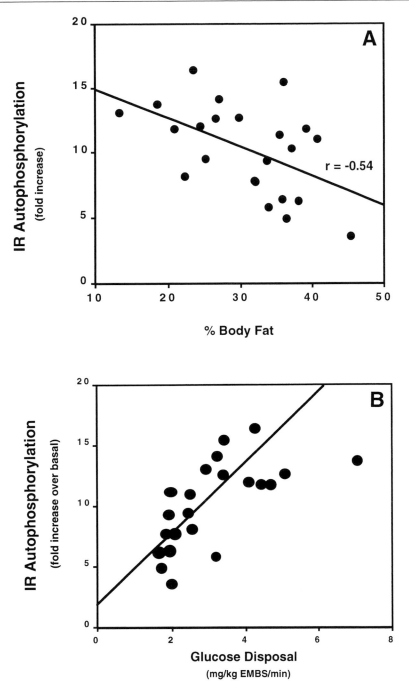

Fig. 4. Interaction between skeletal muscle insulin receptor function, obesity, and insulin resistance in Pima Indians. **(A)** Relationship between skeletal muscle insulin receptor autophosphorylation and percent body fat. Maximal autophosphorylation, determined by ELISA and expressed as the fold increase over basal at 100 nM insulin, declines as function of increasing obesity (r = –0.54, $p < 0.009$). **(B)** Relationship between skeletal muscle insulin receptor autophosphorylation and glucose disposal rates during the hyperinsulinemic glucose clamp (r = 0.62, $p < 0.002$) *(56)*.

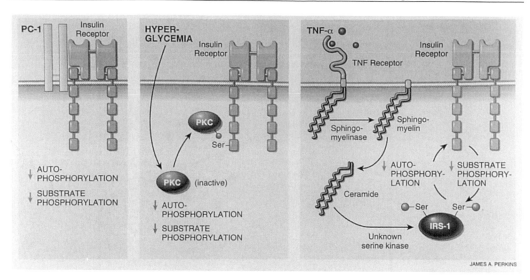

Fig. 5. Proposed mechanisms by which the signaling capability of the intact insulin receptor might be altered. PC-1 is believed to interact directly with the insulin receptor and may interfere with the conformational change necessary for autophosphoryation. Protein kinase C is able to directly phosphorylate regulatory residues on the receptor. The second messanger pathway of the TNF-α receptor serine-phosphorylates IRS-1, which then becomes a less effective substrate for the insulin receptor and can also interact with the receptor, further inhibiting its function. From Science & Medicine 1997;4:18–27.

IRS-1 is able to inhibit insulin receptor substrate kinase activity *(40)*. However, contrary to early reports from studies of obese rodents *(61)*, it has been demonstrated that neutralization of circulating TNFα in humans does not improve insulin sensitivity *(62)*.

Recently, transgenic knockout mice have been developed and studied to examine the role of TNFα in the insulin resistance of obesity *(63)*. Two transgenic strains, which either do not produce TNFα or the TNFα receptor, were either made obese through a high fat diet or crossed with a genetically obese mouse strain. While the absence of the TNFα signaling system seemed to protect against the mild insulin resistance of fat feeding, insulin resistance did develop, though less severely, in the genetically obese, TNFα knockout animals.

Insulin Receptor Splicing

Alternative splicing of the insulin receptor mRNA has been demonstrated, and alterations in the ratio of exon 11^+ to exon 11^- isoforms have been postulated to account for the insulin resistance of Type 2 diabetes *(64)*. It is controversial, however, whether or not the proportion of the exon 11^- isoform is significantly elevated in Type 2 diabetes patients *(65,66)*. In muscle from Pima Indians, insulin resistance is accompanied by an increased proportion of the exon 11^- isoform *(67)*. Importantly, it is not clear that there is a significant functional difference between the two isoforms *(66,68)*. Clearly, much more convincing data must be obtained to make this a viable mechanism to explain insulin resistance.

Membrane Glycoprotein PC-1

Investigation of the plasma membrane glycoprotein PC-1 as an inhibitor of insulin receptor signaling began with a study of fibroblasts derived from an insulin resistant Type

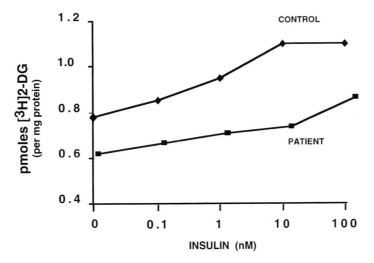

Fig. 6. Impaired insulin action in cells from patient MW. Fibroblast were incubated with insulin and [³H]2-deoxy-D-glucose (2-DG), uptake measured.

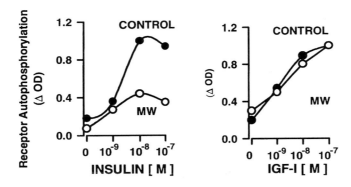

Fig. 7. Stimulation of IR and IGF-I-R β-subunitautophosphorylation in fibroblasts from patient (MW) and a sex- and age-matched control. Fibroblasts were stimulated with insulin or IGF-1. Cells were solubilized and captured on ELISA plates coated with either an insulin antibody (MA20) or an anti-IGF-1 antibody (a-IR3). ELISA plates were washed and probed with an anti-phosphotyrosine kinase antibody and activity measured.

2 diabetes patient (69,70). In her cultured cells, insulin stimulation of biological functions such as glucose transport was impaired (Fig. 6). The insulin receptor content and insulin binding to her fibroblasts was normal, and, when purified, the insulin receptor had normal tyrosine kinase activity. However, these fibroblasts produced a glycoprotein inhibitor of insulin receptor tyrosine kinase that resulted in a decreased whole cell insulin receptor tyrosine kinase activity, while closely related IGF-1 receptor was not affected (Fig. 7). This inhibitor was purified and identified as membrane glycoprotein PC-1. Compared to controls, there was an approximate 10–15-fold increase in the amount of PC-1 in the patient's cells. In addition, PC-1 mRNA was elevated 5–10-fold in cells this patient. Studies of additional Type 2 diabetes patients demonstrated that the PC-1 content is elevated in fibroblasts from the majority of diabetics, and that the cells with elevated PC-1 content have decreased insulin receptor tyrosine kinase activity (Fig. 8).

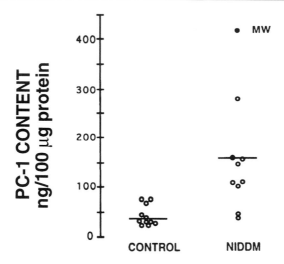

Fig. 8. PC-1 content in dermal fibroblasts from controls and NIDDM patients. Fibroblasts from controls and NIDDM patients were grown then analyzed for PC-1 content by ELISA.

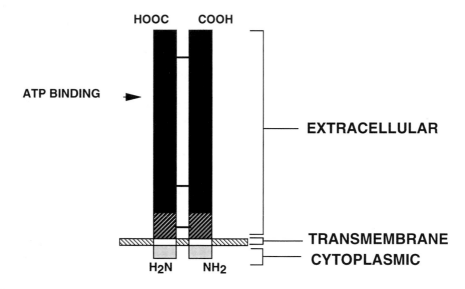

Fig. 9. Schematic structure of PC-1. Major domains of the molecule are shown.

CHARACTERISTICS OF PC-1

PC-1 is a class II transmembrane glycoprotein that is located both on plasma membrane and in the endoplasmic reticulum (Fig. 9). PC-1 is the same protein as liver nucleotide pyrophosphatase/alkaline phosphodiesterase I *(71–79)*. PC-1 is also related to the tumor mobility factor autotaxin, brain specific phosphodiesterase PD-Iα, and the neuroprotein gp130 RB13-6 *(80–82)*. PD-Iα and autotaxin may be the product of the same gene *(80)*. PC-1 has been reported to be expressed in plasma and intracellular membranes of: plasma cells, placenta, the distal convoluted tubule of the kidney, ducts of the salivary gland, epididymis, proximal part of the *vas deferens*, chondrocytes, dermal fibroblasts, skeletal muscle, and adipose tissue *(23,55,78)*. PC-1 exists as a homodimer of 230–260 kDa; the reduced form of the protein has a molecular size of 115–135 kDa, depending on the cell type. Human PC-1 maps to the chromosome location, 6q22–6q23 *(74,76)*. Human and mouse PC-1 are similar; there is an 87% nucleotide and 77% amino acid sequence homology between the two proteins *(74,76)*.

On the basis of studies with monoclonal antibodies it has been suggested that a portion of PC-1 is inserted into the membrane such that there is a small cytoplasmic amino terminus, and a larger extracellular carboxyl terminus *(74,76)* (Fig. 9). In addition, a soluble form of PC-1 has been reported *(83)*. It has been proposed that this soluble form derives from the membrane bound PC-1 form by proteolytic cleavage of a pro-ala sequence. There is an extracellular cysteine-rich domain adjacent to the plasma membrane, and 10 potential N-glycosylation sites. PC-1 has an ATP binding site, an EF-hand motif found in calcium binding proteins and a somatomedin-like region *(74,76)*. The extracellular domain of PC-1 cleaves sugar-phosphate, phosphosulfate, pyrophosphate, and phosphodiesterase linkages *(75,78)*. The active enzyme site for phosphodiesterase and pyrophosphatase contains a key threonine residue *(74,76)*. It has been shown that mutation of this residue does not impair the ability of PC-1 to inhibit IR function *(84)*. Thus the phosphodiesterase activity of PC-1 is not necessary for its ability to inhibit the IR. Just under the plasma membrane is a potential tyrosine phosphorylation site. It has been suggested that PC-1 may have threonine-specific protein kinase activity *(85)*, although it does not have sequence homology to the known threonine kinases.

The physiological function of PC-1 is unknown. It has been proposed that PC-1 may belong to an enzyme cascade system working in concert with other ecto-enzymes that hydrolyze nucleotides and nucleic acids to nucleosides which are then taken up by cells via a nucleoside transporter *(78,79)*. This pathway would allow the salvage of nucleotides from the extracellular fluid, and also allow the uptake of nucleosides by cells that are unable to synthesize purines by the de novo pathway.

PC-1 Overexpression in Muscle and Adipose Tissue of Insulin Resistant Subject

The role of PC-1 in insulin resistance of fat and muscle tissue was investigated in two models of human insulin resistance, the presumed intrinsic insulin resistance of lean, nondiabetic individuals, and the insulin resistance that develops with obesity. In healthy, nondiabetic, nonobese individuals, PC-1 levels were measured in biopsies of either abdominal fat or external oblique muscle *(54,55)*. In these subjects there was a wide range of in vivo insulin sensitivity. There was a significant correlation between muscle PC-1 content and insulin action as measured by the intravenous insulin tolerance test (Fig. 10). PC-1 levels also correlated negatively and significantly with the ability of insulin to stimulate muscle insulin receptor tyrosine kinase in vitro (Fig. 11). In addition, in this population there was a correlation between adipose cell content of PC-1 and in vivo insulin action.

The relationship between PC-1 and the insulin resistance associated with obesity was studied in muscle biopsies from subjects with a wide range of Body Mass Index (BMI) *(23)*. In these subjects, the muscle content of PC-1 was positively correlated with BMI and negatively correlated with the ability of insulin to stimulate glucose transport in muscle strips incubated in vitro (Figs. 12 and 13).

PC-1 Overexpression In Transfected Cells

To demonstrate a causal role for PC-1 in cellular insulin resistance, PC-1 cDNA was transfected into various insulin responsive cell lines *(70)*. MCF-7 cells, a human breast

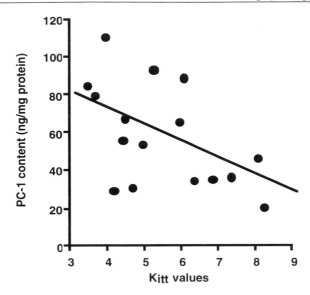

Fig. 10. Relationship between skeletal muscle PC-1 content and insulin sensitivity in lean, non-diabetic subjects. PC-1 content of soluble muscle extracts measured by radioimmunoassay declines with increasing insulin sensitivity, determined during intravenous insulin tolerance test and calculated as K_{itt} values (r = -0.51, p = 0.035) *(54)*.

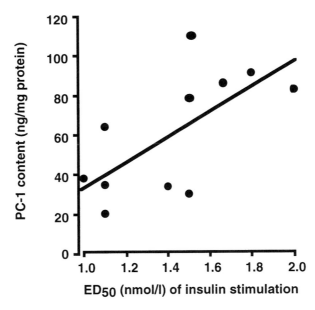

Fig. 11. Relationship between skeletal muscle PC-1 content and insulin receptor function. Muscle PC-1 content positively correlates with insulin receptor insensitivity for insulin, determined as the ED50 for insulin stimulation of receptor tyrosine kinase activity (r = 0.66, p = 0.027) *(54)*.

cancer cell line that normally produces only low levels of PC-1 were studied. Overexpression of this PC-1 in MCF-7 cells did not alter insulin binding. However, as with fibroblasts naturally overexpressing PC-1, increased expression of this protein in

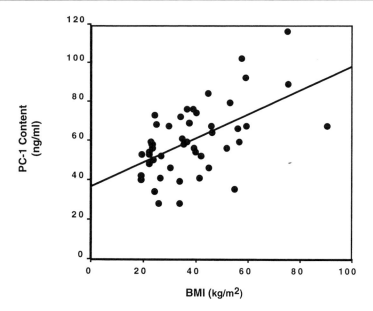

Fig. 12. Correlation between muscle PC-1 content and subject BMI. The content of PC-1 in skeletal muscle biopsies increases as a function of subject BMI ($r = 0.55, p < 0.05$). The PC-1 content of soluble muscle extracts was measured by radioimmunoassay *(23)*.

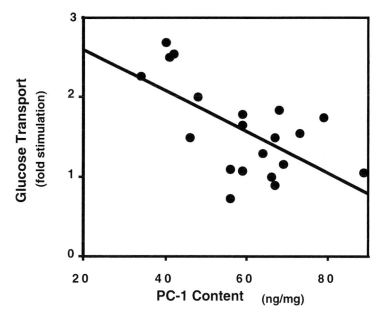

Fig. 13. The relationship between insulin stimulation of muscle glucose transport and muscle PC-1 content. Glucose transport was measured in muscle strips incubated in the presence and absence of 100 n*M* insulin. Insulin stimulation of transport was calculated as the insulin-induced fold increase in [14C] 2-deoxyglucose uptake over basal. The PC-1 content of soluble muscle extract was measured by radioimmunoassay *(23)*.

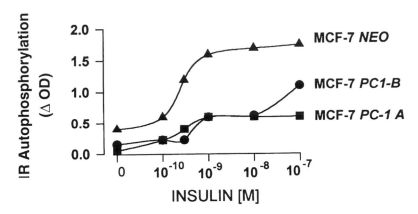

Fig. 14. PC-1 transfection inhibits IR tyrosine kinase activity. Effect of insulin on IR tyrosine kinase activity in MCF-7 NEO controls, and 2 clones of MCF-7-PC-1 cells transfected with PC-1.

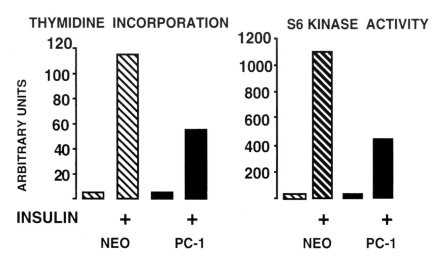

Fig. 15. Effect of insulin on biological functions in MCF-7 cells. MCF-7 NEO cells and MCF-7 PC-1 cells were studied. **(A)** [³H]thymidine incorporation. Cells were incubated for 20 h with insulin and 1 h with [³H]thymidine as described; **(B)** p70 S6 kinase. Cells were incubated 30 min with insulin and S6 kinase measured using shrimp ribosomes.

MCF-7 cells resulted in a marked inhibition of insulin stimulated insulin receptor tyrosine kinase activity (Fig. 14). In addition, various biological effects of insulin were blunted in the transfected cells (Fig. 15). Together, these findings suggest that PC-1 has a direct effect on regulating insulin receptor function, and may play a significant role in human insulin resistant states.

CONCLUSION

Insulin resistance plays a major role in the pathogenesis of Type 2 diabetes. Insulin resistance is a complex phenotype, with both genetic and environmental/lifestyle factors contributing to this trait. The heterogeneous nature of the disease and the incomplete understanding of the intracellular insulin signaling pathway have undoubtedly contributed to the inability to firmly establish the cellular mechanisms of insulin resistance. Defects in insulin receptor signaling capacity remain the most likely cause of diminished insulin action. While defects in the insulin receptor gene account for only a small percentage of the total cases of insulin resistance in humans, the ability of other molecules to modulate the function of the insulin receptor has been demonstrated. The impact of effectors of the insulin receptor such as PC-1, TNFα, and protein kinase C on insulin resistance in humans provides new insights into the causes of insulin resistance.

REFERENCES

1. King H, Rewers M, WHO Ad Hoc Diabetes Reporting Group. Global estimates for the prevelance of diabetes mellitus and impaired glucose tolerance in adults. Diabetes Care 1993;16:137–177.
2. Reaven GM. Role of insulin resistance in human disease. Diabetes 1988;37:1595–1607.
3. Martin BC, Warram JH, Krowlewski AS, Bergman RN, Soelder JS, Kahn CR. Role of glucose and insulin resistence in development of type II diabetes mellitus: results of a 25-year follow-up study. Lancet 1992;340: 925–929.
4. Lillioja S, Mott DM, Howard BV, Bennett PH, Yki-Jarvinen H, Freymond D, Nyomba BL, Zurlo F, Swinburn B, Bogardus C. Impaired glucose tolerance as a disorder of insulin action: longitudinal and cross-sectional studies of Pima Indians. N Engl J Med 1988;318: 1217–1225.
5. Hollenbeck C, Reaven G M. Variations in insulin-stimulated glucose uptake in healthy individuals with normal glucose tolerance. J Clin Endocrinol Metab 1987;64: 1169–1173.
6. Hamman RF. Genetic and environmental determinants of non-insulin-dependent-diabetes mellitus (NIDDM). Diabet Metabol Rev 1992;8:287–338.
7. Bogardus C, Lillioja S, Mott DM, Hollenbeck C, Reaven G M. Relationship between degree of obesity and in vivo insulin action in man. Am J Physiol 1985;248:E286-E291.
8. Vaag A, Henriksen JE, Beck-Nielsen H. Decreased insulin activation of glycogen synthase in skeletal muscles in young non-obese Caucasian first-degree relatives of patients with non-insulin-dependent diabetes mellitus. J Clin Invest 1992;89:782–788.
9. Lillioja S, Mott DM, Zawadzi KK, Young AA, Abbott WGH, Knowler WC, Bennett PH, Moll P, Bogardus C. In vivo insulin action is a familial characteristic in nondiabetic Pima Indians. Diabetes 1987;36:1329–1335.
10. Martin BC, Warram JH, Rosner B, Rich SS, Soeldner JS, Krolewski AS. Familial clustering of insulin sensitivity. Diabetes 1992;41:850–854.
11. Vaag A, Henriksen JE, Madsbad S, Holm, N, Beck-Neilsen H. Insulin secretion, insulin action, hepatic glucose production in identical twins discordant for non-insulin-dependent diabetes mellitus. J Clin Invest 1995;95:690–698.
12. Taylor, SI. Lessons from patients with mutations in the insulin-receptor gene. Diabetes 1992;41:1473.
13. Goldfine, ID. The insulin receptor: molecular biology and transmembrane signaling. Endocr Rev 1987;8:235.
14. Kahn CR, White MF. The insulin receptor and the molecular mechanism of insulin action. J Clin Invest 1988;82:1551.
15. Rosen OM, Herrera R, Olowe Y, Petruzelli LM, Cobb MH. Phosphorylation activates the insulin receptor tyrosine protein kinase. Proc Natl Acad Sci USA 1983;80:3237–3240.
16. Moran ME, Koch CA, Anderson D, Ellis C, England L, Martin GS, Pawson T. Src Homology region 2 domains direct protein-protein—interactions in signal transduction. Proc Natl Acad Sci USA 1990;87:8622–8626.
17. White MF. The IRS-1 signaling system. Curr Opin Genet Devel 1994;4:47–54.
18. Okada ,T, Kamano Y, Sakakibara T, Hazeki O, Ui M. Essential role of phosphotidylinositol 3-kinase in insulin induced glucose transport and antilopolysis in rat adipocytes. J Biol Chem 1994;269:3568–3573.
19. Cheatham B, Vlahos CJ, Cheatam L, Wang L, Blenis J, Kahn CR. (1994) Phosphatidylinositol 3-kinase activation is required for insulin stimulation of pp70 S6 kinase, DNA synthesis and glucose transporter translocation. Mol Cell Biol 14:4902–4911.
20. DeFronzo RA. The triumvirate: B-cell, muscle, liver: a collusion responsible for NIDDM. Diabetes 1988;37:667–687.
21. Reaven GM. The Fourth Muskateer—from Alexandre Dumas to Claude Bernard. Diabetologia 1995;38:3–13.

22. Dohm GL, Tapscott EB, Pories WJ, Dabbs DJ, Flickinger EF, Meelheim D, Fushiki T, Atkinson SM, Elton CW, Dohm GL. An in vitro human muscle preparation suitable for metabolic studies: decreased insulin stimulation of glucose transport in muscle from morbidly obese and diabetic subjects. J Clin Invest 1988;82:486–494.

23. Youngren JF, Maddux BA, Sasson S, Sbraccia P, Tapscott EB, Swanson MS, Dohm GL, Goldfine ID. Skeletal muscle content of membrane glycoprotein PC-1 in obesity: relationship to muscle glucose transport. Diabetes 1996;45:1324–1328.

24. Olefsky JM, Garvey WT, Henry RR, Brillon D, Matthaei S, andFreidenberg GR. Cellular mechanisms of insulin resistance in non-insulin-dependent (type II) diabetes. Am J Med 1988;85(Suppl 5A):86–105.

25. Garvey WT, Maianu L, Huecksteadt TP, Birnbaum MJ, Molina JM, Ciraldi TP. Pretranslational suppression of a glucose transporter protein causes insulin resistance in adipocytes from patients with non-insulin-dependent diabetes mellitus and obesity. J Clin Invest 1991;87:1072–1081.

26. Krentz AJ, Nattrass M. Insulin resistance: a multifacted metabolic syndrome. Insights gained using a low-dose insulin infusion technique. Diabetic Med 1996;13:30–39.

27. Campbell PJ, Carlson MC, Nourijahan, N. Fat metabolism in human obesity. Am J Physiol 1994; E600–E605.

28. Rebrin K, Steil GM, Mittelman SD, Bergman RN. Causal linkage between insulin suppression of lipolysis and suppression of liver glucose output in dogs. J Clin Invest 1996;38:741–749.

29. Randle PJ, Garland PB, Hales CN, Newsholme EA. The glucose fatty acid cycle. Its role in insulin sensitivity and the metabolic disturbance of diabetes mellitus. Lancet 1963;1:785–789.

30. Garvey WT, Maianu L, Huecksteadt TP, Birnbaum MJ, Molina JM, Ciaraldi TP. Pretranslational suppression of a glucose transporter protein causes insulin resistance in adipocytes from patients with non-insulin-dependent diabetes mellitus and obesity. J Clin Invest 1991;87:1072–1081.

31. Pedersen O, Kahn CR, Flier JS, Kahn BB. High fat feeding causes insulin resistance and a marked decrease in the expression of glucose transporters (GLUT4) in fat cells of rats. Endocrinology 1991;129:771–777.

32. Sivitz WI, DeSautel SL, Kayano T, Bell GI, Pessin JE. Regulation of glucose transporter mRNA in insulin-deficient states. Nature 1989;340:72–74.

33. Rodnick KJ, Piper RC, Slot JW, James DE. Interaction of insulin and exercise on glucose transport in muscle. Diabetes Care 1992;15:1679–1689.

34. Youngren JF, Barnard RJ. Effects of acute and chronic exercise on skeletal muscle glucose transport in aged rats. J Appl Physiol 1995;78(5):1750–1756.

35. Pedersen O, Bak JF, Andersen PH, Lund S, Moller DE, Flier JS, Kahn BB. Evidence against altered expression of GLUT1 or GLUT4 in skeletal muscle of patients with obesity or NIDDM. Diabetes 1990;39:865–870.

36. Goodyear LJ, Giorgino F, Sherman LA, Carey J, Smith RJ, Dohm GL. Insulin receptor phosphorylation, insulin receptor substrate-1 phosphorylation, phosphatidylinositol 3-kinase activity are decreased in intact skeletal muscle strips from obese subjects. J Clin Invest 1995;95:2195–2204.

37. Sommercorn J, Fields R, Raz I, Maeda R. Abnormal regulation of ribosomal protein S6 kinase by insulin in skeletal muscle of insulin resistant humans. J Clin Invest 1993;91:509–513.

38. Boulware SD, Tamborlane WV, Rennert NJ, Gesundheit N, Sherwin RS. Comparison of the metabolic effects of recombinant human insulin-like growth factor-I and insulin. Dose-response relationships in healthy young and middle-aged adults. J. Clin. Invest 1994;93:1131–1139.

39. Eldar-Finkelman H, Krebs EG. Phospsorylation of insulin receptor substrate 1 by glycogen synthase kinase 3 impairs insulin action. Proc Natl Acad Sci USA 1997;94:9660–9664.

40. Hotamisiligil GS, Peraldi P, Budavari A, Ellis R, White MF, Spiegelman BM. IRS-1 mediated inhibition of insulin receptor tyrosine kinase activity in TNFα and obesity-induced insulin resistance. Science 1996;271:665–668.

41. Caro JF, Sinha MK, Raju SM, Ittoop O, Pories WJ, Flickinger EG, Meelheim D, Dohm GL. Insulin receptor kinase in human skeletal muscle from obese subjects with and without noninsulin dependent diabetes. J Clin Invest 1987;79:1330–1337.

42. Nyomba BL, Ossowski VM, Bogardus C, Mott DM. Insulin-sensitive tyrosine kinase: relationship with in vivo insulin action in humans. Am J Physiol 1990;258:E964–E974.

43. Grasso G, Frittitta L, Anello M, Russo P, Susti G, Trischitta V. Insulin receptor tyrosine kinase activity is altered in both muscle and adipose tissue from nonobese normoglycemic insulin resistant subjects. Diabetologia. 1995;38:55–61.

44. Handberg A, Vaag A, Vinten J, Beck-Nielsen H. Decreased tyrosine kinase activity in partially purified insulin receptors from muscle of young, nonobese first degree relatives patients with type 2 (non-insulin-depedent) diabetes mellitus. Diabetologia. 1993;36:668–674.

45. Maegawa H, Shigeta Y, Egawa K, Kobayashi M. Impaired otophosphorylation of insulin receptors from abdominal skeletal muscles in non-obese subjects with NIDDM. Diabetes 1991;40:815–819.

46. Obermaier-Kusser B, White MF, Pongratz DE, Su Z, Ermal B, Muhlbacher C, Häring HU. A defective intramolecular autoactivation cascade may cause the reduced kinase activity of the skeletal muscle insulin receptor from patients with non-insulin-depedent diabetes mellitus. J Biol Chem 1989; 264:9497–9504.

47. Scheck SH, Barnard RJ, Lawani LO, Youngren JF, Martin DA, Singh R. Effects of NIDDM on glucose transport system in human skeletal muscle. Diabetes Res 1991;16:111–119.

48. Arner P, Pollare T, Lithell H, Livingston JN. Defective insulin receptor tyrosine kinase in human skeletal muscle in obesity and Type 2. (non-insulin-dependent) diabetes mellitus. Diabetologia 1987; 30:437–440.

49. Nolan JJ, Freidenberg G, Henry R, Reichart D, Olefsky JM. Role of human skeletal muscle insulin receptor kinase in the in vivo insulin resistance of noninsulin-dependent diabetes mellitus and obesity. J Clin Endocrinol Metab 1994;78:471–477.

50. Dunaif A, Xia J, Book, C-B, Schenker E, Tang Z. Excessive insulin receptor serine phosphorylation in cultured fibroblasts and in skeletal muscle: a potential mechanism for insulin resistance in the Polycystic Ovary Syndrome. J Clin Invest 1995;96:801–810.

51. Takayama S, Kahn CR, Kubo K, Foley JE. Alterations in insulin receptor autophosphorylation in insulin resistance: correlation with altered sensitivity to glucose transport and antilipolysis to insulin. J Clin Endocrinol Metab 1987;66:992–999.

52. Klein HH, Vestergaard H, Koetzke G, Pedersen O. Elevation of serum insulin concentration during euglycemic hyperinsulinemic clamp studies leads to similar activation of insulin receptor kinase in skeletal muscle of subjects with and without NIDDM. Diabetes 1995;44:1310–1317.

53. Freidenberg GR, Henry RR, Reichart DR, Olefsky JM. Decreased kinase activity of insulin receptors from adicocytes of non-insulin-dependent diabetic subjects. J Clin Invest 1987;79:240–250.

54. Frittitta L, Youngren JF, Vigneri R, Maddux BA, Trischitta V, Goldfine ID. PC-1 content in skeletal muscle of non-obese, non-diabetic subjects, relationship to insulin receptor tyrosine kinase and whole body insulin sensitivity. Diabetologia 1996;39:1190–1195.

55. Frittitta L, Youngren JF, Sbraccia P, D'Adamo M, Boungiorno A, Vigneri R, Goldfine ID, Trischitta V. Increased adispose tissue PC-1 protein content, but not TNF-α gene expression, is associated to a reduction of both whole body insulin sensitivity and insulin receptor tyrosine kinase activity. Diabetologia 1997;40:282–289.

56. Youngren J.F, Goldfine ID, Pratley RE. Decreased muscle insulin receptor kinase correlates with insulin resistance in normoglycemic Pima Indians. Am J Physiol 1997;273:E276–E283.

57. Moller DE, Chang, P-Y, Yaspelkis III BB, Flier JS, Walberg-Henriksson H, Ivy JL. Transgenic mice with muscle-specific insulin resistance develop increased adiposity, impaired glucose tolerance, dyslipemia. Endocrinology 1996;137:2397–2405.

58. Bollag GE, Roth RA, Beaudoin J, Mochly-Rosen D, Koshland DEJ. Protein kinase C directly phospho-rylates the insulin receptor in vitro and reduces its protein tyrosine kinase activity. Proc Natl Acad Sci USA 1986;83:5822–5824.

59. Kellerer M, Coghlan M, Capp E, Mühlhöfer A, Kroder G, Mosthaf L, Galante P, Siddle K, Häring HU. Mechanism of insulin receptor kinase inhibition in non-insulin-dependent diabetes mellitus patients: phosphorylation of serine 1327 or threonine 1348 is unaltered. J Clin Invest 1995;96:6–11.

60. Kern PA, Saghizadeh M, Ong JM, Bosch RJ, Deem R, Simsolo RB. The expression of tumor necrosis factor in human adipose tissue. Regulation by obesity, weight loss, relationship to liproprotein lipase. J Clin Invest 1995;95:2111–2119.

61. Hotamisiligil GS, Shargill, N.S, Spiegelman BM. Adipose expression of tumor necrosis factor-α: direct role in obesity-linked insulin resistance. Science 1993;259:87–91.

62. Fofei, Hurel S, Newkirk J, Sopwith M, Taylor R. Effects of an engineered human anti-TNF-αlpha antibody (CDP571) on insulin sensitivity and glycemic control in patients with NIDDM. Diabetes 1996;45:881–885.

63. Uysal KT, Wiesbrock SM, Marino MW, Hotamisligil GS. Protection from obesity-induced insulin resistance in mice lacking TNF-α function. Nature 1997;389:610–614.

64. Mosthaf L, Vogt B, Häring HU, Ullrich A. Altered expression of insulin receptor types A and B in the skeletal muscle of non-insulin-dependent diabetes mellitus patients. Proc Natl Acad Sci USA 1991;88:4728–4730.

65. Benecke H, Flier JS, Moller DE. Alternative spliced variants of the insulin receptor protein, expression in normal and diabetic human tissues. J Clin Invest 1992;89:2066–2070.

66. Hansen T, Bjorback C, Vestergaard H, Gronskov K, Bak JF, Pedersen O. Expression of insulin receptor spliced variants and their functional correlates in muscle from patients with non-insulin-dependent diabetes mellitus. J Clin Endocrinol Metab 1993;77:1500–1505.

67. Sell SM, Reese D, Ossowski VM. Insulin-inducible changes in insulin receptor mRNA splice variants. J Biol Chem 1994;269:30769–30772.

68. Kosaki A, Pillay TS, Xu L, Webster, NJ. The B soform of the insulin receptor signals more efficiently than the A isoform in Hep G2 cells. J Biol Chem 1995;270:20816–20823.

69. Sbraccia P, Goodman PA, Maddux BA, Chen Y-DI, Reaven GM, Goldfine ID. Production of an inhibitor of insulin receptor tyrosine kinase in fibroblasts from a patient with insulin resistance and NIDDM. Diabetes 1991;40:295–299.

70. Maddux BA, Sbraccia P, Kumakura S, Sasson S, Youngren J, Fisher A, Spencer S, Grupe A, Henzel W, Stewart TA, Reaven GM, Goldfine ID. Membrane Glycoprotein PC-1 and insulin resistance in non-insulin-dependent diabetes. Nature 1995;373:448–451.

71. Yano T, Funakoshi I, Yamashina I. Purification and properties of nucleotide pyrophosphatase. J Biochem 1985;98:1097–1107.

72. Van Driel IR, Goding JW. Plasma cell membrane glycoprotein PC-1. J Biol Chem 1987;262:4882–4887.

73. Harahap AR, Goding JW. Distribution of PC-1 in non lymphoid tissues. J. Immuno. 1988;141: 2317–2320.

74. Buckley MF, Loveland KA, McKinstry WJ, Garson OM, Goding JW. Plasma cell membrane glycoprotein PC-1 cDNA cloning of the human molecule, amino acid sequence, chromosomal location. J Biol Chem 1990;265:17506–17511.

75. Rebbe, NF, Tong BD, Finley EM, Hickman S. Identification of nucleotide pyrophosphatase/alkaline phosphodiesterase I activity associated with the mouse plasma cell differentiation antigen PC-1. Proc Natl Acad Sci USA 1991;88:5192–5196.

76. Funakoshi I, Kato H, Horie K, Yano T, Hori Y, Kobayashi H, Inoue T, Suzuki H, Fukui S, Tsukahara M, Kajii T, Yamashina I. Molecular cloning of human nucleotide pyrophosphatase. Arch Biochem Biophys 1992;295:180–187.

77. Uriarte M, Stalmans W, Hickman S, Bollen M. Phosphorylation and nucleotide-dependent dephosphorylation of hepatic polypeptides related to the plasma cell differentiation antigen PC-1. Biochem J 1993;293:93–100.

78. Rebbe, NF, Tong BD, Hickman S. Expression of nucleotide pyrophosphatase and alkaline phosphodiesterase I activities of PC-1, the murine plasma cell antigen. Mol Immunol 1993;30:87–93.

79. Yoshida H, Fukui S, Funakoshi I, Yamashina I. Substrate specificity of a nucleotide pyrophosphatase responsible for the breakdown of 3'-phosphoadenosine 5'-phosphosulfate (PAPS) from human placenta. J Biochem 1983;93:1641–1648.

80. Kawagoe H, Soma O, Goji J, Nishimura, N, Narita M, Inazawa J, Nakamura H, Sano K. Molecular cloning and chromosomal assignment of the human brain-type phosphodiesterase I/Nucleotide Pyrophosphotase Gene (PDNP2). Genomics 1995;30:380–384.

81. Murata J, Lee HY, Clair T, Krutzsch HC, Arestad AA, Sobel ME, Liotta LA, Stracke M. cDNA cloning of the human tumor motility-stimulating protein, autotaxin, reveals a homology with phosphodiesterase. J Biol Chem 1994;269:30479–30484.

82. Deisler H, Lottspeich F, Rajewsky MF. Affinity purification and cDNA cloning of rat neural differentiation and tumor cell surface antigen gp130 RB13-6 reveals relationship to human and murine PC-1. J Biol Chem 1995;270:9849–9855.

83. Belli AI, Van Driel IR, Goding JW. Identification and characterization of a soluble form of the plasma cell membrane glycoprotein PC-1 (5'-nucleotide phosphodiesterase) Eur. J Biochem 1993;217:421–428.

84. Grupe A, Alleman J, Goldfine ID, Sadick M, Stewart T. Inhibition of insulin receptor phosphorylation by PC-1 is not mediated by the hydrolysis of Adenosine triphosphate or the generation of Adenosine. J Biol Chem 1995;270:22085–22088.

85. Oda Y, Kuo, M-D, Huang SS, Huang JS. The plasma cell membrane glycoprotein, PC-1, is a threonine specific protein kinase stimulated by acidic fibroblast growth factor. J Biol Chem 1991; 266:16791–16795.

9

NMR Studies on the Mechanism of Insulin Resistance

Gianluca Perseghin, MD, Kitt Falk Petersen, MD, and Gerald I. Shulman, MD, PhD

CONTENTS

INTRODUCTION
BRIEF OVERVIEW OF THE BASIC PRINCIPLES OF NMR SPECTROSCOPY
NMR SPECTROSCOPY OF HUMAN SKELETAL MUSCLE
    IN TYPE 2 DIABETES
NMR SPECTROSCOPY IN HUMAN SKELETAL MUSCLE OF OFFSPRING
    OF TYPE 2 DIABETIC PATIENTS
NMR SPECTROSCOPY IN HUMAN SKELETAL MUSCLE OF OFFSPRING
    OF TYPE 2 DIABETIC PATIENTS: EFFECT OF EXERCISE
NMR SPECTROSCOPY IN HUMAN SKELETAL MUSCLE: INTERACTIONS
    OF GLUCOSE AND LIPID METABOLISM
CONCLUSIONS
REFERENCES

INTRODUCTION

In this chapter we will describe some recent studies in which nuclear magnetic resonance (NMR) spectroscopy has been used to gain new insights into the mechanisms of insulin resistance in man. We will first provide a brief overview of the principles of NMR spectroscopy and then we will focus on the application of the technique to examine insulin regulation of muscle glucose metabolism.

Traditionally, intracellular concentrations of metabolites and enzyme activities have been assessed by the needle biopsy technique and later by radioactive tracer techniques. NMR spectroscopy has several advantages over these techniques in that it is: 1) non-invasive, which allows repeated measurements of metabolite concentrations in tissue over time 2) involves stable isotopes (no ionizing radiation) and 3) it yields chemical information which allow the observer to follow the intracellular fate of a labeled molecule as it is metabolized (e.g., [1-^{13}C] labeled glucose incorporation into glycogen).

From: *Contemporary Endocrinology: Insulin Resistance*
Edited by: G. Reaven and A. Laws © Humana Press Inc., Totowa, NJ

BRIEF OVERVIEW OF THE BASIC PRINCIPLES
OF NMR SPECTROSCOPY

The NMR spectroscopy technique relies on the spin properties of certain atomic nuclei (precession of the nucleus about its own axis), which make them behave like tiny bar magnets. These nuclei are usually oriented randomly in space but when placed in a magnetic field, they behave in a similar fashion to a compass needle and align with or against the direction of the magnetic field, with the two different orientations having slightly different energies. When subjected to electromagnetic energy (a radio-frequency generator sends electromagnetic pulses to a probe located close to the tissue or organ of interest at the frequency at which the nuclei being investigated are oscillating), the nuclei in the tissue absorb some of that energy and move to a higher energy state. When they return to their lower energy states, they give off energy which is collected by the receiver. The higher the magnetic field, the faster the frequency of precession and the greater the difference between the two energy states. The change in energy given off by the nuclei when shifting from a higher to a lower energy spin state is picked up by the probe and the signal is amplified and sent to a computer where the change in energy is transformed into a spectrum. The frequency at which precession occurs depends on the nucleus being analyzed and its molecular environment. Table 1 shows some of the nuclei that can be studied using NMR spectroscopy. Hydrogen nuclei, in the form of protons, when placed in a magnetic field of 1.5 Tesla (T) will precess at 63.9 MHz and when placed in a magnetic field of 2.1 T will precess at 89.5 MHz. The applied magnetic field also induces electronic currents in atoms and molecules which in turn produce a small magnetic field which is dependent upon the electronic environment of the nucleus and therefore in different chemical environments nuclei give rise to signals of slightly different frequencies. The separation of resonance frequencies from an arbitrarily chosen frequency is termed the chemical shift and is expressed in units of part per million (ppm). The intensity of the NMR signals is proportional to the number of contributing nuclei.

^1H is the most sensitive nucleus for NMR studies (Table 1) and for this reason it produces a greater signal-to-noise ratio than any other nucleus. The distinctive features of ^1H-NMR spectroscopy are the complexity of the spectra and the presence of a large solvent peak (H_2O) in spectra of aqueous solutions. The complexity of spectra is due to the ubiquity of hydrogen atoms in biological molecules and interpretation of ^1H spectra is often difficult. The presence of the H_2O peak has been a major disadvantage for in vivo NMR spectroscopy but in more recent years, NMR techniques have been developed to suppress the water signal and detect metabolites that can be present at lower concentrations.

^{31}P is 100% abundant, naturally occurring in all phosphate containing compounds. ^{31}P NMR spectroscopy can be used to quantify high-energy phosphate intermediates as adenosine triphosphate (ATP), adenosine diphosphate (ADP), inorganic phosphate (Pi) and phosphocreatine (PCr). It can also be used to measure tissue concentrations of glucose-6-phosphate (G-6-P) and thus assess the rate controlling steps of glycogen synthesis.

Carbon 13 (^{13}C) comprises only 1.1% of all naturally occurring carbon nuclei; the other natural isotope is carbon 12 (^{12}C), which is NMR "invisible". Due to the low natural abundance, ^{13}C NMR spectroscopy is a relatively insensitive technique (Table 1). However, ^{13}C glycogen can readily be measured in muscle and liver where the glycogen

Table 1
NMR Spectroscopic Properties of the Nuclei Commonly Used in Biology

Nucleus	Spin Quantum Number	Resonance at 1.5T (MHz)	Resonance at 2.1T (MHz)	Natural Abundance (%)	Relative Sensitivity
^1H	1/2	63.9	89.5	99.98	100
^{31}P	1/2	25.9	36.2	100	6.6
^{13}C	1/2	16.0	22.5	1.1	0.016

concentrations are typically >50 mmol/L. Furthermore, the sensitivity of ^{13}C NMR spectroscopy can be improved almost 100-fold by using ^{13}C enriched isotopes. A more detailed review of the basic principles of NMR can be found in references (1,2).

NMR SPECTROSCOPY OF HUMAN SKELETAL MUSCLE IN TYPE 2 DIABETES

Insulin resistance is one of the major features of Type 2 diabetes (3,4). It is present decades before the onset of the disease and it is the best predictor for diabetes occurrence (5,6). Insulin resistance is due to a decrease in insulin-stimulated skeletal muscle glucose uptake; limb balance studies have shown that non-oxidative glucose metabolism is the major pathway accounting for 80–90% of total glucose uptake (7–14). In contrast to these indirect techniques, ^{13}C NMR spectroscopy provides a signal from carbon 1 of glycogen, the size of which corresponds to the concentration of tissue glycogen (15–18). Muscle glycogen has been shown to be 100% visible when comparing ^{13}C NMR spectroscopic measurements with direct biochemical analysis of muscle glycogen obtained by needle biopsy in rabbits and humans (19,20). In the first application of ^{13}C NMR spectroscopy to the study of diabetes and its pathogenesis, the quantitative contribution of muscle glycogen synthesis to whole body glucose uptake was assessed during a hyperglycemic (190 mg/dL)-hyperinsulinemic (70 µU/mL) clamp. Endogenous insulin secretion was inhibited by a concomitant infusion of somatostatin (21) and exogenous insulin was infused at a rate to simulate postprandial conditions. The rate of muscle glycogen synthesis was measured by the increase in the signal of muscle C1-glycogen (Fig. 1A) during the infusion of [1-^{13}C]glucose. During these NMR spectroscopic experiments, the subjects remained in the supine position within the spectrometer and the gastrocnemious muscle of the right leg was positioned at the centre of the magnet (where the magnetic field is most homogeneous) over a ^1H-^{13}C concentric surface coil (21). ^{13}C NMR spectra were acquired in 10-min intervals to monitor muscle glycogen content. This study provided evidence that glycogen synthesis represents the primary pathway for non-oxidative glucose disposal in normal humans (22). In the same study, Type 2 diabetic patients were studied with the same technique and the rate of muscle glycogen synthesis was found to be decreased by 60% compared to healthy subjects. Furthermore glycogen formation represented the major intracellular metabolic defect responsible for the decrease in non-oxidative and whole-body glucose metabolism in subjects with Type 2 diabetes (Fig. 1B).

The defect responsible for the reduction of skeletal muscle glucose metabolism could occur anywhere between glucose uptake into the muscle and glycogen synthase (Fig. 2).

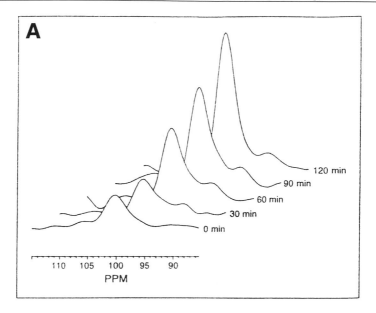

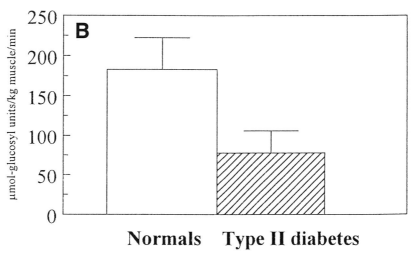

Fig. 1. (A) Typical course of ^{13}C-NMR spectra of muscle glycogen in a normal subject during the hyperglycemic-hyperinsulinemic clamp study. **(B)** Muscle glycogen synthetic rates in normals (open bar) and diabetic subjects (solid bar) during the hyperglycemic-hyperinsulinemic clamp study *(21)*.

Muscle glucose transport and glycogen synthase are both insulin stimulated and each has been suggested to be responsible for the reduced rate of insulin stimulated glucose disposal in patients with Type 2 diabetes mellitus. Synthase activity, measured in biopsy samples, has been shown to be lower in subjects with Type 2 diabetes mellitus than in normal subjects *(23–26)*. Also glucose transport activity has recently been suggested to be impaired in patients with Type 2 diabetes mellitus using different techniques *(27,28)*. As a result of the location of glucose-6-phosphate (G-6-P) between the transport system and glycogen synthase enzymes in the pathway of glycogen synthesis, the concentration

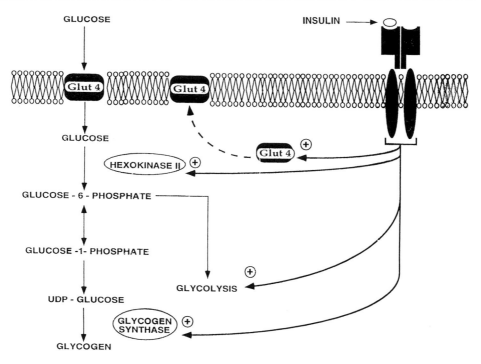

Fig. 2. Schematic representation of the metabolic pathways for intramuscular glucose metabolism. The key insulin-regulated steps of the metabolic pathway are shown, including glucose transport (insulin-dependent glucose transporter *GLUT4*), phosphorylation (hexokinase II) and incorporation into glycogen (glycogen synthase). Decreased activity in any of these steps could be responsible for insulin resistance *(69)*.

of G-6-P is sensitive to the relative activities of these enzymes. However G-6-P measured in human biopsy is likely to be artifactually high because of glycogen breakdown during the delay between sample excision and freezing *(29)*. ^{31}P-NMR spectroscopy is an alternate method of measuring human muscle G-6-P in vivo and does not suffer from autolytic artifacts typical in biopsy specimens *(30,31)*. During the hyperglycemic hyperinsulinemic clamp, ^{31}P NMR spectroscopy was used to monitor the time dependent changes in intramuscular G-6-P concentrations. A baseline spectrum and a spectrum obtained during the study as well as a spectrum of the difference between them are shown in Fig. 3A. In healthy human volunteers it has been observed that under hyperglycemic-hyperinsulinemic conditions the G-6-P concentration increased by approximately 120 μmol/L *(32)*, several times lower than in the biopsy studies, suggesting that the higher concentration in biopsy samples might be caused by glycogen degradation following sample excision. If, under these experimental conditions, glycogen synthase were the only enzyme with reduced activity in Type 2 diabetes mellitus, the initial rate of glucose entry into the G-6-P pool would be the same in normal and diabetic subjects. Thus the delayed removal of G-6-P and the decreased flux through glycogen synthase would result in higher concentrations of G-6-P in Type 2 diabetic patients. In contrast the insulin stimulated increase in intracellular G-6-P was found to be blunted, suggesting an impairment of glucose transport/phosphorylation in the diabetic subjects (Fig. 3B). In those studies *(32)* fasting basal G-6-P concentrations and G-6-P increments during the clamp study

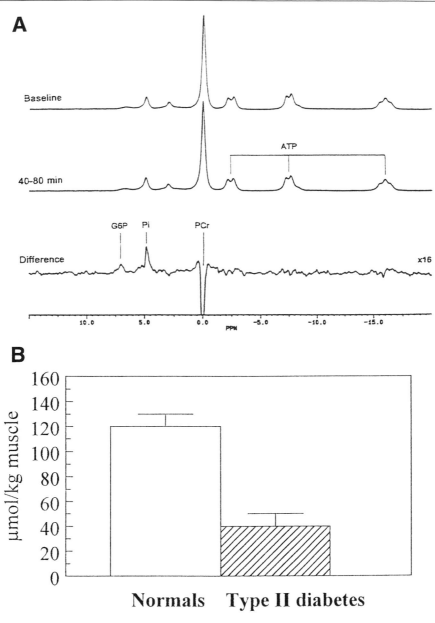

Fig. 3. (A) ^{31}P-NMR spectra of the gastrocnemious muscle of a normal subject. A baseline spectrum and a spectrum acquired over the period of 40–80 min of the insulin clamp are shown as well as the difference spectra. **(B)** Muscle increment of G-6-P concentration in normal (open bar) and diabetic subjects (solid bar) *(32)*.

were lower in diabetic patients compared to healthy subjects, implying that the activity of muscle glucose transport or hexokinase was reduced and it was the most important determinant of the lower rate of insulin stimulated muscle glycogen synthesis in Type 2 diabetes.

These studies demonstrated that Type 2 diabetes is characterized by insulin resistance which is due to reduced insulin-stimulated non-oxidative glucose metabolism primarily caused by impaired muscle glycogen synthesis. The defect responsible for the reduced flux through the glycogen synthetic pathway resides at the level of glucose transport or phosphorylation. The mechanism of insulin resistance in normo-glucose tolerant obese women was also addressed in a recent study *(33)*. Insulin-stimulated muscle glycogen synthesis was measured using ^{13}C NMR spectroscopy during the usual hyperglycemic-hyperinsulinemic clamp and was found to be reduced by 70% in the obese nondiabetic women as compared to the rates in lean controls *(33)*. To determine the biochemical factors underlying the reduced rates of muscle glycogen synthesis ^{31}P NMR spectroscopy was performed simultaneously to measure intracellular G-6-P, interleaving ^{13}C and ^{31}P acquisitions at 10-min intervals during the clamp study. Insulin stimulated increment of muscular G-6-P concentrations were lower in obese as compared to lean controls, suggesting that either glucose transport and or phosphorylation were impaired. These defects in muscle glycogen synthesis and glucose transport/phosphorylation are similar to those observed in subjects with Type 2 diabetes (21) and may reflect a common etiology. Very similar results were obtained in patients with poorly controlled insulin-dependent-diabetes mellitus (Type 1 diabetes). Using comparable experimental designs it was found that insulin resistance in poorly controlled Type 1 diabetic patients was due to lower rates of muscle glycogen synthesis and that defective glucose transport/phosphorylation was the major factor responsible for this alteration *(34)*.

NMR SPECTROSCOPY IN HUMAN SKELETAL MUSCLE OF OFFSPRING OF TYPE 2 DIABETIC PATIENTS

These studies do not address the question as to whether or not the defect in glucose transport or phosphorylation by hexokinase is a primary or secondary defect in the pathogenesis of Type 2 diabetes. Long term exposure to hyperglycemia as shown in poorly controlled Type 1 diabetics may result in reduced transport and hexokinase activity and consequently reduced insulin stimulated muscle glycogen synthesis. In order to answer this question, we examined insulin stimulated muscle glycogen synthesis and the concentration of G-6-P in young, healthy, lean, normo-glycemic offspring of Type 2 diabetic parents. Studies on both families and populations with a high incidence of Type 2 diabetes have found that reduced insulin-dependent glucose metabolism is a common occurrence in nondiabetic first degree relatives *(5,6,12,35–38)*. There are many genetic and environmental risk factors for Type 2 diabetes and they may vary within and between populations; for this reason it has been very difficult to identify a single mechanism responsible for the susceptibility to the disease. By studying a more carefully selected homogeneous population it might be possible to reduce much of the complexity and heterogeneity for Type 2 diabetes in a particular group of patients. Accurate phenotyping for this trait is crucial. Consequently, we studied the distribution of insulin sensitivity in first degree relatives of Type 2 diabetes who have a high likelihood of developing diabetes. Since many factors may contribute to insulin resistance, we screened 49 first degree relatives who were young, healthy, lean, sedentary and had normal glucose tolerance using a euglycemic-hyperinsulinemic clamp *(39)*. As shown in Fig. 4 we found a mixture of three distributions of insulin sensitivity where the offspring of Type 2 diabetic patients might be subdivided in three separate groups: subjects with very low insulin sensitivity (20%),

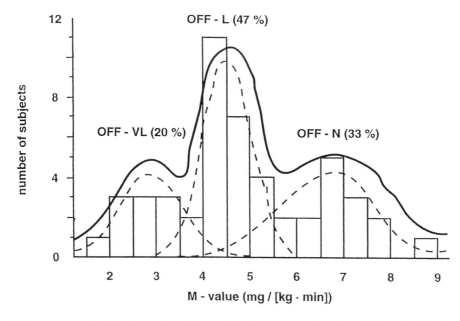

Fig. 4. Frequency distribution of insulin sensitivity among offspring of Type 2 diabetic parents. Best-fitting model to data was mixture of three distributions. Dashed lines represent individual distributions and solid line the sum of the three distributions. OFF-VL represent offspring with very low insulin sensitivity, OFF-L with moderately low insulin sensitivity and OFF-N with normal insulin sensitivity *(39)*.

subjects with moderate impairment of insulin sensitivity (47%) and subjects with insulin sensitivity comparable to normals (33%). A possible interpretation of the data was that insulin action is determined by a single autosomal codominant gene. Although familial clustering of insulin sensitivity has been observed in Pima Indians *(40)* and Caucasian subjects *(41)* these were the first data to suggest that a single gene may be regulating insulin sensitivity in a Caucasian population. This hypothesis has been previously formulated for Pima Indians, an other example of population at very high risk to develop diabetes *(42)*. The novel finding that insulin sensitivity appears to be genetically determined by a single major gene in this population is highly relevant to the pathogenesis of Type 2 diabetes. To test the hypothesis that the abnormality in muscle glycogen synthetic pathway found in Type 2 diabetic patients might be responsible of the reduced insulin sensitivity in the offspring, in particular in that 20% with marked insulin resistance, $^{31}P/^{13}C$ NMR spectroscopy was combined with clamp and indirect calorimetry techniques and used to characterize once more the mechanisms of insulin resistance in this population. The subgroup of very insulin resistant offspring of Type 2 diabetic parents was studied under conditions of hyperglycemia-hyperinsulinemia *(43)* and as shown in their parents they were characterized by reduced rates of insulin stimulated muscle glycogen synthesis and low concentration of intramuscular G-6-P. These data support the hypothesis that the reduction in muscle glucose transport/hexokinase activity is fully expressed prior to the development of diabetes and that it is not secondary to hyperglycemia (glucose toxicity). The presence of this abnormality in subjects at high risk of developing diabetes suggests that abnormal muscle glucose transport/hexokinase activity may be a primary factor in the pathogenesis of Type 2 diabetes mellitus. However, the data cannot be used to distinguish whether the reduced rate of muscle glycogen synthesis in the offspring of Type 2 diabetic parents was due to a reduction in the activity of either glucose transport or hexokinase. Insulin-stimulated muscle glucose transport occurs by facilitated diffusion using the GLUT4 transporter *(44,45)*. In the absence of insulin, GLUT4 is almost completely sequestered in an intracellular compartment. With insulin, this compartment is quickly mobilized to the cell surface, resulting in a substantial increase in both surface GLUT4 levels and glucose transport *(46)*. Measurements of GLUT4 protein and mRNA in the muscle of subjects with Type 2 diabetes have generally shown no difference compared to control subjects *(47)*. However total glucose transporter number may not reflect glucose transport activity, since insulin-stimulated glucose transport also requires the translocation of the transporter to the plasma membrane. Hexokinase has previously been considered insulin independent and therefore not considered as a potential rate-limiting step. However recent studies suggest that in vivo hexokinase activity is insulin dependent and may in some conditions be rate limiting *(48)*. In addition, a reduction in glucose transport may be secondary to impaired glucose and insulin delivery due to reduced muscle capillary density or blood flow *(49,50)*. More recently an increased number of Type IIb muscle fibers in insulin resistant first degree relatives of patients with Type 2 diabetes has been reported *(51)*. Type IIb fibers are associated with a negative correlation with insulin stimulated glucose uptake and whether this finding reflects a reduced physical activity level and fitness in the relatives *(52)* or is of primary genetic origin remains to be determined. All these variables may be involved in the regulation of transport and phosphorylation of glucose at the level of the skeletal muscle, but it is not yet possible to rule out defects in one or the other function. One potential approach to distinguish between abnormalities in glucose transport versus hexokinase contributing to defective insulin stimulated muscle glycogen synthesis in Type 2 diabetes is the measurement of intracellular glucose concentrations using a recently described ^{13}C NMR approach *(53,54)*.

NMR SPECTROSCOPY IN HUMAN SKELETAL MUSCLE OF OFFSPRING OF TYPE 2 DIABETIC PATIENTS: EFFECT OF EXERCISE

As previously discussed, during the hyperglycemic-hyperinsulinemic clamp glucose is predominantly incorporated into muscle glycogen *(21)*. Using ^{13}C NMR spectroscopy it has been shown that after a mixed meal, carbohydrates are incorporated into both liver and skeletal muscle glycogen *(55)*. During exercise muscle glycogen levels decrease according to the type of exercise, workload and rate of muscle contraction. When exercise ceases, the exercised muscles resynthesize glycogen at a rate that is influenced by the post-exercise concentration of intracellular glycogen *(56,57)*. The acute effects of exercise on muscle glucose metabolism can be studied by using exercises that mainly involve isolated muscle groups and monitor muscle glycogen using NMR spectroscopy. In such a setup the muscle group in the contralateral leg can be used as a control. In a study where subjects performed single-leg-toe-raises, the glycogen levels decreased substantially in the gastrocnemious muscle in the exercised leg whereas the glycogen concentration in the resting contralateral leg remained constant and was not affected by the exercise *(58)*. Natural abundance ^{13}C NMR spectroscopy was performed in a 4.7T spectrometer with a 30-cm diameter magnet bore. Subjects remained supine with the right leg posi-

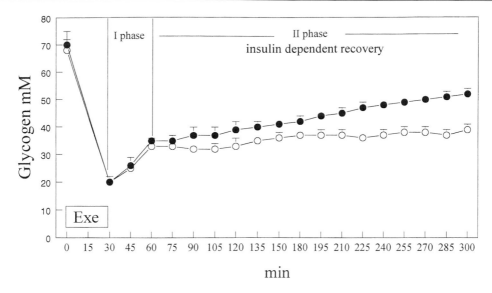

Fig. 5. Time courses of glycogen concentrations during 5-h recovery of glycogen-depleted gastrocnemious muscle. Normal subjects are represented with solid symbols and offspring of NIDDM parents with open symbols *(60)*.

tioned within the homogeneous volume of the magnet and with the calf resting on a surface coil. After the exercise session, the exercising muscles restored the basal level of glycogen concentration over several hours *(58)*. Using this localized exercise protocol in combination with ^{13}C NMR, the combined effect of glycogen concentration and insulin on glycogen resynthesis was studied (59). Subjects performed the single leg-toe-raises to deplete gastrocnemious glycogen to 75, 50 or 25% of resting concentration. The initial resynthesis rate (first hour of the recovery period) was significantly increased when glycogen was depleted to 25% (<35 m*M*) of initial concentration in contrast to 50 or 75% glycogen depletion. After the initial rapid resynthesis phase (1 h), muscle glycogen is replenished at lower rates to reach full recovery in 5–6 h. This is a typical biphasic pattern of glycogen repletion after a glycogen depleting exercise. In normal healthy humans the initial phase of rapid glycogen resynthesis (12–30 m*M*/h) lasting 45 min is followed by a slower phase (3 m*M*/h) which takes hours. The first phase appears to be insulin independent because it was not affected by a somatostatin infusion which suppressed insulin release, whereas the second phase was insulin-dependent as reflected by lower rates of glycogen resynthesis during the somatostatin infusion *(59)*. When insulin resistant offspring of Type 2 diabetic patients performed the same kind of experiment they showed a conserved first phase (insulin-independent) of glycogen repletion and a profound impairment of the second (insulin-dependent) phase (Fig. 5) *(60)*. These findings are in agreement with previous studies in which insulin stimulated muscle glycogen synthesis rates were impaired in offspring of Type 2 diabetic parents *(43)*. In addition ^{31}P NMR spectroscopy was used to measure G-6-P before, immediately after the single leg-toe raises exercise and during the recovery period. The finding was somehow surprising: based on data obtained during the clamp studies (lower intramuscular G-6-P concentrations) in Type 2 diabetic patients suggesting impairment of glucose transport/hexokinase activity, lower G-6-P levels were expected during the insulin-dependent phase; on the contrary, G-6-P levels were normal or slightly higher than in healthy subjects. This set of data (low glycogen synthetic rates in the presence of normal G-6-P concentrations) suggest that both glucose transport/phosphorylation and glycogen synthase activity were reduced in a coordinated manner. The differences observed between the clamp studies and the acute exercise experiments may be due to the fact that insulin and exercise are able to recruit different pools of GLUT4 transporters in the plasma membrane and this effect is additive as already demonstrated (61,62). Due to the positive outcome in cardiac and respiratory performance, aerobic exercise training may be also useful to improve insulin sensitivity in people at high risk for developing diabetes (63–67) and may be a potentially important therapeutic option to prevent or delay the onset of Type 2 diabetes (68). It became important to determine the mechanism by which exercise training improves insulin sensitivity in young, sedentary subjects of normal weight and with normal glucose tolerance who are at high risk for diabetes because they have a strong family history of Type 2 diabetes and because they are insulin resistant. The aim of the study was to assess the effect of one bout of exercise and of a 6 wk-period exercise training on insulin stimulated glycogen synthetic rates (^{13}C NMR spectroscopy) and rate controlling steps (^{31}P NMR spectroscopy) (69). The baseline study (performed before starting any exercise activity) confirmed previous study (43) showing reduced insulin dependent glycogen synthetic rates due to impairment of glucose transport/phosphorylation in the offspring when compared to normal healthy subjects. The same parameters were evaluated 48 h after one bout of exercise constituted by 5-min warm-up, followed by three 15-min sets of stair-climbing exercise performed at 65% of maximal aerobic capacity, with 5 min rest periods allowed between sets. The effect of physical training was evaluated after six wk during which the subjects repeated the exercise protocol four times per each week. The most striking finding of this study was that exercise training resulted in a twofold increase in insulin stimulated muscle glycogen synthesis in the offspring and normal subjects as well (Fig. 6). Because insulin resistance appears to be central to the pathogenesis of Type 2 diabetes, an intervention that improves the action of insulin may be beneficial in preventing or delaying the onset of the disease. Furthermore, the finding that over 60% of the training effect on insulin-stimulated muscle glycogen synthesis was present 48 h after the first exercise session suggests that similar results might be obtained with even fewer weekly exercise session. However the mechanism by which exercise improves insulin sensitivity in humans is unknown, but with the use of ^{31}P NMR spectroscopy, to measure the intramuscular concentration of G-6-P, exercise seems to revert the abnormality of glucose transport/phosphorylation which characterizes the offspring of Type 2 diabetic parents, as reflected by the normalization of the G-6-P concentration during the hyperglycemic-hyperinsulinemic clamp after the exercise (Fig. 7). Nonetheless, despite the normalization of G-6-P, rates of muscle glycogen synthesis were still lower than in the normal subjects, suggesting the existence of a defect in glycogen synthase in addition to the previously described defect in glucose transport/phosphorylation, which exercise was able to unmask. This finding is consistent with the observation that the activity of insulin stimulated glycogen synthase is reduced in skeletal muscle of non-obese first-degree relatives of patients with Type 2 diabetes (70,71). The observation of multiple defects in muscle glycogen metabolism may reflect a common abnormality in the insulin signaling pathway controlling this metabolic pathway (72).

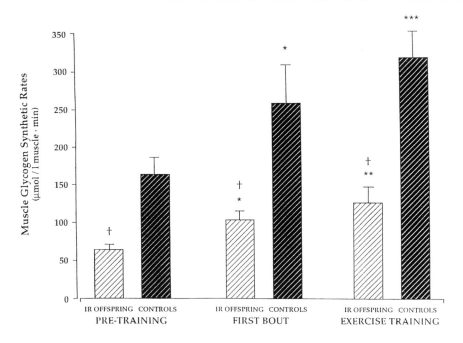

Fig. 6. Muscle glycogen synthetic rates in offspring of Type 2 diabetic parents (light column) and normal subjects (dark column) in the pre-training condition, 48 h after the first bout of exercise and after 6 wk of exercise training *(69)*.

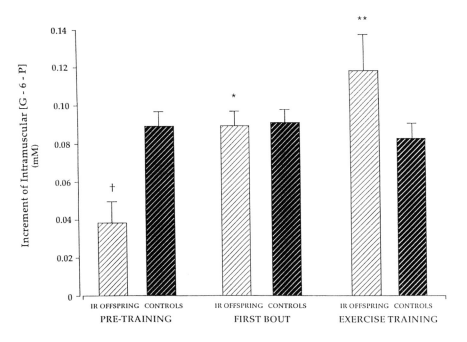

Fig. 7. Increment of intramuscular G-6-P during the hyperglycemic-hyperinsulinemic clamp in offspring of Type 2 diabetic parents (light column) and normal subjects (dark column) in pretraining condition, after the first bout and after 6 wk of physical training *(69)*.

NMR SPECTROSCOPY IN HUMAN SKELETAL MUSCLE:
INTERACTIONS OF GLUCOSE AND LIPID METABOLISM

The experiments previously reviewed using NMR spectroscopic techniques have defined the specific abnormalities in intramuscular glucose metabolism which can explain the mechanisms of insulin resistance in diabetic patients and in their relatives at high risk to develop diabetes, 20–25 yr before they manifest the disease. The similarity of these abnormalities suggests that they may play a primary role in the pathogenesis of Type 2 diabetes mellitus. Among several metabolic parameters free fatty acids (FFA) concentrations have been proposed as an important modulator of insulin action in humans. Our studies demonstrated that FFA concentrations were a reasonable predictor for the degree of insulin resistance in young, healthy offspring of diabetic parents *(39)* and in healthy obese subjects *(33)* suggesting a role of altered FFA metabolism in causing insulin resistance *(73)*. Over 30 yr ago Randle et al. *(74,75)* demonstrated that in isolated rat heart muscle and rat diaphragms, FFA effectively compete with glucose for substrate oxidation and it was therefore suggested that increased fat oxidation might cause the insulin resistance associated with diabetes and obesity. The postulated mechanism has been that increased free fatty acid oxidation causes elevation of intramitochondrial acetyl-CoA/CoA and NADH/NAD- ratios with subsequent inactivation of pyruvate dehydrogenase. This in turn causes citrate concentrations to increase leading to inhibition of phosphofructokinase and subsequent accumulation of G-6-P. In Randle's hypothesis glycogen synthesis was thought to be increased due to availability of substrate (G-6-P), rather than reduced. Finally, increased concentrations of G-6-P would inhibit hexokinase II and result in decreased glucose uptake (Fig. 8). Boden et al (76, 77) provided evidence that a reduction of carbohydrate oxidation was responsible for only one-third of the reduction of insulin-stimulated glucose metabolism in presence of an excess of FFA in humans, whereas impairment of non-oxidative glucose metabolism, which mostly reflecting glycogen synthesis (21), accounted for two-thirds of this fatty acid-dependent reduction in glucose uptake. Roden and coworkers (78) using ^{13}C NMR spectroscopy in combination with the euglycemic-hyperinsulinemic clamp techniques studied the effect of high plasma FFA availability on muscle glycogen synthesis in vivo in human subjects. Each subject was studied with or without lipid substrate (Liposyn and heparin infusion). The observed reduction of non-oxidative glucose metabolism during the infusion of lipid substrate and heparin was paralleled by a reduction in muscle glycogen synthesis (Fig. 9). This effect of FFA *per se* to decrease insulin stimulated glycogen synthesis at plasma concentration of 1.5–2.0 mM takes 3-4 hours to occur. To elucidate the mechanisms behind this reduction in insulin stimulated muscle glycogen synthesis, G-6-P was measured using ^{31}P NMR spectroscopy during the experiment. After 90 min of the lipid infusion, intracellular G-6-P concentration was already reduced compared to the control study, and thereafter continually decreasing to lower levels than in the basal post-absorptive state (<100 M). This finding is consistent with a profound inhibition of the glucose transport/phosphorylation activity. Contrary to the classical mechanism of FFA-induced insulin resistance proposed by Randle in which FFA exert their effect through initial inhibition of pyruvate dehydrogenase, elevation of FFA concentration causes insulin resistance by inhibition of glucose transport/phosphorylation with subsequent reduction in rates of glucose oxidation and muscle glycogen synthesis (Fig. 8). This reduction in insulin inducible glucose transport/phosphorylation is similar to what is observed in patients with Type 2 diabetes

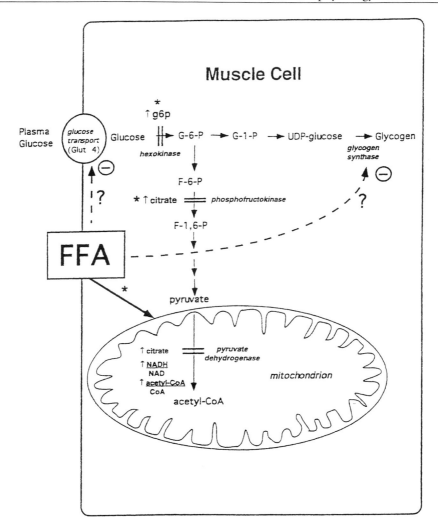

Fig. 8. Schema of potential sites of FFA action on insulin mediated metabolism in skeletal muscle *(78)*.

(21), in their nondiabetic insulin-resistant offspring *(43,69)* and in nondiabetic obese women (33) and further suggests that alterations in intramuscular FFA metabolism may play an important role in the pathogenesis of insulin resistance in Type 2 diabetes *(79–84)*.

CONCLUSIONS

NMR spectroscopy has become a useful tool for investigating muscle glucose metabolism in vivo making a major contribution to the definition of the metabolic defects responsible for insulin resistance in Type 2 diabetes mellitus. By applying this technique it has been possible to demonstrate that muscle glycogen synthesis is the principal pathway for insulin stimulated glucose disposal in both normal and Type 2 diabetic subjects. Furthermore, defects in muscle glycogen synthesis play a predominant role in the insulin resistance that occurs in Type 2 diabetic patients. Additional studies using ^{31}P NMR

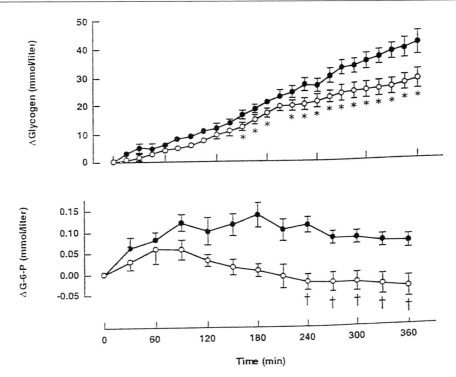

Fig. 9. Increase in calf muscle glycogen (top) and variation in intramuscular G-6-P at low (closed symbols) and elevated plasma free fatty acid concentrations (open symbols) *(78)*.

spectroscopy have shown that the defect in muscle glycogen synthesis is secondary to a defect in glucose transport/phosphorylation. The same defects were found in young, healthy, lean nondiabetic, insulin resistant offspring of Type 2 diabetic patients, suggesting that this defect in glucose transport/phosphorylation may play a primary role in the pathogenesis of Type 2 diabetes. Studies performed immediately after an acute bout of anaerobic exercise or after an aerobic exercise training program highlight the possibility of at least partially reverting these defects in glucose transport/phosphorylation and to improve insulin stimulated glycogen synthesis to levels close to the rates measured in sedentary normal healthy subjects, therefore ameliorating insulin resistance and possibly reducing the risk of developing diabetes. Additional studies to investigate the mechanism of FFA-induced insulin resistance have revealed that a defect in glycogen synthesis rate due to impairment of glucose transport/phosphorylation was inducible by increasing the plasma FFA concentration. The similarity between these defects and those observed in Type 2 diabetes suggests that alteration of lipid metabolism may play an important role in the pathogenesis of insulin resistance observed in Type 2 diabetes.

REFERENCES

1. Gadian DG. An introduction to spectroscopy. In: Nuclear magnetic resonance and its application to living system. Clarendon and Oxford University Press, Oxford and New York, 1992, pp. 1–61.
2. Williams DAR. Background and theory of NMR Spectroscopy. In: Nuclear magnetic resonance spectroscopy. John Wiley & Sons, London, 1986, pp. 1–54.

3. Berson SA, Yalow RS. Insulin antagonists and insulin resistance. In: Ellenberg M and Rifkin H, ed. Diabetes Mellitus: Theory and Practice. McGraw-Hill, New York, 1970, pp. 388–423.

4. De Fronzo RA. Lilly Lecture 1987 (1988). The triumvirate: -cell, muscle, liver. A collusion responsible for NIDDM. Diabetes 37:667–687.

5. Warram JH, Martin BC, Krolewski AS, Soeldner JS, Kahn CR. Slow glucose removal rate and hyperinsulinemia precede the development of type II diabetes in the offspring of diabetic parents. Ann Intern Med 1990;113:909–915.

6. Martin BC, Warram JH, Krolewski AS, Bergman RN, Soeldner JS, Kahn CR. Role of glucose and insulin resistance in development of Type 2 diabetes mellitus: results of a 25-year follow-up study. Lancet 1992;340:925–929.

7. Butterfield WJH, Whichelow MJ. Peripheral glucose metabolism in control subjects and diabetic patients during glucose, glucose-insulin and insulin sensitivity tests. Diabetologia 1965;1:43–53.

8. Jakson RA, Perry G, Rogers J, Advoni U, Pilkington TRE. Relationship between the basal glucose concentration, glucose tolerance and forearm glucose uptake in maturity onset diabetes. Diabetes 1973;22:751–761.

9. Campbell P, Mandarino L, Gerich J. Quantification of the relative impairment in actions of insulin on hepatic glucose production and peripheral glucose uptake in NIDDM. Metabolism 1988;37:15–22.

10. Kelley DE, Mandarino LJ. Hyperglycemia normalizes insulin-stimulated skeletal muscle glucose oxidation and storage in NIDDM. J Clin Invest 1990;86:1999–2007.

11. De Fronzo RA, Gunnarsson R, Bjorkman O, Olsson M, Wahren J. Effects of insulin on peripheral and splanchnic glucose metabolism in NIDDM. J Clin Invest 1985;76:149–155.

12. Eriksson J, Franssila-Kallunki A, Ekstrand A, Saloranta C, Widen E, Schalin C, Groop L. Early metabolic defects in persons at increased risk for non-insulin dependent diabetes mellitus. N Engl J Med 1989;321:337–343.

13. De Fronzo RA, Jacot E, Jequier E, Maeder E, Wahren J, Felber JP. The effect of insulin on the disposal of intravenous glucose: results from indirect calorimetry and hepatic and femoral venous catheterization. Diabetes 1981;30:1000–1007.

14. Golay A, De Fronzo RA, Ferrannini E et al. Oxidative and non-oxidative glucose metabolism in non-obese Type 2 (noninsulin dependent) diabetic patients. Diabetologia 1988;31:585–591.

15. Sillerud GI, Shulman RG. Structure and metabolism of mammalian liver glycogen monitored by carbon-13 nuclear magnetic resonance. Biochemistry 1983;22:1087–1094.

16. Shulman GI, Rothman DL, Chung Y, Petit WA, Barrett EJ, Shulman RG. ^{13}C-NMR studies of glycogen turnover in the perfused rat liver. J Biol Chem 1988;263:5027–5029.

17. Zang LH, Laughton MR, Rothman DL, Shulman RG. ^{13}C-NMR relaxation times of hepatic glycogen in vitro and in vivo. Biochemistry 1990;29:6815–6820.

18. Zang LH, Rothman DL, Shulman RG. ^{1}H NMR visibility of mammalian glycogen in solution. Proc Natl Acad Sci USA 1990;87:1678–1680.

19. Gruetter R, Prolla TA, Shulman RG. ^{13}C-NMR visibility of rabbit muscle glycogen in vivo. Magn Res Med 1991;20:327–332.

20. Taylor R, Price TB, Rothman DL, Shulman RG, Shulman GI. Validation of ^{13}C-NMR measurement of human skeletal muscle glycogen by direct biochemical assay of needle biopsy samples. Magn Reson Med 1992;27:13–20.

21. Shulman GI, Rothman DL, Jue T, Stein P, De Fronzo RA, Shulman RG. Quantitation of muscle glycogen synthesis in normal subjects and subjects with non-insulin-dependent diabetes by ^{13}C nuclear magnetic resonance spectroscopy. N Engl J Med 1990;322:223–228.

22. Bjorntorp P, Sjostrom L. Carbohydrate storage in man: speculation and some quantitative considerations. Metabolism 1978;27(Suppl 2):1853–1865.

23. Roch-Norland AE, Bergstrom J, Hultman E. Muscle glycogen and synthetase in normal subjects g and in patients with diabetes mellitus: effect of intravenous glucose and insulin administration. Scan J Clin Invest 1972;30:77–84.

24. Bogardus C, Lillioja S, Stone K, Mott D. Correlation between muscle glycogen synthase activity and in vivo insulin action in man. J Clin Invest 1984;73:1185–1190.

25. Mandarino LJ, Wright KS, Verity LS, Nichols J, Bell J, Kolterman OG, Beck-Nielsen H. Effects of insulin infusion on human skeletal muscle pyruvate dehydrogenase, phosphofructokinase and glycogen synthase: evidence for their role in oxidative and non-oxidative glucose metabolism. J Clin Invest 1987;80:655–663.

26. Freymond D, Bogardus C, Okubo M, Stone K, Mott D. Impaired insulin stimulated muscle glycogen synthase activation in vivo in man is related to low fasting glycogen synthase phosphatase activity. J Clin Invest 1988;82:1503–1509.

27. Bonadonna RC, Del Prato S, Saccomani MP, Bonora E, Gulli G, Ferrannini E, Bier D, Cobelli C, De Fronzo RA. Transmembrane glucose transport in skeletal muscle of patients with non-insulin dependent diabetes mellitus. J Clin Invest 1993;92:486–494.

28. Kelley DE, Mintun MA, Watkins SC, Simoneau JA, Jadali F, Fredrikson A, Beattie J, Theriault R. The effect of non-insulin-dependent diabetes mellitus and obesity on glucose transport and phosphorylation in skeletal muscle. J Clin Invest 1996;97:2705–2713.

29. Rossetti L, Giaccari A. Relative contribution of glycogen synthesis and glycolysis to insulin mediated glucose uptake: a dose response study. J Clin Invest 1990;85:1785–1792.

30. Godown DG, Radda GK, Richards RE, Seeley PJ. (1979). ^{31}P NMR in living tissue: the road from a promising tool to an important tool in biology. In: Shulman RG, ed. Biological Applications of Magnetic Resonance. Academic Press, New York 463–536.

31. Taylor DJ, Styles P, Matthews PM, Arnold DA, Godown DG, Bore P, Radda GK. Energetics of human muscle: exercise-induced ATP depletion. Magn Reson Med 1986;3:44–54.

32. Rothman DL, Shulman RG, Shulman GI. ^{31}P Nuclear magnetic resonance measurements of muscle glucose-6-phosphate. Evidence for reduced insulin-dependent muscle glucose transport or phosphory-lation activity in non-insulin dependent diabetes mellitus. J Clin Invest 1992;89:1069–1075.

33. Petersen KF, Hendler R, Price TB, Perseghin G, Rothman DL, Held N, Amatruda JM, Shulman GI. ^{13}C/^{31}P NMR studies on the mechanism of insulin resistance in obesity. Diabetes 1998;47:381–386.

34. Cline GW, Magnusson I, Rothman DL, Petersen KF, Laurent D, Shulman GI. Mechanism of impaired insulin-stimulated muscle glucose metabolism in subjects with insulin dependent diabetes mellitus. J Clin Invest 1997;99:2219–2224.

35. Lillioja S, Mott DM, Howard BV, Bennett PH, Yki-Järvinen H, Frimond D, Nyomba BL, Zurlo F, Swinburn B, Bogardus C. Impaired glucose tolerance as a disorder of insulin action. Longitudinal and cross-sectional studies in Pima Indians. N Engl J Med 1988;318:1217–1225.

36. Lillioja S, Mott DM, Spraul M, Ferraro R, Foley JE, Ravussin E, Knowler WC, Bennett PH, Bogardus C. Insulin resistance and insulin secretory dysfunction as precursors of non-insulin-dependent diabetes mellitus. Prospective studies of Pima Indians. N Engl J Med 1993;329:1988–1992.

37. Gulli G, Ferrannini E, Stern M, Haffner S, De Fronzo RA. The metabolic profile of NIDDM is fully established in glucose-tolerant offspring of two Mexican-American NIDDM parents. Diabetes 1992;41:1575–1586.

38. Beck-Nielsen H, Groop LC. Metabolic and genetic characterization of prediabetic states. Sequence of events leading to non-insulin dependent diabetes mellitus. J Clin Invest 1994;94:1714–1721.

39. Perseghin G, Ghosh S, Gerow K, Shulman GI. Metabolic defects in lean nondiabetic offspring of NIDDM parents: a cross-sectional study. Diabetes 1997;46:1001–1009.

40. Lillioja S, Mott DM, Zawadzki JK, Young AA, Abbott WGH, Knowler WC, Bennett PH, Moll P, Bogardus C: In vivo insulin action is familial characteristic in nondiabetic Pima Indians. Diabetes 1987;36:1329–1335.

41. Martin BC, Warram JH, Rosner B, Rich SS, Soeldner JS, Krolewski AS. Familial clustering of insulin sensitivity. Diabetes 1992;41:850–854.

42. Bogardus C, Lillioja S, Nyomba BL, Zurlo F, Swinburn B, Puente ED, Knowler WC, Ravussin E, Mott DM, Bennett PH. Distribution of in vivo insulin action in Pima Indians as a mixture of three normal distributions. Diabetes 1989;38:1423–32.

43. Rothman DL, Magnusson I, Cline G, Gerard D, Kahn CR, Shulman RG, Shulman GI. Decreased muscle transport/phosphorylation is an early defect in the pathogenesis of non-insulin dependent diabetes mellitus. Proc Natl Acad Sci USA 1995;92:983–987.

44. James DE, Piper RC. Insulin resistance, diabetes, and the insulin-regulated trafficking of GLUT4 J Cell Biol 1994;126:1123–1126.

45. Bell GI, Burant CF, Takeda J, Gould GW. Structure and function of mammalian facilitative glucose transporters. J Biol Chem 1993;268:19161–19164.

46. Rea S, James DE. Moving GLUT4. The biogenesis and trafficking of GLUT4 storage vesicles. Diabetes 1997;46:1667–1677.

47. Granner DK, O'Brien RM. Molecular physiology and genetics of NIDDM. Importance of metabolic staging. Diabetes Care 1992;15:369–395.

48. Mandarino LJ, Printz RL, Cusi KA, Kinchington P, O'Doherty RM, Osawa H, Sewell C, Consoli A, Granner DK, De Fronzo RA. Regulation of hexokinase II and glycogen synthase mRNA, protein and activity in human muscle. Am J Physiol 1995;269:E701-E708.

49. Lillioja S, Young AA, Culter CL, Ivy JL, Abbott GH, Zawadzki JK, Yki-Järvinen H, Christin L, Secomb TW, Bogardus C. Skeletal muscle capillary density and fiber type are possible determinants of in vivo insulin resistance in man. J Clin Invest 1987;80:415–424.

50. Laakso M, Edelman SV, Brechtal G, Baron AD. Decreased effect of insulin to stimulate skeletal muscle blood flow in obese man: a novel mechanism for insulin resistance. J Clin Invest 1990; 85:1844–1852.

51. Nyholm B, Qu Zhuqing, Kaal A, Bonnelykke S, Gravholt CH, Andersen JL, Saltin B, Schmitz O. Evidence of an increased number of type IIb muscle fibers in insulin resistant first degree relatives of patients with NIDDM. Diabetes 1997;46:1822–1828.

52. Nyholm B, Mengel A, Nielsen S, Skjoeboek, Moller N, Alberti KGMM, Schmitz O. Insulin resistance in relatives of patients with non-insulin dependent diabetes mellitus: the role of physical fitness and muscle metabolism. Diabetologia 1996;39:813–822.

53. Cline GW, Jucker BM, Rennings A. A novel method to assess intracellular glucose concentration in muscle in vivo. Diabetes 1996;45(Suppl 2):67, 20A.

54. Cline GW, Petersen KF, Krssak M, Shen J, Hundal R, Inzucchi S, Dresner A, Rothman DL, Shulman GI. Glucose transport is rate controlling for insulin stimulated muscle glycogen synthesis in Type 2 diabetes. Diabetes 1998;47(Suppl 1):256, A66.

55. Taylor R, Price TB, Katz LD, Shulman RG, Shulman GI. Direct measurement of change in muscle glycogen concentration after a mixed meal in normal subjects. Am J Physiol 1993;265:E224–E229.

56. Ivy JL, Frishberg BA, Farrell SW, Miller WJ, Sherman WM. Effects of elevated and exercise-reduced muscle glycogen levels on insulin sensitivity. J Appl Physiol 1985;59:154–159.

57. Casey A, Short AH, Hultman E, Greenhaff PL. Glycogen resynthesis in human muscle fibers types following exercise-induced glycogen depletion. J Physiol 1995;483:265–271.

58. Price TB, Rothman DL, Avison MJ, Buonamico P, Shulman RG. ^{13}C-NMR to assess muscle glycogen during low-intensity exercise. J Apll Physiol 1991;70:1836–1844.

59. Price TB, Rothman DL, Taylor R, Avison MJ, Shulman GI, Shulman RG. Human muscle glycogen resynthesis after exercise: insulin dependent and -independent phases. J Apll Physiol 1994;76:104–111.

60. Price TB, Perseghin G, Duleba A, Chen W, Chase J, Rothman DL, Shulman RG, Shulman GI. NMR studies of muscle glycogen synthesis in insulin resistant offspring of parents with non-insulin dependent diabetes mellitus immediately after glycogen depleting exercise. Proc Natl Acad Sci USA 1996;93:5329–5334.

61. Douen AG, Ramlal T, Cartee GD, Klip A. Exercise modulates the insulin-induced translocation of glucose transporters in rat skeletal muscle. FEBS Lett 1990;261:256–260.

62. Goodyear LJ, Hirshman MF, King PA, Horton ED, Thompson CM, Horton ES. Skeletal muscle plasma membrane glucose transport and glucose transporters after exercise. J Appl Physiol 1990;68:193–198.

63. Oshida Y, Yamanouchi K, Hayamizu S, Sato Y. Long term mild jogging increases insulin action despite no influence on body mass index or VO_2max. J Appl Physiol 1989;66:2206–2210.

64. De Fronzo RA, Sherwin RS, Kraemer N. Effect of physical training on insulin action in obesity. Diabetes 1987;36:1379–1385.

65. Tonino RP. Effect of physical training on the insulin resistance of aging. Am J Physiol 1989; 256:E352–E356.

66. Devlin JT, Hirshman M, Horton ED, Horton ES. Enhanced peripheral and splanchnic insulin sensitivity in NIDDM men after single bout of exercise. Diabetes 1987;36:434–439.

67. Segal KR, Edano A, Abalos A et al. Effect of exercise training on insulin sensitivity and glucose metabolism in lean, obese and diabetic men. J Appl Physiol 1991;71:2402–2411.

68. Helmrich SP, Ragland DR, Leung DW, Paffenbarger RS. Physical activity and reduced occurrence of non insulin dependent diabetes mellitus. N Engl J Med 1991;325:147–152.

69. Perseghin G, Price TB, Petersen KF, Roden M, Cline GW, Gerow K, Rothman DL, Shulman GI. Increased glucose transport/phosphorylation and muscle glycogen synthesis after exercise training in insulin resistant subjects. N Engl J Med 1996;335:1357–1362.

70. Schalin-Jännti C, Härkönen M, Groop LC. Impaired activation of glycogen synthase in people at increased risk for developing NIDDM. Diabetes 1992;41:598–604.

71. Vaag A, Henriksen JE, Beck-Nielsen H. Decreased insulin activation of glycogen synthase in skeletal muscle of young non-obese Caucasian first degree relatives of patients with non-insulin dependent diabetes mellitus. J Clin Invest 1992;89:782–788.

72. Kahn CR. Insulin action, diabetogenes and causes of Type 2 diabetes. Diabetes 1994;43:1066–1084.

73. McGarry JD. What if Minkowski had been ageusic? An alternative angle on diabetes. Science 1992;258:766–770.

74. Randle PJ, Garland PB, Hales CN, Newsholme EA. The glucose-fatty acid cycle: its role in insulin sensitivity and the metabolic disturbance of diabetes mellitus. Lancet 1963;i:785–789.

75. Randle PJ, Garland PB, Hales CN, Newsholme EA. The glucose-fatty acid cycle in obesity and maturity onset diabetes mellitus. Ann NY Acad Sci: 1965;131:324–333.
76. Boden G, Jadali F, White J, Liang Y, Mozzoli M, Chen X, Coleman E, Smith C. Effects of fat on insulin stimulated carbohydrate metabolism in normal men. J Clin Invest 1991;88:960–966.
77. Boden G, Chen X, Ruiz J, White JV, Rossetti L. Mechanisms of fatty acid-induced inhibition of glucose uptake. J Clin Invest 1994;93:2438–2446.
78. Roden M, Price TB, Perseghin G, Petersen KF, Rothman DL, Cline GW, Shulman GI. Mechanism of free fatty acid-induced insulin resistance in humans. J Clin Invest 1996;97:2859–2865.
79. Jucker BM, Rennings AJ, Cline GW, Petersen KF, Shulman GI. In vivo NMR investigation of intramuscular glucose metabolism in conscious rat. Am J Physiol 1997;273:E139–E148.
80. Jucker BM, Rennings AJ, Cline GW, Shulman GI. ^{13}C and ^{31}P NMR studies on the effect of increased plasma free fatty acids on intramuscular glucose metabolism in the awake rat. J Biol Chem 1997;272:10464–10473.
81. Schick F, Eismann B, Jung W-I, Bongers H, Bunse M, Lutz O. Comparison of localized proton NMR signals of skeletal muscle and fat tissue in vivo: two lipid compartments in muscle tissue. Magn Reson Med 1993;29:158–167.
82. Stein DT, Dobbins R, Szczepaniak L, Malloy C, McGarry JD. Skeletal muscle triglyceride stores are increased in insulin resistance. Diabetes 1997;46(Suppl 1):23A, 89.
83. Pan DA, Lillioja S, Kriketos AD, Milner MR, Baur LA, Bogardus C, Jenkins AB, Storlien LH. Skeletal muscle triglyceride levels are inversely related to insulin action. Diabetes 1997;46:983–988.
84. Perseghin G, Scifo P De Cobelli F, Vanzulli A, Del Maschio A, Pozza G, Luzi L. Increased muscle triglycerides content in young, non-obese first degree relatives of NIDDM parents: a ^{1}H NMR assessment. Diabetes 1998;47(Suppl 1):A299, 1156.

10

Skeletal Muscle Insulin Resistance in Humans: *Cellular Mechanisms*

Lawrence J. Mandarino, PhD

Contents

Introduction
Insulin Signaling
Glucose Transport
Summary
Acknowledgments
References

INTRODUCTION

The degree of sensitivity of skeletal muscle to insulin is widely variable in humans. Diseases such as non-insulin-dependent diabetes mellitus (NIDDM or Type 2 diabetes) have a characteristic component of muscle insulin resistance. Many obese, nondiabetic individuals are also insulin resistant. However, healthy people who are not overweight also display a spectrum of insulin sensitivity. For example, when the euglycemic, hyperinsulinemic clamp technique is used to measure insulin-stimulated glucose uptake in such healthy individuals, there is a two- to threefold range in glucose uptake. Therefore, some percentage of even lean, healthy people can be said to be insulin resistant. Presumably, the ability of the pancreas to secrete sufficient insulin prevents this insulin resistance from developing into abnormal glucose tolerance.

In all but isolated instances, the molecular or biochemical factors responsible for skeletal muscle insulin resistance are poorly defined. Over and above this, in most cases it is, as yet, not possible to say with any degree of certainty that any particular manifestation of insulin resistance is hereditary or acquired. A number of factors suggest that heredity contributes to muscle insulin resistance: insulin resistance is more common in some populations than in others; insulin resistance tends to run in families; and insulin resistance can be present at a relatively young age before there is time for long-term consequences of environmental factors to have an effect. However, families, and to some extent, populations, also tend to share behaviors and other environmental factors that might cause insulin resistance. Intensive investigation, using candidate gene analysis or genome-wide scanning, has so far not revealed any major genes that are responsible for

From: *Contemporary Endocrinology: Insulin Resistance*
Edited by: G. Reaven and A. Laws © Humana Press Inc., Totowa, NJ

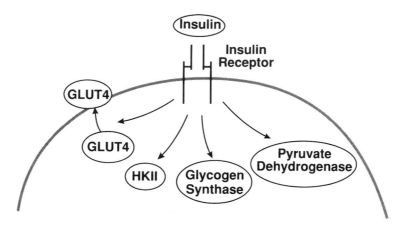

Fig. 1. Potential sites of cellular insulin resistance in skeletal muscle.

even a portion of insulin resistance. This suggests that, although genetic factors clearly play a role in insulin resistance, environmental and behavioral factors (which may in themselves be either acquired or hereditary) must also be important. In the absence of any absolute identification of genes that are clearly responsible for insulin resistance in a large proportion of insulin resistant people, potential genetic and environmental causes and mechanisms of insulin resistance should be given equal attention. This review, therefore, will attempt to distinguish hereditary and environmentally-induced insulin resistance in skeletal muscle and discuss potential mechanisms.

This review will concentrate on the potential cellular mechanisms that might be responsible for insulin resistance. Although there may be contributions of physiological mechanisms, such as alterations in regulation of blood flow, or anatomic mechanisms, such as fiber type composition or capillary density, these will not be discussed here. The potential cellular sites of skeletal muscle insulin resistance are diagrammed in Fig. 1.

INSULIN SIGNALING

Insulin Receptor Binding

Binding of insulin to its receptor is still considered to be the first step in the cellular action of insulin. Although the early finding that binding of insulin to the insulin receptor was reduced in obesity or Type 2 diabetes in tissues such as white blood cells *(1,2)* and adipocytes *(3,4)* generated much interest, most *(5,6)*, but not all *(7)* subsequent studies of insulin receptor binding function in skeletal muscle have not demonstrated decreased insulin binding in insulin resistant conditions. Although a number of naturally occurring mutations that are associated with profound insulin resistance, diabetes, growth and mental retardation have been reported *(8–13)*, few commonly occurring insulin receptor mutations are associated with Type 2 diabetes *(14)*. Mutations affecting a variety of aspects of insulin receptor processing, ligand binding, substrate binding, and tyrosine kinase activity have been described *(8,11)*, but none are associated with common forms of insulin resistance.

Following insulin binding, conformational changes in the β-subunit of the insulin receptor result in activation of an intrinsic tyrosine kinase. The first substrate of the insulin receptor tyrosine kinase appears to be the β-subunit of the insulin receptor itself,

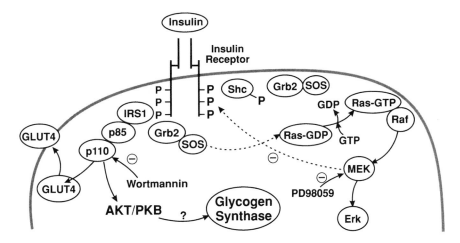

Fig. 2. Outline of insulin signaling pathways.

which becomes phosphorylated on a number of tyrosine residues that are critical for substrate binding. Decreased insulin-stimulated tyrosine phosphorylation of the insulin receptor β-subunit has been reported widely in Type 2 diabetes *(15–19)*, although this has not been a universal finding *(20,21)*. This decrease in phosphorylation could be due to decreased kinase or increased phosphatase activity *(22)*; however, there is another report of decreased tyrosine phosphatase activity in Type 2 diabetes *(23)*. Evidence is accumulating that tyrosine kinase activity of the insulin receptor is reduced in insulin resistance. At least part of the decreased tyrosine kinase activity of the insulin receptor may be acquired as a result of hyperglycemia or tumor necrosis factor α (TNFα). For example, Haring and colleagues showed that high glucose or TNFα inhibit insulin receptor autophosphorylation of the β-subunit of the insulin receptor in Rat1 fibroblasts overexpressing the human insulin receptor *(24)*. The mechanisms of this effect appeared to be different, however, as TNFα, which has been postulated to be involved in the pathogenesis of insulin resistance *(25)*, seemed to act by increasing protein tyrosine phosphatase activity whereas glucose acted through activation of protein kinase C (PKC) *(24)*. Recently, in vitro studies have suggested that a protein kinase C *(26)* and MAP kinase dependent mechanism *(27)* could result in increased serine phosphorylation of the insulin receptor and downregulation of its activity. Whether hyperglycemia in vivo can alter insulin receptor tyrosine kinase activity is unknown; however, hyperglycemia can increase PKC activity *(28)*, and this could in turn lead to serine phosphorylation of the insulin receptor, which could decrease its activity.

Post Receptor Signaling

Intensive investigation over the past decade has led to a more detailed understanding of growth factor receptor signaling in general, and insulin receptor signaling in particular. A detailed review of the current knowledge regarding intracellular signaling is beyond the scope of this review and has been dealt with elsewhere *(29–31)*. Rather, this discussion will focus on the involvement of insulin signaling abnormalities in skeletal muscle insulin resistance. However, for reference, a brief diagrammatic outline of the known elements of insulin signaling is shown in Fig. 2.

Upon activation of the insulin receptor β-subunit tyrosine kinase, several proteins bind to various phosphotyrosine-containing amino acid recognition sequences in the β-subunit. These include, in part, IRS-1/IRS-2 *(32,33)*, Shc *(34,35)*, Grb2 *(36,37)*, and hGrb 10γ*(38)*. At least two divergent, but interacting, signaling pathways lead from the insulin receptor. One depends upon the recognition of phosphotyrosine-containing amino acid sequences (YMXM, YXXM) in IRS1 by SH2 domains in a number of other proteins, including Grb2 and regulatory subunits of the enzyme phosphatidylinositol 3-kinase (PI 3-kinase). With regard to the metabolic action of insulin, of chief importance among the proteins that bind to IRS-1 are these regulatory subunits of PI 3-kinase. The PI 3-kinase catalytic subunit is activated by conformational change through association of its regulatory subunit with IRS-1 *(39)*. Most, if not all, of insulin's metabolic effects, including translocation of GLUT4 transporters *(40,41)* and activation of glycogen synthase *(42,43)* are believed to be mediated by activation of PI 3-kinase because specific inhibitors of PI 3-kinase, such as wortmannin and LY23098 block insulin stimulation of glucose transport or glycogen synthesis. At least one of the transcriptional events influenced by insulin, increased transcription of the hexokinase II (HKII) gene, also is inhibited by wortmannin and presumably depends on insulin activation of PI 3-kinase *(44)*.

The other major signaling pathway activated by the insulin receptor is the "canonical" MAP kinase pathway, leading to phosphorylation and activation of the serine kinases ERK1 and ERK2. The MAP kinase pathway is activated either following Ras direct interaction of Shc with the insulin receptor and subsequent activation of Grb2 and the GTP exchange factor SOS, or activation of Grb2/SOS upon the association of Grb2 with IRS-1/2. Activation of the MAP kinase pathway is a feature shared by the insulin receptor and other growth factor receptors, but its involvement in the well-characterized metabolic effects of insulin is thought to be limited. Neither dominant negative ras mutants *(43)* nor PD 98059, an inhibitor of MEK activation *(41)*, block insulin's ability to translocate GLUT4 vesicles or activate glycogen synthase. The precise function of insulin's activation of the MAP kinase pathway remains to be clarified. Recent work suggests, however, that there is a MEK-dependent, MAP kinase independent mechanism that leads to serine phosphorylation and decreased activity of the insulin receptor *(27)*, while other findings suggest that PKC activity of ERK2 is directly responsible for serine phosphorylation and "desensitization" of IRS1 *(26)*.

There are scant data from in vivo studies regarding insulin signaling in insulin resistant patients. Using skeletal muscle strips from obese subjects, Goodyear and colleagues determined insulin receptor and IRS1 tyrosine phosphorylation and activity of IRS1-associated PI 3-kinase after insulin stimulation and found that all three of these measures of insulin action were decreased in the obese subjects *(45)*. However, the applicability of these data to insulin resistance in general is uncertain because the subjects were morbidly obese (BMI = 52.9), and the skeletal muscle was obtained during abdominal surgery with its attendant potentially confounding factors of stress and anesthesia.

In patients with Type 2 diabetes, there are conflicting data regarding the ability of insulin to activate the β-subunit tyrosine kinase. Olefsky and colleagues reported receptor tyrosine kinase activity following insulin infusion and muscle biopsies in patients with Type 2 diabetes *(17)*. Other investigators have reported similar decreases in β-subunit tyrosine phosphorylation or tyrosine kinase activity *(15,16,18,19)*. Bak *(20)* and Klein *(21)*, on the other hand, found, using techniques similar to these studies, that insulin normally activates the receptor tyrosine kinase in muscle biopsies from patients with

Type 2 diabetes. The reasons for these discrepancies are not known, and this important question awaits further study. However, the preponderance of evidence indicates that the normal insulin-induced increase in insulin receptor tyrosine phosphorylation is attenuated in Type 2 diabetes.

Those few studies that have examined various steps in insulin signaling in muscle from insulin resistant subjects do not provide evidence pertaining to the question of whether these abnormalities might be hereditary or acquired. However, genetic screening of insulin resistant patients using IRS-1 as a candidate gene have revealed several naturally occurring mutations leading to an amino acid sequence change *(46–49)*. In the one study from the UK, no association was found between a Gly(972) Arg substitution and Type 2 diabetes *(49)*, but another study from the UK reported that the prevalence of this allele was greater in insulin resistant (18%) and dyslipidemic subjects (26%) than in controls (11%) *(48)*. A second study confirmed that the IRS1(972) mutation was increased in frequency in patients with Type 2 diabetes *(47)*. The number of subjects remains small, however, and it is unlikely that this mutation can explain the majority of cases of common insulin resistance.

GLUCOSE TRANSPORT

One of the most intensively studied of insulin's metabolic effects is translocation of GLUT4 glucose transporters from an intracellular pool to a site on the plasma membrane that is accessible to extracellular glucose for transport into the cell *(50,51)*. The molecular mechanism responsible for this effect is not completely characterized, but progress is being made in this area. Translocation of GLUT4-containing vesicles to the plasma membrane and fusion of these vesicles with the plasma membrane is under active investigation under the current model of vesicular transport. In this model, proteins called v-SNAREs (vesicular SNAP Receptors) are complementary with t-SNAREs (target-membrane SNAP Receptors), and their interaction is guided by a variety of monomeric guanosine triphosphatase (GTPases) called Rab proteins *(52–54)*. Once target recognition is accomplished, fusion of the vesicle and target membranes is thought to occur when the membrane of the docked vesicle is brought into close apposition with the membrane of the target vesicle by binding of NSF and SNAPs (soluble NSF attachment proteins) to both v-SNAREs and t-SNAREs *(55–57)*. Results of studies using expression or introduction of the cytoplasmic domains of a variety of membrane-associated proteins have identified syntaxin 4 as a t-SNARE and VAMP2 or VAMP3 as v-SNAREs involved in insulin-responsive translocation of GLUT4-containing vesicles to the plasma membrane *(58,59)*. Other investigations have implicated specific Rab GTPases as important recognition proteins *(60,61)*. These findings have not yet been applied to studies designed to assess their role in skeletal muscle insulin resistance in vivo.

Despite the intensive attention that has been paid to glucose transporter translocation using in vitro systems, quantification of glucose transport in vivo in human muscle has remained a difficult issue. Until recently, many investigators have inferred that there are abnormalities in glucose transport from the results of studies using techniques that measure the intracellular pathways of glucose metabolism in skeletal muscle. The major pathways are glucose storage (glycogen synthesis) and glycolysis, which can be further subdivided into glucose oxidation and release of the glycolytic products lactate and pyruvate, along with alanine, which equilibrates relatively rapidly with pyruvate. When these pathways all have been found to be reduced similarly, the conclusion has been that there is an upstream defect that accounts for the similar reductions. Because glucose transport often has been assumed to determine the rate of glucose uptake under most conditions, an abnormality in glucose transport therefore has been inferred. Recently, however, new methods have been developed that promise to shed light directly on this issue. Techniques now exist for modeling either glucose tracer bolus injection and wash-out curves in the human forearm *(62–64)* or positron emission tomograph data obtained using radiolabeled fluorodeoxyglucose *(65,66)* to obtain estimates of the rate of transport of glucose, independent of its further metabolism. These techniques have been used to show that insulin-stimulated rates of glucose transport are decreased in forearm or leg muscle of patients with Type 2 diabetes *(64,66)*. However, studies using muscle biopsy specimens to measure GLUT4 protein or mRNA content have found no difference in the expression of the GLUT4 proteins in Type 2 diabetes *(67,68)*, and there are no common mutations in the GLUT4 gene that are associated with Type 2 diabetes *(69)*. These data have led to the conclusion that decreased insulin-induced translocation of the GLUT4 transporter to the cell surface is responsible for the decreased rate of glucose transport observed in Type 2 diabetes. This has yet to be satisfactorily demonstrated in vivo in human muscle, however, mainly because of the difficulties in subfractionating skeletal muscle membrane in general and in small needle muscle biopsy specimens in particular. Two approaches have been taken to circumvent these problems. First, Klip and colleagues have devised a method to subfractionate muscle membranes from 200–400 mg of muscle *(70)*. They have used this technique in ~500 mg biopsies of the vastus lateralis muscle taken before and during euglycemic hyperinsulinemic clamps to demonstrate and quantify a shift in GLUT4 protein from an intracellular membrane fraction to a membrane fraction enriched in plasma membrane markers *(70)*. This plasma membrane fraction also exclusively contained the dihydropyridine receptor, a transverse tubule marker. When they applied this technique to muscle from patients with Type 2 diabetes *(71)*, they found that hyperinsulinemia failed to normally translocate GLUT4 protein to the sarcolemma. A similar approach has been taken by Goodyear, et al. *(67)*. The disadvantage of this approach is the rather large size of the biopsies necessitates either multiple needle passes or an open biopsy *(72)*, so the applicability of this technique is limited. Another approach uses confocal laser microscopy and immunofluorescence staining to examine localization changes of GLUT4 staining *(73)*. This approach has the advantage of not requiring the difficult and subcellular fractionation process, but suffers somewhat from uncertainties regarding quantification. Quantification of immunofluorescence staining is difficult and is an uncertainty shared by most immunofluorescence techniques. Regardless, using this technique, GLUT4 immunostaining associated with muscle sarcolemma after in vivo insulin stimulation also was found to be decreased in patients with Type 2 diabetes *(66)*. Since these studies were performed in patients who also underwent estimation of muscle glucose transport rates using PET scanning, it was possible to demonstrate that the reduction in the rate of glucose transport was correlated with reduced sarcolemmal GLUT4 immunostaining *(66)*.

In summary, there is good evidence from in vivo studies that the insulin-stimulated rate of glucose transport is decreased in muscle from insulin resistant patients and it is likely that this results from decreased insulin-induced translocation of GLUT4 vesicles to the plasma membrane. Genetic screening has not demonstrated an association of any GLUT4 allele with insulin resistance nor a decreased expression of GLUT4, but it has not been determined whether there are genetic abnormalities in the vesicular trafficking proteins involved in glucose transport. On the other hand, there also is little evidence that environmental factors are involved. Studies from the laboratory of Klip, have provided evidence that the GLUT4 translocation system may respond to high glucose concentrations by decreasing the stimulation of GLUT4 translocation by insulin *(70)*. This important issue needs more investigation, especially with respect to its mechanism.

Glucose Phosphorylation and Hexokinase

The phosphorylation of glucose to form glucose-6-phosphate (G-6-P) is the first irreversible step in glucose metabolism, and in skeletal muscle the rate of glucose uptake is thought to equal the rate of phosphorylation of glucose. The glycolytic intermediate G-6-P sits at a crossroad in glucose metabolism. It can be converted to glucose 1-phosphate and enter the pathway to glycogen synthesis or be converted to fructose 6-phosphate and enter the glycolytic pathway. Despite this critical position in glucose metabolism, little recent work has addressed the question of how insulin regulates hexokinase activity in skeletal muscle. The tools of molecular biology recently have provided the reagents required to answer questions about the role of hexokinase in insulin resistance in human skeletal muscle *(74,75)*. Two isoforms of hexokinase are expressed in skeletal muscle: hexokinase I (HKI) and hexokinase II (HKII). These closely related genes highly similar in primary sequence; however, their regulation in skeletal muscle has distinct features. Insulin induces the transcription of the HKII gene in vitro *(74)* and in vivo in rats *(76)* and increases HKII mRNA content in human skeletal muscle exposed in vivo to insulin during a euglycemic, hyperinsulinemic clamp *(77)*. In contrast, HKI transcription or mRNA level is unaffected by insulin *(77)*. In insulin resistant humans, there have been very few attempts to quantify the hexokinase step in vivo. The forearm tracer washout modeling technique *(63)* and PET scanning *(66)* afford the opportunity to measure the rate of insulin-stimulated glucose phosphorylation independently of glucose transport. Results from studies using either technique indicate that the rate of glucose phosphorylation is decreased in insulin resistant patients with Type 2 diabetes *(64,66)*. Furthermore, these models indicate that the abnormality in glucose phosphorylation is independent of the defect in glucose transport.

In vitro date using human skeletal muscle is generally confirmative of the in vivo modeling data. Bak and colleagues reported that HKII expression was reduced in skeletal muscle of patients with Type 2 diabetes who were studies in the postabsorptive state *(78)*. Pendergrass et al. *(79)* extended this observation by demonstrating that in patients with obesity or Type 2 diabetes, the ability of physiological insulin concentrations to increase HKII mRNA in skeletal muscle was completely abolished, and this was accompanied by decreased HKII activity as well as decreased leg muscle glucose uptake. From these data it is possible to speculate that insulin maintains the basal level of HKII expression and that it is conceivable that this reduced level of HKII activity in Type 2 diabetes may be involved in the abnormality in muscle glucose phosphorylation observed using tracer washout modeling *(64)* or PET imaging *(66)*.

Regardless of the abnormalities in insulin-stimulated HKII expression in insulin resistant patients, insulin acutely (within minutes) increases glucose transport and phosphorylation, yet only increases HKII expression after 2 to 4 h in vivo in humans *(77,79)*, and after 6 to 12 h in the rat *(76)*. Therefore, there must be another mechanism by which insulin acutely regulates hexokinase activity in skeletal muscle. Many years ago, Bessman proposed that one mechanism used by insulin to increase glucose metabolism might be an induction of association of

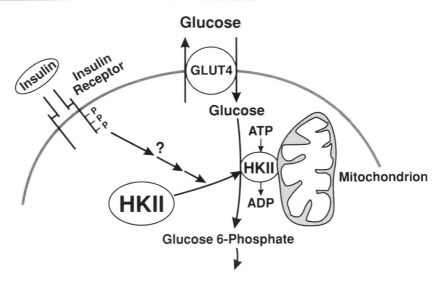

Fig. 3. Model of insulin-stimulated translocation of hexokinase II from a cytosolic compartment to the outer mitochondrial membrane.

hexokinase with mitochondria, in close proximity to a source of ATP *(80)*. Molecular evidence that this is indeed the case has emerged from identification of porin as the mitochondrial binding site for HK *(81)*, and characterization of the amino acid sequence determinants in HKII that are involved I mitochondrial binding *(82)*. Although there are conditions where the binding of hexokinase to mitochondria is regulated by factors other than insulin in insulin insensitive tissues *(83)*, the evidence that insulin regulated hexokinase in muscle in this manner was meager *(84,85)*. Recently, Vogt et al. *(86)*, using the glucose clamp technique and muscle biopsies, showed that 30 min of insulin infusion in healthy volunteers was associated with a shift in the subcellular distribution of HKII, but not HKI, from a cytosolic site to a particulate-bound fraction enriched in mitochondria. Taken together, these findings have led to a model whereby insulin directs the intracellular trafficking of HKII to the mitochondrial membrane, where its binding brings it in close proximity to high concentrations of ATP and increases its activity by increasing the substrate concentration (*see* Fig. 3). It will be important to address this in insulin resistant patients.

Because of the defects in HKII activity and expression in Type 2 diabetes, the HKII locus has been a focus of investigation as a candidate gene for insulin resistance. At least four studies have failed to find an association of variant HKII alleles with insulin resistance *(75,87–89)*. A common missense mutation resulting in the amino acid substitution Gln142H is present in 15–20% of patients with Type 2 diabetes and in nondiabetics, and is not correlated with insulin resistance. Other alleles exist with lower frequencies, but none are associated with insulin resistance. The finding that HKII activity in inversely correlated with fasting blood glucose levels has led to the suggestion that defects in HKII activity might be secondary to metabolic abnormalities, rather than being a direct hereditary abnormality *(75)*. This issue warrants further investigation.

Glycogen Synthesis

By far the most extensively examined site for insulin resistance in skeletal muscle is the pathway of glycogen synthesis. Depending upon the insulin concentration, during a euglycemic, hyperinsulinemic clamp 50 to 80% of glucose taken up by muscle is stored as glycogen *(90)*, so quantitatively, this pathway is of primary importance. Decreased insulin-stimulated glycogen synthesis in vivo was the first intracellular pathway of glucose metabolism that was shown to be reduced in obese subjects *(91)* or patients with Type 2 diabetes *(92)*. Furthermore, insulin activation of the rate-limiting enzyme in this pathway, glycogen synthase, has proven to be the most reliable and reproducible measurement of insulin action in muscle biopsies taken during euglycemic clamp studies in humans. Moreover, insulin activation of glycogen synthase is significantly correlated with systemic *(93–95)* or muscle *(90)* glucose storage. Such findings prompted intense interest in glycogen synthase as a candidate gene for muscle insulin resistance. Both basal and insulin-stimulated glycogen synthase activities have been consistently reported to be decreased in obesity and Type 2 diabetes *(93,95–97)*, and there is one report of reduced basal glycogen synthase mRNA and protein in muscle biopsies taken from patients with Type 2 diabetes *(98)*, although there is no evidence that physiological hyperinsulinemia regulates the expression of the glycogen synthase gene in vivo in humans *(77,98)*.

Nevertheless, even though insulin does not appear to induce glycogen synthase gene expression in skeletal muscle in humans, there are clear effects of insulin to dephosphorylate and activate glycogen synthase in vivo. Although the signaling pathway leading from the insulin receptor to dephosphorylation of glycogen synthase has not been delineated, it is wortmannin sensitive and MAP kinase independent (see above), indicating the involvement of insulin activation of PI 3-kinase. More distally, characterization of glycogen binding proteins such as PPP1R3 ("G_m") and PPP1R5 that bring protein phosphatase 1 in proximity to glycogen synthase has opened a new path of potential investigation into reduced glycogen synthase activation by insulin *(99,100)*. If there were abnormalities in expression or regulation of these regulatory proteins in diabetes or obesity, it could be possible to explain the reduction in insulin stimulation of dephosphorylation of glycogen synthase. There is a single report that did not find a widespread relationship between mutants of PPP1R3 and Type 2 diabetes *(101)*.

There is evidence for and against a hereditary origin of the abnormality in glycogen synthase regulation in insulin resistance. Studies in first degree relatives of patients with Type 2 diabetes have uniformly suggested that insulin-stimulated glucose storage and glycogen synthase activity are decreased before the development of Type 2 diabetes *(102–104)*. This is true regardless of the techniques used; NMR spectroscopy *(102)* or euglycemic clamps and muscle biopsies *(103,104)*. It seems evident that this abnormality is not a product of hyperglycemia as these individuals have been studied while they were euglycemic and had not progressed to impaired glucose tolerance. This does not automatically imply that the defect in insulin-stimulated glucose metabolism is a primary genetic defect, however. Many of the first degree relatives of patients with Type 2 diabetes are themselves obese and hyperinsulinemic, and hyperinsulinemia, produced experimentally in lean healthy volunteers, can also reproduce the abnormality in insulin-stimulated glycogen synthesis *(105)*. On the other hand, Henry and Ciaraldi cultured myoblasts obtained from patients with Type 2 diabetes and insulin-sensitive controls *(106)*. Under appropriate conditions, these myoblasts fuse in culture to form myotubes that express a striated, multinucleated skeletal muscle phenotype. These investigators have found the myotubes cultured from muscle obtained from patient with Type 2 diabetes that were grown in 5 m*M* glucose and low insulin retained their characteristic insulin resistance compared to myotubes from control muscle cultured under the same conditions; insulin-stimulated glycogen synthase activity was significantly reduced in the cells cultured from the diabetic muscle *(106)*. These data suggest that there is a primary genetic component to the reduction in insulin-stimulated glycogen synthesis in Type 2 diabetes. However, environmental factors may also be playing a role. Using the same system of cultured myotubes, Henry and Ciaraldi showed that either high glucose or high insulin concentrations in culture can produce insulin resistance *(107)*, and experimental hyperinsulinemia in vivo can produce defects in insulin stimulated glucose uptake, transport, and glycogen synthesis *(105,108,109)*. The mechanism by which hyperinsulinemia produces this abnormality is unknown. However, hyperglycemia has been shown to reduce insulin-stimulated glycogen synthesis by virtue of its metabolism to glucosamine *(110)*. Recent attention has been paid to this pathway as a potential mechanism for so-called "glucose toxicity," but its role in insulin resistance in Type 2 diabetes is still poorly defined. Hyperglycemia could also activate protein kinase C and induce MAP kinase mediated serine phosphorylation of the insulin receptor or IRS1, as discussed above.

The glycogen synthase locus has drawn attention as a candidate gene in the search for polymorphisms that could be responsible for insulin resistance. Initial intense interest was generated by the finding of a common allele at this locus that was associated with Type 2 diabetes in the Finnish population *(111)*. This mutation was in an intron, so it did not affect the primary amino acid sequence of the protein, but there were reduced glycogen synthase protein levels in these patients. In the Pima Indians, who obviously are genetically distinct from the Finnish population, there is an association of Type 2 diabetes with glycogen synthase alleles that are also present in noncoding regions *(112)*. In this population there is no decrease in glycogen synthase mRNA, but protein content is decreased *(112)* as in the Finnish sample. However, these investigators concluded that alterations in the glycogen synthase gene probably were not responsible for the association with Type 2 diabetes, but that there may be a nearby locus on chromosome 19 that is contributing a genetic element to the disease *(112)*.

Glucose Oxidation

The final fate of glucose to be discussed is that of oxidation. Glucose that undergoes glycolysis in muscle can either be reduced to lactate and released or can enter the Krebs cycle and be oxidized. Pyruvate dehydrogenase (PDH) is a complicated multienzyme complex that catalyzes the reaction converting pyruvate to acetyl-CoA and CO_2 *(113)*. The regulation of this enzyme in diabetics drew attention from two perspectives. First, inhibition of PDH by products of fatty acid oxidation formed the cornerstone of the Randle Cycle, whereby increased fat oxidation in diabetics was postulated to inhibit glucose metabolism *(114,115)*. Second, if PDH were inhibited in Type 2 diabetes, this would favor the conversion of pyruvate to lactate, and excessive lactate released from skeletal muscle could potentially provide substrate for increased gluconeogenesis in Type 2 diabetes, possibly contributing to fasting hyperglycemia *(116)*.

The regulation of PDH by insulin, glucose, and Type 2 diabetes, like glycogen synthase, has been studied using the glucose clamp technique and muscle biopsies *(94)*. Insulin increases the activity of PDH in muscle biopsies taken from lean, insulin-sensitive control subjects *(94,117,118)*. However, insulin stimulation of PDH activity appears to be very labile, as it is lost in older, slightly heavier but otherwise healthy sedentary control subjects who appear to have intact the response of glycogen synthase to insulin *(117)*.

Patients with Type 2 diabetes exhibit a different and somewhat surprising phenomenon. When these patients underwent muscle biopsies under postabsorptive, hyperglycemia conditions after being withdrawn from sulfonylurea therapy, PDH activity in the muscle biopsies was increased relative to either age- and BMI-matched controls or lean subjects, rather than being decreased *(96)*, and insulin had no additional effect to increase PDH activity in the diabetics. This was surprising in light of the observation that patients with Type 2 diabetes have low to normal *(92,96)* rates of glucose oxidation measured using systemic indirect calorimetry. This seemed counter-intuitive in light of the Randle Cycle. It could be argued, however, that under resting, postabsorptive conditions, skeletal muscle glucose oxidation represents a minor portion of systemic glucose oxidation. Therefore, measurements of systemic glucose oxidation might mislead with respect to muscle fuel selection. Kelley and Mandarino used local indirect calorimetry across the leg in an effort to circumvent this problem *(97)*. They found that the rate of glucose oxidation across the leg was increased, rather than decreased, in patients with Type 2 diabetes, and the increase in glucose oxidation was associated with increased leg muscle PDH activity *(97)*. Since muscle glucose uptake was not increased basally in the diabetics, increased glycogenolysis fueled the increase in glucose oxidation. A potential explanation for the increase in PDH activity is that increased glycogenolysis provided increased glycolytic substrates, such as pyruvate, which acts to inhibit PDH kinase and thus shift PDH to a less phosphorylated, more active, form.

Increased muscle PDH activity under basal conditions in Type 2 diabetes is likely to be an acquired, rather than a genetic abnormality. Experimental hyperglycemia was produced in lean and obese nondiabetic subjects by use of a combined infusion of glucose and somatostatin to block insulin secretion (119). Insulin, glucagon, and growth hormone were infused to replace basal levels, in an example of the so-called pancreatic clamp. Under these conditions, leg muscle glucose oxidation and PDH activity rose to near the level of the patients with Type 2 diabetes, and the increase was greater in the obese than in the lean control subjects *(119)*. Therefore, short-term experimental hyperglycemia could perfectly reproduce the changes seen in muscle from patients with Type 2 diabetes. Conversely, when euglycemia was produced in the diabetics with a low-dose, overnight insulin infusion that suppressed hepatic glucose production without increasing muscle glucose uptake, PDH activity was reduced *(97)* The subunit complexity of the PDH holoenzyme complex has made this enzyme an unattractive target for genetic investigation, but to date no alleles in the gene coding for the decarboxylase activity have been reported to be associated with insulin resistance or Type 2 diabetes.

SUMMARY

The potential biochemical or molecular sites of insulin resistance are summarized in Table 1, along with studies that have provided evidence for the existence of acquired or common genetic determinants of abnormalities. From this review it should be apparent that there are many cellular abnormalities that could contribute to insulin resistance in skeletal muscle from patients with obesity or Type 2 diabetes. It is not yet clear to what extent any of these abnormalities is responsible for insulin resistance. It is possible that any of these defects alone might not be sufficient to seriously affect insulin sensitivity, but in combination with another abnormality could be produce insulin resistance. It is also possible that different individuals, families, or populations might have different molecular causes of muscle insulin resistance. A clearer definition of the sites of

Table 1
Potential Biochemical and Molecular Determinants of Muscle Insulin Resistance

Site	Acquired	Hereditary	References
Insulin signaling			
Insulin receptor tyrosine kinase	+	+	*8,11,15–22*
IRS-1	?	—	*45,46–49*
PI 3-kinase	?	?	—
Glucose transport			
GLUT4 sequence	n/a	—	*69*
GLUT4 expression	+	—	*67,68*
GLUT4 translocation	?	?	*62–67,71*
Glucose phosphorylation			
HKII	+	—	*64,66,75,78,79,87-89*
Glycogen synthesis			
Glycogen synthase	+	—	*90–97,102–107,110–112*
PP1	?	—	—
Glycogen binding proteins	?	?	*101*
Glucose oxidation			
PDH activity	+	?	*96,119*

insulin resistance and their acquired or hereditary nature is needed to design and direct appropriate therapies.

ACKNOWLEDGMENTS

The expert secretarial assistance of Marilyn Cannefax and Jerry Lynn Beesley is gratefully acknowledged.

REFERENCES

1. Bar RS, Gorden P, Roth J, Kahn CR, DeMeyts P. Fluctuations in the affinity and concentration of insulin receptors on circulating monocytes of obese patients. J Clin Invest 1976;58:1123–1135.
2. Beck-Nielsen H. The pathogenic role of an insulin receptor defect in diabetes mellitus of obese. Diabetes 1978;17:1175–1181.
3. Olefsky JM. Decreased insulin binding to adipocytes and circulating monocytes from obese subjects. J Clin Invest 1976;57:1165–1172.
4. Kolterman O, Gray R, Griffin J, Bernstein P, Insel J, Scarlett J, Olefsky J. Receptor and postreceptor defects contribute to the insulin resistance in non-insulin dependent diabetes mellitus. J Clin Invest 1981;68:957–969.
5. Bak J, Jacobsen U, Jorgensen F, Pedersen O. Insulin receptor function and glycogen synthase activity in skeletal muscle biopsies from patients with insulin-dependent diabetes mellitus: effects of physical training. J Clin Endocrinol Metab 1989;69:158–164.
6. Damsbo P, Hother Nielsen O, Beck-Nielsen H. Reduced glycogen synthase activity in skeletal muscle from obese patients with and without Type 2 (non-insulin-dependent) diabetes mellitus. Diabetologia 1991;34:239–245.
7. Dohm GL. Insulin receptor kinase in human skeletal muscle from obese patients with and without noninsulin-dependent diabetes mellitus. J Clin Invest 1987;79:1330–1337.
8. Taylor SI. Lilly Lecture: molecular mechanisms of insulin resistance. Lessons from patients with mutations in the insulin-receptor gene. Diabetes 1992;41:1473–1490.
9. Krook A, Kumar S, Laing I, Boulton AJ, Wass JA, O'Rahilly S. Molecular scanning of the insulin receptor gene in syndromes of insulin resistance. Diabetes 1994;43:357–368.

10. Wertheimer E, Litvin Y, Ebstein RP, Bennet ER, Barbetti F, Accili D, Taylor SI. Deletion of exon 3 of the insulin receptor gene in a kindred with a familial form of insulin resistance. J Clin Endocrinol Metab 1994;78:1153–1158.

11. Krook A, O'Rahilly S. Mutant insulin receptors in syndromes of insulin resistance. Baillières Clin Endocrinol Metab 1996;10:97–122.

12. Rouard M, Macari F, Bouix O., Lautier C, Brun JF, Lefebvre P, Renard E, Bringer J, Jaffiol C, Grigorescu F. Identification of two novel insulin receptor mutations, Asp59Gly and Leu62Pro, in type A syndrome of extreme insulin resistance. Biochem Biophys Res Comm 1997;234:764–768.

13. Kadowaki H, Takahashi Y, Ando A, Momomura K, Kaburagi Y, Quin JD, MacCuish AC, Koda N, Fukushima Y, Taylor SI, Akanuma Y, Yazaki Y, Kadowaki T. Four mutant alleles of the insulin receptor gene associated with genetic syndromes of extreme insulin resistance. Biochem Biophys Res Comm 1997;237:516–520.

14. 't Hart LM, Stolk RP, Heine RJ, Crobbee DE, van der Does FE, Massen JA. Association of the insulin-receptor variant Met-985 with hyperglycemia and non-insulin-dependent diabetes mellitus in the Netherlands: a population based study. Am J Hum Genetics 1996;59:1119–1125.

15. Caro JF, Sinha MK, Raju SM, Ittoop O, Pories WJ, Flickinger EG, Meelheim D, Dohm GL. Insulin receptor kinase in human skeletal muscle from obese subjects with and without non-insulin dependent diabetes. J Clin Invest 1987;79:1330–1337.

16. Obermaier-Kusser B, White MF, Pongratz DE, Su Z, Ermel B, Muhlbacher C, Haring HU. A defective intramolecular autoactivation cascade may cause the reduced kinase activity of the skeletal muscle insulin receptor from patients with non-insulin-dependent mellitus. J Biol Chem 1989; 264:9497–9504.

17. Nolan JJ, Freidenberg G, Henry R, Reichart D, Olefsky JM. Role of human skeletal muscle insulin receptor kinase in the in vivo insulin resistance of noninsulin-dependent diabetes mellitus and obesity. J Clin Endocrinol Metab 1994;78:271–277.

18. Kellerer M, Coghlan M, Capp E, Muhlhofer A, Kroder G, Mosthaf L, Galante P, Siddel K, Haring HU. Mechanism of insulin receptor kinase inhibition in non-insulin-dependent diabetes mellitus patients. Phosphorylation of serine 1327 or threonine 1348 is unaltered. J Clin Invest 1995;96:6–11.

19. Nolan JJ, Ludvik B, Baloga J, Reichart D, Olefsky JM. Mechanisms of the kinetic defect in insulin action in obesity and NIDDM. Diabetes 1997;46:994–1000.

20. Pedersen O, Hother-Nielson O, Bak J, Hjollund E, Beck-Nielsen H. Effects of sulfonylureas on adipocyte and skeletal muscle insulin action in patients with non-insulin-dependent diabetes mellitus. Am J Med 1991;90:22S–28S.

21. Klein HH, Vestergaard H, Kotzke G, Pedersen O. Elevation of serum insulin concentration during euglycemic hyperinsulinemic clamp studies leads to similar activation of insulin receptor kinase in skeletal muscle of subjects with and without NIDDM. Diabetes 1995;44:1310–1317.

22. McGuire MC, Fields RM, Nyomba BL, Raz I, Bogardus C, Tonks NK, Sommercorn J. Abnormal regulation of protein tyrosine phosphatase activities in skeletal muscle of insulin-resistant humans Diabetes 1991;40:939–942.

23. Worm D, Vinten J, Staehr P, Henriksen JE, Handberg A, Beck-Nielsen H. Altered basal and insulin-stimulated phosphotyrosine phosphatase (PTPase) activity in skeletal muscle from NIDDM patients compared with control subjects. Diabetologia 1996;39:1208–1214.

24. Kroder G, Bossenmaier B, Kellerer M, Capp E, Stoyanov B, Muhlhofer A, Berti L, Horikoshi H, Ullrich A, Haring H. Tumor necrosis factor-alpha- and hyperglycemia-induced resistance. Evidence for different mechanisms and different effects on insulin signaling. J Clin Invest 1996;97:1471–1477.

25. Hoffman C, Lorenz K, Braithwaite S, Colea J, Palazube B, Hotamsligil G, Spiegelman B. Altered gene expression for tumor necrosis factor-α and its receptors during drug and dietary modulation of insulin resistance. Endocronology 1994;134:264–270.

26. DeFea K, Roth R. Modulation of insulin receptor Substrate-1 tyrosine phosphorylation and function by mitogen-activated protein kinase. J Biol Chem 1997;272:31400-1406.

27. Chin JE, Liu F, Roth RA. Activation of protein kinase c alpha inhibits insulin-stimulated tyrosine phosphorylation of insulin receptor substrate-1. Mol Endocrinol 1994;8:51–58.

28. Craven P, Derubertis F. Protein kinase C is activated in glomeruli from streptozotocin diabetic rats. Possible mediation by glucose. J Clin Invest 1989;83:1667–1675.

29. White MF, Kahn CR. The insulin signaling system. J Biol Chem 1994;269:1–4.

30. Yenush L, White MF. The IRS-signaling system during insulin and cytokine action. Bioessays 1997;19:491–500.

31. Saltiel AR. Diverse signaling pathways in the cellular actions of insulin. Am J Physiol 1996; 270:E375–E385.

32. Tanasijevic MJ, Myers MG Jr., Thomas RS, Crimmins DL, White MF, Sacks DB. Phosphorylation of the insulin receptor substrate IRS-1 by casein kinase II. J Biol Chem 1993;268:18157–18166.

33. Patti M, Sun X, Bruening J, Araki E, Lipes M, White M, Kahn CR. 4PS/IRS-2 is the alternative substrate of the insulin receptor in IRS-1 deficient mice. J Biol Chem 1995;270:24670–24673.

34. Sasaoka T, Rose DW, Jhun BH, Saltiel AR, Draznin B, Olefsky JM. Evidence for a functional role of Shc proteins in mitogenic signaling induced by insulin-like growth factor-1, and epidermal growth factor. J Biol Chem 1994;269:13689–13694.

35. Kao AW, Waters SB, Okada S, Pessin JE. Insulin stimulated the phosphorylation of the 66- and 52-kilodalton Shc isoforms by distinct pathways. Endocrinology 1997;138:2474–2480.

36. Skolnik EY, Lee CH, Batzer A, Vicentini LM, Zhou M, Daly R, Myers MJ Jr., Backer JM, Ullrich A, White MF. The SH2/SH3 domain-containing protein GRB2 interacts with tyrosine-phosphorylated IRS-1 and Shc: implications for insulin control of ras signaling. EMBO J 1993;12:1929–1936.

37. Myers MG Jr., Wang LM, Sun XJ, Zhang Y, Yenush L, Schlessinger J, Pierce JH, White MF. Role of IRS-1-GRB-2 complexes in insulin signaling. Mol Cell Biol 1994;14:3577–3587.

38. Dong LQ, Du H, Porter SG, Kolakowski LF, L AV, Mandarino LJ, Fan J, Yee D, Liu F. Cloning, chromosome localization, expression, and characterization of an Src homology 2 and pleckstrin homology domain-containing insulin receptor binding protein hGrb10γ. J Biol Chem 1997; 272:29104–29112.

39. Backer JM, Myers MG Jr., Sun XJ, Chin DJ, Shoelson SE, Miralpeix M, White MF. Association of IRS-1 with the insulin receptor and the phosphatidylinositol 3'-kinase. Formation of binary and ternary signaling complexes in intact cells. J Biol Chem 1993;268:8204–8212.

40. Cheatham B, Vlahos C, Cheatham L. Phosphatidylinositol 3-kinase is required for insulin stimulation of pp70 s6 kinase, DNA synthesis and glucose transporter translocation. Mol Cell Biol 1994;14:4902–4911.

41. Kanai F, Todaka M, Hayashi H, Kamohara S, Ishii K, Okada T, Hazeki O, Ui M, Ebina Y. Insulin-stimulated GLUT4 translocation is relevant to the phosphorylation of IRS-1 and the activity of PI 3-kinase. Biochem Biophys Res Commun 1993;195:762–768.

42. Cross D, Alessi D, Vandenheede J, McDowell H, Hundal H, Cohen P. The inhibition of glycogen synthase kinase–3 by insulin or insulin-like growth factor 1 in the rat skeletal muscle cell line L6 is blocked by wortmannin but not rapamycin. Biochem J 1994;303:21–26.

43. Dorrestjin J, Ouwens D, Van Den Berghe N, Bos J, Maassen J. Expression of a dominant-negative Ras mutant does not affect stimulation of glucose uptake and glycogen synthesis by insulin. Diabetologia 1996;39:558–563.

44. Osawa H, Sutherland C, Robey R, Printz R, Granner D. Analysis of the signaling pathway involved in the regulation of hexokinase II gene transcription by insulin. J Biol Chem 1996;271:16690–16694.

45. Goodyear L, Giorgino F, Sherman L, Carvey J, Smith R, Dohm GL. Insulin receptor phosphorylation, insulin receptor substrate-1 phosphorylation, and phosphatidylinositol 3-kinase activity are decreased in intact skeletal muscle strips from obese subjects. J Clin Invest 1995;95:2195–2204.

46. Imai Y, Fuysco A, Suzuki Y, Lesniak MA, D'Alfonzo R, Sesti G, Bertoli A, Lauro R, Accili D, Taylor SI. Variant sequences of insulin receptor substrate-1 in patients with noninsulin-dependent diabetes mellitus. J Clin Endocrinol Metab 1994;79:1655–1658.

47. Armstrong M, Haldane F, Taylor RW, Humpriss D, Berrish T, Stewart MW, Turnbull DM, Alberti KG, Walker M. Human insulin receptor substrate-1: variant sequences in familial non-insulin-dependent diabetes mellitus [published erratum appears in Diabetic Med 1996 May;13(5): 397]. Diabetic Med 1996;13:133–138.

48. Zhang Y, Wat N, Stratton IM, Warren-Perry MG, Orho M, Groop L, Turner RC. UKPDS 19: heterogeneity in NIDDM: separate contributions of IRS-1 and beta 3-adrenergic-receptor mutations to insulin resistance and obesity respectively with no evidence for glycogen synthase gene mutations. UK Prospective Diabetes Study. Diabetologia 1996;39:1505–1511.

49. Armstrong M, Haldane F, Avery PJ, Mitcheson J, Stewart MW, Turnbull DM, Walker M. Relationship between insulin sensitivity and insulin receptor substrate-1 mutations in non-diabetic relatives of NIDDM families. Diabetic Med 1996;13:341–345.

50. Cushman S, Wardzala L. Potential mechanism of insulin action on glucose transport in the isolated rat adipose cell. J Biol. Chem 1980;255:4578–4762.

51. Suzuki K, Kono T. Evidence that insulin causes translocation of glucose transport activity to the plasma membrane from an internal storage site. Proc Natl Acad Sci USA 1980;77:2542–2545.

52. Goud B. Small GTP-binding proteins as compartmental markers. Semin Cell Biol 1992;3:301–307.

53. Lombardi D, Soldati T, Riederer MA. Rab9 functions in transport between late endosomes and the trans Golgi network. EMBO J 1993;12:677–682.

54. Marsh M, Cutler D. Membrane traffic: taking the Rabs off endocytosis. Curr Biol 1993;3:30–33.

55. Waters MG, Griff IC, Rothman JE. Proteins involved in vesicular transport and membrane fusion. Curr Opin Cell Biol 1991;3:615–620.

56. Sztul ES, Melancon P, Howell KE. Targeting and fusion in vesicular transport. Trends Cell Biol 1992;2:381–386.

57. Zimmerberg J, Vogel SS, Chernomordik LV. Mechanisms of membrane fusion. Ann Rev Biophys Biomol Struct 1993;22:433–466.

58. Cheatham B, Volchuk A, Kahn CR, Want L, Rhodes CJ, Klip A. Insulin-stimulated translocation of GLUT 4 glucose transporters requires SNARE-complex proteins. Proceedings of the National Academy of Sciences of the United States of America 1996;93:15169–15173.

59. Olson AL, Knight JB, Pessin JE. Syntaxin 4, VAMP2, and/or VAMP3/cellubrevin are functional target membrane and vesicle SNAP receptors for insulin-stimulated GLUT4 translocation in adipocytes. Mol Cell Biol 1997;17:2425–2435.

60. Shisheva A, Doxsey SJ, Buxton JM, Czech MP. Pericentriolar targeting of GDP-dissociation inhibitor isoform 2. European J Cell Biol 1995;68:143–158.

61. Shisheva A, Czech MP. Association of cytosolic Rab4 with GDI isoforms in insulin-sensitive 3T3-L1 adipocytes. Biochem 1997;36:6564–6570.

62. Saccomani MP, Bonadonna RC, Bier DM, DeFronzo RA, Cobelli C. A model to measure insulin effects on glucose transport and phosphorylation in muscle: a three-tracer study. Am J Physiol 1996;270:E170–E185.

63. Bonadonna R, Del Prato S. Saccomani M, Bonora E, Gulli G, Ferrannini E, Bier D, Cobelli C, DeFronzo R. Transmembrane glucose transport in skeletal muscle of patients with non-insulin-dependent diabetes mellitus. J Clin Invest 1993;92:486–494.

64. Bonadonna RC, Del Prato S, Bonora E, Saccomani MP, Gulli g, Natali A, Frascerra S, Pecori N, Ferrannini E, Bier D, Cobelli C, DeFronzo RA. Roles of glucose transport and glucose phosphorylation in muscle insulin resistance of NIDDM. Diabetes 1996;45:915–925.

65. Raitakari M, Nuutila P, Ruotsalainen U, Laine H, Teras M, Iida H, Makimattila S, Utriainen T, Oikonen V, Sipila H, Haaparanta M, Solin O, Wegelius U, Knuuti J, Yki-Jarvinen H. Evidence for dissociation of insulin stimulation of blood flow and glucose uptake in human skeletal muscle: studies using [150]H2O, [18F]fluoro–2-deoxy-D-g;lucose, and positron emission tomography. Diabetes 1996; 45:1471–1477.

66. Kelley DE, Mintun MA, Watkins SC, Simoneau JA, Jadali F, Frederickson A, Beattie J, Theriault R. The effect of non-insulin-dependent diabetes mellitus and obesity on glucose transport and phosphorylation in skeletal muscle. J Clin Invest 1996;97:2705–2713.

67. Pedersen O, Bak JF, Andersen PH, Lund S, Moller DE, Flier JS, Kahn BB. Evidence against altered expression of GLUT1 or GLUT4 in skeletal muscle of patients with obesity or NIDDM. Diabetes 1990;39:865–870.

68. Garvey WT, Maianu L, Hancock J, Golichowski A, Baron A. Gene expression of GLUT4 in skeletal muscle from insulin-resistant patients with obesity, IGT, GDM, and NIDDM. Diabetes 1992;41:465–475.

69. Buse JB, Yasuda K, Lay TP, Seo TS, Olson AL, Pessin JE, Karam JH, Seino S, Bell GI. Human GLUT4/muscle-fat glucose-transporter gene. Characterization and genetic variation. Diabetes 1992;41:1436–1445.

70. Guma A, Zierath H, Wallberg-Henrickson H, Klip A. Insulin induces translocation of GLUT–4 glucose transporters in human skeletal muscle. Am. J Physiol 1995;268:E613–E622.

71. Zierath JR, He L, Guma A, Odegaard WE, Klip A, Wallberg-Henriksson H. Insulin action on glucose transport and plasma membrane GLUT4 content in skeletal muscle from patients with NIDDM. Diabetologia 1996;39:1180–1189.

72. Goodyear LJ, Hirshman MF, King PA, Thompson CM, Horton ED, Horton ES. Skeletal muscle plasma membrane glucose transport and glucose transporters after exercise. J Appl Physiol 1990;68:193–198.

73. Watkins SC, Frederickson A, Theriault R, Korytkowski M, Turner DS, Kelley DE. Insulin-stimulated Glut 4 translocation in human skeletal muscle: a quantitative confocal microscopic assessment. Histochemical J 1997;29:91–96.

74. Printz RL, Koch S, Potter LR, O'Doherty RM, Tiensinga JJ, Moritz S, Granner DK. Hexokinase II mRNA and gene structure, regulation by insulin, and evolution. J Biol Chem 1993;268:5209–5219.

75. Lehto M, Huang X, Davis EM, LeBeau MM, Laurila E, Eriksson KF, Bell GI, Groop L. Human hexokinase II gene: exon-intron organization, mutation screening in NIDDM, and its relationship to muscle hexokinase activity. Diabetologia 1995;38:1466–1474.

76. Burcelin R, Printz R, Kande J, Assan R, Granner D, Girard J. Regulation of glucose transporter and hexokinase II expression in tissues of diabetic rats. Am J Physiol 1993;265:E392–E401.

77. Mandarino LJ, Printz RL, Cusi KA, Kinchington P, O'Doherty R, Osawa H, Sewell C, Consoli A, Granner DK, DeFronzo RA. Regulation of hexokinase II and glycogen synthase mRNA, protein, and activity in human muscle. Am J Physiol 1995;269:E701–E708.

78. Vestergaard H, Bjorbaek C, Hansen T, Larsen FS, Granner DK, Pedersen O. Impaired activity and gene expression of hexokinase II in muscle from non-insulin-dependent diabetes mellitus patients. J Clin Invest 1995;96:2639–2645.

79. Pendergrass M, Koval J, Vogt C, Yki-Jarvinen H, Iozzo P, Pipek R, Ardehali H, Printz R, Granner D, DeFronzo RA, Mandarino LJ. Insulin-induced hexokinase II expression is reduced in obesity and non-insulin-dependent diabetes mellitus. Diabetes 1998;47:387–394.

80. Bessman B, Geiger P. Compartmentation of hexokinase and creatine phosphokinase, cellular regulation, and insulin action. Curr Topics Cell Reg 1980;16:55–86.

81. Laursen S, Belknap J, Sampson K, Knull H. Hexokinase redistribution in vivo. Biochem Biophys Acta 1990;1034:118–121.

82. Ardehali H, Yano Y, Printz RL, Koch S. Whitesell RR, May JM, Granner DK. Functional organization of mammalian hexokinase II. Retention of catalytic and regulatory functions in both the NH2-and COOH-terminal halves. J Biol Chem 1996;271:1849–852.

83. Laursen SE, Belknap JK, Sampson KE, Knull HR. Hexokinase redistribution in vivo. Biochem Biophys Acta 1989;1084:118–121.

84. Chen-Zion M, Bassukevitz Y, Beitner R. Sequence of insulin effects on cytoskeletal and cytosolic phosphofructokinase, mitochondrial hexokinase, glucose 1,6-bisphosphate and fructose 2,6-bisphosphate levels, and the antagonistic action of calmodulin inhibitors on diaphragm muscle. Int J Biochem 1992;24:1661–1667.

85. Russell RR III, Mrus JM, Mommessin JL, Taegtmeyer H. Compartmentation of hexokinase in rat heart. J. Clin Invest 1992;90:1972–1977.

86. Vogt C, Yki-Jarvinen H, Iozzo P, Pipek R, Pendergrass M, Koval J, Ardehali H, Printz R, Granner D, DeFronzo RA, Mandarino LJ. Effects of insulin on subcellular localization of hexokinase II in human skeletal muscle in vivo. J Clin Endocrinol Metab 1997;83:1–5.

87. Laakso M, Malkki M, Deeb SS. Amino acid substitutions in hexokinase II among patients with NIDDM. Diabetes 1995;44:330–334.

88. Vidal-Puig A, Printz RL, Stratton IM, Granner DK, Moller DE. Analysis of the hexokinase II gene in subjects with insulin resistance and NIDDM and detection of a Gln142 → His substitution. Diabetes 1995;44:340–346.

89. Taylor RW, Printz RL, Armstrong M, Granner DK, Alberti KG, Turnbull DM, Walker M. Variant sequences of the Hexokinase II gene in familial NIDDM. Diabetologia 1996;39:322–328.

90. Kelley D, Reilly J, Veneman T, Mandarino LJ. Effect of insulin on skeletal muscle glucose storage, oxidation, and glycolysis in humans. Am J Physiol 1990;258:E923–E929.

91. Boden G, Ray TK, Smith RH, Owen OE. Carbohydrate oxidation and storage in obese non-insulin-dependent diabetic patients. Diabetes 1983;32:982–987.

92. Thiebaud D, Jacot E, DeFronzo RA, Maeder E, Jequier E, Felber JP. The effect of graded doses of insulin on total glucose uptake, glucose oxidation, and glucose storage in man. Diabetes 1982;31:957–963.

93. Bogardus C, Lillioja S, Stone K, Mott D. Correlation between muscle glycogen synthase activity and in vivo insulin action in man. J Clin Invest 1984;73:1185–1190.

94. Damsbo P, Hother-Nielsen O, Beck-Nielsen H. Reduced glycogen synthase activity in skeletal muscle from obese patients with and without Type 2 (non-insulin-dependent) diabetes mellitus. Diabetologia 1991;34:239–245.

95. Thorburn AW, Gumbiner B, Bulacan R, Brechtel G, Henry RR. Multiple defects in muscle glycogen synthase activity contribute to reduced glycogen synthesis in non-insulin dependent diabetes mellitus. J Clin Invest 1991;87:489–495.

96. Mandarino LJ, Consoli A, Kelley DE, Reilly JJ, Nurjhan N. Fasting hyperglycemia normalized oxidative and nonoxidative pathways of insulin-stimulated glucose metabolism in non-insulin-dependent diabetes mellitus. J Clin Endocrinol Metab 1990;71:1544–1551.

97. Kelley D, Mandarino L. Hyperglycemia normalizes insulin-stimulated skeletal muscle glucose oxidation and storage in non-insulin-dependent diabetes mellitus. J Clin Invest 1990;86:1999–2007.

98. Vestergaard H, Bjorbaek C, Andersen P, Bak J, Pedersen O. Impaired expression of glycogen synthase mRNA in skeletal muscle of NIDDM patients. Diabetes 1991;40:1740–1745.

99. Chen YH, Hansen L, Chen MX, Bjorbaek C, Vestergaard H, Hansen T, Cohen PTW, Pedersen O. Sequence of the human glycogen-associated regulatory subunit of type I protein phosphatase and analysis of its coding region and mRNA level in muscle from patients with NIDDM. Diabetes 1994;43:1234–1241.

100. Brady MJ, Printen JA, Mastick CC, Saltiel AR. Role of protein targeting to glycogen (PTG) in the regulation of protein phosphatase–1 activity. J Biol Chem 1997;272:20198–20204.

101. Chen YH, Hansen L, Chen MX, Bjorbaek C, Vestergaard H, Hansen T, Cohen PT, Pedersen O. Sequence of the human glycogen-associated regulatory subunit of type 1 protein phosphatase and analysis of its coding region and mRNA level in muscle from patients with NIDDM. Diabetes 1994;43:1234–1241.

102. Rothman D, Magnusson I, Cline G, Gerard D, Kahn CR, Shulman R, Shulman G. Decreased muscle glucose transport/phosphorylation is an early defect in the pathogenesis of non-insulin-dependent diabetes mellitus. Proc Natl Acad Sci 1995;92:983–987.

103. Vaag A, Henriksen J, Beck-Nielsen H. Decreased insulin activation of glycogen synthase in skeletal muscle in young non-obese Caucasian first-degree relatives of patients with non-insulin-dependent diabetes mellitus. J Clin Invest 1992;89:782–788.

104. Gulli G, Ferrannini E, Stern M, Haffner S, DeFronzo RA. The metabolic profile of NIDDM is fully established in glucose-tolerant offspring of two Mexican-American NIDDM parents. Diabetes 1992;41:1575–1586.

105. Del Prato S, Leonetti F, Simonson DC, Sheehan P, Matsuda M, DeFronzo RA. Effect of sustained physiologic hyperinsulinemia and hyperglycemia on insulin secretion and insulin sensitivity in man. Diabetologia 1994;37:1025–1035.

106. Henry R, Ciaraldi T, Abrams-Carter L, Mudalie S, Park KS, Nikoulina S. Glycogen synthase activity is reduced in cultured skeletal muscle cells of non-insulin-dependent diabetes mellitus subjects. J Clin Invest 1996;98:1231–1236.

107. Henry R. Ciaraldi T, Mudaliai S, Abran L, Nikonlira S. Acquired defects of glycogen synthase activity in cultured human skeletal muscle cells. Diabetes 1996;45:400-407.

108. Mandarino LJ, Baker B, Rizza R, Genest J, Gerich J. Infusion of insulin impairs human adipocyte glucose metabolism in vitro without decreasing adipocyte insulin receptor binding. Diabetologia 1984;27:358–363.

109. Rizza RA, Mandarino LJ, Genest J, Baker BA, Gerich JE. Production of insulin resistance by hyperinsulinaemia in man. Diabetologia 1985;28:70–75.

110. Crook E, Zhou J, Daniels M, Neidigh H, McClain D. Regulation of glycogen synthase by glucose, glucosamine, and glutamine: fructose–6-phosphate aminotransferase. Diabetes 1995;44:314–320.

111. Groop L, Kankuri M, Schalin-Jantti C, Eckstrand A, Nikula-Ijas P, Wilder E, Kuismanen E, Eriksson J, Fransilla-Kallunki A, Saloranta C, Koskimies S. Association between polymorphism of the glycogen synthase gene and non-insulin-dependent diabetes mellitus. New Eng J Med 1993, 328:10–14.

112. Majer M, Mott DM, Mochizuki H, Rowles JC, Pedersen O, Knowler WC, Bogardus C, Prochazka M. Association of the glycogen synthase locus on 19q13 with NIDDM in Pima Indians. Diabetologia 1996;39:314–321.

113. Wieland O. The mammalian pyruvate dehydrogenase complex: structure and regulation. Rev Physiol Biochem Pharmacol 1983;96:123–170.

114. Randle PJ, Garland PB, Hales CN, Newsholme EA. The glucose fatty-acid cycle. Its role in insulin sensitivity and the metabolic disturbances of diabetes mellitus. The Lancet 1963; I:7285–289.

115. Randle PJ. Fuel selection in animals. Biochem Soc Trans 1986;14:799–806.

116. Consoli A, Nurjhan N, Capani F, Gerich J. Predominant role of gluconeogenesis in increased hepatic glucose production in NIDDM. Diabetes 1989;38:550–557.

117. Mandarino LJ, Wright KS, Verity LS, Nichols J, Bell JM, Kolterman OG, Beck-Nielsen H. Effects of insulin infusion on human skeletal muscle pyruvate dehydrogenase, phosphofructokinase and glycogen synthase. J Clin Invest 1987;80:655–663.

118. Mandarino LJ, Consoli A, Jain A, Kelley DE. Differential regulation of intracellular glucose metabolism by glucose and insulin in human muscle. Am J Physiol 1993;265:E898–E905.

119. Mandarino LJ, Consoli A, Jain A, Kelley DE. Interaction of carbohydrate and fat fuels in human skeletal muscle; impact of obesity and NIDDM. Am J Physiol 1996;270:E463–E470.

11

The Role of the Liver in Insulin Action and Resistance

Jerry Radziuk, PhD, MD, CM, FRCP and Susan Pye, MSc

CONTENTS

INTRODUCTION
THE LIVER AND GLUCOSE FLUXES
INSULIN AND HEPATIC GLUCOSE FLUXES
HEPATIC INSULIN RESISTANCE AND TYPE 2 DIABETES
SUMMARY: *HEPATIC EFFECTS OF INSULIN*
HEPATIC MODULATION OF INSULIN ACTION
REFERENCES

INTRODUCTION

The phenotypic expression of non-insulin-dependent diabetes (NIDDM or Type 2 diabetes) and its associated syndrome (Syndrome X, insulin resistance syndrome [IRS]) has given rise to a great deal of debate on what is inherited and what is acquired in the pathogenesis of this disease state *(1)*. In particular, the tissues or metabolic processes involved have all been implicated as primary sites in its evolution.

Established Type 2 diabetes is characterized by defects in both insulin secretion and action *(2–4)*. Low insulin response to intravenous glucose *(5)* and therefore impaired secretion has been considered as a characteristic of the prediabetic state. Inadequate insulin responses have been found in subjects with impaired glucose tolerance *(4)*. This could arise due to altered *(7)* or disordered *(8–11)* secretory patterns in relatives of patients with Type 2 diabetes. Loss of the first-phase insulin response is another lesion that occurs early in the natural history of Type 2 diabetes *(12,13)*. The resulting hyperglycemia is initially compensated for by a hypersecretion of insulin *(4,15)*, although this may not be as large as originally thought *(14)*. It is commonly held that impairment of the second phase of insulin secretion comprises an important part of the decompensation which leads to clinical diabetes in genetically-predisposed individuals *(4,15–17)*.

Various aspects of the insulin secretory response to glucose have thus been implicated as genetically programmed defects in the pathogenesis of Type 2 diabetes.

From: *Contemporary Endocrinology: Insulin Resistance*
Edited by: G. Reaven and A. Laws © Humana Press Inc., Totowa, NJ

Nevertheless, it is most frequently insulin resistance that is considered the primary lesion which underlies the potential development of Type 2 diabetes. It has been shown to predict the development of hyperglycemia in genetically prone individuals *(18)*. It has been shown in longitudinal studies and in a number of prediabetic populations that insulin resistance at the level of the skeletal muscle is an early event in the etiology of the disease which exists well before metabolic derangements occur *(18–30)*, and is considered to be inherited *(26)*.

The liver is the other major organ involved in glucose homeostasis. Insensitivity of the liver to insulin has also been cited as a major contribution to etiology of both glucose intolerance and subsequently Type 2 diabetes *(6,31,32)*. Although the methodology of measurement of hepatic glucose production has been questioned *(30,33)*, in general, there appears to be a correlation between fasting blood glucose and hepatic glucose production *(34)*. Similarly, at an earlier stage of development, the degree of glucose intolerance can be related to the lack of suppression of endogenous glucose production after meals (or glucose loads) *(6,35)*. In nondiabetic first-degree relatives of patients with Type 2 diabetes, impaired hepatic glucose production rather than disposal may be an early defect *(36)*. It has therefore been suggested that abnormal hepatic glucose production is the major factor responsible for both fasting and postprandial hyperglycemia *(37)* and may therefore precede the development of peripheral insulin resistance. Similarly in rats with newly-induced streptozotocin-diabetes, increased glucose production and therefore hepatic insulin resistance is the major cause of hyperglycemia *(38)*.

Clearly, defects in insulin secretion and both peripheral and hepatic insulin resistance play a role in the etiology of Type 2 diabetes. With current knowledge, it is difficult to assign precedence to any particular process. Rather there exists a network of interrelated metabolic defects, which in association with impaired insulin secretion eventually cause a fundamental disruption of glucose homeostasis *(39)*. Increasingly, multiple impairments are reported *(40–42)* and at earlier stages *(6)*, consistent with the notion of Type 2 diabetes as a disease precipitated by environmental factors superimposed on a polygenic susceptibility background *(43)*.

On the other hand, it has also been suggested that most of the described defects are not genetic but secondary to the disease process *(40,44)*. Indeed, glucotoxicity *(45)* arising from a chronic hyperglycemia could induce both impairments in GLUT4-mediated glucose transport in muscle *(46,47)* and in insulin secretion *(48,49)*. It could be said however, that the liver is exempt from the effects of hyperglycemia since this should not in itself, increase glucose production.

A unifying hypothesis for the etiology of Type 2 diabetes is nevertheless an attractive goal and would reconcile the disparate potential etiologies. It would be expected that such a common pathway would occur at the molecular level. It also suggests parallelism in the development of defects in insulin secretion *(50)* and glucose production *(34)*, as fasting blood glucose increases. In the specific instance of some families with maturity-onset diabetes of the young (MODY) mutations in the glucokinase gene yielded an enzyme with a lower affinity for glucose and resulted in impaired glucose-stimulated insulin secretion *(51)*. Simultaneously, impaired hepatic glucose metabolism is seen with decreased glycogen synthesis and increased gluconeogenesis *(52)*. The parallel defects in insulin secretion and glucose production are thus, in this instance, seen to have a molecular basis.

It has been suggested that Type 2 diabetes could be "restructured" as a disease of lipid metabolism *(53,54)* and increased lipid levels could explain both resistance of glucose metabolism to the action of insulin and β-cell dysfunction. Certainly free fatty acids (FFA) have long been implicated in the overproduction and decreased peripheral utilization of glucose *(55–59)*. They also stimulate insulin secretion *(60)* and are, in fact, essential to glucose-stimulated secretion *(61)*, although prolonged exposure *(62,63)* could cause an impairment.

These potential systemic mediators may be reflected intracellularly by specific molecular signals. An elegant hypothesis put forward by Prentki and Corkey *(64)* links the multiple defects of obesity and Type 2 diabetes with altered insulin secretion using the concept of glucolipoxia, a general metabolic disease with multiple clinical manifestations. This is mediated by changes in intracellular long-chain acyl-CoA (LC-acylCoA) and malonyl CoA which are signals of metabolic abundance and link carbohydrate and lipid metabolism in the β-cell as well as muscle, liver and adipose tissue. Alterations in enzymatic signal generation or tissue-specific effector sensitivity which synthesize the effects of environment and genetics could then contribute to the pleiotropic expressions of the general metabolic disorder.

Certain molecules can therefore integrate metabolic information. It can be further suggested that organs, and specifically the liver may play an analogous role. The liver is anatomically located in a strategic position—between the splanchnic and the peripheral circulations. It therefore receives unattenuated signals from the pancreas and indeed, is a primary target for pancreatic hormones. Simultaneously, it is the major site for removal and degradation of insulin *(65–67)* and is thus in a position to modulate the pancreatic insulin signal and therefore to influence its peripheral action. Both aspects of the potential role of the liver in the pathogenesis of insulin resistance will be briefly explored here.

THE LIVER AND GLUCOSE FLUXES

The (now) classical concept of the role of the liver in glucose metabolism can be summarized *(68)* as follows. During the absorptive period following meals, the liver takes up glucose and stores it as glycogen. Postabsorptively, the glycogen is released in the process of glycogenolysis, and as glycogen stores are depleted, a gradual increase in new glucose synthesis from glucogenic substrates takes place, so that the rate of glucose production is maintained. The liver is ideally situated to function in this buffering capacity vis-à-vis the periphery since it is interposed between the splanchnic and peripheral circulations. The great improvement in tolerance to glucose when it was administered orally vs intravenously was well known and attributed to two mechanisms: (i) an augmentation of insulin secretion (the incretin effect, *69–72*), mediated by intestinal factors *(73–75)* and (ii) the conversion of a net hepatic glucose production which maintains glycemia during the fasting period to a net hepatic glucose uptake. In particular, a large fraction of newly-absorbed glucose was deemed to be taken up by the liver on a first-pass basis *(76,77)*. Using splanchnic arterio-venous difference in humans, Felig and colleagues *(78)* estimated this fraction to be 40–60% of ingested glucose. It was furthermore suggested that glucose intolerance arose from a decrease in this uptake by the liver and a resulting decrease in the filtering of newly-absorbed glucose prior to its appearance in the systemic circulation *(79)*. Since insulin secretion also takes place into the portal vein, it could be surmised that the maintenance of normal glucose tolerance was dependent on the primary action of newly released insulin, which converted net glucose output to uptake.

The use of tracers in estimating the first-pass hepatic extraction somewhat altered this picture *(80,81)*. An intravenously infused glucose tracer was used to determine the continuously changing systemic metabolic clearance and appearance rates of glucose prior to and during an oral glucose load. Labeling the glucose load with a second tracer, allowed the separate determination of the systemic appearance of the ingested glucose. By subtracting the appearance of ingested glucose from its total systemic appearance, it was found that endogenous glucose production was suppressed by 60 to 80%, depending on the size of the glucose load. Simultaneously, it was shown that a minimum of 92–95% of the ingested glucose entered the systemic circulation precluding a "filtering" function for the liver whereby it would retain a large fraction of newly absorbed glucose and thus delay its entry into the peripheral circulation. Small extraction rates of 5% or less were corroborated across the splanchnic bed in humans *(82)* and across the liver in pigs *(81)*. Since glucose absorption was extended over approximately four hours, it could be shown that this absorption rate corresponded to approximately one-fifth of the total glucose inflow to the liver (i.e., from absorption and from the mesenteric circulation). Thus, a small extraction rate could lead to a significant total uptake of glucose by the liver. This was estimated at approximately 25–30 g, following the ingestion of 100 g of glucose.

Sufficient glucose could therefore be sequestered by the liver to provide substrate for the synthesis of glycogen in amounts previously described after a meal either by biopsy *(83,84)* or subsequently by nuclear magnetic resonance (NMR) *(85)*. Moreover, this flux represents approximately one-quarter of the ingested amount and could well be regulated by portal insulin.

In order to directly assess the amount of glycogen formed from glucose in the human liver after a glucose meal, this glycogen was mobilized immediately post-absorptively using an intravenous infusion of glucagon *(86,87)*. By measuring the amount of ingested glucose label which was released from the liver in this way, it was demonstrated that only a small amount *(8 ± 1 g out of 100 g)* of the stimulated glucose production could be attributed to glycogen formed directly from ingested glucose during the absorptive period *(86)*. This estimate rose to 9.5 ± 1.2 g when the circulating pool of unlabeled glucose, present prior to the load was also taken into account *(87)*.

These data suggested an alternate source of substrate for glycogen formation, namely, glucogenic precursors. This possibility was also assessed in humans using $^{14}CO_2$ delivered as intravenous bicarbonate during the absorptive period, as a marker for glucose and glycogen synthesis from pyruvate-level substrates by gluconeogenic processes *(88–90)*. This label was again mobilized postabsorptively from glycogen stores as ^{14}C-glucose using a glucagon infusion. Incorporation of ^{14}C from $^{14}CO_2$ into glycogen was well above what could be accounted for by circulating labeled glucose or by the stimulation of gluconeogenesis by the glucagon infusion *(88–90)*. Using corrections for tricarboxylic acid (TCA) cycle label dilution *(88,91)*, it was estimated that approximately 14.7 ± 4.5 g of glycogen was synthesized by gluconeogenetic pathways. This dual route for glycogen synthesis is consistent with other early work in rats *(92,93)*. The simultaneous suppression of the delivery of gluconeogenic product to the circulation and its entry into glycogen suggests its diversion away from release into the circulation and into storage *(90,92)*.

Two alternative tracers which label the substrates for the gluconeogenetic process were also used to estimate glycogen synthesis by this route using an otherwise identical protocol *(90)*. ^{14}C-U-lactate was used to track conversion of circulating lactate to glyco-

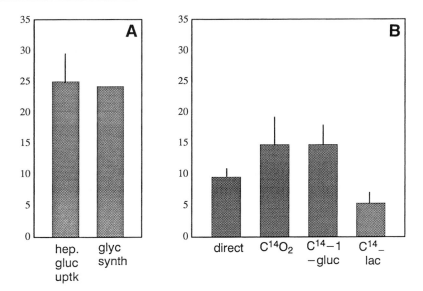

Fig. 1. The hepatic disposal of glucose following a 100 g glucose load is summarized. **(A)** An average of 5% of absorbed glucose is taken up on a first-pass basis *(80,81)*. Taking recirculating glucose into account yields an estimate of 25–30 g total uptake over the absorption period *(80,81)*. **(B)** Synthesis of glycogen directly from circulating glucose was 9.5 g *(86,87,89)*. Using $C^{14}O_2$ and recycled C^{14}-1-glucose as labels 14.7 g of glycogen was calculated to be formed by gluconeogenic pathways *(89,90)*. Using C^{14}-U-lactate as a label, 5.3 g of glycogen formation was estimated. The difference in the two estimates can be accounted for by dilution of lactate label by the formation of unlabeled lactate from glucose by the gut and by recycling of glucose via pyruvate within the liver (the 'indirect' pathway).

gen and recycling of ^{14}C from the first to the 6th position of the glucose molecule was used to track conversion of ^{14}C-1-glucose to ^{14}C-3-lactate prior to its reconstitution to glycogen. Interestingly, the estimate of gluconeogenetic glycogen synthesis obtained from the recycling of label was 14.7 ± 3.2 g, essentially identical to that calculated using the $^{14}CO_2$ label *(90)*. Synthesis of glycogen from circulating lactate however amounted to only 5.3 ± 1.4 g or 36% of the total gluconeogenetic flux to glycogen *(90)*.

Estimates of hepatic glucose uptake and glycogen synthesis by way of the different pathways are summarized in Fig. 1. Total glycogen synthesis, estimated by adding the separately estimated direct and gluconeogenic components of glycogen synthesis, is nearly identical to that seen after a mixed meal with similar carbohydrate content, detected using nmr *(85)*. The caveat to all these measurements *(94)* is that simultaneous glycogen synthesis and breakdown has also been demonstrated *(95,96)* so that amounts measured by both these methods are more representative of a net glycogen synthesis. Since both processes take place simultaneously, however, either could be the target of regulation by insulin.

The amount of hepatic glucose uptake and total glycogen synthesis are very similar (Fig. 1), a situation which was subsequently described in dogs *(92)*. This was attributed to an intrahepatic cycling of glucose, via pyruvate, to glycogen *(88,92,98)*. It has thus been suggested that all liver glycogen is formed from glucose taken up by the liver without (direct pathway) or with (indirect pathway) cycling through pyruvate *(88,92)*. Although this may take place to some extent, it is clearly not the only pathway followed, given the incorporation of circulating ^{14}C-lactate into glycogen *(90)*. The flux from circulating substrates into glycogen, specifically from lactate, is also likely to be essential to an efficient synthesis of this molecule. The inhibition of phosphoenolpyruvate-carboxykinase (PEPCK) using 3-mercaptopicolinic acid *(99,100)* minimized hepatic glycogen synthesis following glucose loading. In the perfused rat liver, the extent of such synthesis was also shown to quantitatively depend upon lactate uptake from the perfusate, independently of ambient glucose concentrations *(101,102)*.

The difference between the estimates based on ^{14}C-lactate and recycled ^{14}C-glucose or [14]CO_2 incorporation is however consistent with the existence of such an indirect pathway. This difference can also arise secondary to a dilution of lactate label in the portal vein due to metabolism of circulating (and unlabeled) glucose to lactate in the gut. That this occurs has been shown in the pig *(81)* and in humans *(103)*. Moreover, even in dogs, whose livers produce lactate during glucose loading, significant amounts of labeled lactate *(104)* are simultaneously extracted. The results are therefore also compatible with a metabolic zonation of the liver *(105,106)* where periportal hepatocytes are more glucogenic and perivenous cells more glycolytic. Simultaneous glycolysis and gluconeogenesis could therefore take place, but the glycolytic activity contributes primarily to circulating lactate. As previously reviewed *(81,104)*, it is not only the gut that may contribute to lactate production after glucose loading. Other tissues include the CNS, the erythrocytes, as well as the skin *(107)*, subcutaneous *(108)* and visceral fat. Interestingly, the muscle contributes little lactate *(109,110)* under these circumstances.

The discussion above was not intended to be comprehensive but rather to identify the critical fluxes which are coordinated in the systemic supply of glucose postabsorptively and in the hepatic disposition of glucose postprandially. These fluxes are summarized below and in Fig. 2.

A. Hepatic glucose uptake/output
    (1) Phosphorylation (glucokinase)
    (2) Dephosphorylation (glucose-6-phosphatase)
B. Glycogen metabolism
    (3) Synthesis (synthase)
    (4) Glycogenolysis (phosphorylase)
C. Glycolysis/gluconeogenesis
    (5) Gluconeogenesis
    (6) Glycolysis
    (7) Oxidation
D. Substrate supply
    (8) Lactate, alanine, etc.

INSULIN AND HEPATIC GLUCOSE FLUXES

During the absorption of a carbohydrate meal, insulin is the principal hormone which promotes the disposition of glucose. Intestinal hormones enhance its secretion when glucose is ingested, relative to the response when it is administered intravenously. The resulting increase in insulin concentrations is responsible for the improvement in glucose tolerance which is seen after oral (vs intravenous) glucose administration. The decrease in glycemia is considered to arise primarily from a systemic action of insulin on glucose removal, with the bulk of this occurring in the peripheral tissues *(80,110,111)*. As discussed above however, the liver likely accounts for approximately 25% of the glucose

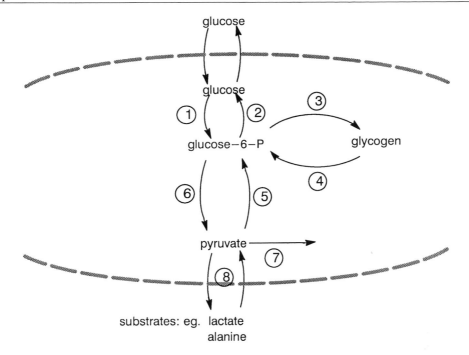

Fig. 2. An overall perspective on the critical metabolic fluxes in the liver which are involved in the provision of glucose postabsorptively and in the disposition of glucose postprandially. Numbers refer to the listing in the text and outline potential targets of insulin action.

disposal. This fraction has been estimated by some investigators to be even higher. It might be expected therefore that insulin would be a major contributor to the regulation of postprandial metabolite fluxes in the liver. Other hormones such as glucagon and perhaps gut hormones or leptin would also participate in this regulation. The level of glycemia itself is known to influence the liver's action on glucose. Perhaps more importantly, other metabolites such as glucogenic substrate and FFA, whose concentrations may be determined peripherally under the influence of insulin, could be considered as the immediate mediators of insulin's effect on the liver. This partition of control of hepatic glucose metabolism by insulin between the immediate portal effects and those mediated via its primary peripheral effects has been formalized as the "direct" and "indirect" effects of insulin.

Direct and Indirect Effects of Insulin

The direct effects of insulin comprise its effects on enzyme activities and synthesis. The indirect effects include those on the provision of substrate for liver gluconeogenesis and changes in FFA levels induced by insulin. Ashmore and Weber *(112)* proposed rapid actions of insulin which were mediated by a reduction in intracellular cAMP and a decrease in FFA levels, which would stimulate enzymes promoting glycogen synthesis and glycolysis and inhibit enzymes mediating glycogen breakdown and gluconeogenesis. Longer-term action on glycolysis and gluconeogenesis would be mediated by new enzyme biosynthesis.

A decrease in the provision of glucogenic substrates to the liver has not been seen in the context of glucose loading with its concurrent hyperinsulinemia *(113)*, suggesting that insulin is not likely to act by suppressing the overall peripheral mobilization of substrate. Moreover, lactate is generally increased following glucose loading and may arise peripherally as well as in the gut both in the pig *(81)* and in the human *(103)* indicating rather, an increase in substrate availability. If the decrease in substrate availability was due to an insulin-induced decrease in their peripheral generation from glucose (the Cori cycle), this is not compatible with a liver response curve to insulin which is well to the left (ED_{50} ~25–50 µU/mL) relative to the peripheral dose response (ED_{50} ~60 µU/mL) *(114,115)*. Finally, in the face of varying availability of glucogenic substrates or glycogen, hepatic autoregulation *(116–118)* adjusts the flux to glucose from glycogenolysis and gluconeogenesis from different substrates in order to maintain a constant production of glucose. This would further obscure an effect of insulin on an individual flux of a glucogenic substrate.

FFA, on the other hand, are produced primarily by hydrolysis, from adipose tissue and circulating triglycerides. The production, and the removal of the FFA are hormonally controlled. It has been suggested, *(119,120)* in a dog model, that circulating FFA are at least partial if not primary *(121)* determinants of the insulin effect on the liver. This is consistent with the parallel decreases in both FFA and hepatic glucose production (as well as increases in peripheral glucose uptake) in response to insulin *(121)*. In contrast to peripheral glucose metabolism which supplies substrate for gluconeogenesis via the Cori and glucose-alanine cycles, the ED_{50}'s for lipolysis and the oxidation of circulating FFA and tissue lipid (15–45 µU/mL, *122,123*) bracket that for the suppression of hepatic glucose production by insulin. These data are also compatible with an FFA-mediated effect of insulin on the liver.

In humans however, observations have been less consistent. Increasing FFA with lipid/heparin infusions was shown, in some studies, both to increase glucose production during a relative insulinopenia *(124,125)* and to impair its suppression during a hyperinsulinemic euglycemic clamp *(126–128)*. Other work however, failed to demonstrate a stimulation of glucose production when FFA were raised with lipid/heparin infusions in normal subjects *(129–131)*. Inhibition of lipolysis in healthy fasted volunteers in one study *(132)*, moreover, led to a stimulation of hepatic glucose production (HGP). This is consistent with early work in dogs demonstrating an inhibitory effect of elevated FFA on HGP *(133,134)*. This discussion is not meant to be exhaustive, but only to illustrate the complex nature of the interaction of insulin and FFA in the regulation of carbohydrate metabolism and therefore of the role the latter may play in insulin resistance.

The direct effects of insulin on hepatic glucose metabolism are necessarily bounded by its relationship to fasting glucose and to the metabolic responses to a meal. As already described above, one of the major components of this response is the inhibition of HGP. This appears to be primarily mediated by an increased flux of glucose-6-phosphate (G-6-P) to glycogen and towards glycolysis. There is no indication of a decrease in gluconeogenetic flux towards G-6-P itself. Recent work *(135)* in the perfused rat liver may help to clarify to what extent these changes are in fact mediated by insulin. Isolated rat livers from 20h-fasted rats were perfused with donor blood and a continuous infusion of lactate. Under basal conditions with no hormone added, much of this lactate is converted to glucose. With the addition of insulin maintained at approximately the ED_{50} for the liver, hepatic glucose output was indeed suppressed (relative to controls) by at least 50%. Glycogen content of the livers simultaneously increased. Analysis of the perfusate label (C14-lactate and -glucose) concentrations provided a strong indication that gluconeogenic flux had, if anything, increased rather than fallen. The parallels between the postprandial fluxes in vivo and those seen in a well-defined in vitro system, strongly suggest that the direct effects of insulin play a principal role in redirecting carbon fluxes so as to minimize glycemia. Since fatty acids were excluded from this system, they could not mediate the effects. Moreover, gluconeogenesis which is considered the major target of FFA in the liver *(136)* is not decreased, emphasizing the direct effects of insulin.

Direct and rapidly-occurring effects of insulin on the liver have been described for a long time. For example the administration of low dose insulin led to an immediate (<10 min) decrease in hepatic glucose output measured using balance techniques in a dog model *(137)*. This was corroborated by a large amount of data in both humans and animal models, using both splanchnic balance and tracer techniques which indicated that insulin acts on the liver and acts rapidly suggesting a direct action *(138–142)*. Finally, a large number of effects of insulin on the activity of enzymes involved in hepatic glucose metabolism have been described *(143)*. A number of these changes take place very rapidly *(144)*, again indicating a direct action of insulin in the liver.

It can be seen that the interaction between different metabolite fluxes and their regulatory hormones is complex. It may be difficult therefore to precisely define "direct" and "indirect" effects of insulin of these fluxes.

Hepatic Effects of Insulin: Actions on Enzymes

Although far from unanimously, the liver has been implicated as a major site for insulin resistance *(35–37, but 30–33)* in Type 2 diabetes. The implication is that it is also a major site of insulin action. In the context of meals, other contenders in regulating the hepatic response include glucose, as well as the indirect pathways of insulin action, with FFA in particular. That the insulin effect is primary, has however been suggested by a number of investigators *(141,145)*.

Since the transport of glucose across the hepatic membrane is not rate limiting *(146)*, the regulation of hepatic glucose output and uptake, occurs at the level of the gluconeogenetic, glycolytic and glycogen synthetic fluxes. In particular, it is localized to the substrate cycles which comprise these pathways *(143)*. Substrate cycles are an efficient mechanism for increasing the sensitivity of the regulation of flux through a metabolic pathway *(147)*. Two non-equilibrium and chemically distinct reactions occurring in opposite directs can yield large changes in the net flux through this cycle with only small changes in either (or both) of the component reactions. This clearly yields dramatic increases in sensitivity since for example, 10% changes in enzyme activity or activation can yield fold changes in flux, even reversing its direction. Moreover, the sensitivity is determined by the rate of cycling and is proportional to the ratio of cycling rate to flux. These cycles include:

A. Hepatic glucose uptake/output
  (1) Glucose cycle (glucokinase (GK)/glucose-6-phosphatase (G6Pase))
B. Glycogen metabolism
  (2) Glycogen cycle (synthase/phosphorylase)
C. Glycolysis/gluconeogenesis
  (3) Phosphofructokinase/fructose-1,6-diphosphatase cycle
  (4) Pyruvate/phosphoenolpyruvate cycle (phosphoenolpyruvate carboxykinase (PEPCK)/pyruvate kinase (PK))

Fluxes through these cycles have been shown to occur continuously. For example glycogen synthesis occurs during fasting *(148)* and glycogenolysis during meal absorp-

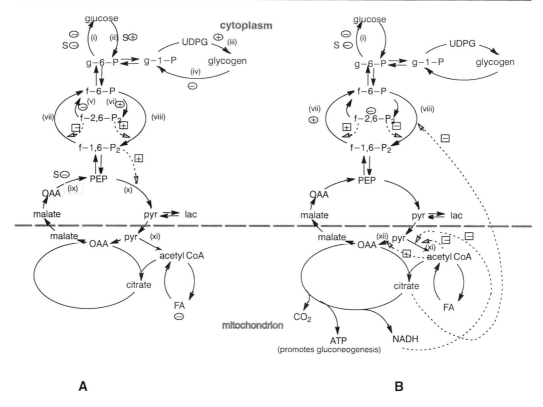

A   **B**

Fig 3. (A) Effects of insulin on metabolic pathways in the liver. Inhibitory effects on enzyme activities or substrate concentrations are indicated with (–) and stimulatory effects with (+). Primary effects are indicated by circles and secondary effects by boxes. Effects on new enzyme synthesis are preceded by an 'S'. **(B)** Effects of FFA on metabolic pathways are noted in the same way as described above. Insulin decreases FFA concentrations. Therefore the effects of insulin would be the opposite of what is indicated for FFA. [Key: (i) glucose-6-phosphatase, (ii) glucokinase, (iii) glocogen synthase, (iv) glycogen phosphorylase, (v) fructose-2,6-diphosphatase, (vi) 6-phosphofructose-2-kinase, (vii) fructose-1,6-diphosphatase, (viii) 6-phosphofructose-1-kinase, (ix) phosphoenolpyruvatecarboxykinase, (x) pyruvate kinase, (xi) pyruvate dehydrogenase, (xii) pyruvate carboxylase.]

tion *(95,96)*. Glucose uptake (and detritiation of [2-H^3] glucose) occurs continuously during net glucose production *(135)*. Similarly, although not part of a substrate cycle, gluconeogenesis occurs even when there is no net glucose output *(81)*. Since regulation occurs at the level of these substrate cycles, these are the most likely loci for insulin action. The metabolic pathways for glucose are therefore redrawn in Fig. 3A with this in mind, and the principal sites of insulin action indicated. Fig. 3B shows the parallel influences of FFA, which may mediate at least to some extent the indirect actions of insulin.

A. Glucose Uptake/Output

The relative activity of the GK and G6Pase in this substrate cycle, determines both the flux and its direction through this reaction. Inhibition of flux through G6Pase was shown after carbohydrate meals in rats *(149)*, by a decrease in the relative loss of [^{3}H] from

[2-^{3}H] glucose as well as in the hepatic concentrations of G-6-P. This suggested a role for the enzyme in the action of insulin on the liver, which was subsequently demonstrated by Barrett and colleagues *(150)*. Euglycemic hyperinsulinemia in rats completely suppressed glucose production and decreased hepatic [G-6-P] whereas insulin suppressed G6Pase in liver homogenates and isolated microsomes. Taken together, the evidence indicates that G6Pase is involved in HGP suppression as part of a coordinated network of insulin effects *(150)*. Other studies *(151)* demonstrated an acute 23% decrease in G6Pase activity in rats in vivo in the presence of insulin, parallel to the inhibitory effect of the hormone on HGP. Finally, a decrease in FFA oxidation induced by etomoxir, reduced the activity (and the gene expression) of G6Pase, suggesting that this enzyme too, may be influenced by insulin via indirect pathways *(152,220)*.

Physiological doses of insulin suppress HGP *(135–138)* and increase hepatic glucose uptake in a net sense *(135,137,153)*. This suggests a concomitant increase in (at least the relative) activity of GK. A decrease of 40% in K_m for GK was documented in normal rats during euglycemic hyperinsulinemic clamps *(151)* and this was accompanied by a doubling of V_{max} in diabetic (90% pancreatectomized) rats. This increase in activity may be mediated by translocation of glucokinase from intracellular binding sites to sites which may, for example, be contiguous with glycogen molecules thus favouring the glycogen synthetic pathway *(154)*.

Interestingly, recent work *(155)* has demonstrated that mutations in the glucokinase gene result in a familial subtype of Type 2 diabetes characterized by an early age of onset (MODY: maturity onset diabetes of the young). Such mutations lead both to impairment in the inhibition of HGP in response to carbohydrate meals *(156)* and decreased glycogen synthesis *(157)* in addition to the well-known deterioration in glucose-mediated insulin secretion. Any insulin resistance present in these patients appeared to be primarily due to effects of the resulting hyperglycemia *(158)*. A similar picture was obtained using glucosamine to inhibit GK activity *(159)*. On the other hand, expression of the glucokinase gene in transgenic streptozotocin-diabetic mice induced hepatic glycolysis and a normalization of glycemia *(159)* underlining the importance of stimulation of GK synthesis by insulin *(160,161)*. Defects in G6Pase and GK have also been manifested as alterations in the glucose cycle. Glucose cycling was increased in Type 2 diabetes *(162,163)* during the post-prandial and post-absorptive states albeit not to a great extent. An elevated rate of glucose cycling could contribute to a decreased net hepatic glucose uptake since more newly phosphorylated glucose would be immediately dephosphorylated. It could thus be a contributor to hepatic insulin resistance. On the other hand, cycling is *decreased* in glucokinase-deficient MODY patients where liver defects are known to be present *(156)*. Taken together, these observations suggest that G6Pase and GK are likely involved in the pathogenesis of hepatic insulin resistance but their contribution may be minor relative to the remainder of the interacting metabolic reactions which may contribute to abnormal liver glucose metabolism.

B. Glycogen Metabolism

Hepatic G-6-P levels are determined from the balance of fluxes which replenish it (glucokinase, gluconeogenesis, glycogenolysis) and which deplete it (G-6-Pase, glycolysis and glycogen synthase). Increases in liver G-6-P concentrations could therefore provide a "push" mechanism for the stimulation of net glycogen synthesis which could be at least partially mediated by insulin. Although the sources of G-6-P for glycogen

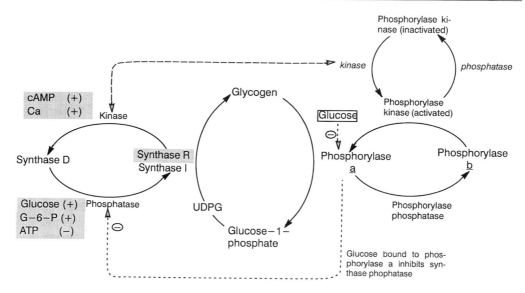

Fig. 4. Scheme describing the regulatory interactions in the synthesis and breakdown of hepatic glycogen.

synthesis were not considered to be as numerous as they now are, this mechanism is equivalent to that originally described by Soskin (164) with circulating glucose as the principal source of G-6-P. In 1967 DeWulf and Hers (165) demonstrated a rapid decrease in UDP-glucose and G-6-P in mice which were administered glucose, strongly suggesting that glucose controlled glycogen deposition by stimulating synthase and therefore by a "pull" mechanism. Glucose was the dominant regulatory factor, thus extending the mass effect of Soskin to this regulatory scheme. This evolved into the concepts illustrated in Fig. 4 (166–169): glucose binds to phosphorylase a which inhibits its activity, rendering it more susceptible to inactivation by phosphorylase phosphatase. Phosphorylase a was considered a strong inhibitor of synthase phosphatase. When a sufficient amount of the phosphorylase was inactivated, there was less inhibition of the synthase phosphatase with a resulting increase in synthase I activity and the net synthesis of glycogen.

This scheme provided an elegant switching mechanism by which the liver could be converted from an organ of net glucose output to net glucose uptake and storage. This mechanism however has needed significant modification. Synthase was shown to be activated before (170) or without (171,172) any reduction in phosphorylase a, during, for example, the absorption of a glucose load. As reviewed in (169) it was shown that glucose stimulated synthase phosphatase directly but with a very high activator constant (25 mM). G-6-P however stimulated this phosphatase at physiological levels (173), leading to the concept that glucose has to be phosphorylated prior to this action (174). The independence of phosphorylase deactivation and synthase activation is also compatible with glycogen turnover which, if anything, is accentuated during glucose loading (95,96). Interestingly, synthase activation during the fed to fasted transition responds almost as an on-off switch (175) suggesting a similar response to that previously proposed for glucose, but with an effector which would be expected to some extent, to parallel glucose levels although it can also be altered by inputs mediated for example, by insulin. This effector can convert the liver from net glycogen breakdown to net synthesis. Although the role of insulin in the promotion of glycogen deposition is not completely clear, a number of studies have indicated its potential importance. In cultured chicken embryo hepatocytes *(176)*, the presence of insulin was a prerequisite for maximal glycogen formation and insulin-stimulated synthase activity whereas glucose alone did not exert such an effect. In primates, *(177)* during a euglycemic hyperinsulinemic clamp, there was a simultaneous deactivation of phosphorylase and activation of synthase which however, was independent of a falling concentration of G-6-P. There was also no net synthesis of glycogen and an actual decrease in content over time. Similar results were obtained in rats *(178,179)* with no changes in synthase or phosphorylase. An allosteric inhibition of phosphorylase by insulin was noted in postabsorptive rats which partially explained the suppression of HGP *(180)*. Most of these data do suggest that insulin sets up the enzymatic conditions for net glycogen synthesis but that this does not occur unless substrate (glucose) is added, such as under hyperglycemic, hyperinsulinemic conditions *(176)*.

Other mechanisms by which insulin may contribute to increases in glycogen synthesis could occur via the accumulation of G-6-P. As already discussed, glucokinase and G6Pase activities may be influenced by insulin. G-6-P levels would rise secondary to the maintenance of gluconeogenic flux while, for example, G6Pase was inhibited. Alternatively, gluconeogenic flux could, somewhat paradoxically, increase. This type of mechanism has been suggested by recent data *(135)* in perfused livers, with apparent increases in gluconeogenic flux accompanying decreased HGP and increased glycogen synthesis. These data are compatible with a previous demonstration that glucose and lactate taken up by the liver promote glycogenesis by different mechanisms *(101,102)*. When glucose and lactate were added to a (recirculating) fasted livers perfusion, it appeared that glucose (and therefore presumably the G-6-P arising from it) does not in itself determine the amount of glycogen synthesized—it only sets the range within which this synthesis may take place. On the other hand, the availability of lactate or its uptake by the liver determines the rate of glycogen synthesis—within the range set by the glucose concentration. Moreover, the effect of the glucogenic flux from lactate is saturable *(102)*, with respect to glycogen synthesis but not with respect to HGP. This suggests that levels of G-6-P from lactate would be increasing proportionately to the flux from lactate but their effect would saturate. Decreasing lactate uptake and glucogenic flux (while increasing lactate concentrations) using metformin in the same system, decreased glycogen synthesis *(181)*. All these observations taken together with the finding that glucogenic flux is essential to net glycogen synthesis, suggest that the glucogenic flux itself determines the rate of glycogen synthesis (within the limits set by glucose) or that G-6-P derived from this flux is different from the G-6-P derived from glucose and thus exerts its effects differently. This hypothesis would be analogous to the finding that G-6-P produced by glucokinase overexpressed in rat primary hepatocytes stimulates glycogen synthesis whereas G-6-P from overexpressed hexokinase does not *(182)*. The translocation of glucokinase may be involved in juxtaposing substrate and enzyme in the regulation of glycogen synthesis *(154)*. Finally fluxes from glucogenic substrates, with lactate in particular, and from glucose could have different effects in the different metabolic zones of the liver. Thus, when glucose was the only exogenous substrate in a perfused liver, glycogen was formed primarily in the perivenous areas and with gluconeogenic precursors as substrate, glycogen synthesis was primarily periportal *(183)*.

Much of the just discussed data does not bear specifically in the mechanisms of regulation of glycogen synthesis by insulin, but does suggest novel loci for this regulation and ways in which hepatic insulin resistance may be manifested.

Little is known about the potential contributions of impaired glycogen synthesis to hepatic insulin resistance and in particular of the role of FFA in mediating it. It might be anticipated that decreases in net glycogen formation with increases in glycogenolysis following meals could lead to the impaired suppression of HGP and to the generalized decrease in glucose storage. A decrease in hepatic glycogen content in the immediate postabsorptive period was indeed visualized by nmr *(184)* in patients with Type 2 diabetes. However, as already seen, a lower rate of glycogen synthesis could arise secondary to deficiencies in other enzymes such as glucokinase. Furthermore, by using the acute glucose response to glucagon administration as a measure of hepatic glycogen content, and comparing normal and Type 2 diabetes subjects after a 64-h fast, Clore et al. *(185)* concluded that liver glycogen can be *increased* in Type 2 diabetes. Similarly, in overnight-fasted obese patients *(186)* liver glycogen measured by biopsy was also significantly increased. In both cases gluconeogenesis was found to be increased. In patients with Type 2 diabetes, basal HGP was elevated whereas in the obese subjects it was not, suggesting an impairment in hepatic autoregulation in the former case. Nevertheless the elevated glycogen levels could arise from an accelerated gluconeogenetic rate which could both contribute to the G-6-P pool and, as already discussed, independently contribute to an increased rate of glycogen synthesis. This would be further accentuated by a potentially attenuated rate of insulin-stimulated glycolysis.

The higher glycogen levels could then lead to increased rates of glycogenolysis which in turn, contribute to an elevated HGP (e.g., *187*). Finally, the presence of high glycogen levels would impair further glycogen deposition. Animal studies suggest that it is under these circumstances that increases in FFA would be most likely to impair the suppression of HGP by insulin *(188)*. It can be concluded therefore that liver glycogen accumulation is an insulin-dependent process and therefore likely to be impaired under conditions of insulin resistance. The network of other interactions however could preclude clear observations of this impairment.

C. Gluconeogenesis and Glycolysis

Increased rates of gluconeogenesis could not only lead to elevated glycogen levels but also contribute significantly to increased basal glucose production and decreased suppression of this rate following meals or in the presence of insulin. Because of the degree of autoregulation it might be expected that elevated rates of gluconeogenesis might be compensated by decreased rates of glycogenolysis *(116–118,189)*. Could insulin resistance at the level of HGP then be manifested as increased gluconeogenetic rates for which compensation remains incomplete? That the answer is "yes," can be inferred from studies in transgenic rats *(190)* where a noninsulin responsive PEPCK gene was overexpressed. In this model gluconeogenesis was increased and glucose tolerance impaired *(191)*. Moreover, chronically increased gluconeogenesis can result in an elevated rate of glucose production. This was demonstrated in NZO diabetic mice *(192)* where obesity resulted in accelerated lipolysis with increased glycerol as substrate and FFA-mediated increase in the activities of pyruvate carboxylase and fructose-1, 6-bisphosphatase.

An increase in gluconeogenesis is the most frequently cited reason for increased basal glucose production rates as well as inadequate suppression in this rate during meal absorption (decreased suppression). The hepatocytes from insulin-resistant genetically obese *fa/fa* rat demonstrate a lack of responsiveness of gluconeogenesis to insulin *(193)* compared to the lean *(Fa/-)* rats. In the diabetic rat under hyperinsulinemic conditions, hyperglycemia stimulates glycogen synthesis in the liver but primarily by the gluconeogenic pathway *(194)*. In the same vein, gluconeogenesis measured using the incorporation of labeled precursors into glucose has been found to be increased *(195–197)*. Indeed Consoli et al *(198)* have suggested that the entire increase in glucose output in Type 2 diabetes was due to an increase in gluconeogenesis (Fig. 5), as has also been suggested by nmr measurements *(184)*. The concept has been extended since increased glucose production *(32)* due to gluconeogenesis has been found as an early defect in Type 2 diabetes prior to the development of overt fasting hyperglycemia. Accelerated glucose turnover was, moreover, found in first-degree relatives of patients with Type 2 diabetes *(36)*. Impaired suppression of glucose production *(6)* presumably at the level of gluconeogenesis was also seen by some investigators *(6,41)*. More recent work has also demonstrated that insulin's restraining action on basal glucose production is impaired in Type 2 diabetes. In the presence of hyperinsulinemia however, although the output rates continue to be higher than normal, the absolute suppression of glucose production is normal *(199)*.

It should be reemphasized that a decreased gluconeogenic flux, appearing systemically in response to insulin, is not necessarily an indicator of a decreased flux from glucogenic substrates towards glucose-6-phosphate since the latter can be directed towards glycogen, as already discussed. Glucose-6-phosphate can also be depleted when glycolysis is stimulated. This stimulation has been implicated as a major action of insulin in the liver *(179,200)* under conditions of euglycemic hyperinsulinemia. This could lead to an increase in the carbon cycling which has been suggested to occur between pyruvate and glucose-6-phosphate *(98,201)*. This concept is supported to some extent in dogs by a simultaneous net production of lactate and glycogen synthesis via both direct and gluconeogenic pathways, the total of which is quantitatively equivalent to liver glucose uptake *(97)*. Similarly, the bidirectional exchange of C14 between glucose and lactate in a recirculating perfused liver increases in the presence of insulin *(135)*. On the other hand, in the dog model, labeled lactate extraction by the liver is approximately 20% and continues at this rate during glucose loading with its concomitant hyperinsulinemia *(104)*. In the liver perfusions, lactate uptake is also maintained at a high rate. Medium or circulating lactate therefore appears to be involved to a significant extent as substrate for liver glucogenic fluxes. At the organ level therefore, increased liver glycolysis with maintenance of the uptake of extra-hepatic substrates could therefore increase gluconeogenic flux. However, intracellulary, increased glycolytic activity would be expected to be coupled with a decrease in gluconeogenic activity, consistent with an increase, following insulin or meals, in fructose-2,6-diphosphate *(179,200)*. This intermediate is a major control element for switching between glycolysis and gluconeogenesis, particularly in the liver *(202)*.

The rapid action of insulin on liver gluconeogenesis and glycolysis under physiological circumstances therefore directly implicates the bifunctional enzyme 6-phosphofructo-2-kinase-fructose-2,6-diphosphatase which determines the synthesis/degradation of fructose-2, 6-diphosphate *(179)*. This compound then allosterically activates 6-phosphofructo-1-kinase and inhibits fructose-1, 6-diphosphatase, thus inhibiting gluconeogensis and generating glycolytic glucose-1, 6-diphosphate. The latter intermediate then stimulates PK further along the glycolytic pathway. Pyruvate carboxy-

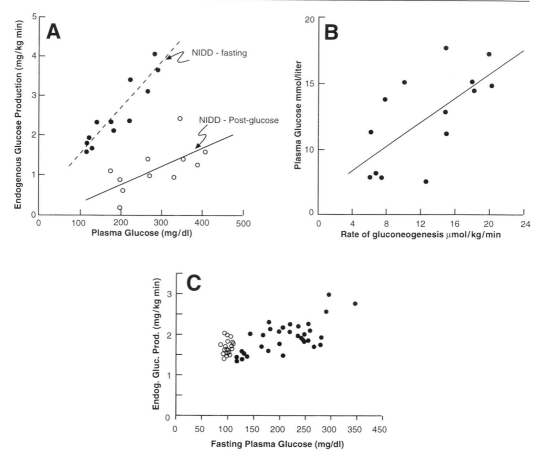

Fig. 5. (A) Relationship between endogenous glucose production and plasma glucose concentration in the fasting state and following oral glucose administration in subjects with Type 2 diabetes (Metabolism 1988;37:78). **(B)** Relationship between fasting plasma glucose concentrations and the rate of gluconeogenesis in Type 2 diabetes subjects estimated using [6-^{3}H] glucose and [2-^{14}C] acetate (Diabetes 1989;38:550). **(C)** Relationship between glucose production and fasting plasma glucose concentration in control subjects and patients with Type 2 diabetes estimated using an extended tracer infusion (Diabetes 1994;43:1440).

lase does not appear to be directly regulated by insulin *(203)*. Decreases in PEPCK activity occur more slowly with a decay in the amount of enzyme present secondary to a relatively rapid inhibition in its synthesis *(204)* and a slower degradation process *(205)*. In summary, therefore, insulin stimulates flux through the pyruvate-phosphoenolpyruvate cycle, thus diverting intermediates away from the gluconeogenetic pathway (*see* Fig. 3A), in counterpoint to the glucagon-mediated inhibition of PK and therefore, of this substrate cycle.

Effects of insulin may also be mediated indirectly by suppression of FFA oxidation. This reduces pyruvate carboxylase (PC) activity since levels of mitochondrial acetyl CoA, a major allosteric effector of PC decrease. This also increases fructose-2, 6-diphosphate, decreasing gluconeogenic efficiency *(206)* and stimulating glycolysis *(179,207)*. The presence of unoxidized FFA, independently of its oxidation rate may also enhance the production of fructose-2, 6-diphosphate, potentially accentuating the effect of inhibitors of its oxidation in increasing glycolysis and decreasing gluconeogenesis *(208)*.

Interestingly, in a mouse model of Type 2 diabetes (the obese NZO mouse) it was concluded that increased glucose production resulted from an increase in PC and fructose-1, 6-diphosphatase activity which was strongly suggested to arise respectively from increased FFA oxidation and availability, secondary to an obesity-related increase in lipolysis *(192)*. In hepatocytes from obese (vs lean) *fa/fa* Zucker rats, responsiveness of fructose-2, 6-diphosphate levels as well as of 6-phosphofructo-2-kinase and PK to insulin were all impaired *(193)*. In addition to acetyl CoA, fatty acid oxidation also leads to an accumulation of NADH. Both inhibit pyruvate dehydrogenase (via PDH kinase). Mitochrondrial citrate also increases and inhibits 6-phosphofructo-1-kinase, slowing down glycolysis *(55)*. A decrease in fatty acid oxidation induced by insulin will therefore reverse these effects, stimulating glycolysis. All these data suggest that defects in insulin action at the level of gluconeogenesis and glycolysis contribute to hepatic insulin resistance. Some of these effects may be at least partly mediated by alterations in FFA concentrations and oxidation.

We have seen that glucose production and uptake by the liver is regulated by a vast and intricate network of interacting influences be they hormonal or metabolic. The overall effect however is a constant rate of postabsorptive glucose production and meal-related suppression of this production accompanied by a net uptake of glucose by the liver.

HEPATIC INSULIN RESISTANCE AND TYPE 2 DIABETES

Although this has been argued, the normal liver appears to be exquisitely sensitive to insulin. This was demonstrated in animals directly *(136,137)*. In parallel studies in humans, tolbutamide was infused at such a dose that only a small increase in insulin secretion was seen (as C-peptide changes) but not enough to detectably alter peripheral insulin levels *(209)*. Under these circumstances both glucose production and glucose concentrations decreased. The change in glucose concentrations in these studies was necessarily small in order to avoid counter-regulatory influences. The change in HGP was however implicitly in response to portal insulin levels. These observations are supported by a dose-response curve for hepatic insulin effects which is well to the left of that for its peripheral effects *(139)*. With this sensitivity to portal insulin, it could be anticipated that small defects in the insulin secretory response could have major effects on hepatic glucose output. This would link the etiological hypotheses based on liver resistance to insulin *(35–42)* and those based on β-cell defects *(7–14,210,211)* as has been suggested by for example, Mitrakou and coworkers *(6)*, Prentki and Corkey *(64)* and others. An early β-cell defect would therefore lead to increased glucose production. This would likely initially occur in the stimulated system (postprandially) and eventually under basal conditions. Support for this is seen in the tightly correlated increases in HGP and fasting plasma glucose *(4,31,212)* which are illustrated in Fig. 5A. In addition, experimentally induced early phase defects in insulin secretion appear to specifically affect HGP *(13)*. An alternative argument entails a primary defect at the liver with hyperinsulinemia arising specifically as a compensation for the increased glucose production. Whatever the mechanism, at least a relative hyperglycemia results. This leads to glucose toxicity *(45)* which would cause both a peripheral resistance to insulin *(45–47)* and β-cell dysfunction *(48,49)*. The insulin resistance both at peripheral and hepatic sites would contribute to the early compensatory hyperinsulinemia seen and, combined with the glucose toxic effects, eventually to beta cell failure.

It is interesting that an analogous sequence of events has been attributed to the development of insulin resistance in the case of MODY. The peripheral insulin resistance present in this state was inferred to be secondary to the hyperglycemia which follows from the β-cell (and likely liver) enzyme defects *(213)*. Also interesting however is the fact that the insulin resistance seen in MODY, as well as in transgenic rats with PEPCK overexpression *(191)* is mild. This suggests that these defects may be insufficient to cause severe diabetes.

A large number of studies however suggest that the extension can be made from milder forms of diabetes where the metabolic function of the liver is known to be impaired to more severe forms of the disease. Thus, fasting hyperglycemia, perhaps the hallmark of decompensating diabetes, has been related to increases in basal glucose production *(32–38,212,214)*. These increases also appear to be present at an earlier stage of the pathogenesis of Type 2 diabetes *(32,36)* and may be related to subtle changes in insulin secretion *(6,211)*. Interestingly, the etiological basis of the hyperglycemia in both the diabetic GK *(42)* and the streptozotocin-induced diabetic rat *(38)* appears to be related to changes in liver glucose metabolism in the face of β-cell defects rather than in peripheral insulin action. Similarly, suppression of glucose production following meals may also be impaired *(6,35)* although this impairment is not always found *(199)*. Overall, a strong case may be made for impaired liver glucose metabolism which is resistant to both basal and stimulated insulin. The basis for this resistance may be due both to molecular defects and inappropriate insulin secretion patterns.

Caveats however can be made based on the methodologies for measuring glucose production *(30,33,215)*. These have been based on infusions of glucose tracers, following a priming injection. Basal glucose production is determined from tracer and glucose samples after a steady-state of the tracer concentration is presumed to have been reached. It has been argued that given the impaired metabolic clearance of glucose also present in Type 2 diabetes, the amount of primer may have been inappropriate so that steady-states were not likely to have been reached in many experiments. It may be added that what may often be seen in such studies is "pseudoplateaux" both of tracer and glucose concentrations. These drift gradually in time, yielding varying estimates of basal turnover. Improved approaches, based on more appropriate primers or extended tracer infusions, lead to quite a different picture of the relationship between glucose production and levels in normal subjects and diabetic patients (Fig. 5C) *(216)*. Similarly, some measurements of suppression of production and first-pass uptake following glucose ingestion, may also have methodological difficulties because of their nonsteady-state nature leading to significant variances in the results. These observations suggest a smaller role for hepatic insulin resistance in the phenotypic expression of the diabetic process. When coupled with the many observations in first-degree relatives of individuals with Type 2 diabetes, which demonstrate specific, early peripheral lesions in insulin action particularly in the muscle *(18–22,30,56,217)* a strong case may also be made for the periphery as the primary site of insulin resistance.

Likely however, both are true (e.g., *34,218)* and the progression of the disease is based on the complex set of metabolic, hormonal and likely neural interactions previously cited *(39)*. Moreover, it can be argued that the final expression of Type 2 diabetes develops incrementally. For example, a small deficit in insulin secretion would lead to a small increase in HGP which in turn produces a small increase in overall ambient glycemia. Assuming that glucose toxicity is a continuous process, changes in peripheral insulin action could take place which would lead to further changes in glycemia, glucose toxicity, β-cell impairment, glucose production and peripheral action. This argument can however be initiated anywhere in the sequence, underlining the difficulty in identifying the initial lesion.

Roles of Lipid Metabolism

Carbohydrate and lipid metabolism are intimately and intricately interrelated. Each affects the other, is regulated by insulin while simultaneously contributing to the determination of the rate of its secretion, and each may alter the way in which insulin acts, or the sensitivity of various metabolic processes to insulin. The picture is evidently not that simple since many other factors: hormonal, neural and metabolic may further modulate these interactions. It can be illustrated in Type 2 diabetes by the circadian rhythms seen in both circulating cortisol and FFA levels and rates of HGP which are completely out of phase with the latter, suggesting a regulatory relationship with cyclic changes in insulin sensitivity *(219)*. Considerations such as these help in explaining the variety of results obtained on the effects of lipids on carbohydrate metabolism and its regulation by insulin, particularly in the liver.

As has already been discussed, FFA can be shown to affect a large number of processes and their regulation by insulin *(220)* in the generation of a net glucose output by the liver. Studies in a dog model have even led to the suggestion that FFA is the principal, if not the only mediator of insulin effects on the liver *(121)*. These results are not entirely consistent with those in humans. Increases in circulating FFA with infusions of Intralipid and heparin during insulinopenia and hypoglycemia were shown to increase HGP *(124,125,221)*. Others demonstrated no changes in the basal HGP in response to increased FFA, although increases in gluconeogenesis with reciprocal changes in glycogenolysis (hepatic autoregulation) could explain this *(122,131,189)*. Similarly, during insulin infusion, suppression of lipolysis using Acipimox or increases in circulating FFA levels were shown to alter the suppression of HGP by insulin *(126,128,224)* or not *(124,223)*. The variability of the results obtained could depend on whether elevations or decreases in FFA were induced *(230)*, and the length and timing of the treatments *(231)*.

They could also result from the sources of the FFA—whether circulating or intracellular. It has for example, been suggested that the triglyceride effect on the suppressibility of HGP is induced by way of triglyceride hydrolysis and increases in the intracellular FFA pool without interference from the circulating FFA *(225,226)*. Similarly, as already discussed, FFA concentrations themselves and FFA oxidation may have different effects contributing to HGP. In particular, gluconeogenesis from alanine and pyruvate was stimulated by an increase in FFA oxidation, whereas that from lactate was increased by FFA without a change in its oxidation *(227)*. Hypertriglyceridemia itself could be considered as a contributing factor in the etiology of insulin resistance since it is closely associated with it. This has however, not been borne out in studies which lowered triglycerides with gemfibrozil *(228)*. The data on the interactions between lipid and carbohydrate metabolism in the etiology of insulin resistance in the liver remain incomplete and await further clarification. As an illustration of these issues, metformin has been shown to be associated with lower circulating FFA *(229,232)* in Type 2 diabetes. In one study, measurements suggested an improvement in HGP and hepatic insulin sensitivity *(232)*. In the other, changes in circulating FFA were related only to alterations in the metabolic clearance of glucose *(229)*.

SUMMARY: *HEPATIC EFFECTS OF INSULIN*

Although lipotoxicity undoubtedly contributes to insulin resistance *(233)* and, in particular, hepatic insulin resistance, it is likely not the underlying cause. For example, visceral adipose tissue has long been considered metabolically active and resistant to insulin, thus providing an excess of FFA to the portal vein (when it, itself, is in excess). This has been implicated in the etiology of the hepatic insensitivity to insulin seen in Type 2 diabetes *(234)*. Other studies however, have demonstrated portal FFA levels which are not significantly higher than peripheral in morbidly obese subjects *(236)*. In fact, enhanced sensitivity of abdominal fat to insulin has also been shown *(237,238)*. This would improve uptake of FFA and storage of triglyceride in this tissue. Such an observation would be consistent with a paradoxically impaired FFA metabolism in muscle in parallel with that of glucose in abdominally obese women *(239)*. The impairment in its peripheral metabolism would then result in FFA which would be available for storage in visceral tissue. With observations such as these, it seems less likely that FFA *mediates* insulin sensitivity or insulin resistance.

The large amount of evidence demonstrating that FFA affects insulin sensitivity however, strongly suggests that they may *modulate* insulin action in the liver as well as in other tissues. Thus, under different metabolic circumstances, increased FFA and their increased oxidation could alter hepatic insulin action whether it is basal or stimulated, or not. This suggests a modulatory effect, particularly when coupled with the evidence indicating direct effects of insulin on the activities and expression of a number of enzymes involved in hepatic glucose metabolism. These would presumably be mediated by way of established signalling pathways. In this way, insulin might be expected to "set up" the machinery for an appropriate hepatic response. The particular set of metabolic circumstances which prevail at the time would then dictate the exact nature of the response.

We have already seen that FFA can alter the response. The glycogen content of the liver can further influence this modulation *(187,188)*. Similarly, Sacca et al. *(141)* concluded that the suppressive effect of hyperglycemia on HGP is strictly dependent on the degree of hepatic insulinization. In addition, hyperglycemia without insulin is totally unable to activate the process of hepatic glucose uptake. In subjects with Type 2 diabetes, after a very low energy diet, HGP and glucose levels decreased. After refeeding, HGP increased *(240)*. All these data suggest that glucose too, can modulate insulin's effect on the liver.

The arterial-portal glucose gradient has been postulated to be important in determining the degree of glucose uptake by the liver *(241)*. Interestingly, in a bivascularly perfused liver, an arterial-portal gradient does not itself change the net rate of glucose production. Only the addition of insulin converts the net production to a net uptake *(242)*, again suggesting that insulin creates the enzymatic conditions for uptake. The degree to which this occurs is determined by the gradient. Hormones such as glucagon, cortisol, leptin may also have similar modulatory influences on insulin action as may drugs such as metformin or the thiazolidinediones.

HEPATIC MODULATION OF INSULIN ACTION

As the periphery may modulate hepatic insulin action, there is evidence that the liver may modulate the action of insulin on peripheral tissues.

The liver is not only a target of insulin action, as already discussed, but a principal regulator of peripheral insulin concentrations. It extracts a large fraction, varying between 20 and 80%, of the insulin presented to it *(65–67)*. This extraction is variable *(243)* and may be regulated acutely by, for example, glucose *(244)* and FFA *(245)* suggesting a linkage to peripheral indicators of the efficiency of insulin action. It is also altered in chronic disease states such as liver cirrhosis *(246–248)*. Portal shunting or hepatocellular

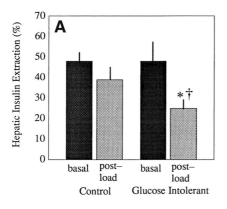
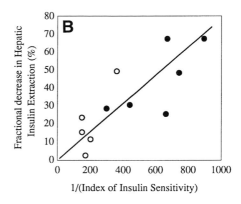

Fig. 6. (A) Hepatic insulin extraction in control and glucose intolerant subjects under basal conditions and following glucose loading expressed as means ±SEM (*$p < 0.05$) when compared to basal, (†, $p < 0.05$) when compared to the corresponding control measurement. **(B)** Correlation between the percent decrease in hepatic insulin extraction following glucose loading and 1/ISI where ISI is an index of insulin sensitivity defined by the product of the glucose and insulin areas ($r = 0.81$, $p = 0.0028$). (Endocrinol and Metabol 1996;3:265 ©1996 W. B. Saunders Company, Limited, London, by permission.)

damage decrease insulin extraction in this disease state which is simultaneously characterized by a peripheral hyperinsulinemia and insulin resistance *(248)*.

The hyperinsulinemia has been deemed to arise both from the decreased insulin uptake and from a hypersecretion of the hormone *(249–251)*. The latter would be secondary to a decreased insulin sensitivity, which could in turn arise partly from downregulation of receptors due to hyperinsulinemia, and partly due to other metabolic abnormalities *(252)*

Hyperinsulinemia is also characteristic of the compensated stage of Type 2 diabetes *(4)* and has been most frequently considered to be due to a hypersecretory response to systemic insulin resistance. However in patients who are obese *(253)*, and particularly abdominally obese *(254)*, it was suggested that there may also be a decrease in the metabolic clearance rate (MCR) of insulin, due primarily to a decrease in its hepatic removal.

The question was therefore asked, whether in patients with glucose intolerance, a decrease in the hepatic uptake of insulin could be a primary lesion, contributing to the hyperinsulinemia and insulin resistance of the diabetic state *(255)*. To assess this issue, non-obese subjects with normal fasting glucose and insulin but significant glucose intolerance were selected. Fasting insulin secretion and post-hepatic insulin appearance were determined using injections of C-peptide and labeled insulin respectively *(256,257)*. From this, a basal hepatic extraction of insulin was calculated and was found to be identical: $48 \pm 5\%$ and $48 \pm 9\%$ in the control and glucose intolerant subjects. Using the basal characterization of the subjects' insulin kinetics and the assumption that changes in the MCR of insulin were proportional to those in its hepatic extraction, it was found that following an oral glucose load, the hepatic insulin extraction decreased disproportionately (Fig. 6A) in the glucose intolerant subjects (to $25 \pm 4\%$ vs $39 \pm 6\%$, $p < 0.05$). This indicated that the elevated postprandial insulin concentrations were in fact primarily due to a decreased efficiency of hepatic removal, at least in this subgroup of patients. Moreover, a correlation was seen (Fig. 6B) between the decrease in insulin removal and an index of insulin resistance (defined as the inverse of the product of insulin and glucose areas during the oral glucose tolerance test). Decreases in circulating FFA were almost identical in the two cases, suggesting that the changes in hepatic insulin uptake precede changes in the sensitivity of lipolysis to insulin which could potentially affect liver insulin removal *(245)*. This would occur by way of FFA from visceral fat depots, released into the portal vein and selectively affecting this function of the liver *(245)*. Both in vitro and in vivo evidence however, militates against this hypothesis *(258–260)* since metabolic clearance of insulin was found to be unaffected by fatty acids. It is furthermore, consistent with the concept that splanchnic obesity is a result, not a cause of insulin resistance *(239,261,262)*.

The correlation (Fig. 6B) seen, between the decrease in insulin removal and an index of insulin resistance, suggests that the two may be linked. As pointed out, it appears unlikely that the impairments in insulin removal and insulin sensitivity are related by a common cause, such as increased FFA. The concept was therefore entertained, that a decrease in hepatic insulin removal could be directly causative of a systemic insulin resistance. Such a decrease could be experimentally induced by diverting the pancreatic venous drainage around the liver *(263)*, thus reducing hepatic insulin uptake at least by the amount which would occur on first passage through the liver.

Interestingly, the clinical experiment has been frequently performed in the context of pancreas and more recently, islet, transplantation. The venous drainage of pancreas transplants has usually been into iliac vessels and therefore peripheral *(264)* although portal anastomoses have been performed *(265,266)*. Systemic hyperinsulinemia is indeed, frequently found in patients who have had heterotopic pancreas or pancreatic segment transplantation and in animal models *(265,267–274)*, although this is not always the case *(275–278)*. The hyperinsulinemia, in conjunction with an often normal tolerance to glucose, is suggestive of a degree of insulin resistance.

In order to isolate the question of the site of pancreatic venous drainage from those of decreased β-cell pancreatic denervation, immunosuppressive therapy, and renal function (since kidneys are often transplanted simultaneously with the pancreas), the pancreaticoduodenal and splenic veins were anastomosed to the inferior vena cava or back to the portal vein (controls) in dogs. This maintained the integrity of the entire pancreas as well as of its innervation. Systemic versus portal venous drainage then became the only factor which was altered in the comparison of the effect of the two sites of insulin delivery on carbohydrate metabolism and peripheral insulinemia. Fasting insulin concentrations doubled following diversion of the pancreatic venous drainage to the inferior vena cava. They remained unchanged compared to preoperative levels when venous drainage remained portal. A euglycemic hyperinsulinemic clamp, with insulin concentrations near 35 µU/mL was used to assess insulin sensitivity, estimated as the tracer-determined metabolic clearance rate of glucose divided by the insulin concentration. Insulin sensitivity fell by over 60% following systemic diversion of the pancreatic venous outflow (Fig. 7). The dose-response curve of metabolic glucose clearance versus insulin concentrations was shifted to the right *(279)*. The responsiveness, or response to saturating insulin concentrations, was also decreased, consistent with the decrease in muscle GLUT4 seen by Elahi and colleagues *(280)*.

We have suggested above that insulin may "set up" the response of the liver to a particular set of metabolic circumstances. A number of factors including glucose, FFA and the CNS may then modulate this response. The data following pancreatic venous diversion to the systemic circulation strongly suggest that, in an analogous fashion, the

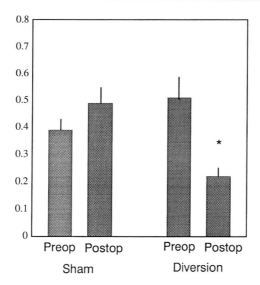

Fig. 7. Index of insulin sensitivity calculated as a change in the metabolic clearance of glucose divided by the corresponding change in insulin concentrations during a hyperinsulinemic euglycemic clamp study in dogs with their pancreatic venous drainage diverted to the inferior vena cava or reanastomosed to the portal vein (shams). In Diversion Postop, $p < 0.05$ vs Diversion Preop and Sham (J Clin Invest 1993; 92: 1713).

liver may modulate both the insulin response and the response to insulin following a metabolic challenge. This modulation is specifically related to the uptake of insulin since altering this uptake by removing the first-pass component, decreases insulin sensitivity by more than 50%. A possible mechanism for this is suggested by the fact that the systemic response is highly sensitive to the profile of the insulin levels—e.g., the presence of an acute phase response, and the magnitude of the early response *(281)* and the pulsatility of insulin secretion *(282)*. All these can be altered, damped or enhanced by the liver. Alternative mechanisms by which the liver modulates peripheral insulin sensitivity could also be humoral or neural. Finally, as already mentioned, metabolic and other factors, could alter the effect of the liver. For example, both glucose and FFA have been implicated, although not universally, in changing the liver's uptake of insulin. Increased lactate concentrations have recently been suggested to increase the extraction *(283)* although this is not entirely consistent with previous data demonstrating an unaltered MCR with lactate infusion in humans *(284)*. Interestingly, the liver's effect on the systemic response to insulin has been shown in cats *(285)* and rats *(286)* to be dependent on some function of the hepatic parasympathetic nerves. Hepatic denervation was associated with a decreased sensitivity to injected insulin which was reversed by intraportal acetylcholine administration. Vagotomy in humans with parasympathetic denervation of both liver and pancreas however, did not alter the insulin response or the MCR of glucose following an oral glucose load *(287,288)*. Similarly, the glycemic and insulinemic responses to intraduodenal glucose in hepatic-denervated and -innervated dogs were not different *(289)*, indicating identical systemic sensitivities to insulin. It could be concluded that the variability in the observed changes due to metabolic or neural interventions, depending on species or metabolic circumstances, imply their modulatory nature on an underlying hepatic process. They also underline the existence of this process and the importance of the portal site of insulin entry in generating its entire response *(290)*.

In summary, it may be suggested that the central effect of insulin on the liver is direct. This effect may however be modified by a large number of factors, emanating from the periphery or the splanchnic bed. Similarly, although the principal effects of insulin on peripheral tissues are also clearly direct, they may be modulated by an array of similar factors. It is suggested however that this modulation may to an important extent, be mediated by the liver. Many loci are therefore available for the generation of insulin resistance, both hepatic and peripheral. Their multifactional nature contributes to their elusiveness.

REFERENCES

1. Cerasi E, Luft R. "What is inherited—what is added" hypothesis for the pathogenesis of diabetes mellitus. Diabetes 1967;16:615.
2. Banting FG, Best CH. The internal secretion of the pancreas. J Lab Clin Med 1922;7:251.
3. Himsworth HP. Diabetes mellitus: its differentiation into insulin-sensitive and insulin-insensitive types. Lancet 1936;1:127.
4. DeFronzo R, Bonadonna R, Ferrannini E. Pathogenesis of NIDDM: A balanced overview. Diabetes Care 1992;15:318.
5. Efendic S, Grill V, Luft R, Wajngot A. Low insulin response: A marker of prediabetes. Adv Exp Med Biol 1988;246:167–174.
6. Mitrakou A, Kelley D, Mokan M, Veneman T, Pangburn T, Reilly J, Gerich J. Role of reduced suppression of glucose production and diminished early insulin release in impaired glucose tolerance. N Engl J Med 1992;326:22–29.
7. Reaven GM, Shen SW, Silvers A, Farquhar JW. Is there a delay in the plasma insulin response of patients with chemical diabetes mellitus? Diabetes 1971;20:416.
8. Lang DA, Matthews DR, Peto J, Turner RC. Cyclic oscillations of basal plasma glucose and insulin concentrations in human beings. N Engl J Med 1979;301:1023–1027.
9. O'Rahilly S, Turner RC, Matthews DR. Impaired pulsatile secretion of insulin in relatives of patients with non-insulin-dependent diabetes. New Engl J Med 1988;318:1225–1230.
10. O'Meara NM, Sturis J, Van Cauter E, Polonsky KS. Lack of control by glucose of ultradian insulin secretory oscillations in impaired glucose tolerance and in non-insulin-dependent diabetes mellitus. J Clin Invest 1993;92:262–271.
11. Kudva YC, Butler PC. Insulin secretion in Type 2 diabetes mellitus. In: Draznin B and Rizza R, eds. Clinical Research in Diabetes and Obesity II. Diabetes and Obesity. Humana, Totowa, NJ, 1997, pp. 119–136.
12. Simpson RG, Benedetti A, Grodsky GM, Karam JH, Forsham PH. Early phase of insulin release. Diabetes 1968;17:684–692.
13. Luzi L, DeFronzo R. Effect of loss of first-phase insulin secretion on hepatic glucose production and tissue glucose disposal in humans. Am J Physiol 1989;257:E241–E246.
14. Temple R, Carrington C, Luzio S, Owens D, Schneider A, Sobey W, Hales C. Insulin deficiency in non-insulin-dependent diabetes. The Lancet 293–295, February 11, 1989.
15. Reaven GM. Role of insulin resistance in the pathophysiology of non-insulin dependent diabetes mellitus. Diabetes/Metabolism Reviews 1997;9(Suppl 1):55–125.
16. Bogardus C, Lillioja S, Howard BV, Reaven G, Mott D. Relationships between insulin secretion, insulin action, and fasting plasma glucose concentration in nondiabetic and noninsulin dependent diabetic subjects. J Clin Invest 1984;74:1238–46.
17. Polonsky KS, Sturis J, Bell GI. Non-insulin dependent diabetes mellitus—a genetically programmed failure of the beta cell to compensate for insulin resistance. New Eng J Med 1996;334:777–783.
18. Warram JH, Martin BH, Krolewski AS, Soeldner JS, Kahn CR. Slow glucose removal rate and hyperinsulinemia precede the development of type II diabetes in the offspring of diabetic patients. Ann Intern Med 1990;113:909–915.
19. Sicree RA, Zimmet PZ, King HOM, Coventry JS. Plasma insulin response among Nauruans: prediction of deterioration in glucose tolerance over 6 years. Diabetes 1987;36:179–186.

20. Haffner SM, Stern MP, Hazuda HP, Pugh JA, Patterson JK. Hyperinsulinemia in a population at high risk for non-insulin-dependent diabetes mellitus. N Eng J Med 1986;315:220–224.

21. Lillioja S, Mott DM, Howard BV, Bennett PH, Yki-Järvinen H, Freymond D, Nyomba BL, Zurlo F, Swinburn B, Bogardus C. Impaired glucose tolerance as a disorder of insulin action. Longitudinal and cross-sectional studies in Pima Indians. N Engl J Med 1988;318:1217–1225.

22. Eriksson J, Franssila-Kallunki A, Ekstrand A, Saloranta C, Widen E, Schalin C, Groop L. Early metabolic defects in persons at increased risk for non-insulin-dependent diabetes mellitus. N Engl J Med 1989;321:337–343.

23. Kida Y, Esposito-Del Puente A, Bogardus C, Mott DM. Insulin resistance is associated with reduced fasting and insulin-stimulated glycogen synthase phosphatase activity in human skeletal muscle. J Clin Invest 1990;85:476–481.

24. Katz A, Bogardus C. Insulin-mediated increase in glucose 1,6-biphosphate is attenuated in skeletal muscle of insulin-resistant man. Metabolism 1990;39:1300–1304.

25. Kida Y, Nyomba BI, Bogardus C, Mott DM. Defective insulin response of cyclic adenosine monophosphate-dependent protein kinase in insulin resistant humans. J Clin Invest 1991;87:673–679.

26. Vaag A, Henriksen JE, Beck-Nielsen H. Decreased insulin activation of glycogen synthase in skeletal muscles in young non-obese caucasian first-degree relatives of patients with non-insulin-dependent diabetes mellitus. J Clin Invest 1992;89:782–788.

27. Schalin-Jäntti C, Härkönen M, Groop LC. Impaired activation of glycogen synthase in people at increased risk for developing NIDDM. Diabetes 1992;41:598–604.

28. Kida Y, Raz I, Maeda R, Nyomba BL, Stone K, Bogardus C, Sommercorn J, Mott DM. Defective insulin response of phosphorylase phosphatase in insulin-resistant humans. J Clin Invest 1992; 89:610–617.

29. Häring Hu, Mehnert H. Pathogenesis of Type 2 (non-insulin-dependent) diabetes mellitus: candidates for a signal transmitter defect causing insulin resistance of the skeletal muscle. Diabetologia 1993;36:176–182.

30. Beck-Nielsen H, Hother-Nielsen O, Vaag A, Alford F. Pathogenesis of Type 2 (non-insulin-dependent) diabetes mellitus: the role of skeletal muscle glucose uptake and hepatic glucose production in the development of hyperglycaemia. A critical comment. Diabetologia 1994;37:217–221.

31. Consoli A. Role of liver in pathophysiology of NIDDM. Diabetes Care 1992;15:430–441.

32. Perriello G, Pampanelli S, Del Sindaco P, Lalli C, Ciofetta M, Volpi E, Santeusanio F, Brunetti P, Bolli, G. Evidence of increased systemic glucose production and gluconeogenesis in an early stage of NIDDM. Diabetes 1997;46:1010–1016.

33. Chen Y-DI, Swislocki ALM, Jeng C-Y, Juang J-H, Reaven GM. Effect of time on measurement of hepatic glucose production. J Clin Endocrinol Metab 1988;67:1084–1088.

34. DeFronzo RA. The triumvirate: β-Cell, muscle, liver. A collusion responsible for NIDDM. Diabetes 1988;37:667–687.

35. Ferrannini E, Simonson D, Katz L, Reichard G, Bevilacqua S, Barrett E, Olsson M, DeFronzo RA. The disposal of an oral glucose load in patients with non-insulin-dependent diabetes. Metabolism 1988;47:79–85.

36. Osei K. Increased basal glucose production and utilization in nondiabetic first-degree relatives of patients with NIDDM. Diabetes 1990;39:597–601.

37. Gerich JE. Is muscle the major site of insulin resistance in Type 2 (non-insulin-dependent) diabetes melltius? Diabetologia 1991;34:607–610.

38. Burcelin R, Eddouks M, Maury J, Kande J, Assan R, Girard J. Excessive glucose production, rather than insulin resistance, accounts for hyperglycaemia in recent-onset streptozotocin-diabetic rats. Diabetologia 1995;38:283–290.

39. Bonadonna RC. In vivo metabolic defects in non-insulin-dependent diabetes mellitus. Horm Res 1993;39(Suppl 3):102–106.

40. Vaag A, Henriksen J, Madsbad S, Holm N, Beck-Nielsen H. Insulin secretion, insulin action, and hepatic glucose production in identical twins discordant for non-insulin-dependent diabetes mellitus. J Clin Invest 1995;95:690–698.

41. Turk D, Alzaid A, Dinneen S, Nair KS, Rizza R. The effects of non-insulin-dependent diabetes mellitus on the kinetics of onset of insulin action in hepatic and extrahepatic tissues. J Clin Invest 1995;95:755–762.

42. Picarel-Blanchot F, Berthelier C, Bailbé D, Portha B. Impaired insulin secretion and excessive hepatic glucose production are both early events in the diabetic GK rat. Am J Physiol 1996;271 (Endocrinol Metab 34): E755–E762.

43. McCarthy MI, Froguel P, Hitman GA. The genetics of non-insulin-dependent diabetes mellitus: tools and aims. Diabetologia 1994;37:959–968.
44. Hales CN, Barker DJP. Type 2 (non-insulin-dependent) diabetes mellitus: the thrifty phenotype hypothesis. Diabetologia 1992;35:595–601.
45. Rossetti L, Giaccari A, DeFronzo RA. Glucose toxicity. Diabetes Care 1990;13:610–630.
46. Zierath JR, Galuska D, Nolte LA, Thörne A, Kristensen J, Wallberg-Henriksson H. Effects of glycaemia on glucose transport in isolated skeletal muscle from patients with NIDDM: in vitro reversal of muscular insulin resistance. Diabetologia 1994;37:270–277.
47. Ramlal T, Rastogi S, Vranic M, Klip A. Decrease in glucose transporter number in skeletal muscle of mildly diabetic (streptozotocin-treated) rats. Endocrinology 1989;125:890–897.
48. Leahy JL, Bonner-Weir S, Weir GC. Minimal chronic hyperglycemia is a critical determinant of impaired insulin secretion after an incomplete pancreatectomy. J Clin Invest 1988,81:1407–1414.
49. Leahy J. Natural history of β-cell dysfunction in NIDDM. Diabetes Care 1990;13:992–1010.
50. Ward WK, Bolgiano DC, McKnight B, Halter JB, Porte D Jr. Diminished β-cell secretory capacity in patients with non-insulin-dependent diabetes mellitus. J Clin Invest 1984;74:1318–1328.
51. Froguel P, Vaxillaire M, Sun F. Close linkage of glucokinase locus on chromosome 7p to early-onset noninsulin dependent diabetes mellitus. Nature 1992;36:162–164.
52. Velho G, Petersen K, Perseghin G, Hwang J-H, Rothman D, Pueyo M, Cline G, Froguel P, Shulman G. Impaired hepatic glycogen synthesis in glucokinase-deficient (MODY–2) subjects. J Clin Invest 1996;98:1755–1761.
53. McGarry JD. What if Minkowski had been ageusic? An alternative angle on diabetes. Science 1992;258:766–770.
54. Reaven GM. The fourth musketeer: from Alexandre Dumas to Claude Bernard. Diabetologia 1995;38:3–13.
55. Randle PJ, Garland PB, Hales CN, Newsholme EA. The glucose fatty-acid cycle: its role in insulin sensitivity and the metabolic disturbances of diabetes mellitus. Lancet 1963;i:785–789.
56. Reaven GM. Role of insulin resistance in the pathophysiology of non-insulin dependent diabetes mellitus. Diabetes/Metab Rev 1993;9(Suppl 1):55–125.
57. Ferrannini E, Barrett EJ, Bevilacqua S, DeFronzo RA. Effect of fatty acids on glucose production and utilization in man. J Clin Invest 1983;72:1737–1747.
58. Boden G, Jadali F, White J, Liang Y, Mozzoli M, Chen X, Coleman E, Smith C. Effects of fat on insulin-stimulated carbohydrate metabolism in normal men. J Clin Invest 1991;88:960–966.
59. Boden G, Chen X. Effects of fat on glucose uptake and utilization in patients with non-insulin-dependent diabetes. J Clin Invest 1995;96:1261–1268.
60. Malaisse WJ, Malaisse-Lagae F. Stimulation of insulin secretion by non-carbohydrate metabolites. J Lab Clin Med 1968;72:438–448.
61. Stein DT, Esser V, Stevenson BE, Lane KE, Whiteside JH, Daniels MB, Chen S, McGarry JD. Essentiality of circulating fatty acids for glucose-stimulated insulin secretion in the fasted rat. J Clin Invest 1996;97:2728–2735.
62. Zhou Y-P, Grill VE. Long-term exposure of rat pancreatic islets to fatty acids inhibits glucose-induced insulin secretion and biosynthesis through a glucose fatty acid cycle. J Clin Invest 1994;93:870–876.
63. Milburn JL Jr, Hirose H, Lee YH, Nagasawa Y, Ogawa A, Ohneda M, Beltrandel H, Newgard CB, Johnson JH, Unger RH. Pancreatic β-cells in obesity: evidence for induction of functional, morphological and metabolic abnormalities by increased long chain fatty acids. J Biol Chem 1995;270:1295–1299.
64. Prentki M, Corkey B. Are the β-cell signaling molecules malonyl-CoA and cytosolic long-chain acyl-CoA implicated in multiple tissue defects of obesity and NIDDM? Diabetes 1996;45:273–283.
65. Field JB. Extraction of insulin by liver. Ann Rev Med 1973;24:309–314.
66. Ferrannini E, Cobelli C. The kinetics of insulin in man. II. Role of the liver. Diabetes Metab Rev 1987;3:365–397.
67. Pye S, Watarai T, Davies J, Radziuk J. Comparison of the continuously calculated fractional hepatic extraction of insulin with its fractional extraction using a new double tracer technique. Metabolism 1993;42:145–153.
68. Ruderman NB. Muscle amino acid metabolism and gluconeogenesis. Ann Rev Med 1975;26:245–258.
69. McIntyre N, Holdsworth CD, Turner DS. Intestinal factors in the control of insulin secretion. J Clin Endocrinol Metab 1965;25:1317–1324.
70. Perley MJ, Kipnis DM. Plasma insulin response to oral and intravenous glucose: studies in normal and diabetic subjects. J Clin Invest 1967;46:1954–1562.

71. Erlick H, Stimmler L, Hlad CJ Jr. Plasma insulin responses to oral and intravenous glucose administration. J Clin Endocrinol Metab 1964;24:1076–1082.

72. Buchanan KD, McKiddie MT. The insulin response to glucose: A comparison between oral and intravenous tolerance tests. J Endocrinol 1967;39:13–20.

73. Dupré J, Curtis JD, Unger RH. Effects of secretin pancreozymin or gastrin on the response of the endocrine pancreas to administration of glucose or arginine in man. J Clin Invest 1969; 48:745–757.

74. Unger RH, Eisentraut AM. Enteroinsular axis. Arch Int Med 1969;123:261–266.

75. Brown JC, Dryburgh JR, Ross SA, Dupré J. Identification and actions of gastric inhibitory polypeptide. Rec Prog Horm Res 1975;31:487–532.

76. Scow RO, Cornfield J. Quantitative relations between the oral and intravenous glucose tolerance curves. Am J Physiol 1954;179:435–438.

77. James RG, Osborn JO. The analysis of glucose measurements by computer simulation. J Physiol 1965;181:59–67.

78. Felig P, Wahren J, Hendler R. Influence of oral glucose ingestion on splanchnic glucose and gluconeogenic substrate metabolism in man. Diabetes 1975;24:468–475.

79. Felig P, Wahren J, Hendler R. Influence of maturity-onset diabetes on splanchnic glucose balance after oral glucose ingestion. Diabetes 1978;27:121–126.

80. Radziuk J, McDonald TJ, Rubenstein D, Dupré J. Initial splanchnic extraction of ingested glucose in normal man. Metabolism 1978;27:657–669.

81. Radziuk J. Tracer methods and the metabolic disposal of a carbohydrate load in man. Diabetes/Metab Rev 1987;3:231–267.

82. Ferrannini E, Wahren J, Felig P, DeFronzo RA. The role of fractional glucose extraction in the regulation of splanchnic glucose metabolism in normal and diabetic man. Metabolism 1980;29:28–35.

83. Nilsson LH, Hultman E. Liver glycogen in man—the effect of total starvation on a carbohydrate-poor diet followed by carbohydrate refeeding. Scand J Clin Lab Invest 1973;32:325–330.

84. Nilsson LH, Hultman E. Liver and muscle glycogen in man after glucose and fructose infusion. Scand J Clin Lab Invest 1974;33:5–10.

85. Taylor R, Magnussen I, Rothman DL, Cline GW, Caumo A, Cobelli C, Shulman GI. Direct assessment of liver glycogen storage by ^{13}C-nuclear magnetic resonance spectroscopy and regulation of glucose homeostasis after a mixed meal in normal subjects. J Clin Invest 1996;97:126–132.

86. Radziuk J. Hepatic glycogen formation by direct uptake of glucose following oral glucose loading in man. Can J Physiol Parmacol 1979;57:1196–1199.

87. Radziuk J. Hepatic glycogen in humans. I. Direct formation after oral and intravenous glucose or after a 24-h fast. Am J Physiol 1989;257:E145–E157.

88. Radziuk J. Glucose and glycogen metabolism following glucose ingestion: a turnover approach. In: Cobelli C, Bergman R, eds. Carbohydrate Metabolism. Quantitative Physiology and Modelling. J. Wiley and Sons, London, 1981, pp. 239–266.

89. Radziuk J. Source of carbon in hepatic glycogen synthesis during absorption of an oral glucose load in humans. Fed Proc 1982;41:88–90.

90. Radziuk J. Hepatic glycogen in humans. II. Gluconeogenetic formation after oral and intravenous glucose. Am J Physiol 1989;257:E158–E169.

91. Hetenyi G Jr. Correction factor for the estimation of plasma glucose synthesis from the transfer of C^{14} atoms from labelled substrate in vivo: a preliminary report. Can J Physiol Pharmacol 1979;57:767–770.

92. Shikama H, Ui M. Glucose load diverts hepatic glucogenic product from glucose to glycogen in vivo. Am J Physiol 1978;235:E354–E360.

93. Baer A, Radziuk J. Sources of hepatic glycogen formation in conscious rats during intraduodenal glucose loading. Clin Res 1980;28:385A.

94. Barrett E, Bevilacqua S, DeFronzo R, Ferrannini E. Glycogen turnover during refeeding in the postabsorptive dog: Implications for the estimation of glycogen formation using tracer methods. Metabolism 1994;43:285–292.

95. David M, Petit W, Laughlin M, Shulman R, King J, Barrett E. Simultaneous synthesis and degradation of rat liver glycogen. J Clin Invest 1990;86:612–617.

96. Shulman GI, Rothman DL, Chung Y, Rossetti L, Petit WA, Barrett EJ, Shulman RG. ^{13}C NMR studies of glycogen turnover in the perfused rat liver. J Biol Chem 1988;263:5027–5029.

97. Moore MC, Cherrington AD, Cline G, Pagliassoti MJ, Jones EM, Neal DW, Badet C, Shulman GI. Sources of carbon for hepatic glycogen synthesis in the conscious dog. J Clin Invest 1991;88:578–87.

98. Agius J, Tosh D, Peak M. The contribution of pyruvate cycling to loss of [6-³H] glucose during conversion of glucose to glycogen in hepatocytes: effects of insulin, glucose and acinar origin of hepatocytes. Biochem J 1993;238:255–262.

99. Sugden MC, Watts DI, Palmer TN, Myles DD. Direction of carbon flux in starvation and after refeeding: in vitro and in vivo effects of 3-mercaptopicolinate. Biochem Intern 1983;7:329–37.

100. Newgard CB, Moore SV, Foster DW, McGarry JD. Efficient hepatic glycogen synthesis in refeeding rats requires continued carbon flow through the gluconeogenic pathway. J Biol Chem 1984;259:6958–63.

101. Zhang Z, Radziuk J. Effects of lactate on pathways of glycogen formation in the perfused rat liver. Biochem J 1991;280:419.

102. Zhang Z, Radziuk J. The coordinated regulation of hepatic glycogen formation in the perfused rat liver by glucose and lactate. Am J Physiol 1994;266:E583–E591.

103. Bjorkman O, Eriksson LS, Nyberg B, Wahren J. Gut exchange of glucose and lactate in basal state and after oral glucose in postoperative patients. Diabetes 1990;39:747–751.

104. Radziuk J, Pye S, Zhang Z. Substrates and the regulation of hepatic glycogen metabolism. In: Östenson CG, Efendic S, Vranic M, ed. Advances in Experimental Medicine & Biology. Plenum, New York, 1993, pp. 235–252.

105. Jungermann K, Katz N, Teutsch H, Sasse D. Possible metabolic zonation of liver parenchyma into glucogenic and glycolytic hepatocytes. In: Thurman RG, Williamson JR, Drott HR, Chance B, eds. Alcohol and Aldehyde Metabolizing Systems. Academic Press, New York, 1977.

106. Jungermann K, Katz N. Functional hepatocellular heterogeneity. Hepatology 1982;2:385–395.

107. Johnson JA, Fusaro RM. The role of skin in carbohydrate metabolism. Advances in Metabolic Disorders 1972;6:1–55.

108. Jansson PA, Smith U, Lönnroth P. Evidence for lactate production by human adipose tissue in vivo. Diabetologia 1990;33:253–256.

109. Jackson RA, Peters N, Advani U, Perry G, Rogers J, Brough WH, Pilkington TR. Forearm glucose uptake during the oral glucose tolerance test in normal subjects. Diabetes 1973;22:442–458.

110. Radziuk J, Inculet R. The effects of ingested and intravenous glucose on forearm uptake of glucose and glucogenic substrate in normal man. Diabetes 1983;32:977–981.

111. DeFronzo RA, Jequier ELE, Maeder E, Wahren J, Felber JP. The effect of insulin on the disposal of intravenous glucose. Results from indirect calorimetry and hepatic and femoral venous catheterization. Diabetes 1981;30:1000–1007.

112. Ashmore J, Weber G. Hormonal control of carbohydrate metabolism in liver. In: Dickens F, Randle PJ, Whelan WJ, eds. Liver in Carbohydrate Metabolism and Its Disorders, Vol I. Academic Press, London, 1968, pp. 335–374.

113. Felig P, Wahren J. Influence of endogenous insulin secretion on splanchnic glucose and amino acid metabolism in man. J Clin Invest 1971;10:1702–1711.

114. Rizza RA, Mandarino LJ, Gerich JE. Dose-response characteristics for effects of insulin on production and utilization of glucose in man. Am J Physiol 1981;240:E630–E639.

115. Yki-Järvinen H, Young AA, Lamkin C, Foley JE. Kinetics of glucose disposal in the whole body and across the forearm in man. J Clin Invest 1987;79:1713–1719.

116. Jahoor F, Peters EJ, Wolfe RR. The relationship between gluconeogenic substrate supply and glucose production in humans. Am J Physiol 1990;258:E288–E296.

117. Jenssen T, Nurjhan N, Consoli A, Gerich JE. Failure of substrate-induced gluconeogenesis to increase overall glucose appearance in normal humans. J Clin Invest 1990;85:489–497.

118. Clore JN, Glickman PS, Nestler JE, Blackard WG. In vivo evidence for hepatic autoregulation during FFA-stimulated gluconeogenesis in normal humans. Am J Physiol 1991;261:E425–E429.

119. Sindelar DK, Balcom JH, Chu CA, Neal DW, Cherrington AD. A comparison of the effects of selective increases in peripheral or portal insulin on hepatic glucose production in the conscious dog. Diabetes 1996;45:1594–1604.

120. Lewis GF, Zinman B, Groenewoud Y, Vranic M, Giacca A. Hepatic glucose production is regulated both by direct hepatic and extrahepatic effects of insulin in humans. Diabetes 1996;45:454–462.

121. Rebrin K, Steil GM, Getty L, Bergman RN. Free fatty acid as a link in the regulation of hepatic glucose output by peripheral insulin. Diabetes 1995;44:1038–1045.

122. Bonadonna RC, Groop LC, Zych K, Shank M, DeFronzo RA. Dose-dependent effect of insulin on plasma free fatty acid turnover and oxidation in humans. Am J Physiol 1990;259:E736–E750.

123. Groop LC, Bonadonna RC, Simonson DC, Petrides AS, Shank M, DeFronzo RA. Effect of insulin on oxidative and nonoxidative pathways of free fatty acid metabolism in human obesity. Am J Physiol 1992;263:E79–E84.

124. Ferrannini E, Barrett EJ, Bevilacqua S, DeFronzo RA. Effect of fatty acids on glucose production and utilization in man. J Clin Invest 1983;72:1737–1747.

125. Boden G, Jadali F. Effects of lipid on basal carbohydrate metabolism in normal men. Diabetes. 1991;40:686–692.

126. Saloranta C, Koivisto V, Widen E, Falholt K, DeFronzo RA, Harkonen M, Groop L. Contribution of muscle and liver to glucose-fatty acid cycle in humans. Am J Physiol 1993;264:E599–E605.

127. Lee KU, Lee HK, Koh CS, Min HK. Artificial induction of intravascular lipolysis by lipid-heparin infusion leads to insulin resistance in man. Diabetologia 1988;31:285–290.

128. Bevilacqua S, Bonadonna RC, Boni C, Ciociaro D, Maccari F, Giorico MA, Ferrannini E. Acute elevation of free fatty acid levels leads to hepatic insulin resistance in obese subjects. Metabolism 1987;36:502–506.

129. Boden G, Jadali F, White J, Liang Y, Mozzoli M, Chen X, Coleman E, Smith C. Effects of fat on insulin-stimulated carbohydrate metabolism in normal men. J Clin Invest 1991;88:960–966.

130. Groop LC, Bonadonna RC, Shank M, Petrides AS, DeFronzo RA. Role of free fatty acids and insulin in determining free fatty acid and lipid oxidation in man. J Clin Invest 1991;87:83–89.

131. Johnston P, Hollenbeck C, Sheu W, Chen YD, Reaven GM. Acute changes in plasma non-esterified fatty acid concentration do not change hepatic glucose production in people with Type 2 diabetes. Diabetic Medicine 1990;7:871–875.

132. Fery F, Plat M, Baleriaux M, Balasse EO. Inhibition of lipolysis stimulates whole body glucose production and disposal in normal postabsorptive subjects. J Clin Endo Metab 1997;82:825–830.

133. Seyffert WA, Madison LL. Physiological effects of metabolic fuels on carbohydrate metabolism. I. Acute effects of elevation of plasma free fatty acids on hepatic glucose output, peripheral glucose utilization, serum insulin and plasma glucagon levels. Diabetes 1967;16:765–776.

134. Wolfe RR, Shaw JHF. Inhibitory effect of plasma free fatty acids on glucose production in the conscious dog. Am J Physiol 1984;246:E181–E186.

135. Zhang Z, Radziuk J. Insulin effects on hepatic glucose production: extent and pathways. Diabetologia 1997;40(Supp 1):979, A249.

136. Madison LL, Combes B, Adams R, Strickland B. The physiological significance of the secretion of endogenous insulin into the portal circulation. III. Evidence for a direct immediate effect of insulin on the balance of glucsoe across the liver. J Clin Invest 1960;39:507–522.

137. Madison LL. Role of insulin in the hepatic handling of glucose. Archives of Internal Medicine 1969;123:284–292.

138. Steele R. Influences of glucose loading and of injected insulin on hepatic glucose output. Annals of the New York Academy of Sciences 1959;82:420–430.

139. Firth R, Bell P, Rizza R. Insulin action in non-insulin-dependent diabetes mellitus: the relationship between hepatic and extrahepatic insulin resistance and obesity. Metab: Clin Exp 1987;36:1091–1095.

140. Kolterman OG, Gray RS, Griffin J, Burstein P, Insel J, Scarlett JA, Olefsky JM. Receptor and postreceptor defects contribute to the insulin resistance in non-insulin-dependent diabetes mellitus. J Clin Invest 1981;68:957–969.

141. Sacca L, Cicala M, Trimarco B, Ungaro B, Vigorito C. Differential effects of insulin on splanchnic and peripheral glucose disposal after an intravenous glucose load in man. J Clin Invest 1982;70:117–126.

142. DeFronzo R, Ferrannini E, Hendler R, Felig P, Wahren J. Regulation of splanchnic and peripheral glucose uptake by insulin and hyperglycemia in man. Diabetes 1983;32:35–45.

143. Pilkis SJ, Claus TH. Hepatic gluconeogenesis/glycolysis: regulation and structure/function relationships of substrate cycle enzymes. Annual Review of Nutrition 1990;11:465–515.

144. Barrett E, Liu Z. Hepatic glucose metabolism and insulin resistance in NIDDM and obesity. Baillière's Clinical Endocrinology and Metabolism 1993;7:875–901.

145. Felig P, Wahren J. Influence of endogenous insulin secretion on splanchnic glucose and amino acid metabolism in man. J Clin Invest 1971;50:1702–1711.

146. Hetenyi G Jr, Kopstick FX, Retlstorf LJ. The effect of insulin on the distribution of glucose between the blood plasma and the liver in alloxan-diabetic and adrenalectomized rats. Can J Biochem Physiol 1963;41:2431–2439.

147. Newsholme EA, Crabtree B. Substrate cycles in metabolic regulation and heat generation. Biochem Soc Symp 1976;41:61–110.

148. Hellerstein MK, Neese RA, Linfoot P, Christiansen M, Turner S, Letscher A. Hepatic gluconeogenic fluxes and glycogen turnover during fasting in humans. A stable isotope study. J Clin Invest 1997;100:1305–1319.

149. Newgard CB, Foster DW, McGarry D. Evidence for suppression of hepatic glucose–6-phosphatase with carbohydrate feeding. Diabetes 1984;33:192–195.

150. Gardner L, Liu Z, Barrett E. The role of glucose–6-phosphatase in the action of insulin on hepatic glucose production in the rat. Diabetes 1993;42:1614–1620.

151. Barzilai N, Rossetti L. Role of glucokinase and glucose–6-phosphatase in the acute and chronic regulation of hepatic glucose fluxes by insulin. J Biol Chem 1993;268(33): 25019–25025.

152. Blackard WG, Clore JN. Insulin effects on substrate metabolism. In: Draznin B, Rizza R, ed. Clinical Research in Diabetes and Obesity, Part I: Methods, Assessment, and Metabolic Regulation. Humana, Totowa, NJ, 1997, 205–220.

153. Pagliassotti M, Holste L, Moore M, Neal D, Cherrington A. Comparison of the time courses of insulin and the portal signal on hepatic glucose and glycogen metabolism in the conscious dog. J Clin Invest 1996;97:81–91.

154. Agius D, Peak M. Intracellular binding of glucokinase in hepatocytes and translocation by glucose, fructose and insulin. Biochem J 1993;296:785–796.

155. Vionnet N, Stoffel M, Takeda J, Yasuda K, Bell GI, Zouali H, Lesage S, Velho G, Iris F, Passa Ph, Froguel Ph, Cohen D. Nonsense mutation in the glucokinase gene causes early-onset non-insulin-dependent diabetes mellitus. Nature 1992;356:721–722.

156. Tappy L, Dussoix P, Iynedjian P, Henry S, Schneiter P, Zahnd G, Jequier E, Philippe J. Abnormal regulation of hepatic glucose output in maturity-onset diabetes of the young caused by a specific mutation of the glucokinase gene. Diabetes 1997;45:204–208.

157. Velho G, Petersen KF, Perseghin G, Hwang J-H, Rothman DL, Pueyo ME, Cline GW, Froguel P, Shulman GI. Impaired hepatic glycogen synthesized glucokinase-deficient (MODY–2) subjects. J Clin Invest 1996;98:1755–1761.

158. Clément K, Pueyo ME, Vaxillaire M, Rakotoambinina B, Thuillier F, Passa Ph, Froguel Ph, Robert J-J, Velho G. Assessment of insulin sensitivity in glucokinase-deficient subjects. Diabetologia 1996;39:82–90.

159. Barzilai N, Hawkins M, Angelov I, Hu M, Rossetti L. Glucosamine-induced inhibition of liver glucokinase impairs the ability of hyperglycemia to suppress endogenous glucose production. Diabetes 1996;45:1329–1335.

160. Ferre T, Pyol A, Riu E, Bosch F, Valera A. Correction of diabetic alterations by glucokinase. Proc Natl Acad Sci 1996;93:7225–7230.

161. Vaulont S, Kahn A. Transcriptional control of metabolic regulation genes by carbohydrates. FASEB J 1994;8:28–35.

162. Efendic S, Karlander S, Vranic M. Mild Type 2 diabetes markedly increases glucose cycling in the postabsorptive state and during glucose infusion irrespective of obesity. J Clin Invest 1988;81:1953–1961.

163. Rooney DP, Neely RDG, Beatty O, Bell NP, Sheridan B, Atkinson AB, Trimble ER, Bell PM. Contribution of glucose/glucose 6-phosphate cycle activity to insulin resistance in Type 2 (non-insulin-dependent) diabetes mellitus. Diabetologia 1993;36:106–112.

164. Soskin S. The liver and carbohydrate metabolism. Endocrinology 1940;26:297–308.

165. DeWulf H, Hers HG. The stimulation of glycogen synthesis and of glycogen synthetase in the liver by the administration of glucose. Eur J Biochem 1967;2:50–56.

166. Stalmans W, DeWulf H, Hue L, Hers HG. The sequential inactivation of glycogen phosphorylase and activation of glycogen synthetase after the administration of glucose to mice and rats. The mechanism of the hepatic threshold to glucose. Eur J Biochem 1974;41:117–134.

167. Hers HG. The control of glycogen metabolism in the liver. Ann Rev Biochem 1976;45:167–189.

168. van de Werve G, Jeanrenaud B. Liver glycogen metabolism: an overview. Diabetes/Metab Rev 1987;3:47–78.

169. Nutall FQ, Gilboe DP, Gannon MC, Niewohner CB, Tan AWH. Regulation of glycogen synthesis in the liver. Am J Med 1988;85(Suppl 5A):77–85.

170. Nuttall FQ, Gannon MC, Larner J. Oral glucose effect on glycogen synthetase and phosphorylase in heart, muscle and liver. Physiol Chem Phys 1972;4:497–515.

171. Niewoehner CB, Gilboe DP, Nuttall FQ. Metabolic effects of oral glucose in the liver of fasted rats. Am J Physiol 1984;246:E89–E94.

172. Ciudad CJ, Massague J, Guinovart JJ. The inactivation of glycogen phosphorylase in rats is not a prerequisite for the activation of liver glycogen synthase. FEBS Lett 1979;99:321–324.
173. Gilboe DP, Nuttall FQ. Stimulation of liver glycogen particle synthase D phosphatase activity by caffeine, AMP and glucose–6-phosphate. Arch Biochem Biophys 1982;19: 179–185.
174. Carabaza A, Ciudad CJ, Baque S, Guinovart JJ. Glucose has to be phosphorylated to activate glycogen synthase, but not to inactivate glycogen phosphorylase in hepatocytes. FEBS Lett 1992;296:211–214.
175. Fernandez-Novell JM, Roca A, Bellido D, Vilaró S, Guinovart JJ. Translocation and aggregation of hepatic glycogen synthase during the fasted to refed transition in rats. Eur J Biochem 1996; 238:570–575.
176. Parkes JL, Grieninger G. Insulin, not glucose, controls hepatocellular glycogen deposition. J Biol Chem 1985;260:8090–8097.
177. Ortmeyer H, Bodkin N, Hansen B. Insulin regulates liver glycogen synthase and glycogen phosphorylase activity reciprocally in rhesus monkeys. Am J Physiol 1997;272:E133–E138.
178. Kruszynska YT, Home PD, Albert KGMM. In vivo regulation of liver and skeletal muscle glycogen synthase activity by glucose and insulin. Diabetes 1986;35:662–667.
179. Terrettaz J, Assimacopoulos-Jeannet F, Jeanrenaud B. Inhibition of hepatic glucose production by insulin in vivo in rats: contribution of glycolysis. Am J Physiol 1986;250:E346–E351.
180. Liu Z, Gardner L, Barrett E. Insulin and glucose suppress hepatic glycogenolysis by distinct enzymatic mechanisms. Metabolism 1993;42(12):1546–1551.
181. Radziuk J, Pye S, Zhang Z, Wiernsperger N. Effects of metformin on lactate uptake and gluconeogenesis in the perfused rat liver. Diabetes 1997 46:1406–1413.
182. Seoane J, Gómez-Foix AM, O'Doherty RM, Gómez-Ara C, Newgard CB, Guinovart JJ. Glucose 6-phosphate produced by glucokinase, but not hexokinase I, promotes the activation of glycogen synthesis. J Biol Chem 1996;271:23756–23760.
183. Bartels H, Vogt B, Jungermann K. Glycogen synthesis from pyruvate in the periportal and from glucose in the perivenous zone in perfused livers from fasted rats. FEBS Lett 1987;221:277–283.
184. Magnusson I, Rothmann DL, Katz LD, Shulman RG, Shulman GI. Increased rate of gluconeogenesis in type II diabetes mellitus. A ^{13}C nuclear magnetic resonance study. J Clin Invest 1992;90:1323–1327.
185. Clore JN, Post EP, Bailey J, Nestler JE, Blackard WG. Evidence for increased liver glycogen in patients with noninsulin-dependent diabetes mellitus after a 3-day fast. J Clin Endocrinol Metab 1992;74:660–666.
186. Müller C, Assimacopoulos-Jeannet F, Mosimam F, Schneiter Ph, Riou JP, Pachiaudi C, Felber JP, Jequier E, Jeanrenaud B, Tappy L. Endogenous glucose production, gluconeogenesis and liver glycogen concentration in obese nondiabetic patients. Diabetologia 1997;40:463–468.
187. Wise S, Nielsen M, Rizza R. Effects of hepatic glycogen content on hepatic insulin action in humans: Alteration in the relative contributions of glycogenolysis and gluconeogenesis to endogenous glucose production. J Clin Endoc Metab 1997;82:1828–1833.
188. Kruszynska YT, McCormack JG, McIntyre N. Effect of glycogen stores and nonesterified fatty acid availability on insulin-stimulated glucose metabolism and tissue pyruvate dehydrogenase activity in the rat. Diabetologia 1991;34:205–211.
189. Puhakainen I, Yki-Järvinen H. Inhibition of lipolysis decreases lipid oxidation and gluconeogenesis from lactate but not fasting hyperglycemia or total hepatic glucose production in NIDDM. Diabetes 1993;42:1694–1699.
190. Rosella G, Zajac J, Kaczmarczyk S, Andrikopoulos S, Proietto J. Impaired suppression of gluconeogenesis induced by overexpression of a noninsulin-responsive phosphoenolpyruvate carboxykinase gene. Molec Endocrinol 1993;7:1456–1462.
191. Rosella G, Zajac JD, Baker L, Kaczmarczyk SJ, Andrikopoulos S, Adams TE, Proietto J. Impaired glucose tolerance and increased weight gain in transgenic rats overexpressing a noninsulin-responsive phosphoenolpyruvate carboxykinase gene. Mol Endocrenol 1995;9(10):1396–1404.
192. Andrikopoulos S, Proietto J. The biochemical basis of increased hepatic glucose production in a mouse model of type 2 (non-insulin-dependent) diabetes mellitus. Diabetologia 1995;38:1389–1396.
193. Sánchez-Gutiérrez J, Sánchez-Arias J, Lechuga C, Valle J, Samper B, Feliu J. Decreased responsiveness of basal gluconeogenesis to insulin action in hepatocytes isolated from genetically obese (fa/fa) Zucker rats. Endocrinology 1994;134:1868–1873.
194. Giaccari A, Rossetti L. Predominant role of gluconeogenesis in the hepatic glycogen repletion of diabetic rats. J Clin Invest 1992;89:36–45.
195. DeMeutter RC, Shreeve WW. Conversion of DL-lactate [2-C14] or [3-C14] or pyruvate [2–14C] to blood glucose in humans: effects of diabetes, insulin, tolbutamide, and glucose load. J Clin Invest 1963;42:525–533.

196. Zawadski J, Wolfe R, Mott D, Lillioja S, Howard B, Bogardus C. Increased rate of Cori cycle in obese subjects with NIDDM and effects of weight reduction. Diabetes 1988;37:154–159.

197. Comstock J, Ellerhorst J, Garber A. Effect of sulfonylurea therapy on glucose-alanine precursor-product interrelationship in NIDDM. Diabetes 1987;36(Suppl 1):4A.

198. Consoli A, Nurijhan N, Capani F, Gerich J. Predominant role of gluconeogenesis in increased hepatic glucose production in NIDDM. Diabetes 1989;38:550–57.

199. Katz H, Homan M, Jensen M, Caumo A, Cobelli C, Rizza R. Assessment of insulin action in NIDDM in the presence of dynamic changes in insulin and glucose concentration. Diabetes 1994;43:289–296.

200. Halimi S, Assimacopoulos-Jeannet F, Terrettaz J, Jeanrenaud B. Differential effect of steady-state hyperinsulinaemia and hyperglycaemia on hepatic glycogenolysis and glycolysis in rats. Diabetologia 1987;30:268–272.

201. Phillips J, Clark D, Henly D, Berry M. The contribution of glucose cycling to the maintenance of steady-state levels of lactate by hepatocytes during glycolysis and gluconeogenesis. Eur J Biochem 1995;227:352–358.

202. Hue L, Rider M. Role of fructose 2, 6-biphosphate in the control of glycolysis in mammalian tissues. Biochem J 1987;245:313–324.

203. Peret J, Chanez M. Influence of diet, cortisol and insulin on the activity of pyruvate carboxylase and phosphoenolpyruvate carboxykinase in the rat liver. J Nutr 1976;106:103–110.

204. O'Brien RM, Granner DK. PEPCK gene as model of inhibitory effects of insulin on gene transcription. Diabetes Care 1990;13:327–329.

205. Exton JH, Harper SC, Tucker AL, Ho RJ. Effects of insulin on gluconeogenesis and cyclic AMP levels in perfused livers from diabetic rats. Biochimica et Biophysica Acta 1973;329:23–40.

206. Clore JN, Stillman JS, Helm ST, Blackard WG. Evidence for dissociation of gluconeogenesis stimulated by non-esterified fatty acids and changes in fructose 2, 6-biphosphate in cultured rat hepatocytes. Biochem J 1992;288:145–148.

207. Hue L, Maisin L, Rider M. Palmitate inhibits liver glycolysis. Involvement of fructose 2, 6-bisphosphate in the glucose/fatty acid cycle. Biochem J 1988;251:541–545.

208. Blackard W, Clore J, Powers L. A stimulatory effect of FFA on glycolysis unmasked in cells with impaired oxidative capacity. Am J Physiol 1990;259:E451–E456.

209. Maheux P, Chen Y-D, Polonsky K, Reaven G. Evidence that insulin can directly inhibit hepatic glucose production. Diabetologia 1997;40:1300–1306.

210. Chen K-W, Boyko E, Bergstrom R, Leonetti D, Newell-Morris L, Wahl P, Fujimoto W. Earlier appearance of impaired insulin secretion than of visceral adiposity in the pathogenesis of NIDDM. Diabetes Care 1995;18:747–753.

211. Porte D, Kahn S. The key role of islet dysfunction in Type 2 diabetes mellitus. Clin Invest Med 1995;18:247–254.

212. Féry F. Role of hepatic glucose production and glucose uptake in the pathogenesis of fasting hyperglycemia in Type 2 diabetes: normalization of glucose kinetics by short-term fasting. J Clin Endocrinol Metab 1994;78:536–542.

213. Clément K, Pueyo ME, Vaxillaire M, Rakotoambinina B, Thuillier F, Passa Ph, Froguel Ph, Robert J-J, Velko G. Assessment of insulin sensitivity in glucokinase-deficient patients. Diabetologia 1996;39:82–90.

214. Dinnen S, Gerich J, Rizza R. Carbohydrate metabolism in non-insulin-dependent diabetes. N Eng J Med 1972;327:717–713.

215. Hother-Nielsen O, Beck-Nielsen H. Insulin resistance, but normal basal rate of glucose production in patients with newly diagnosed mild diabetes mellitus. Acta Endocrinol (Copenhagen) 1995;124:637–645.

216. Jeng C-Y, Sheu NH-H, Fuh MM-T, Chen Y-DI, Reaven GM. Relationship between hepatic glucose production and fasting plasma glucose concentration in patients with non-insulin-dependent diabetes mellitus. Diabetes 1994;43:1440–1444.

217. Groop LC, Kankuri M, Schalin-Jäntti C, Estrand A, Nikula-Ijäs P, Widen E, Kuismanen E, Eriksson J, Franssila-Kallunki A, Saloranta C, Koskimies S. Association between polymorphism of the glycogen synthase gene and non-insulin-dependent diabetes mellitus. N Eng J Med 1993;328:10–14.

218. Firth R, Bell P, Rizza R. Insulin action in non-insulin-dependent diabetes mellitus: The relationship between hepatic and extrahepatic insulin resistance and obesity. Metabolism 1987;36:1091–1095.

219. Boden G, Chen X, Urbain JL. Evidence for a circadian rhythm of insulin sensitivity in patients with NIDDM caused by cyclic changes in hepatic glucose production. Diabetes 1996;45:1044–1050.

220. Oakes N, Cooney G, Camilleri S, Chisholm D, Kraegen E. Mechanisms of liver and muscle insulin resistance induced by chronic high-fat feeding. Diabetes 1997;46:1768–1774.

221. Baron AD, Brechtel G, Edelman SV. Effects of free fatty acids and ketone bodies on in vivo non-insulin-mediated glucose utilization and production in humans. Metabolism 1989;38:1056–1061.

222. Clore JN, Glickman PS, Helm ST, Nestler JE, Blackard WG. Evidence for dual control mechanism regulating hepatic glucose output in nondiabetic men. Diabetes 1991;40:1033–1040.

223. Yki-Järvinen H, Puhakainen I, Koivisto VA. Effect of free fatty acids on glucose uptake and nonoxidative glycolysis across human forearm tissues in the basal state and during insulin stimulation. J Clin Endocrinol Metab 1991;72:1268–1277.

224. Lee K-U, Park J, Kim C, Hong S, Suh K, Park KS, Park SW. Effect of decreasing plasma free fatty acids by Acipimox on hepatic glucose metabolism in normal rats. Metab: Clin Exp 1996;45:1408–1414.

225. Piatti PM, Monti LD, Baruffaldi L, Magni F, Paroni R, Fermo I, Costa S, Santambrogio G, Nasser R, Marchi M, Galli-Kienle M, Pontiroli A, Pozza G. Effects of an acute increase in plasma triglyceride levels on glucose metabolism in man. Metab: Clin Exp 1995;44:883–889.

226. Yki-Järvinen H, Puhakainen I, Saloranta C, Taskinen M-R. Demonstration of a novel feedback mechanism between FFA oxidation from intracellular and intravascular sources. Am J Physiol 1991;260:680–689.

227. Blumenthal SA. Stimulation of gluconeogenesis by palmitic acid in rat hepatocytes: Evidence that this effect can be dissociated from the provision of reducing equivalents. Metabolism 1983;32:971–976.

228. Sane T, Knudsen P, Vuorinen-Markkola H, Yki-Järvinen H, Taskinen M-R. Decreasing triglyceride by gemfibrozil therapy does not affect the glucoregulatory or antilipolytic effect of insulin in nondiabetic subjects with mild hypertriglyceridemia. Metabolism 1995;44:589–596.

229. Abbasi F, Kamath V, Rizvi AA, Carantoni M, Chen Y-DI, Reaven GM. Results of a placebo-controlled study on the metabolic effects of the addition of metformin to sulforylurea-treated patients: evidence for a central role of adipose tissue. Diabetes Care 1997;201:1863–1869.

230. Saloranta C, Franssila-Kallunki A, Ekstrand A, Taskinen M-R, Groop L. Modulation of hepatic glucose production by non-esterified fatty acids in type 2 (non-insulin-dependent) diabetes mellitus. Diabetologia 1991;34:409–415.

231. Saloranta C, Taskinen M-R, Widén E, Härkönen M, Melander A, Groop L. Metabolic consequences of sustained suppression of free fatty acids by Acipimox in patients with NIDDM. Diabetes 1993;42:1559–1566.

232. Perriello G, Misericordia P, Volpi E, Santucci A, Santucci C, Ferrannini E, Ventura MM, Santeusanio F, Brunetti P, Bolli GB. Acute antihyperglycemic mechanisms of metformin in NIDDM: evidence for suppression of lipid oxidation and hepatic glucose production. Diabetes 1994;43:920–928.

233. Unger R. Lipotoxicity in the pathogenesis of obesity-dependent NIDDM. Genetic and clinical implications. Diabetes 1995;44:863–870.

234. Martin ML, Jensen MD. Effects of body fat distribution on regional lipolysis in obesity. J Clin Invest 1991;88:609–613.

235. Bjorntorp P. Metabolic implications of body fat distribution. Diabetes Care 1991;14:1132–1143.

236. Blackard WG, Clore JN, Glickman PS, Nestler JE, Kellum JM. Insulin sensitivity of splanchnic and peripheral adipose tissue in vivo in morbidly obese man. Metabolism 1993;42:1195–1200.

237. Rebutte-Scrive M, Anderson B, Olbe L, Bjorntorp P. Metabolism of adipose tissue in intraabdominal depots in severely obese men and women. Metabolism 1990;39:1021–1025.

238. Smith U, Hammersten J, Bjorntorp P, Kral JG. Regional differences and effect of weight reduction on human fat cell metabolism. Eur J Clin Invest 1979;9:327–332.

239. Colberg SR, Simoneau J-A, Thaete FL, Kelley DE. Skeletal muscle utilization of FFA in women with visceral obesity. J Clin Invest 1995;95:1846–1853.

240. Henry RR, Scheaffer L, Olefsky JM. Glycemic effects of intensive caloric restriction and isocaloric refeeding in noninsulin-dependent diabetes mellitus. J Clin Endocrinol Metab 1985;61:917–925.

241. Adkins BA, Myers SR, Hendrick GK, Stevenson RW, Williams PE, Cherrington AD. Importance of the route of intravenous glucose delivery to hepatic glucose balance in the conscious dog. J Clin Invest 1987;79:557–565.

242. Gardemann A, Strulik H, Jungermann K. A portal-arterial glucose concentration gradient as a signal for an insulin-dependent net glucose uptake in perfused rat liver. FEBS Lett 1986;202:255–259.

243. Morishima T, Bradshaw C, Radziuk J. Measurement using tracers of steady-state turnover and metabolic clearance of insulin in dogs. Am J Physiol 1985;248: E203-E208.

244. Kaden M, Harding P, Field JB. Effect of intraduodenal glucose administration on hepatic extraction of insulin in the anesthetized dog. J Clin Invest 1973;52: 2016–2028.

245. Svedberg J, Strömblad G, Wirth A, Smith U, Björntorp P. Fatty acids in the portal vein of the rat regulate hepatic insulin clearance. J Clin Invest 1991;88:2054–2058.
246. Marchesini G, Zoli M, Dondi C, Angiolini A, Forlani G, Melli A, Bianchi FB, Pisi E. Blood glucose and glucoregulatory hormones in liver cirrhosis: a study of 24 h profiles and of the role of portal-systemic shunting. Gastroenterologie Clinique et Biologique 1982;6:272–278.
247. Petrides AS, DeFronzo RA. Glucose and insulin metabolism in cirrhosis. J Hepatol (Amsterdam) 1989;8:107–114.
248. Kruszynska YT, Home PD, McIntyre N. Relationship between insulin sensitivity, insulin secretion and glucose tolerance in cirrhosis. Hepatology 1991;14:103–111.
249. Proietto J, Dudley FJ, Aitken P, Alford FP. Hyperinsulinemia and insulin resistance of cirrhosis: the importance of insulin hypersecretion. Clin Endocrinol 1984;21:657–663.
250. Kasperska-Czyzykowa T, Heding LG, Czyzyk A. Serum levels of true insulin: C-peptide and proinsulin in peripheral blood of patients with cirrhosis. Diabetologia 1983;25:506–509.
251. Ballmann M, Hartmann H, Deacon CF, Schmidt WE, Conlon JM, Creutzfeldt W. Hypersecretion of proinsulin does not explain the hyperinsulinaemia of patients with liver cirrhosis. Clin Endocrinol 1986;25:351–361.
252. Cavallo-Perin P, Cassader M, Bozzo C. Mechanism of insulin resistance in human liver cirrhosis: evidence of a combined receptor and postreceptor defect. J Clin Invest 1985;75:1659–1665.
253. Faber OK, Christensen K, Kehlet H, Madsbad S, Binder C. Decreased insulin removal contributes to hyperinsulinemia in obesity. J Clin Endocrinol Metab 1981;53:618–621.
254. Peiris AN, Mueller RA, Smith GA, Struve MF, Kissebah AH. Splanchnic insulin metabolism in obesity: influence of body fat distribution. J Clin Invest 1986;78:1648–1657.
255. Wasilewska M, Pye S, Braaten J, Radziuk J. Hepatic insulin removal following oral glucose loading in nonobese subjects with glucose intolerance and mild Type 2 diabetes. Endocrinol and Metab 1996;3:265–274.
256. Morishima T, Pye S, Polonsky K, Radziuk J. The measurement and validation of nonsteady-state rates of C-peptide appearance in the dog. Diabetologia 1986;29:440–446.
257. Morishima T, Bradshaw C, Radziuk J. Measurement using tracers of steady-state turnover and metabolic clearance of insulin in dogs. Am J Physiol 1985; 248:E203–E208.
258. Kolaczynski JW, Boden G. Effects of oleate and fatty acids from omental adipocytes on insulin uptake in rat liver cells. Endrocinology 1993;133:2871–2874.
259. Boden G, Chen X, Ruiz J, White JV, Rossetti L. Mechanisms of fatty acid-induced inhibition of glucose uptake. J Clin Invest 1994;93:2438–2446.
260. Boden G, Chen X. Effects of fat on glucose uptake and utilization in patients with non-insulin-dependent diabetes. J Clin Invest 1995;96:1261–1268.
261. Blackard WG, Clore JN, Glickman PS, Nestler JE, Kellum JM. Insulin sensitivity of splanchnic and peripheral adipose tissue in vivo in morbidly obese man. Metabolism 1993;42:1195–1200.
262. Henry RR. Impaired muscle fat metabolism: a cause or effect of visceral obesity? J Clin Invest 1995;95:1427–1428.
263. Radziuk J, Barron P, Najm H, Davies J. The effect of systemic drainage of the pancreas on insulin sensitivity. J Clin Invest 1993;92(4):1713–1721.
264. Squifflet J-P. Pancreas Transplantation: Experimental and Clinical Studies. Karger, Basel, Switzerland, 1990.
265. Rosenlof LK, Earnhardt RC, Pruett TL, Stevenson WC, Douglas MT, Cornett GC, Hanks JB. Pancreas transplantation: an initial experience with systemic and portal drainage of pancreatic allografts. Am Surg 1992;215:586–595.
266. Shokouh-Amiri MH, Gaber AO, Gaber LW, Jensen SL, Hughes TA, Elmer D, Britt LG. Pancreas transplantation with portal venous drainage and enteric exocrine diversion: a new technique. Transplant Proc 1992;24:776–777.
267. Katz H, Holman M, Velosa J, Robertson P, Rizza R. Effects of pancreas transplantation on postprandial glucose metabolism. N Engl J Med 1991;325:1278–1283.
268. Van Der Burg, MPM, Gooszen HG, Guicherit OR, Jansen JBMJ, Frolich M, Van Haastert FA, Lamers CBHW. Contribution of partial pancreatectomy, systemic hormone delivery, and duct obliteration to glucose regulation in canine pancreas: importance in pancreas transplantation. Diabetes 1989;38:1082–1089.
269. Sells RA, Calne RY, Hadjiyanakis V, Marshall VC. Glucose and insulin metabolism after pancreas transplantation. BMJ 1972;3:678–681.

270. Osei K, Cottrell DA, Henry ML, Tesi RJ, Ferguson RM, O'Dorisio TM. Insulin insensitivity and glucose effectiveness in type I diabetic allograft recipients. Transplant Proc 1992;24:828–830.

271. Earnhardt RC, Kindler DD, Weaver AM, Cornett G, Elahi D, Veldhuis JD, Hanks JB. Hyperinsulinaemia after pancreatic transplantation prediction by a novel computer model and in vivo verification. Ann Surg 1993;218:428–443.

272. Diem P, Abid M, Redmon JB, Sutherland DER, Robertson P. Systemic venous drainage of pancreas allografts as independent cause of hyperinsulinaemia in Type 1 diabetic recipients. Diabetes 1990;39:534–540.

273. Pozza G, Bosi E, Secchi A, Piatti PM, Touraine JL, Gelet A, Pontiroli AE, Dybernard JM, Traeger J. Metabolic control of Type 1 (insulin-dependent) diabetes after pancreas transplantation. BMJ 1985;291:510–513.

274. Östman J, Bolinder J, Gunnarsson R, Brattström C, Tyden G, Wahren J, Groth C-G. Metabolic effects of pancreas transplantation: effects of pancreas transplantation on metabolic and hormonal profiles in IDDM patients. Diabetes 1989;38(Suppl 1):88–93.

275. Luzi L, Secchi A, Facchini F, Battezzati A, Staudacher C, Spotti D, Castoldi R, Ferrari G, Di Carlo V, Pozza G. Reduction of insulin resistance by combined kidney-pancreas transplantation in Type 1 (insulin-dependent) diabetic patients. Diabetologia 1990;33:549–556.

276. Krusch DA, Brown KB, Cornett G, Freedlender AE, Kaiser DL, Hanks JB. Insulin-dependent and insulin-independent effects after surgical alterations of the pancreas. Surgery (St. Louis) 1989;106:60–68.

277. Christiansen E, Andersen HB, Rasmussen K, Christensen NJ, Olgaard K, Kirkegaard P, Tronier B, Vølund A, Damsbo P, Burcharth F, Madsbad S. Pancreatic β-cell function and glucose metabolism in human segmental pancreas and kidney transplantation. Am J Physiol 1993;264:E441–E449.

278. Pozza G, Traeger J, Dubernard JM, Secchi A, Pontiroli AE, Bosi E, Malik MC, Ruitton A, Blanc N. Endocrine responses of Type 1 (insulin-dependent) diabetic patients following successful pancreas transplantation. Diabetologia 1983;24:244–248.

279. Barron P, Zhi R, Davies J, Welsh L, Radziuk J. Sensitivity and responsiveness of glucose removal to insulin decrease following systemic pancreatic venous drainage. Transplantation Proceedings 1995;27:3038–3039.

280. Elahi D, McAloon-Dyke M, Clark BA, Kahn BB, Weinreb JE, Minaker KL, Wong GA, Morse LA, Brown RS, Shapiro ME, Gingerich RL, Rosenlof LK, Pruett TL, Andersen DK, Hanks JB. Sequential evaluation of islet cell responses to glucose in the transplanted pancreas in humans. Am J Surg 1993;165:15–22.

281. Kendall D, Sutherland D, Najarian J, Goetz F, Robertson R. Effects of hemipancreatectomy on insulin secretion and glucose tolerance in healthy humans. N Engl J Med 1990;322:898–903.

282. Goodner CJ, Walibe BC, Koerker DJ, Ensinck JW, Brown AC, Chickedel EW, Palmer J, Kalnasy L. Insulin, glucagon and glucose exhibit synchronous, sustained oscillations in fasting monkeys. Science 1977;195:177–179.

283. Pagano C, Rizzato M, Lombardi AM, Fabris R, Favaro A, Federspil G, Vettor R. Effect of lactate on hepatic insulin clearance in perfused rat liver. Am J Physiol (Regulatory Integrative Comp Physiol 39) 1996;270:R682–R687.

284. Ferrannini E, Natali A, Brandi LS, Bonadonna R, Vigili de Kreutzemberg S, DelPrato S, Santoro D. Metabolic and thermogenic effects of lactate infusion in humans. Am J Physiol 1993;265:E504–E512.

285. Xie H, Lautt WW. Insulin resistance of skeletal muscle produced by hepatic parasympathetic interruption. Am J Physiol 1996;270:E858–E863.

286. Xie H, Lautt WW. Insulin resistance caused by hepatic cholinergic interruption and reversed by acetylcholine administration. Am J Physiol 1996;271:E587–E592.

287. Corssmit EPM, Van Lanschot JJB, Romijn JA, Endert E, Sauerwein HP. Truncal vagotomy does not affect postabsorptive glucose metabolism in humans. J Appl Physiol 1995;79:97–101.

288. Fabris SE, Thorburn A, Litchfield A, Proietto J. Effect of parasympathetic denervation of liver and pancreas on glucose kinetics in man. Metabolism 1996;45:987–991.

289. Moore MC, Shulman GI, Giaccari A, Pagliassotti MJ, Cline G, Neal D, Rossetti L, Cherrington AD. Effect of hepatic nerves on disposition of an intraduodenal glucose load. Am J Physiol 1993;265:E487–E496.

290. Radziuk J, Barron P. Does pancreatic portal venous drainage matter? Diabetes Annual 1995;9:141–157.

12

The Pathophysiological Consequences of Adipose Tissue Insulin Resistance

Gerald M. Reaven, MD

CONTENTS

INTRODUCTION
IS THE ADIPOSE TISSUE "INSULIN RESISTANT"?
WHAT ARE THE CONSEQUENCES OF ADIPOSE TISSUE
   INSULIN RESISTANCE?
CONCLUSION
REFERENCES

INTRODUCTION

The relationship between insulin resistance and adipose tissue is exceedingly complex. At the simplest level, as discussed in the subsequent section, even the meaning of "insulin resistance" in this context is not totally clear. In order to focus this review on the relationship between adipose tissue and insulin resistance, it will be organized as an answer to the two following fundamental questions: 1) Do differences in the ability of insulin to regulate adipose tissue exist between individuals? and 2) If so, what are the metabolic consequences of these differences in insulin action on adipose tissue?

IS THE ADIPOSE TISSUE "INSULIN RESISTANT"?

Although the phrase "insulin resistance" is widely used, its precise meaning is rarely defined. In the vast majority of cases, the phrase insulin resistance describes a decrease in the ability of insulin to stimulate whole body glucose disposal. This function is most often assessed under steady-state infusion conditions, using either the insulin suppression test or the euglycemic, hyperinsulinemic clamp technique *(1,2)*. These approaches, as conventionally employed, provide an excellent method for assessing the ability of insulin to stimulate muscle glucose uptake, but an insensitive measure of insulin action on adipose tissue. This state of affairs obtains for two reasons. In the first place, adipose tissue consumes relatively little glucose *(3)*; its primary physiological function is to store energy in the form of triglyceride in order to supply the fuel needed to sustain life between meals. Thus, any observed decrease in whole body glucose uptake in response to an insulin infusion will primarily be a reflection of a defect in muscle glucose disposal.

From: *Contemporary Endocrinology: Insulin Resistance*
Edited by: G. Reaven and A. Laws © Humana Press Inc., Totowa, NJ

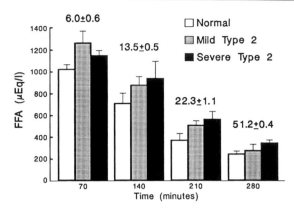

Fig. 1. Relationship between increases in plasma insulin concentration and suppression of FFA level during 70-min sequential infusion studies. Plasma FFA concentrations at 70, 140, 210, and 280 min are displayed on the vertical axis. The numbers of above the bars are the mean insulin concentration at the end of each 70-min infusion. Results of studies in normal subjects, patients with mild Type 2 diabetes, and patients with severe Type 2 diabetes are shown. (Reprinted from Diabetologia 1995;38:3. Copyright © 1995 Springer-Verlag-Heidelberg.)

Secondly, and more importantly, adipose tissue is extremely insulin sensitive as compared to muscle. For example, the results of sequential insulin infusion studies *(4)* shown in Fig. 1 indicate that plasma free fatty acid (FFA) concentrations are approximately half-maximally suppressed in nondiabetic and diabetic subjects when plasma insulin concentrations are increased from ~6 to ~20 μU/mL. Thus, small changes in plasma insulin concentrations have profound effects on plasma FFA concentrations. Furthermore, it can also be seen that plasma FFA concentrations are essentially maximally suppressed at plasma insulin concentrations of approximately 50 μU/mL irrespective of metabolic state. Since most studies of "insulin resistance" are performed at steady-state insulin concentrations >50 μU/mL, individual differences in the ability of insulin to suppress plasma FFA concentrations will be dampened, and the presence of adipose tissue insulin resistance extremely hard to discern. On the other hand, when insulin infusion studies are performed at lower insulin concentrations in nondiabetic volunteers (Fig. 2), it has been shown that the ability of insulin to stimulate glucose disposal by muscle and suppress plasma FFA concentrations are highly correlated *(5)*.

The results shown in Fig. 2 indicate that the ability of insulin to suppress FFA release from adipose tissue varies approximately fourfold from person to person in nondiabetic individuals, and that this defect parallels the decrease in insulin-mediated glucose uptake by muscle SSPG concentration. This phenomenon is not confined to healthy volunteers, but also can be seen in patients with Type 2 diabetes *(6)*. An illustration of this is shown in Fig. 3, in which the relationship in patients with Type 2 diabetes between insulin-mediated glucose disposal by muscle and insulin suppression of plasma FFA is illustrated. It should be emphasized that the studies quantifying insulin resistance in muscle were performed at steady-state insulin concentrations of ~60 μU/mL, as compared to insulin concentration of ~10 μU/mL for estimating FFA suppression.

In summarizing this section it seems evident that the answer to the rhetorical question raised at the beginning is "yes" and that insulin resistance at the level of adipose tissue can be detected in both nondiabetic volunteers and patients with noninsulin-dependent

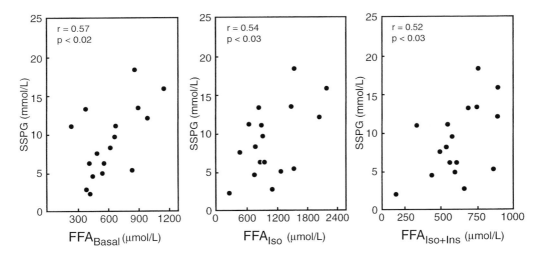

Fig. 2. Relationship between insulin resistance (SSPG values) and mean plasma FFA concentrations during basal insulin replacement (left panel), in response to isoproterenol (Iso) infusion (middle panel), and in response to isoproterenol (Iso) plus insulin (Ins; right panel). The correlation coefficients (r) between the two variables are shown in the upper left corner of each panel. (Reprinted from ref. 5. © The Endocrine Society.)

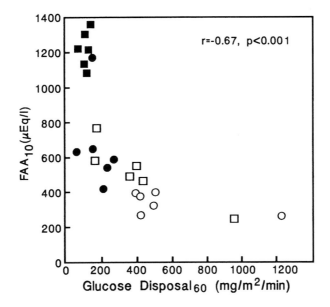

Fig. 3. Relationship ($r = -0.67$; $p < 0.001$) between glucose disposal (horizontal axis) at an insulin concentration ~60 µU/mL and plasma FFA concentration (vertical axis) at an insulin concentration ~10 µU/mL in four different groups. ○ = non-obese, normal; ● = non-obese, Type 2; □ = obese, normal; ■ = obese, Type 2. (Reprinted from J Clin Endocrinol Metab 1987;64:17 © The Endocrine Society.)

diabetes mellitus (Type 2 diabetes). Furthermore, the magnitude of the defect in insulin regulation of muscle and adipose tissue appears to be highly correlated. In the next section the implication of adipose tissue insulin resistance will be explored.

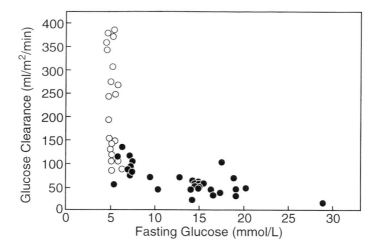

Fig. 4. Relationship between fasting plasma glucose concentration and glucose metabolic clearance rates observed during hyperinsulinemic, glucose clamp studies in 20 nondiabetic subjects (○) and 30 patients with Type 2 diabetes (●). The clamp studies were performed over a 120-min period, with a steady-state plasma insulin concentration of approximately 100μU/mL. (Reprinted from Diabetologia 1995;38:3. Copyright © 1995 Springer-Verlag-Heidelberg.)

WHAT ARE THE CONSEQUENCES OF ADIPOSE TISSUE INSULIN RESISTANCE?

Development of Hyperglycemia

Although muscle insulin resistance is a common finding in patients with Type 2 diabetes *(2,6–8)*, this defect, by itself, cannot account for the development of hyperglycemia. For example, resistance to insulin-mediated glucose disposal by muscle is not limited to patients with Type 2 diabetes, and muscle insulin resistance is a common finding *(9,10)* in nondiabetic subjects with impaired glucose tolerance (IGT). Resistance to insulin-mediated glucose disposal by muscle can also be demonstrated in nondiabetic first degree relatives of patients with Type 2 diabetes *(11,12)*. Finally, significant differences in the ability of insulin to stimulate glucose disposal by muscle are present in individuals with normal glucose tolerance *(13,14)* and in a significant number of these individuals the magnitude of their defect in insulin-mediated glucose disposal approximates that of patients with Type 2 diabetes. The implications of these observations can be easily seen in Fig. 4 which illustrates the relationship between insulin-stimulated glucose disposal by muscle (estimated by the glucose clamp technique) and fasting plasma glucose concentration in a series of non-obese individuals (15). It is obvious from these data that there was not a simple relationship between insulin resistance and fasting plasma glucose concentration. More specifically, a normal fasting plasma glucose concentration could be maintained by individuals who were essentially as insulin resistant as many patients with frank Type 2 diabetes. In addition, once fasting hyperglycemia supervened, significantly higher fasting plasma glucose concentrations were seen with relatively small decreases in insulin-mediated muscle glucose disposal. Consequently, it seems reasonable to conclude that resistance to insulin-mediated muscle glucose uptake by muscle is present in the great majority of individuals with glucose

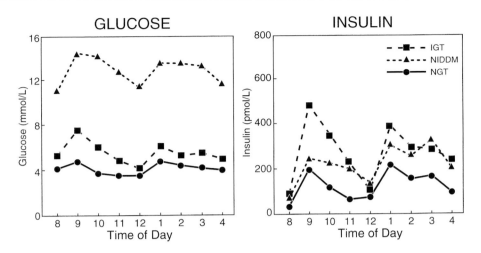

Fig. 5. Plasma glucose and insulin concentrations in non-obese subjects with normal glucose tolerance (NGT, ●), impaired glucose tolerance (IGT ■), or noninsulin-dependent diabetes (Type 2 diabetes (▲) measured hourly from 8 AM to 4 PM. Breakfast at 8 AM and lunch at noon. Reprinted from the J Clin Endo and Metab 76:44-1993 with permission of the journal and the authors.

intolerance, but that this defect, by itself, can neither account for the development of significant hyperglycemia in patients with Type 2 diabetes, nor for the severity of fasting hyperglycemia in these individuals.

The ability of individuals with muscle insulin resistance to maintain normal glucose tolerance depends on the capacity of their pancreatic β-cells to overcome this defect. Significant hyperglycemia only develops when the insulin secretory response is not sufficient to overcome the defect in insulin action on muscle. Evidence for this point of view is shown in Fig. 5, which illustrates day-long plasma glucose and specifically determined insulin concentrations in non-obese, normal volunteers, individuals with IGT, and patients with frank Type 2 diabetes measured hourly from 8 AM to 4 PM, before and after meals (breakfast at 8 AM, lunch at 12 noon). Essentially identical relationships were seen in obese individuals. These results *(16)* clearly show that the development of significant hyperglycemia in patients with Type 2 diabetes is associated with ambient plasma insulin concentrations much lower in absolute terms than in individuals with IGT, and slightly higher than in the normal volunteers. However, despite the relatively small differences in circulating insulin level between the normal subjects, and patients with Type 2 diabetes, plasma glucose concentrations were increased approximately threefold in the patients. In other words, dramatic changes in level of glycemia are associated with relatively minor quantitative changes in day long circulating insulin concentrations. What metabolic changes could occur as a result of the observed differences in circulating insulin level to account for the development of fasting hyperglycemia? In this context, resistance to insulin regulation at the level of the adipose tissue appears to offer a reasonable explanation. Specifically, adipose tissue is extremely insulin sensitive as shown in Fig. 1, and as emphasized previously, regulation of the release of FFA from adipose tissue occurs over a relatively narrow range of plasma insulin concentrations. It is also apparent from the results in Figs. 2 and 3 that muscle and adipose tissue insulin resistance are highly correlated. Based upon these considerations, it seems reasonable to propose that the ability of insulin to normally suppress FFA release from adipose tissue is the fundamental change that occurs when insulin secretory function begins to decline in insulin resistant individuals, and that the subsequent increase in circulating FFA concentrations is primarily responsible for the development of significant hyperglycemia. Thus, we will now turn our attention to the pathophysiological events that contribute to the deterioration of glucose tolerance.

β-CELL FUNCTION

Although it has been apparent for some time that plasma FFA concentrations increase in patients with Type 2 diabetes as β-cell function begins to decline *(17)*, the notion that the consequent increase in plasma FFA concentration may further suppress glucose-stimulated insulin secretion is of quite recent vintage. Specifically, considerable evidence has been published in the past that FFA's acutely stimulate insulin secretion *(18–20)*. However, recent reports from Grill's research group *(21–24)* have emphasized that chronic FFA elevations, both in vitro and in vivo, can suppress glucose-stimulated insulin secretion. These data raise the possibility that elevated FFA levels may act as a positive feedback mechanism in patients with Type 2 diabetes, and that their increase acts to further depress glucose-stimulated β-cell function in patients with Type 2 diabetes. The studies from Grill's laboratory performed in normal rats have been extended by Unger and colleagues in Zucker diabetic fatty (ZDF) rats. The results of these efforts have been recently summarized *(25)*, and suggest that the changes seen in islets from diabetic ZDF rats, i.e., a decrease in glucose-induced insulin secretion, GLUT 2 loss, and increased TG concentration, are most likely related to elevated FFA concentrations.

Based upon the above considerations, it seems obvious that the role of elevated FFA concentrations in regulation of β-cell function is worthy of increased attention. In particular, it is important to distinguish between a primary role of elevated plasma FFA concentrations as a cause of the initial decline in β-cell function that leads to the loss of β-cell compensation in insulin resistant individuals, as differentiated from a secondary effect that acts in a positive feedback manner to further impair β-cell secretory function.

MUSCLE GLUCOSE UPTAKE

In 1963, the hypothesis that there is substrate competition between glucose and FFA for glucose disposal by muscle was introduced *(26)*. The existence of a glucose-fatty acid cycle was postulated, and it was argued that elevations in plasma FFA concentration lead to enhanced muscle FFA uptake and oxidation which, in turn, inhibit muscle glucose uptake. This notion has received considerable attention since its introduction, and there is ample evidence that acute elevations in plasma FFA concentrations will decrease insulin-stimulated glucose uptake by muscle in normal subjects and patients with Type 2 diabetes *(27–31)*.

On the other hand, existence of a glucose fatty acid cycle, and the fact that increases in plasma FFA concentration can inhibit muscle glucose uptake, does not mean that elevated FFA levels are the primary cause of insulin resistance in patients with Type 2 diabetes. In the first place, substantial increases in plasma FFA concentrations are necessary in order to demonstrate an inhibitory effect on insulin-mediated glucose disposal. It could be argued that this may be true of acute FFA elevations, but that lesser increases in plasma FFA levels could have a similar effect under chronic conditions. However, a significant degree of insulin resistance and hyperglycemia can exist in nondiabetic individuals, at a time when plasma FFA concentrations are only marginally increased *(32)*.

Furthermore, it is obvious from the results shown in Fig. 4, that there is only a modest increment in insulin resistance as patients with Type 2 diabetes progress from a moderate to a severe degree of fasting hyperglycemia. Since this is when the greatest increases in circulating FFA concentrations occur (17), it does not seem reasonable to conclude that the change in FFA concentration is responsible for the development of fasting hyperglycemia. In support of this notion is the result of a recent study by Boden and Chen (33) indicating that the major part of muscle insulin resistance in patients with Type 2 diabetes was unlikely to be a simple function of increased FFA concentrations. Thus, although increases in plasma FFA concentration may contribute to the insulin resistance present in patients with Type 2 diabetes and fasting hyperglycemia, it does not appear that this change in the primary reason why fasting hyperglycemia develops.

HEPATIC GLUCOSE PRODUCTION (HGP)

An increase in plasma FFA flux to the liver, secondary to higher plasma FFA concentrations, will stimulate hepatic glucose production (HGP). The link between increased FFA flux to the liver and HGP is most likely related to the stimulation of hepatic FFA oxidation that occurs when plasma FFA concentrations become elevated. The biochemical changes that follow an increase in hepatic FFA oxidation have been the subject of a recent thoughtful review, and there is abundant evidence to support the view that hepatic FFA oxidation and gluconeogenesis are directly related (34). I believe it most likely that it is this effect of FFA on hepatic intermediary metabolism that plays a crucial role in the development of fasting hyperglycemia in patients with Type 2 diabetes.

Perhaps the most controversial issue concerning the development of hyperglycemia in Type 2 diabetes is the role played by the liver. It has become dogma that hyperglycemia in patients with Type 2 diabetes is directly related to increases in HGP (35–39). However, it has recently been argued (40–43) that the tracer techniques used these earlier studies overestimated HGP, secondary to the enlarged glucose pool size in patients with fasting hyperglycemia and the consequent inability to reach isotopic steady-state. In contrast, when HGP was measured under conditions in which isotopic steady-state was reached, it seemed to be quite similar in absolute terms to values observed in nondiabetic individuals (42–44). For example, the data shown in Fig. 6 are the results of measures of HGP made in 51 individuals, (18 normal and 33 with Type 2 diabetes) using steady-state isotopic conditions (44). In this study, patients with Type 2 diabetes were divided into three groups (on the basis of their fasting glucose concentration (FPG): DM-1 (FPG < 10 mmol/L): DM-2 (FPG > 10 < 13 mmol/L): and DM-3 (FPG > 13 mmol/L), and Fig. 6 displays the mean FPG and HPG values for these four groups. It can be seen that the FPG values increased progressively from normal subjects to the DM-3 group, but that this was not true of the measurements of HPG. Indeed, HPG was not increased above normal in the DM-1 groups (FPG > 10 mmol/L), and was only increased by approximately 30% in the patients with the highest FPG (<13.0 mmol/L). These results differ substantially from the vast majority of previous studies in that the increase in HGP in patients with the most severe degree of fasting hyperglycemia was only 30% higher than normal values, not two to three times higher.

The implication of these findings raises an important issue concerning the role of the liver in the pathogenesis of hyperglycemia in patients with Type 2 diabetes. At the simplest level, the observation that values for HPG are similar in hyperglycemic patients with Type 2 diabetes does not mean that the liver is acting normally in these individuals.

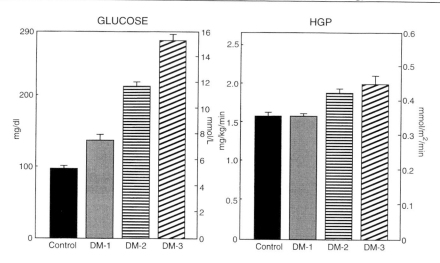

Fig. 6. Fasting plasma glucose concentration and hepatic glucose production (HGP) in control subjects (n = 11) and three groups of patients with Type 2 diabetes (DM-1, DM-2, and DM-3). The patients with Type 2 diabetes were divided into three groups of 11 each on the basis of their fasting plasma glucose concentration: DM-1, <180 mg/dL; DM-2, 180-250 mg/dL; and DM-3, >250 mg/dL. (Reprinted from Diabetes 1994;48:1440. With permission of the journal and the authors.)

Indeed, it appears that the liver in patients with Type 2 diabetes is not responding appropriately, e.g., HGP is not suppressed by the hyperglycemia. This seems to me to represent the most reasonable description of these events, and I believe that the inability of the liver to be suppressed normally to hyperglycemia is secondary to the increase in FFA flux to the liver, and it is the continued secretion of a "normal" amount of glucose into an expanded plasma glucose pool that sustains the state of fasting hyperglycemia.

In summary, there are defects of comparable severity in the ability of insulin to regulate muscle glucose uptake and suppress adipose tissue lipolysis in the majority of patients with Type 2 diabetes. Although the defect in insulin-mediated glucose disposal by muscle is considered to be necessary for the development of Type 2 diabetes, it, by itself, can not account for the appearance of fasting hyperglycemia. Frank decompensation of glucose homeostasis only supervenes when circulating plasma insulin concentrations fall to a level which is no longer able to suppress FFA release from adipose tissue. As plasma FFA concentrations increase, a vicious cycle is likely to be initiated, in which the elevated FFA concentrations act to further inhibit glucose-stimulated insulin secretion and insulin-stimulated glucose disposal, as well as maintaining a normal HGP in the face of a greatly expanded plasma glucose pool. As such, it appears that loss of the normal ability of insulin to regulate lipolysis occupies a central role in the development of hyperglycemia in patients with Type 2 diabetes.

Hypertriglyceridemia

FFA derived from the plasma serves as the major substrate for the synthesis of very low density lipoprotein (VLDL)—triglyceride (TG) by the liver. In the most general sense, the higher the plasma FFA concentration, and the more the FFA delivery to the liver, the greater the increase in hepatic VLDL-TG secretion and plasma TG concentration. This relation is shown in Fig. 7, which represents the results of a series of experi-

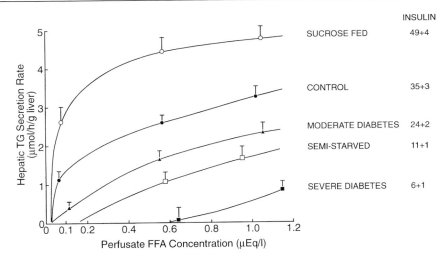

Fig. 7. Effect of differences in in vivo ambient insulin concentration on the relationship between perfusate FFA concentration and hepatic TG secretion rate by perfused rat liver. The data points depict mean (±SEM) values. Mean (±SEM) pre-existing insulin levels in each animal model are displayed to the right of each dose-response curve. (Reprinted from Horm Metab Res 1984;16:230. With permission of the journal and the authors.)

ments in which the ability of increases in perfusate FFA concentration to stimulate TG secretion was determined in perfused livers obtained from different groups of experimental rats *(45)*. In these experiments various manipulations were performed in order to create a series of animal models with insulin resistance, but over a wide range of ambient plasma insulin concentrations. In general, these results show that the higher the perfusate FFA concentration, the greater the increase in hepatic TG secretion. However, it is apparent that the shape of the FFA-hepatic TG secretion dose response curve differs substantially as a function of the in vivo insulin concentrations of the experimental models. Thus, the dose response curve is shifted far to the right in perfused livers from rats made insulin resistant and insulin deficient by streptozotocin injection (severe diabetes). At the other extreme is the curve observed when livers from sucrose-fed, insulin resistant, and hyperinsulinemic rats are perfused, and it is clear that in this case the dose response curve is shifted far to the left. In other words, although an increase in FFA perfusate concentration stimulated the liver to synthesize and secrete more TG, the ambient insulin concentration present in the donor of the liver regulated the magnitude of the livers response. Based upon the insights gained from these relationships shown in Fig. 7, a series of studies have been performed in both animals and humans aimed at defining the relationships between ambient plasma concentrations of insulin and FFA and hepatic VLDL-TG secretion and/or circulating TG concentrations in situations characterized by muscle and adipose tissue insulin resistance. In this section, three different, somewhat prototypic, clinical situations will be described emphasizing the varying role that elevated FFA concentrations play in regulation of VLDL metabolism.

Insulin Resistant, Hypoinsulinemic Individuals

Patients with Type 1 diabetes, in poor glycemic control have muscle and adipose tissue insulin resistance. Fasting plasma glucose and FFA concentrations in such patients, in

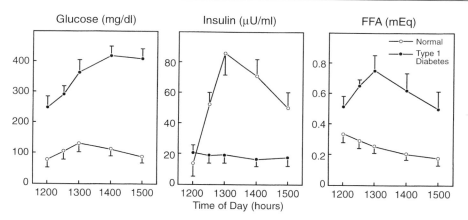

Fig. 8. Mean (±SEM) plasma glucose, free insulin, and FFA concentrations before and after a meal at 1200 h in normal individuals and patients with Type 1 diabetes. ○ normal: ● Type 1 diabetes. (Adapted from Diabetes 1981;30[Suppl 2]:66. With permission of the journal and authors.)

fair glycemic control, are much higher than in normal subjects, whereas their free insulin concentrations are not. The results in Fig. 8 compare plasma glucose free insulin, and FFA concentration in such subjects and in normal volunteers when measurements were made before lunch (1200 h) and at hourly intervals until 1500 h *(46,47)*. It can be seen that insulin-treated patients with Type 1 diabetes had greatly increased plasma glucose and FFA concentrations, but that their ambient postprandial-free insulin levels were much lower.

Based upon the dose-response relationship between hepatic VLDL-TG secretion and perfusate FFA concentrations and ambient insulin levels shown in Fig. 7, high FFA concentrations in the presence of absolutely low plasma insulin concentrations, should minimally, if at all, stimulate hepatic VLDL-TG secretion, and plasma TG concentrations should not be higher than normal under these conditions. This prediction has been validated by kinetic studies demonstrating that hepatic VLDL-TG secretion and plasma TG concentrations in these patients with Type 1 diabetes were no higher than in the control population *(46,47)*.

INSULIN RESISTANT, NORMOINSULINEMIC INDIVIDUALS

As described previously, patients with Type 2 diabetes and fasting hyperglycemia have both muscle and adipose tissue insulin resistance, with increases in plasma glucose and FFA concentrations, and plasma insulin concentrations that are similar in absolute terms to values seen in normal volunteers. Plasma glucose, insulin, and FFA concentrations in normal volunteers and hyperglycemic patients with Type 2 diabetes, before and for 3 h after lunch, are shown in Fig. 9 *(46,47)*. It can be seen from these results that plasma glucose and FFA concentrations were significantly higher than normal in the diabetic patients, reflecting muscle and adipose tissue resistance, whereas plasma insulin levels (in absolute terms) were similar to those of the normal subjects *(46,47)*. Given the combination of normal ambient insulin levels and higher FFA concentrations, the relationship obtained in the perfused liver (Fig. 7) would predict that patients with Type 2 diabetes would have higher than normal values for both TG secretion and TG concentration. In other words, since these patients have normal ambient insulin levels, the FFA-hepatic TG

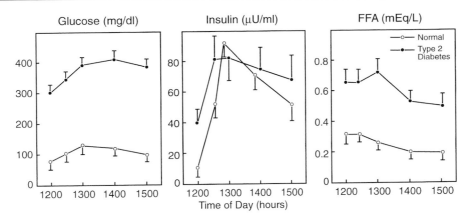

Fig. 9. Mean (±SEM) plasma glucose, insulin, and FFA concentrations before and after a meal at 1200 hours in normal individuals and patients with Type 2 diabetes. ○ normal; ● Type 2 diabetes. (Adapted from Diabetes 1981;30[Suppl 2]: 66. With permission of the journal and the authors.)

secretion dose response curve will be "normal" and the higher FFA levels should increase hepatic VLDL-TG secretion, and plasma TG concentration; a prediction confirmed by experiments in both animal models of Type 2 diabetes and patients with the clinical syndrome (46,47).

INSULIN RESISTANT, HYPERINSULINEMIC INDIVIDUALS

Muscle and adipose tissue insulin resistance are present in nondiabetic individuals, with hypertriglyceridemia (HTG). Plasma glucose, insulin, FFA, and glycerol concentrations from 8 AM to 4 PM in insulin resistant subjects with HTG and insulin sensitive individuals with normal TG concentrations are shown in Fig. 10 (32). These results demonstrate that plasma levels of glycerol, FFA, and insulin were higher in the HTG subjects. When correlation coefficients between these variables were calculated, significant relationships between degree of hypertriglyceridemia and day long plasma glycerol, FFA, and insulin concentrations were observed. To evaluate the role of these changes in regulation of plasma TG concentrations, multiple regression analysis was performed. When this was done, statistically significant relationships were seen between both FFA and insulin levels and plasma TG concentrations. Furthermore, it has been shown that HTG is the result of an increase in hepatic VLDL-TG secretion. Taking into account the relationship between perfusate FFA levels and ambient insulin concentrations observed in the perfused liver (Fig. 7), the increase in hepatic TG secretion in nondiabetic subjects is secondary to both an insulin-related shift to the left of the FFA-hepatic TG dose response curve and an increase in FFA flux to the liver (46,47).

In summary, both muscle and adipose tissue insulin resistance appear to be necessary for hypertriglyceridemia to develop. Adipose tissue insulin resistance leads to increased lipolysis and higher circulating FFA and glycerol concentrations. As long as plasma insulin concentrations are maintained at normal concentrations in absolute terms, the increase in ambient plasma FFA concentrations will stimulate hepatic TG secretion and increase plasma TG concentrations. Furthermore, the higher the plasma insulin concentration, the greater the ability of a given increase in plasma FFA concentration to stimulate hepatic TG secretion.

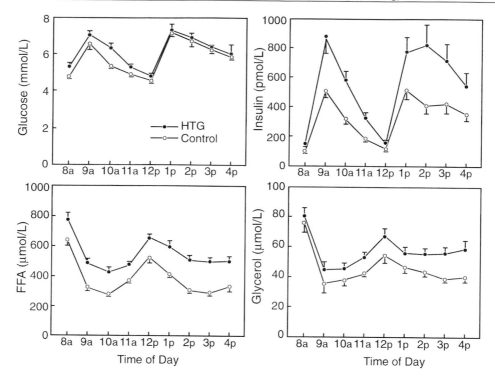

Fig. 10. Plasma glucose, insulin, FFA and glycerol concentrations in response to meals in hypertriglyceridemic (HTG ●) and control subjects (control ○) measured hourly from 8 AM to 4 PM. Breakfast at 8 am and lunch at noon. (Reprinted from Endocrinol Metab 1994;1:15. With permission of the journal and the authors.)

CONCLUSION

The population at large differs enormously in the ability of insulin to stimulate muscle glucose disposal and inhibit adipose tissue lipolysis. Defects in insulin-mediated glucose disposal by muscle are associated with parallel abnormalities in regulation of FFA release from adipose tissue. As long as the pancreatic β-cell is capable of secreting enough insulin to maintain plasma FFA concentrations which are only moderately elevated, gross decompensation of glucose homeostasis is prevented and the only untoward consequence of adipose tissue insulin resistance will be an increase in hepatic TG secretion and hypertriglyceridemia. When the pancreas loses the ability to maintain the requisite degree of hyperinsulinemia, plasma FFA and glycerol levels increase precipitously, HGP rates are no longer suppressed normally by an increase in plasma glucose pool size, and unequivocal fasting hyperglycemia supervenes. In addition, the increase in plasma FFA and glycerol concentration will stimulate hepatic VLDL-TG secretion, and render such individuals at risk of developing hypertriglyceridemia, and a series of associated changes in lipoprotein concentration and composition. As such, it seems quite apparent that adipose tissue insulin resistance plays a crucial role in the pathogenesis of both hyperglycemia and hypertriglyceridemia.

REFERENCES

1. DeFronzo RA, Tobin J, Andres R. The glucose clamp technique. A method for quantifying insulin secretion and resistance. Am J Physiol 1979;237:214–223.

2. Greenfield MS, Doberne L, Kraemer FB, Tobey TA, Reaven GM. Assessment of insulin resistance with the insulin suppression test and the euglycemic clamp. Diabetes 1981;30:387–392.

3. Björntorp P, Sjöström L. Carbohydrate storage in man: speculations and some quantitative considerations. Metabolism 1978;27(Suppl 2):1853–1865.

4. Swislocki ALM, Chen Y-DI, Golay A, Chang M-O, Reaven GM. Insulin suppression of plasma-free fatty acid concentration in normal individuals and patients with Type 2 (non-insulin-dependent) diabetes. Diabetologia 1987;30:622–626.

5. Pei D, Chen Y-DI, Hollenbeck CB, Bhargava R, Reaven GM. Relationship between insulin-mediated glucose disposal by muscle and adipose tissue lipolysis in healthy volunteers. J Clin Endocrinol Metab 1995;80:3368–3372.

6. Chen Y-DI, Golay A, Swislocki ALM, Reaven GM. Resistance to suppression of plasma free fatty acid concentrations and insulin stimulation of glucose uptake in non-insulin-dependent diabetes mellitus. J Clin Endocrinol Metab 1987;64:17–21.

7. Ginsberg H, Kimmerling G, Olefsky JM, Reaven GM. Demonstration of insulin resistance in untreated adult onset diabetic subjects with fasting hyperglycemia. J Clin Invest 1975;55:454–461.

8. Reaven GM. Insulin resistance in non-insulin-dependent diabetes mellitus. Does it exist and can it be measured? Am J Med 1983;74:3–17.

9. Shen S-W, Reaven GM, Farquhar JW. Comparison of impedance to insulin mediated glucose uptake in normal and diabetic subjects. J Clin Invest 1970;49:2151–2160.

10. Ginsberg H, Olefsky JM, Reaven GM. Further evidence that insulin resistance exists in patients with chemical diabetes. Diabetes 1974;23: 674–678.

11. Laws A, Stefanick ML, Reaven GM. Insulin resistance and hypertriglyceridemia in nondiabetic relatives of patients with non-insulin-dependent diabetes mellitus. J Clin Endocrinol Metab 1989;69: 343–347.

12. Ho LT, Chang ZY, Wang JT, Li SH, Liu YF, Chen Y-DI, Reaven GM. Insulin insensitivity in offspring of parents with Type 2 diabetes mellitus. Diabetic Med 1990;7:31–34.

13. Hollenbeck CB, Reaven GM. Variations in insulin stimulated glucose uptake in healthy individuals with normal glucose tolerance. J Clin Endocrinol Metab 1987;64:1169–1173.

14. Reaven GM, Brand RJ, Chen Y-DI, Mathur AK, Goldfine I. Insulin resistance and insulin secretion are determinants of oral glucose tolerance in normal individuals. Diabetes 1993;42:1324–1332.

15. Reaven GM, Hollenbeck CB, Chen Y-DI. Relationship between glucose tolerance, insulin secretion, and insulin action in non-obese individuals with varying degrees of glucose tolerance. Diabetologia 1989;32:52–55.

16. Reaven GM, Chen Y-DI, Hollenbeck CB, Sheu WHH, Ostrega D, Polonsky KS. Plasma insulin, C-peptide, and proinsulin c concentrations in obese and nonobese individuals with varying degrees of glucose tolerance. J Clin Endocrinol Metab 1993;76:44–48.

17. Reaven GM, Hollenbeck CB, Jeng C-Y, Wu MS, Chen Y-DI. Measurement of plasma glucose, free fatty acid, lactate, and insulin for 24 h in patients with NIDDM. Diabetes 1988;37:1020–1024.

18. Pelkonen R, Miettinen A, Taskinen M-R, Nikkila EA. Effect of acute elevation of plasma glycerol, triglyceride and FFA levels on glucose utilization and plasma insulin. Diabetes 1968;17:76–82.

19. Malaisse WJ, Malaisse-Lagae F. Stimulation of insulin secretion by non-carbohydrate metabolites. J Lab Clin Med 1968;72:438–448.

20. Crespin SR, Greenough WB, Steinberg D. Stimulation of insulin secretion by long-chain free fatty acids. J Clin Invest 1973;52:1979–1984.

21. Sako Y, Grill V. A 48-h lipid infusion in the rat time-dependently inhibits glucose-induced insulin secretion and β-cell oxidation through a process likely coupled to fatty acid oxidation. Endocrinology 1990;127:1580–1589.

22. Zhou YP, Grill V. Long-term exposure of rat pancreatic islets to fatty acids inhibits glucose-induced insulin secretion and biosynthesis through a glucose fatty acid cycle. J Clin Invest 1994;93:870–876.

23. Zhou YP, Grill V. Long-term exposure to fatty acids and ketones inhibits B-cell functions in human pancreatic islets of Langerhans. J Clin Endocrinol Metab 1995;80:1575–1560.

24. Zhou YP, Grill V. Palmitate-induced β-cell insensitivity to glucose is coupled to decreased pyruvate dehydrogenase activity and enhanced kinase activity in rat pancreatic islets. Diabetes 1995;44:394–399.

25. Unger RH. Lipotoxicity in the pathogenesis of obesity-dependent NIDDM. Genetic and clinical implications. Diabetes 1995;44:863–870.

26. Randle PJ, Garland PB, Hales CN, Newsholme EA. The glucose-fatty acid cycle: its role in insulin sensitivity and the metabolic disturbances of diabetes mellitus. Lancet 1963;1:785–789.

27. Thiébaud D, De Fronzo RA, Jacot E, et al. Effect of long-chain triglyceride infusion on glucose metabolism in man. Metabolism 1982;31:1128–1136.
28. Ferrannini E, Barret EJ, Bevilacqua S, DeFronzo RA. Effect of fatty acids on glucose production and utilization in man. J Clin Invest 1983;72: 1737–1747.
29. Bevilacqua S, Buzzigoli G, Bonadonna R, Brandi S, Oleggini M, Boni C, Geloni M, Ferrannini E. Operation of Randle's cycle in patients with NIDDM. Diabetes 1990;39:383–389.
30. Boden G, Chen X, Ruiz J, White JV, Rossetti L. Mechanisms of fatty acid-induced inhibition of glucose uptake. J Clin Invest 1994;93:2438–2446.
31. Boden M, Price TB, Perseghin G, et al. Mechanism of free fatty acid-induced insulin resistance in humans. J Clin Invest 1996;97:2859–2865.
32. Jeng C-Y, Fuh MM-T, Sheu WH-H, Chen Y-DI, Reaven GM. Hormone and substrate modulation of plasma triglyceride concentration in primary hypertriglyceridemia. Endocrinol Metab 1994;1:15–21.
33. Boden G, Chen X. Effects of fat on glucose uptake and utilization in patients with non-insulin-dependent diabetes. J Clin Invest 1995;96:1261–1268.
34. Foley JE. Rationale and application of fatty acid oxidation inhibitors in treatment of diabetes mellitus. Diabetes Care 1992;15:773–781.
35. DeFronzo RA, Simonson D, Ferrannini E. Hepatic and peripheral insulin resistance: a common feature of Type 2 (non-insulin-dependent) and Type 1 (insulin dependent) diabetes mellitus. Diabetologia 1982;23:313–319.
36. Nankervis A, Proietto J, Aitken P, Harewood M, Alford F. Differential effects of insulin therapy on hepatic and peripheral insulin sensitivity in Type 2 (non-insulin-dependent) diabetes. Diabetologia 1982;23:320–325.
37. Best J, Judzewitsch R, Pfeifer M, Beard J, Kolter J, Porte Jr D. The effect of chronic sulfonylurea therapy on hepatic glucose production in noninsulin dependent diabetes. Diabetes 1982;31:333–338.
38. Firth RG, Bell PM. Marsh HM, Hansen I, Rizz RA. Postprandial hyperglycemia in patients with non-insulin-dependent diabetes mellitus. Role of hepatic and extra hepatic tissues. J Clin Invest 1986;77:1525–1532.
39. Campbell PJ, Mandarino LJ, Gerich JE. Quantification of the relative impairment in actions of insulin on hepatic glucose production and peripheral glucose uptake in non-insulin-dependent diabetes mellitus. Metabolism 1988;37:15–21.
40. Chen Y-DI, Jeng C-Y, Hollenbeck CB, Wu M-S, Reaven GM. Relationship between plasma glucose and insulin concentration, glucose production, and glucose disposal in normal subjects and patients with non-insulin-dependent diabetes. J Clin Invest 1988;82:21–15.
41. Chen Y-DI, Swislocki ALM, Jeng C-Y, Juang J-H, Reaven GM. Effect of time on measurement of hepatic glucose production. J Clin Endocrinol Metab 1988;67:1084–1088.
42. Hother-Nielsen O, Beck-Nielsen H. On the determination of basal glucose production rate in patients with Type 2 (non-insulin-dependent) diabetes mellitus using primed-continuous 3-^{3}H-glucose infusion. Diabetologia 1990;33:603–610.
43. Hother-Nielsen O, Beck-Nielsen H. Insulin resistance, but normal basal rates of glucose production in patients with newly diagnosed mild diabetes mellitus. Acta Endocr 1991;124:637–645.
44. Jeng C-Y, Sheu WH-H, Fuh MM-T, Chen Y-DI, Reaven GM. Relationship between hepatic glucose production and fasting plasma glucose concentration in patients with non-insulin-dependent diabetes mellitus. Diabetes 1994;48:1440–1444.
45. Reaven GM, Mondon CE. Effect of in vivo plasma insulin levels on the relationship between perfusate free fatty acid concentration and triglyceride secretion by perfused rat livers. Horm Metab Res 1984;16:230–232.
46. Greenfield M, Koltermann O, Olefsky J, Reaven GM. Mechanism of hypertriglyceridemia in diabetic patients with fasting hyperglycemia. Diabetologia 1980;18:441–446.
47. Reaven GM, Greenfield MS. Diabetic hypertriglyceridemia: evidence for three clinicals syndromes. Diabetes 1981;30:66–75.

13 Insulin Action and Endothelial Function

Alain D. Baron, MD
and Michael J. Quon, MD, PhD

CONTENTS

INTRODUCTION
IN VIVO PERSPECTIVE
IN VITRO PERSPECTIVES
CLINICAL IMPLICATIONS OF ENDOTHELIAL DYSFUNCTION
    IN STATES OF INSULIN RESISTANCE
ACKNOWLEDGMENTS
REFERENCES

INTRODUCTION

The endothelium is a diaphanous cellular monolayer lining the lumen of the vasculature throughout the body and weighs approximately 1.8 kg in a 70 kg man. This large organ has long been recognized for its barrier and transport functions and is thought to be mostly passive in these capacities. In the last decade the endothelium has been shown to have many other diverse biological functions. These include the active control of vascular tone *(1–3)*, regulation of blood fluidity *(4)*, modulation of monocyte adhesion *(5,6)*, and lipid peroxidation *(7–10)*, to name but a few. More recently, the endothelium is also being recognized as an endocrine and humoral-responsive organ. Indeed, the endothelium produces a variety of hormones acting in a paracrine fashion to regulate vascular tone as well as growth and remodeling of the vascular wall *(11–14)*. In addition, the endothelium possesses receptors for humoral ligands. These receptors, whose predominant role was thought to be transendothelial transfer of hormones are now known to have downstream signal transduction mechanisms resident in the endothelium.

Relevant to the syndrome of insulin resistance, this chapter will discuss the evidence and functional implications of the endothelium as a target tissue for insulin action. We will present both in vivo and in vitro evidence that the vascular endothelium responds to insulin by increasing the release of nitric oxide and that this action is impaired in states of insulin resistance. The pathophysiological implications of these observations to the

From: *Contemporary Endocrinology: Insulin Resistance*
Edited by: G. Reaven and A. Laws © Humana Press Inc., Totowa, NJ

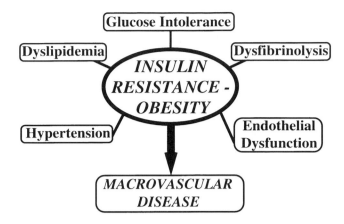

Fig. 1. Conceptual representation of the syndrome of insulin resistance. Insulin resistance is associated with a clustering of cardiovascular risk factors. These risk factors are: increased blood pressure, dyslipidemia, glucose intolerance, dysfibrinolysis, and endothelial dysfunction.

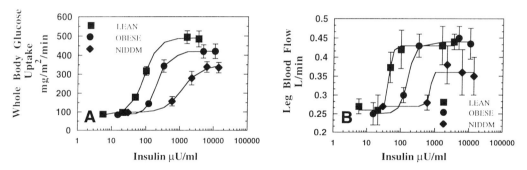

Fig. 2. Rates of whole body glucose uptake **(A)** and leg blood flow **(B)** as a function of prevailing serum insulin level during euglycemic clamp studies in lean (closed squares), obese nondiabetic subjects (closed circles), and patients with non insulin-dependent diabetes (Type 2 diabetes; closed diamonds). Note the log scale on the abscissa. (Reprinted with permission from ref. *16*.)

increased risk of macrovascular disease associated with insulin resistance will be discussed (Fig. 1).

IN VIVO PERSPECTIVE

Dose-Dependent Effects of Insulin on Vasodilation in Skeletal Muscle Vasculature

Insulin has a dose-dependent effect to vasodilate skeletal muscle vasculature *(15)*. This vasodilation occurs at physiological insulin concentrations with an EC_{50} (concentration to reach half-maximal effect) of 44 μU/mL and with a t1/2 (time to reach half-maximal vasodilation) of approximately 35 min *(16)*. Figure 2 illustrates the effect of physiologic concentrations of insulin to cause an approximately twofold increase in leg blood flow above baseline in lean insulin-sensitive individuals (measured by thermodilution). Because these studies were performed during euglycemic clamp conditions it follows that this insulin effect is independent of changes in glycemia. The magnitude of

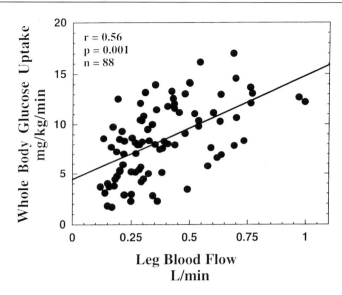

Fig. 3. Correlation between rates of whole body glucose uptake and rates of leg blood flow in lean and obese nondiabetic subjects measured during euglycemic hyperinsulinemic clamp studies over a wide range of steady state serum insulin concentrations. (Reprinted with permission from ref. *17.*)

the vasodilation appears related not only to the insulin concentration but also to the rate of insulin stimulated glucose metabolism. This is illustrated by the robust correlation between the rate of insulin-stimulated glucose uptake and the extent of vasodilation in Fig. 3 *(17).*

Resistance to insulin's action to stimulate glucose metabolism which characterizes clinical states of obesity, Type 2 diabetes, and hypertension is associated with impaired insulin-mediated vasodilation *(1,16).* As illustrated in Fig. 2A, the relationship between dose response curves for insulin-mediated glucose uptake in subjects of varying degrees of insulin resistance are largely paralleled by the relationship between dose response curves for insulin's action to vasodilate (Fig. 2B). That is, the most insulin-resistant subjects display the greatest impairment in insulin-mediated vasodilation. Insulin administration is also accompanied by important increases in cardiac output and a modest fall in mean arterial blood pressure consistent with an effect of insulin to reduce systemic vascular resistance. The fall in systemic vascular resistance is modest (~15%) compared to the reduction in leg vascular resistance (~40%) suggesting a differential and specific effect of insulin to dilate skeletal muscle vasculature *(18).*

In summary, insulin's action to vasodilate skeletal muscle vasculature varies as a function of its action to stimulate glucose metabolism and occurs predominantly at the level of resistance vessels. Thus, it appears that insulin-mediated vasodilation and insulin-sensitivity vis-à-vis its action to stimulate glucose metabolism are tightly coupled in some yet to be determined fashion.

Nitric Oxide and Insulin-Mediated Vasodilation

Nitric oxide (NO) is a gas that is continuously released from the endothelium where it is synthesized from the precursor L-arginine in a reaction catalyzed by nitric oxide

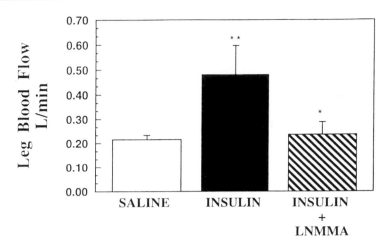

Fig. 4. Effect of intrafemoral artery infusion of the nitric oxide synthase inhibitor N^G-monomethyl-L-arginine (L-NMMA; 16 mg/min) on leg blood flow during hyperinsulinemic ($120 \, mU/m^2/min$) euglycemic clamp studies. $*p < 0.05$, $**p < 0.01$. (Adapted from J Clin Invest 1994;94:1175. Used with permission.)

synthase (eNOS isoform in endothelium). NO released from the endothelium diffuses via the subendothelial space to the smooth muscle where it binds to the heme group of guanylate cyclase and stimulates the generation of cyclic GMP which then transduces its effects to cause smooth muscle relaxation and resulting vasodilation (See In Vitro Perspective for more detail). In vivo, one can probe 1) endothelium-dependent vasodilation by the use of agents which cause the release of NO from the endothelium such as the muscarinic agonist methacholine chloride; 2) endothelium-independent vasodilation by the use of NO donor compounds such as sodium nitroprusside and, 3) NO-dependent vascular tone with the use of an inhibitor of NO synthase such as the arginine analog N^G-monomethyl-L-arginine (L-NMMA). Vascular responses to infusing these agents directly into the femoral artery can be assessed by measuring changes in limb blood flow. These methods allow one to assess endothelial-dependent and -independent vasodilation as well as NO-dependent vascular tone in humans.

To determine whether insulin-mediated vasodilation is dependent on the release of endothelium-derived NO, intrafemoral artery infusions of the NO synthase inhibitor L-NMMA were performed after a period of euglycemic hyperinsulinemia designed to cause maximal vasodilation. As illustrated in Fig. 4, infusion of L-NMMA completely abrogated the insulin induced vasodilation, suggesting that insulin-mediated vasodilation is entirely NO-dependent. Other studies have confirmed the NO dependency of insulin-mediated vasodilation in the forearm (19). To further test whether insulin-mediated vasodilation occurs via a direct effect of insulin to enhance the release of NO from vascular endothelium rather than merely enhancing the action of NO on the vascular smooth muscle cell, other experimental approaches have been taken. One approach is to examine the effects of subvasodilatory insulin doses (~25 μU/mL) to enhance the vasodilatory response to an endothelium-dependent vasodilator such as methacholine chloride (20). Studies performed in the leg and forearm have shown that endothelium-dependent vasodilation is enhanced in the presence of insulin (20,21). In contrast, the response to the NO donor sodium nitroprusside was unaltered by co-infusion of insulin, suggesting that insulin is sensitizing the endothelial response to the endothelium-dependent vasodilator methacholine chloride *(20,22)*. To more definitively establish that insulin increases NO release from endothelium, studies were recently undertaken to measure femoral venous efflux of the stable oxidative end products of nitric oxide, nitrate (NO_3) and nitrite (NO_2) together (commonly referred to as NOx). NOx concentrations were measured by a chemiluminescence technique and NOx flux was calculated as the product of the NOx concentration × the rate of leg blood flow. Femoral venous NOx fluxes were measured under basal conditions and after a period of euglycemic hyperinsulinemia designed to stimulate NO production. Insulin was found to cause a net increase in NOx release from the leg *(23)*. Moreover, when L-NMMA was infused concomitantly with insulin, venous NOx flux fell rapidly and could not be overcome by continued hyperinsulinemia *(23)*.

Together, these data suggest that insulin vasodilates skeletal muscle vasculature via the net release of endothelium-derived NO. While it is possible that insulin is causing the production of NO via the stimulation of NOS isoforms residing in cells other than the endothelium *(23,24)*, this is unlikely as vasodilation in response to intra-arterial methacholine chloride (an endothelium-dependent vasodilator) was enhanced by insulin *(25)* but had no effect on the response to sodium nitroprusside. Together these data are consistent with a direct in vivo effect of insulin to stimulate NO release from the endothelium.

Skeletal Muscle Vasodilation, Tissue Perfusion, and Insulin Sensitivity

Given the importance of tissue perfusion for substrate and hormonal delivery, it is reasonable to examine the contribution of insulin-mediated vasodilation to insulin's overall effect to stimulate glucose uptake into skeletal muscle. To this end, euglycemic hyperinsulinemic clamp studies achieving high, but physiologic, prevailing insulin levels (~75 μU/mL) were performed in lean healthy subjects. Leg glucose uptake (LGU) was measured 1) under near steady-state conditions after 4 h of hyperinsulinemia during which rates of insulin stimulated glucose uptake and vasodilation were fully expressed and 2) during a subsequent 30 min intrafemoral artery infusion of L-NMMA designed to inhibit NO production and reduce leg blood flow rates back to basal rates. LGU was calculated by the balance technique, LGU = Femoral arteriovenous glucose difference × Flow or LGU = AVGΔ × F. L-NMMA infusion caused a complete abrogation of the insulin-mediated vasodilation, thus returning rates of leg blood flow back to baseline values. With the reduction in limb blood flow (LBF), glucose extraction (AVGΔ) rose approximately 50% from ~30 mg/dL to 44 mg/dL. However, this rise in extraction was not sufficient to overcome the fall in perfusion rate and LGU decreased by ~25%, $p < 0.001$ *(26)* (Fig. 5). Thus, insulin-mediated vasodilation appears to augment insulin's action to stimulate skeletal muscle glucose uptake and may account for ~ one-fourth of insulin's overall stimulatory effect on glucose uptake. The corollary of this finding is that impairment of insulin's normal ability to vasodilate could in turn contribute to insulin resistance. Such a mechanism has been proposed to account for the insulin resistance associated with essential hypertension occurring independent of other factors such as obesity *(1)*.

Insulin Sensitivity and Nitric Oxide Production

We have already established that insulin-mediated vasodilation is NO dependent and that insulin-mediated vasodilation is impaired in states of insulin resistance. Thus, it

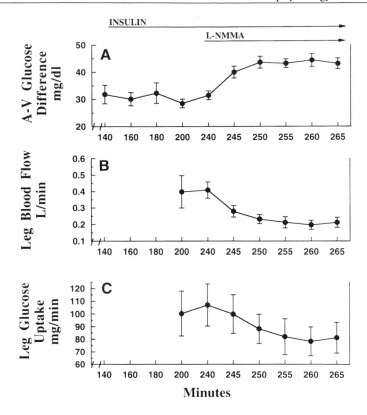

Fig. 5. Arteriovenous glucose difference **(A)**, leg blood flow **(B)** and leg glucose uptake **(C)** in lean insulin sensitive subjects during a euglycemic hyperinsulinemic (40 mU/m^2/min) clamp and during a superimposed intraarterial infusion of L-NMMA (16 mg/min) for 30 min.

follows logically that insulin-mediated NO release may be impaired in states of insulin resistance. To test this idea, recent studies have examined the effects of maximally effective doses of insulin to stimulate femoral venous NOx flux in subjects exhibiting a wide range of insulin sensitivity *(23)*. Basal NOx flux rates were not different between subject groups exhibiting insulin-stimulated rates of whole-body glucose uptake ranging from 4 mg/kg/min in obese Type 2 diabetic subjects to 15 mg/kg/min in endurance trained athletes. In contrast, during insulin stimulation, athletes exhibited a significant 130% increase in NOx production above baseline while diabetic subjects exhibited no change in NOx production above basal. Thus, the data are consistent with the notion that insulin-mediated NO production occurs as a function of insulin sensitivity with insulin resistant subjects exhibiting reduced NO production. In sum, insulin resistance is associated with impairment of the endothelial NO system as reflected by reduced stimulated NOx production and thus, may also be associated with more generalized endothelial dysfunction.

Insulin Sensitivity and Endothelial Function

To test whether insulin resistance is associated with more generalized endothelial dysfunction, studies have examined endothelial-dependent vasodilation to various endothelial-dependent vasodilators *(20)* and flow mediated vasodilation *(27)* in insulin resistant states. As illustrated in Fig. 6, endothelium-dependent vasodilation to the agent

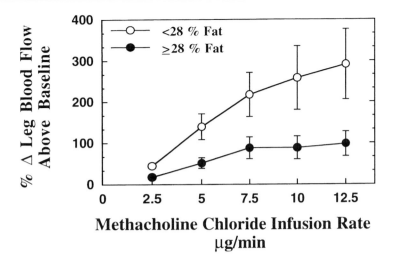

Fig. 6. Leg Blood flow increments relative to baseline (Δ% LBF) in response to a graded intrafemoral artery infusion of the endothelium-dependent vasodilator, methacholine chloride, under basal (saline) conditions in control and obese subjects as defined by percent fat content (control: < 28%, obese: ≥ 28%). (Adapted from J Clin Invest 1996;97:2604. Used with permission.)

methacholine chloride is markedly impaired in obese insulin resistant subjects (≥28% body fat) compared to lean insulin sensitive subjects (<28% body fat). This endothelial dysfunction was independent of factors known to be associated with endothelial impairment such as high blood pressure, elevations in low density lipoprotein (LDL) or total cholesterol, and smoking, suggesting that the simple state of obesity/insulin resistance is associated with endothelial dysfunction. It is important to point out that more recent data suggest that the relationship between obesity and endothelial dysfunction is stronger in men than in premenopausal women *(28)*. Interestingly, obese subjects of either gender, with Type 2 diabetes exhibit endothelial dysfunction which is similar to obese male nondiabetic counterparts. Vasodilatory responses to the administration of intra-arterial sodium nitroprusside were identical in lean, obese, and Type 2 diabetic subjects indicating normal endothelium-independent vasodilation *(20)*. Thus, simple obesity/insulin resistance is associated with marked endothelial dysfunction independent of hyperglycemia. In summary, obesity/insulin resistance is associated with endothelial dysfunction independent of other known clinical factors which modulate endothelial function. Importantly, hyperglycemia does not appear to further impair endothelial function over that observed with simple obesity/insulin resistance alone. Hyperglycemia *per se* has been shown to impair endothelium-dependent vasodilation in animal models *(29,30)* and humans *(31)*. Therefore, the mechanism(s) for insulin resistance and hyperglycemia-induced endothelium dysfunction do not appear additive and may be quite different.

Potential Mechanisms for Endothelial Cell Dysfunction Associated with Insulin Resistance

ROLE OF FATTY ACIDS

Recent studies have explored potential mechanisms linking insulin resistance (independent of hyperglycemia, hypertension, and hypercholesterolemia) with endothelial dysfunction. Subjects with insulin resistance exhibit impaired antilipolytic actions of

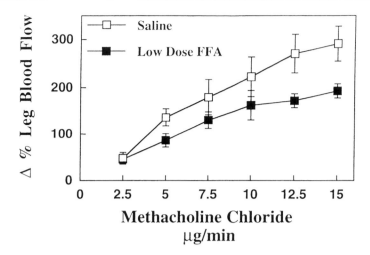

Fig. 7. Leg Blood flow increments relative to baseline (Δ% LBF) in response to a graded intrafemoral artery infusion of the endothelium-dependent vasodilator, methacholine chloride, during infusion of saline or 20% intralipid emulsion (45cc/h) plus heparin (0.2 U/kg/min) designed to increase systemic FFA level two to threefold (~1200 μ*M*).

insulin and, thus, exhibit day-long elevation of circulating concentrations of free fatty acids (FFA) *(32)*. Based on in vitro data suggesting that FFA impair NO synthase activity in cultured endothelial cells *(33)*, we tested the idea that elevated circulating FFA levels can impair endothelial cell function in vivo. To this end, graded intrafemoral artery infusions of methacholine chloride were performed to establish the full dose-response curve for endothelium-dependent vasodilation during an infusion of either saline or two hours of a lipid emulsion in conjunction with heparin to enhance hydrolysis of the triglyceride particle and elevate circulating FFA concentrations to approximately 1200 μ*M*. As illustrated in Fig. 7, raising FFA concentrations caused a marked impairment of endothelium-dependent vasodilation. Similar endothelial dysfunction was also induced by inhibition of endogenous insulin secretion with somatostatin, thereby enhancing the release of endogenous FFA to achieve circulating levels approximating those achieved with exogenous infusions. Thus, elevating circulating FFA concentrations from both endogenous or exogenous sources causes marked endothelial cell dysfunction. Given that insulin resistance is associated with day-long elevations in FFA, it is logical to suggest that chronic elevations of these substrates may be instrumental in causing endothelial dysfunction in states of insulin resistance.

ROLE OF ALTERED INSULIN SIGNALING

The precise defects in insulin signal transduction pathways underlying insulin resistance in common diseases such as diabetes, obesity and hypertension have not been elucidated for the majority of patients. However, it is clear that abnormalities in signaling molecules involved with metabolic insulin signaling pathways can cause insulin resistance. For example, many patients with syndromes of extreme insulin resistance have been found to have functionally significant mutations in their insulin receptor gene *(34)*. Similarly, transgenic mice homozygous for a null allele of the insulin receptor substrate-1 (IRS-1) gene are mildly insulin resistant *(35,36)*, and transgenic mice heterozygous for null alleles of both the insulin receptor and IRS-1 develop diabetes *(37)*. Since there is a clear relationship between insulin sensitivity with respect to glucose metabolism and insulin sensitivity with respect to vasodilation, it is conceivable that metabolic insulin signaling pathways share elements in common with insulin signaling pathways in endothelium involved with vasodilator actions. Thus, signaling defects that contribute to insulin resistance with respect to glucose metabolism may also impact on the vasodilator actions of insulin. This would provide a plausible mechanism linking insulin resistant diseases such as diabetes and obesity with defects in the vasodilator actions of insulin and endothelial dysfunction that may predispose to macrovascular disease and hypertension.

IN VITRO PERSPECTIVES

Regulated Production of NO in Endothelium

The major isoform of NO synthase expressed in endothelium is endothelial nitric oxide synthase (eNOS). eNOS is a heme-containing enzyme that catalyzes the synthesis of NO by hydroxylation of the substrate L-arginine to N^G- hydroxy-L-arginine followed by oxidation of this intermediate to the products NO and L-citrulline (for review see 38). Cofactors that participate in the transfer of electrons required for the production of NO by eNOS include NADPH, FAD, FMN, tetrahydrobiopterin, and molecular oxygen. The eNOS protein contains a linker region with a calmodulin binding site that joins the amino-terminal oxygenase domain (containing heme and binding sites for L-arginine and tetrahydrobiopterin) with the carboxy terminal reductase domain (containing FAD, FMN, and NADPH binding sites homologous to P450 reductase). Treatment of endothelial cells with classical cholinergic agonists such as acetylcholine causes an influx of calcium mediated by activation of the acetylcholine receptor (a seven transmembrane G protein-coupled receptor) that results in stimulation of eNOS activity via interaction of calcium/calmodulin with the calmodulin binding site on eNOS. Endothelial-derived NO diffuses into vascular smooth muscle cells causing vasorelaxation. The importance of eNOS to the regulation of vascular tone and hemodynamics has been unequivocally demonstrated by the presence of hypertension in transgenic mice that are homozygous for a null allele of the eNOS gene (39).

Insulin Signaling Pathways Related to Production
of NO in Endothelium

In vivo studies implicate endothelial-derived NO as a mediator of vasodilator actions of insulin (25). Most, if not all, of the biological actions of insulin are initiated by the binding of insulin to its cell surface receptor (40). The insulin receptor belongs to a large family of receptor tyrosine kinases. Cytokines and other growth factors that signal through tyrosine kinase dependent mechanisms are known to greatly induce transcription of the iNOS isozyme found in macrophages (resulting in increased production of NO for cytotoxic functions) (41). However, a clearly defined mechanism linking signaling by tyrosine kinase receptors such as the insulin receptor with activation of eNOS in endothelial cells has not been well established.

It has been appreciated for some time that insulin receptors are expressed at low levels in endothelial cells (~40,000 receptors/cell) (42,43). One function of endothelial insulin receptors is to transport insulin across the endothelium to classical targets such as muscle, adipose tissue, and liver where insulin can exert its metabolic effects (44). It is also possible that signal transduction by endothelial insulin receptors plays an important physiological role and contributes to metabolic effects of insulin. Endothelial cells themselves are not very responsive to insulin with respect to glucose uptake because they do not express the insulin responsive glucose transporter GLUT4. However, if activation of the insulin receptor mediates production of NO in endothelium, this may contribute to whole body glucose disposal by resulting in increased blood flow to muscle (a major determinant of glucose uptake). Furthermore, this would imply that defects in insulin-stimulated production of NO are capable of contributing to insulin resistance with respect to glucose metabolism.

In order to elucidate specific insulin signal transduction pathways responsible for the production of NO in endothelial cells, it is necessary to investigate this novel action of insulin at the cellular and molecular level. Because NO has a short half-life (~5 s) and is present at nanomolar concentrations in vivo, it has been difficult to establish methods for directly measuring NO in cell culture models that are amenable to cellular and molecular manipulations. Recently, a commercially available NO-selective amperometric electrode has been used to directly measure NO production in response to insulin in primary cultures of human umbilical vein endothelial cells (HUVEC) *(43)*. This has made it possible to begin the characterization of insulin signal transduction pathways related to production of NO in a physiologically relevant cell type.

Insulin causes a dose-dependent, saturable increase in the production of NO in HUVEC (Fig. 8B) *(43)*. Of note, the production of NO in response to insulin is an acute effect that occurs within a few min. This is in contrast to the vasodilator effects of insulin in vivo which occur on a time scale of 15–20 min to hours *(15,45)*. This discrepancy between the time scale for in vitro endothelial NO production and in vivo vasodilator response suggests that other effects of insulin may also be contributing to the hemodynamic actions of insulin. For example, insulin may stimulate the release of compounds such as endothelin that may oppose effects of NO *(46)*. In addition, activation of sympathetic activity by insulin may also modulate vasodilator responses *(47)*. Finally, because vasodilation appears to be coupled to the rate of insulin-stimulated glucose uptake (which during insulin infusions occurs with a time course of hours), it follows that insulin's in vivo vasodilatory effects parallel the time course of insulin's action on glucose metabolism.

The concentrations of insulin required to stimulate the production of NO in vitro are significantly higher than those required for vasodilator effects of insulin in vivo. This is likely due to technical limitations of the direct measurement method. For example, the in vitro experiments are carried out at room temperature because the NO electrode is extremely sensitive to temperature variations and it is difficult to carry out experiments at physiological temperature (37°C). Furthermore, HUVEC may not be as sensitive to insulin with respect to production of NO as endothelial cells from small vessels perfusing the muscle beds. Finally, it is possible that the NO electrode is simply not sensitive enough to detect significant production of NO in response to insulin concentrations in the low physiological range. Nevertheless, this model system has proven useful for understanding insulin signal transduction pathways related to production of NO.

Similar to the vasodilator response in vivo, insulin-stimulated production of NO in HUVEC can be completely blocked by preincubation of cells with L-NAME (a competitive inhibitor of eNOS). Furthermore, preincubation of the cells with genestein (a tyrosine kinase inhibitor) also completely blocks the production of NO in response to insulin. Taken together, these data suggest a necessary role for the receptor tyrosine kinase in activation of eNOS by insulin. More direct evidence that the insulin receptor

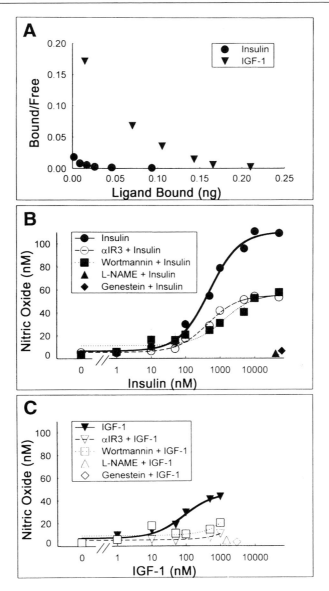

Fig. 8. Differential effects of insulin and IGF-1 on production of NO in HUVEC. **(A)** Scatchard analysis of insulin and IGF-1 binding studies. From this experiment we estimated that there are approximately 10X as many IGF-1 receptors as insulin receptors on HUVEC. **(B)** Production of NO from HUVEC in response to insulin in the presence or absence of various inhibitors. Data shown are the mean ± SEM of n independent experiments. Insulin alone, (closed circles), n = 12; pretreatment with 1 mM L-NAME for 1 h, (closed upright triangle), n = 7; pretreatment with 25 μ*M* genestein for 15 min, (closed diamond), n = 3; pretreatment with 500 n*M* wortmannin for 40 min, (closed square), n = 4; pretreatment with 25 n*M* (IR-3 for 5 min, (open circles), n = 5. **(C)** Production of NO from HUVEC in response to IGF-1 in the presence or absence of various inhibitors. IGF-1 alone, (closed inverted triangle), n = 13; pretreatment with 1 mM L-NAME for 1 h, (open upright triangle), n = 3; pretreatment with 25 μ*M* genestein for 15 min, (open diamond), n = 4; pretreatment with 500 n*M* wortmannin for 40 min, (open square), n = 4; pretreatment with 25 n*M* (IR-3 for 5 min, (open inverted triangle), n = 4.

tyrosine kinase is necessary to mediate the effect of insulin on production of NO has been obtained using HUVEC that were transfected with either wild-type insulin receptors or kinase-deficient mutant insulin receptors *(48)*. Overexpression of wild-type insulin receptors leads to a threefold increase in the level of NO produced in response to maximal insulin stimulation while cells overexpressing kinase-deficient insulin receptors respond like the untransfected control cells.

Interestingly, the number of insulin receptors present in HUVEC is ~10 times less than the number of related insulin growth factors (IGF-1) receptors (Fig. 8A) *(43)*. The binding affinity of insulin for the IGF-1 receptor is ~100 times less than for the insulin receptor. Therefore, it is possible that high concentrations of insulin may signal, in part, through the more abundant IGF-1 receptor. However, the level of NO produced in response to a maximally stimulating concentration of insulin is approximately twice that seen with maximal IGF-1 stimulation (Fig. 8B,C). In addition, incubating HUVEC with a blocking antibody against the IGF-1 receptor only partially inhibits the production of NO in response to insulin while completely blocking the response to IGF-1. Therefore, while some of insulin's effects on production of NO may be mediated through the IGF-1 receptor, there is a significant effect mediated specifically by the insulin receptor.

Parallels Between Metabolic Insulin Signaling Pathways and Insulin Signaling Pathways Related to Production of NO in Endothelium

After the binding of insulin to its receptor and activation of the receptor tyrosine kinase, cellular substrates such as IRS-1, -2, -3, -4, and Shc are phosphorylated *(49–55)*. Phosphotyrosine motifs on these substrates then engage and activate multiple downstream signaling molecules *(40)*. In some cases, specific downstream signaling molecules have been associated with particular biological actions of insulin. For example, phosphatidylinositol 3-kinase (PI3K) has been shown to be a necessary mediator of metabolic actions of insulin such as the translocation of the insulin responsive glucose transporter GLUT4 to the cell surface in adipose cells *(56)*. Interestingly, wortmannin (an inhibitor of PI3K) is able to partially block the production of NO in response to insulin in HUVEC (Fig. 8B) *(43)*. Therefore, insulin signaling pathways involved with production of NO in endothelium may share elements in common with insulin signaling pathways related to glucose transport in classical insulin target cells. These data also imply that defects in signaling resulting in insulin resistance with respect to glucose metabolism have the potential to cause insulin resistance with respect to vasodilator actions of insulin. Thus, insulin resistance may contribute to a relative increase in peripheral vascular tone. This is an attractive hypothesis that provides a mechanism to relate insulin resistance and diabetes with commonly associated diseases such as hypertension and abnormalities associated with endothelial dysfunction. Indeed, consistent with this hypothesis is the in vivo observation that insulin sensitivity with respect to glucose metabolism is positively correlated with insulin sensitivity with respect to vasodilator actions of insulin *(1,15,16,18)*.

Another parallel between metabolic insulin signaling pathways in classical insulin targets such as adipose cells and insulin signaling pathways related to production of NO in endothelium is the fact that activation of PI3K *per se* is not sufficient to elicit an insulin-like response. For example, stimulation of adipose cells with platelet-derived growth factor (PDGF) results in activation of PI3K at a level comparable to that seen with insulin stimulation but does not result in the translocation of GLUT4 *(57,58)*. Similarly, PDGF stimulation of endothelial cells results in activation of PI3K *(59)* but does not result in measurable production of NO *(43)*. These results suggest that the biological specificity of insulin action is dependent on more than simply activating a particular signaling molecule. Perhaps subcellular localization of signaling molecules or the formation of specific signaling complexes are contributing to specificity.

As progress is made in the elucidation of insulin signaling pathways related to production of NO in endothelium, it will be interesting to determine the extent of overlap between metabolic signaling pathways in classical insulin targets such as muscle and adipose tissue and signaling pathways related to production of NO in endothelium. For example, a physiological role for Akt (a serine-threonine kinase downstream of PI3K) in insulin-stimulated translocation of GLUT4 was recently identified in rat adipose cells *(60)*. Does Akt also play a role in insulin-stimulated production of NO in endothelium or will this represent a point of divergence in the insulin signaling pathway? Another important avenue of investigation that remains is to determine mechanisms linking insulin signaling pathways with the activation of eNOS. Recently, tyrosine phosphorylation of eNOS was reported in endothelial cells treated with phosphatase inhibitors *(61)*. However, the physiological significance of this phenomenon and its relationship to insulin signaling are unclear. Other recent studies demonstrating interactions of calmodulin with IRS-1 and PI3K are also intriguing since calmodulin is a major regulator of eNOS activity *(62,63)*. Although there is still a great deal to be learned, it is clear that insulin signal transduction pathways in endothelium are mediating important and novel physiological actions related to the regulation of hemodynamics and metabolism.

CLINICAL IMPLICATIONS OF ENDOTHELIAL DYSFUNCTION IN STATES OF INSULIN RESISTANCE

Over a decade ago, Gerald Reaven coined Syndrome X or the Insulin Resistance Syndrome (IRS) *(64)*. While the definition of this syndrome is one of debate and in constant evolution, there is much consensus about its existence and its core features (Fig. 1). The greater than chance clustering of insulin resistance (particularly in the context of central obesity) with elevated FFA, elevated triglycerides and reduced high-density lipoprotein (HDL), elevated fasting glucose (also known as impaired fasting glucose or dysglycemia), impaired glucose tolerance, abnormalities in blood fluidity, and elevations of blood pressure is a common clinical finding *(65)*. The syndrome's clinical importance stems from the consistent observation that IRS is associated with a 2–3 fold increased risk of coronary heart disease mortality *(64,66)*. That insulin resistance is the central factor accounting for the clustering of cardiovascular risk factors is suggested by numerous studies demonstrating amelioration of these risk factors with therapeutic maneuvers directed at improving insulin sensitivity such as weight reduction *(67,68)* and exercise *(69,70)*. Perhaps some of the most compelling evidence that insulin resistance is central to the syndrome comes from studies utilizing the insulin action enhancing drug troglitazone in obese patients with impaired glucose tolerance who exhibit many features of the syndrome *(71)*. Troglitazone therapy was shown to enhance (but not normalize) insulin sensitivity in these patients and this effect was accompanied by moderate but significant reductions in circulating triglyceride, elevations in HDL and lowering of blood pressure independent of changes in weight or adiposity. Thus, while a number of issues remain to be resolved about the genetics, molecular, biochemical and metabolic basis of IRS, features of the syndrome appear to be at least partially reversible with therapeutic strategies directed at reversing the abnormality in insulin action.

It is important to underline that the cardiovascular risk factors (abnormal lipoproteins, blood pressure, dysglycemia) associated with insulin resistance do not fully account for the increase in cardiovascular risk. Therefore, other factors associated with insulin resistance are likely to be at play. The endothelium plays a critical role at maintaining the health of the vascular wall, blood pressure, blood fluidity, and redox state (72). In turn, endothelial dysfunction is suspected to play a critical and initiating role in the pathogenesis of the atherosclerotic plaque (73–76). Through the coordinate production of vasodilating and growth inhibiting factors and counterbalancing vasoconstricting growth promoting factors, the endothelium plays a key role in maintaining the health of the vascular wall (11,12). For example, NO decreases vascular smooth muscle cell proliferation and lowers vascular resistance (77) while endothelin I promotes smooth muscle cell growth and increases vascular tone (77). In addition, NO inhibits monocyte adhesion to endothelial cells, enhances fibrinolysis, reduces platelet adhesiveness, reduces lipid peroxidation thus protecting the vascular wall from plaque formation (11). Given that insulin resistance is associated with dysfunction of the endothelium derived NO system, it follows logically that endothelial dysfunction likely contributes significantly to the increased risk of macrovascular disease in insulin resistant states. Dysfunction of the endothelium derived NO system has been shown to be associated with accelerated atherosclerosis in a variety of animal models (78,79). Conversely, maneuvers directed at elevating endothelium derived NO production appear to protect against atherosclerotic plaque formation (80–82). Thus, it follows logically from these lines of evidence that endothelial dysfunction may represent an early and central pathogenetic event leading to macrovascular disease in patients with insulin resistance. This hypothetical construct will undoubtedly be the focus of much future research.

ACKNOWLEDGMENTS

Dr. Alain Baron wishes to thank all previous co-authors that have contributed to this work, in particular, Dr. Helmut Steinberg and Ginger Brechtel-Hook, Research Nurse. This work has been supported in part by grants DK42469, MO1-RR750 and DK 20542 from the NIH, a Veterans Affairs Merit Review Award, and a Grant-in-Aid A3392 from the American Heart Association awarded to Dr. Alain Baron. The in vitro work described in this chapter has been supported in part by a Research Award grant from the American Diabetes Association to Dr. Michael J. Quon.

REFERENCES

1. Baron AD, Brechtel-Hook G, Johnson A, Hardin D. Skeletal muscle blood flow. A possible link between insulin resistance and blood pressure. Hypertension 1993;21:129–135.
2. Vallance P, Collier J, Moncada S. Effects of endothelium-derived nitric oxide on peripheral arteriolar tone in man. Lancet 1989;2:997–1000.
3. Stammler JS, Loh E, Roddy M-A, Currie KE, Creager MA. Nitric oxide regulates basal systemic and pulmonary vascular resistance in healthy humans. Circulation 1994;89:2035–2040.
4. Wu KK, Thiagarajan P. Role of endothelium in thrombosis and hemostasis. Annu Rev Med 1996;47:315–331.
5. Adams MR, McCredie R, Jessup W, Robinson J, Sullivan D, Celermaje DS. Oral L-arginine improves endothelium-dependent dilatation and reduces monocyte adhesion to endothelial cells in young men with coronary artery disease. Atherosclerosis 1997;129:261–269.

6. Lefer AM. Nitric Oxide: nature's naturally occuring leukocyte inhibitor. Circulation 1997;95:553–554.

7. Bruckdorfer KR, Jacobs JM, Rice-Evans C. Endothelium-derived relaxing factor (nitric oxide), lipoprotein oxidation and atherosclerosis. Biochem Soc Trans 1990;18:1061–1063.

8. Hogg N, Kalyanaraman B, Joseph J, Struck A, Parthasarathy S. Inhibition of low-density lipoprotein oxidation by nitric oxide. FEBS Lett. 1993;334:170–174.

9. Jessup W, Dean RT. Autoinhibition of murine macrophage mediated oxidation of low density lipoprotein by nitric oxide synthesis. Atherosclerosis 1997;101:145–155.

10. Jessup W. Cellular modification of low-density lipoproteins. Biochem Soc Trans 1993;21:321–325.

11. Moncada S, Higgs A. The L-arginine—nitric oxide pathway. N Engl J Med 1993;329:2002–2012.

12. Cooke JP, Tsao PS. Endothelium-derived relaxing factor. In Sowers JR, ed. Endocrinology of the Vasculature. Humana, Totowa, NJ, 1996, pp. 3–20.

13. Cohen RA. The role of nitric oxide and other endothelium-derived vasoactive substances in vascular disease. Prog Cardiovasc Dis 1995;38:105–128.

14. Lloyd-Jones DM, Bloch KD. The vascular biology of nitric oxide and its role in atherogenesis. Annu Rev Med 1996;47:365–375.

15. Laakso M, Edelman SV, Brechtel G, Baron AD. Decreased effect of insulin to stimulate skeletal muscle blood flow in obese man: A novel mechanism for insulin resistance. J Clin Invest 1990;85:1844–1852.

16. Laakso M, Edelman SV, Brechtel G, Baron AD. Impaired insulin mediated skeletal muscle blood flow in patients with NIDDM. Diabetes 1992;41:1076–1083.

17. Baron AD. Insulin and the vasculature-old actors, new roles. J Invest Med 1996;44:406–412.

18. Baron AD, Brechtel G. Insulin differentially regulates systemic and skeletal muscle vascular resistance. Am J Physiol 1993;265:E61–E67.

19. Scherrer U, Randin D, Vollenweinder P, Vollenweinder L, Nicod P. Nitric oxide release accounts for insulin's vascular effects in humans. J Clin Invest 1994;94:2511–2515.

20. Steinberg H, Chaker H, Leaming R, Johnson A, Brechtel G, Baron AD. Obesity/insulin resistance is associates with endothelial dysfunction. Implications for the syndrome of insulin resistance. J Clin Invest 1996;97:2601–2610.

21. Taddei S, Virdis A, Mattei P, Natali A, Ferrannini E, Salvetti A. Effects of insulin on acetylcholine-induced vasodilation in the forearm of normotensive subjects. Hypertension 1995;25:552 (Abstract).

22. Nagao T, Illiano S, Vanhoutte PM. Heterogeneous distribution of endothelium-dependent relaxations resistant to Ng-nitro-L-arginine in rats. Am J Physiol 1992;263:H1090–H1094.

23. Steinberg HOECressman YWu GHook JCronin AJohnson, ADBaron. Insulin mediated nitric oxide production is impaired in insulin resistance. Diabetes 1997;46(Suppl 1):24A (Abstract).

24. Madar Z, Zierrath J, Nollte L, Thorne A, Voet H, Wallberg-Henriksson H. Human skeletal muscle nitric oxide synthase-characterization and its activity in obese subjects. Diabetes 1997;46(Suppl 1):24A (Abstract).

25. Steinberg HO, Brechtel G, Johnson A, Fineberg N, Baron AD. Insulin mediated skeletal muscle vasodilation is nitric oxide dependent. A novel action of insulin to increase nitric oxide release. J Clin Invest 1994;94:1172–1179.

26. Baron AD, Steinberg HO, Chaker H, Leaming R, Johnson A, Brechtel G. Insulin-mediated skeletal muscle vasodilation contributes to both insulin sensitivity and responsiveness in lean humans. J Clin Invest 1995;96:786–792.

27. Natali A, Taddei S, Galvan AQ, Camastra S, Baldi S, Frascerra S, Virdis A, Sudano I, Salvetti A, Ferrannini E. Insulin sensitivity, vascular reactivity, clamp-induced vasodilatation in essential hypertension. Circulation 1997;96:849–855.

28. Steinberg HO, Hook G, Cronin J, Johnson A, Baron AD. Endothelial function is preserved in obese premenopausal women but not in obese men. Hypertension 1997;30(3):503 (Abstract).

29. Bohlen HG, Lash JM. Topical hyperglycemia rapidly suppresses EDRF-mediated vasodilation of normal rat arterioles. Am J Physiol 1993;265:H219–H225.

30. Jin JS, Bohlen HG. Non-insulin-dependent diabetes and hyperglycemia impair rat intestinal flow-mediated regulation. Am J Physiol 1997;272:H728–H734.

31. Williams SB, Cusco JA, Roddy M-A, Johnstone, MACreager MT. Impaired nitric oxide-mediated vasodilation in non-insulin-dependent diabetes. Circulation 1994;90:I–513 (Abstract).

32. Jeng C-Y, Fuh MM-T, Sheu WH-H, Chen Y-DI, Reaven GM. Hormone and substrate modulation of plasma triglyceride concentration in primary hypertriglyceridaemia. Endocrinol Metab 1994;1:15–21.

33. Davda RK, Stepniakowski KT, Lu G, Ullian E, Goodfriend TL, Egan BM. Oleic acid inhibits endothelial nitric oxide synthase by a protein kinase C-independent mechanism. Hypertension 1995;26:764–770.

34. Taylor SI. Lilly Lecture: Molecular mechanisms of insulin resistance. Lessons from patients with mutations in the insulin-receptor gene. Diabetes 1992;41:1473–1490.

35. Araki E, Lipes MA, Patti M-E, Brüning JC, Haag B III, Johnson RS, Kahn CR. Alternative pathway of insulin signalling in mice with targeted disruption of the IRS-1 gene. Nature 1994;372:186–190.

36. Tamemoto H, Kadowaki T, Tobe K, Yagi T, Sakura H, Hayakawa T, Terauchi Y, Ueki K, Kaburagi Y, Satoh S, Sekihara H, Yoshioka S, Horikoshi H, Furuta Y, Ikawa Y, Kasuga M, Yazaki Y, Aizawa S. Insulin resistance and growth retardation in mice lacking insulin receptor substrate-1. Nature 1994;372:182–186.

37. Bruning JC, Winnay J, Bonner-Weir S, Taylor SI, Accili D, Kahn CR. Development of a novel polygenic model of NIDDM in mice heterozygous for IR and IRS-1 null alleles. Cell 1997;88:561–572.

38. Stuehr DJ. Structure-function aspects in the nitric oxide synthases. [Review] [95 refs]. Annu Rev Pharmacol Toxicol 1997;37:339–359.

39. Huang PL, Huang Z, Mashimo H, Bloch KD, Moskowitz MA, Bevan JA, Fishman MC. Hypertension in mice lacking the gene for endothelial nitric oxide synthase. Nature 1995;377:239–242.

40. Quon MJ, Butte AJ, Taylor SI. Insulin signal transduction pathways. Trends Endocrin Metab 1994;5:369–376.

41. Nathan C, Xie QW. Nitric oxide synthases: roles, tolls, controls. [Review] [30 refs]. Cell 1994; 78:915–918.

42. Bar RS, Hoak JC, Peacock ML. Insulin receptors in human endothelial cells: identification and characterization. J Clin Endocrinol Metab 1978;47:699–702.

43. Zeng G, Quon MJ. Insulin-stimulated production of nitric oxide is inhibited by wortmannin. Direct measurement in vascular endothelial cells. J Clin Invest 1996;98(4):894–898.

44. King GL, Johnson SM. Receptor-mediated transport of insulin across endothelial cells. Science 1985;227:1583–1586.

45. Baron AD. Hemodynamic actions of insulin. Am J Physiol 1994;267:E187–E202.

46. Ferri C, Pittoni V, Piccoli A, Laurenti O, Cassone MR, Bellini C, Properzi G, Valesini G, De Mattia G, Santucci A. Insulin stimulates endothelin-1 secretion from human endothelial cells and modulates its circulating levels in vivo. J Clin Endocrinol Metab 1995;80:829–835.

47. Saruta T, Kumagai H. The sympathetic nervous system in hypertension and renal disease. Curr Opin Neph Hypert 1996;5:72–79.

48. Zeng GB, Clinton K, Kirby M, Mostowski H, Quon MJ. Tyrosine kinase-deficient mutant insulin receptors overexpressed in vascular endothelial cells fail to mediate production of nitric oxide. Hypertension 1997;30:504 (Abstract).

49. Myers MG Jr, White MF. Insulin signal transduction and the IRS proteins. Annu Rev Pharmacol Toxicol 1996;36:615–658.

50. Sun XJ, Wang LM, Zhang Y, Yenush L, Myers MG Jr, Lane WS, Pierce JH, White MF. Role of IRS-2 in insulin and cytokine signalling. Nature 1995;377:173–177.

51. Lavan BE, Lane WS, Lienhard GE. The 60-kDa phosphotyrosine protein in insulin-treated adipocytes is a new member of the insulin receptor substrate family. J Biol Chem 1997;272:11439–11443.

52. Holgado-Madruga M, Emlet DR, Moscatello DK, Godwin AK, Wong AJ. A Grb2-associated docking protein in EGF- and insulin-receptor signalling. Nature 1996;379:560–564.

53. Ricketts WA, Rose DW, Shoelson S, Olefsky JM. Functional roles of the Shc phosphotyrosine binding and Src homology 2 domains in insulin and epidermal growth factor signaling. J Biol Chem 1996;271:26165–26169.

54. Sasaoka T, Draznin B, Leitner JW, Langlois WJ, Olefsky JM. Shc is the predominant signaling molecule coupling insulin receptors to activation of guanine nucleotide releasing factor and p21ras-GTP formation. J Biol Chem 1994;269:10734–10738.

55. Lavan BE, Fantin VR, Chang ET, Lane WS, Keller SR, Lienhard GE. A novel 160-kDa phosotyrosine protein in insulin treated embryonic kidney cells is a new member of the insulin receptor substrate family. J Biol Chem 1997;272:21403–21407.

56. Quon MJ, Chen H, Ing BL, Liu ML, Zarnowski MJ, Yonezawa K, Kasuga M, Cushman SW, Taylor SI. Roles of 1-phosphatidylinositol 3-kinase and ras in regulating translocation of GLUT4 in transfected rat adipose cells. Mol Cell Biol 1995;15:5403–5411.

57. Quon MJ, Chen H, Lin CH, Zhou L, LIng B, Zarnowski MJ, Kazlauskas A, Cushman SW, Taylor SI. Effects of overexpressing wild-type and mutant PDGF receptors on translocation of GLUT4 in transfected rat adipose cells. Biochem Biophys Res Commun 1996;226:587–594.

58. Isakoff SJ, Taha C, Rose E, Marcusohn J, Klip A, Skolnik EY. The inability of phosphatidylinositol 3-kinase activation to stimulate GLUT4 translocation indicates additional signaling pathways are required for insulin-stimulated glucose uptake. Proc Natl Acad Sci USA 1995;92:10247–10251.

59. Wennstrom S, HawkinsP, Cooke F, Hara K, Yonezawa K, Jackson T, Claesson-Welsh L, Stephens L. Activation of phosphoinositide 3-kinase is required for PDGF-stimulated membrane ruffling. Curr Biol 1994;4:385–393.

60. Cong L, Chen H, Li Y, Zhou L, McGibbon MA, Taylor SI, Quon MJ. Physiologic role of Akt in insulin-stimulated translocation of GLUT 4 in transfected rat adipose cells. Mol Endocrinol 1997; 11:1881–1890.

61. Garcia-Cardena G, Fan R, Stern DF, Liu J, Sessa WC. Endothelial nitric oxide synthase is regulated by tyrosine phosphorylation and interacts with caveolin-1. J Biol Chem 1996;271:27237–27240.

62. Munshi HG, Burks DJ, Joyal JL, White MF, Sacks DB. Ca2+ regulates calmodulin binding to IQ motifs in IRS-1. Biochemistry 1996;35:15883–15889.

63. Joyal JL, Burks DL, Pons S, Matter WF, Vlahos CJ, White MF, Sacks DB. Calmodulin activates phosphatidylinositol 3 kinase. J Biol Chem 1997;272:28183–28186.

64. Reaven GM. Role of insulin resistance in human disease. Diabetes 1988;37:1595–1607.

65. Chen Y-DI, Reaven GM. Insulin resistance and atherosclerosis. Diabetes Rev 1997;5(4):331–342.

66. Laakso M, Lehto S. Epidemiology of macrovascular disease in diabetes. Diabetes Rev 1997;5(4):294–315.

67. Henry RR, Wallace P, Olefsky JM. Effects of weight loss on mechanisms of hyperglycemia in obese non-insulin dependent diabetes mellitus. Diabetes 1986;35:990–998.

68. Henry RR, Gumbiner B. Benefits and limitations of very-low-calorie diet therapy in obese NIDDM. [Review] [151 refs]. Diabetes Care 1991;14:802–823.

69. Devlin JT. Effects of exercise on insulin sensitivity in humans. [Review] [25 refs]. Diabetes Care 1992;15:1690–1693.

70. Holloszy JO, Schultz J, Kusnierkiewicz J, Hagberg JM, Ehsani AA. Effects of exercise on glucose tolerance and insulin resistance. Brief review and some preliminary results. [Review] [25 refs]. Acta Medica Scand—Supplementum 1986;711:55–65.

71. Nolan J, Ludvik B, Beerdsen P, Joyce M, Olefsky J. Improvement in glucose tolerance and insulin resistance in obese subjects treated with troglitazone. N Engl J Med 1994;331:1188–1193.

72. Hsueh WA, Quinones MJ, Creager MA. Endothelium in insulin resistance and diabetes. Diabetes Rev 1997;5(4):343–352.

73. Von der Leyen HE, Gibbons GH, Morishita R, Lewis NP, Zhang L, Nakajima M, Kaneda Y, Cooke JP, Dzau VJ. Gene therapy inhibiting neointimal vascular lesion: In vivo transfer of endothelial cell nitric oxide synthase gene. Proc Natl Acad Sci USA 1995;92:1137–1141.

74. Marks DS, Vita JA, Folts JD, Keaney JF Jr, Welch GN. Inhibition of neointimal proliferation in rabbits after vascular injury by a single treatment with a protein adduct of nitric oxide. J Clin Invest 1995;96:2630–2638.

75. De Caterina R, Libby P, Peng HB, Thannickal VJ, Gimbrone MA Jr, Shin WS, Liao JK. Nitric oxide decreases cytokine-induced endothelial activation. Nitric oxide selectively reduces endothelial expression of adhesion molecules and proinflammatory cytokines. J Clin Invest 1995;96:60–68.

76. Zeiher AM, Fisslthaler B, Schray-Utz B, Busse R. Nitric oxide modulates the expression of monocyte chemoattractant protein 1 in cultured human endothelial cells. Circ Res 1995;76:980–986.

77. Vanhoutte PM, Rubanyi GM, Miller VM, Houston DS. Modulation of vascular smooth muscle contraction by the endothelium. [Review] [97 refs]. Ann Rev Physiol 1986;48:307–320.

78. Cayatte AJ, Palacino JJ, Horten K, Cohen RA. Chronic inhibition of nitric oxide production accelerates neointima formation and impairs endothelial function in hypercholesterolemic rabbits. Arterioscl Thromb 1994;14:753–759.

79. Naruse K, Shimizu K, Muramatsu M, Toki Y, Miyazaki Y, Hashimoto H, Ito T. Long-term inhibition of NO synthesis promotes atherosclerosis in the hypercholesterolemic rabbit thoracic aorta. PGH2 does not contribute to impaired endothelium-dependent relaxation [see comments]. Arterioscl Thromb 1994;14:746–752.

80. Girerd XJ, Hirsch AT, Cooke JP, Dzau VJC. L-arginine augments endothelium-dependent vasodilation in cholesterol-fed rabbits. Circ Res 1990;67:1301–1308.

81. Cooke JP, Singer AH, Tsao P, Zera P, Rowan RA. Antiatherogenic effects of L-arginine in the hypercholesterolemic rabbit. J Clin Invest 1992;90:1168–1172.

82. Tsao PS, McEvoy LM, Drexler H, Butcher EC, Cooke JP. Enhanced endothelial adhesiveness in hypercholesterolemia is attenuated by L-arginine. Circulation 1994;89:2176–2182.

III CLINICAL SYNDROMES ASSOCIATED WITH INSULIN RESISTANCE

14

Insulin Resistance and Dyslipidemia: *Implications for Coronary Heart Disease Risk*

Ami Laws, MD

CONTENTS

INTRODUCTION
INSULIN RESISTANCE DEFINED
INSULIN RESISTANCE AND ABNORMALITIES OF FASTING LIPIDS
    AND LIPOPROTEINS
INSULIN RESISTANCE AND ABNORMALITIES OF POSTPRANDIAL LIPIDS
    AND LIPOPROTEINS: *IMPLICATIONS FOR ATHEROGENESIS*
SUMMARY
REFERENCES

Tissue resistance to insulin-stimulated glucose uptake and to insulin suppression of nonesterified fatty acid levels (NEFA) is related to numerous lipid and lipoprotein abnormalities that increase coronary heart disease (CHD) risk. This chapter will review recent advances in understanding these associations.

INTRODUCTION

Researchers have begun focusing increased attention to the role of the metabolic defects of insulin resistance in the etiology of atherosclerosis *(1–7).* Research investigating the link between insulin resistance and atherogenesis was initially motivated by a desire to understand the strong relationship between non-insulin-dependent diabetes (NIDDM or Type 2 diabetes) and increased risk of CHD *(8–19).*

More recently, it has been recognized that metabolic abnormalities associated with insulin resistance exist in a far greater proportion of the population than that comprised of patients with Type 2 diabetes. Hence the relevance of understanding the relations of these metabolic abnormalities to CHD has acquired broader significance.

Resistance to insulin-mediated glucose uptake is present in normoglycemic obese and/or sedentary persons *(20,21),* in persons with impaired glucose tolerance [IGT] *(22,23),*

From: *Contemporary Endocrinology: Insulin Resistance*
Edited by: G. Reaven and A. Laws © Humana Press Inc., Totowa, NJ

in normoglycemic persons with a family history of Type 2 diabetes (24,25) and in normoglycemic patients with hypertension (26,27). Certain ethnic groups, including Mexican-Americans (28), Native Americans (29), and persons from the South Asian subcontinent (30,31) also demonstrate high prevalences of resistance to insulin-mediated glucose uptake. Thus, broad segments of the population are affected by insulin resistance. These nondiabetic persons are at increased risk for CHD on the basis of the atherogenic lipid and lipoprotein changes related to insulin resistance that will be discussed in this chapter. The specific relation of Type 2 diabetes to CHD risk will not be reviewed here since it has been previously extensively discussed (8–19).

INSULIN RESISTANCE DEFINED

The actions of insulin that impact lipid and lipoprotein concentrations are twofold: 1) stimulation of glucose uptake by peripheral (primarily muscle) cells; and 2) suppression of plasma nonesterified fatty acid (NEFA) levels.

Resistance to Insulin Medicated Glucose Uptake

Muscle tissue resistance to insulin-stimulated glucose uptake in persons with normal glucose tolerance (NGT) and normal pancreatic function leads to circulating hyper-insulinemia as the pancreas attempts to compensate for decreased peripheral glucose uptake. Thus, in persons with intact pancreatic secretory function, directly measured tissue insulin resistance and insulin levels are highly correlated (32,33).

In persons who are susceptible to developing the spectrum of disorders of carbohydrate metabolism that comprise insulin resistance (viz. impaired glucose tolerance and Type 2 diabetes), the pancreas begins to lose its ability to generate sufficiently high insulin levels to maintain normal plasma glucose levels. Thus, persons with impaired glucose tolerance (IGT) have insulin levels that are higher than normal, but still insufficient to overcome tissue insulin resistance. IGT is therefore characterized by both high insulin and high glucose levels. Because of the relative failure of pancreatic insulin secretion, insulin levels are less strongly correlated with directly measured tissue insulin resistance in persons with IGT than in persons with NGT (32,33).

Both resistance to insulin-stimulated glucose uptake (34–38) and hyperinsulinemia (39,40) have been shown in numerous studies to be related to abnormal levels of lipids and lipoproteins. The metabolic basis for these relationships will be discussed subsequently.

Resistance to Insulin Suppression of Nonesterified Fatty Acid Levels (NEFA)

NEFA are present in plasma primarily as the products of lipolysis of triglyceride stored in adipose tissue (Fig. 1). They are the main substrates for energy metabolism in the fasting state when insulin and glucose levels are relatively low. Circulating NEFA are also the major substrates for liver triglyceride synthesis (41–44).

Increases in insulin concentrations such as occur in the fed state normally suppress plasma NEFA primarily by inhibiting hormone-sensitive lipase, the enzyme responsible for lipolysis (Fig. 1). Insulin may also decrease plasma NEFA by promoting their re-esterification in adipose cells for storage as triglyceride (45,46).

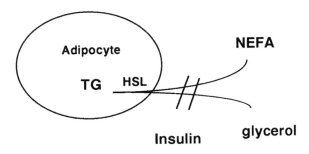

Fig. 1. Adipocyte lipolysis. Hormone sensitive lipase (HSL) causes breadkown of adipocyte triglyceride (TG) into NEFA and glycerol. Insulin inhibits this process.

In persons resistant to the suppressive effect of insulin on adipose tissue lipolysis, NEFA levels are elevated.

Impaired NEFA suppression by insulin has been demonstrated to occur in the same groups that have resistance to insulin-stimulated glucose uptake. In epidemiologic studies, Byrne et al. *(22)* and Laws et al. *(23)* showed that NEFA suppression is impaired in persons with IGT compared to those with NGT despite the fact that this group has higher insulin levels *(23)*. In metabolic studies, Pei et al. (1995) demonstrated that in nondiabetic subjects, resistance to insulin-mediated glucose uptake was accompanied by impairment of insulin inhibition of isoproterenol-stimulated lipolysis *(47)*. Yki-Jarvinen and Taskinen showed parallel impairment in insulin-stimulated glucose uptake and insulin suppression of lipolysis in hypertriglyceridemic diabetic and nondiabetic subjects (48). Roust and Jensen demonstrated that following a mixed meal, lipolysis was suppressed less in women with upper body (or abdominal) obesity than in women with lower body obesity or non-obese women *(49)*. This was despite higher insulin levels in the upper body obese women who have been shown to have resistance to insulin-stimulated glucose uptake. Finally, a defect in insulin suppression of NEFA levels in persons with Type 2 diabetes has been extensively documented *(50–53)*.

Only one exception to the parallel occurrence of resistance to insulin-stimulated glucose uptake and resistance to insulin suppression of NEFA has been demonstrated. McKeigue et al. *(54)* and Laws et al. *(23)* have recently shown that compared to women, men have impaired NEFA suppression following glucose challenge *(23,54)*, despite similar capacities for insulin-mediated glucose uptake *(23)*. Impaired NEFA suppression in men was explained in part by the gender difference in central obesity as measured by waist-hip ratio (WHR) *(23,54)*. Impaired suppression of NEFA in men in these studies was significantly associated with elevated triglyceride and apolipoprotein B (apoB) levels *(23,54)*. This gender difference in NEFA suppression and its relation to triglyceride and apoB concentrations may explain in part the higher CHD risk in men vs women.

In addition to the role elevated NEFA levels play in initiating atherogenic lipid and lipoprotein changes discussed below, they may have a direct role in atherogenesis.

Direct effects of elevations of NEFA on formation of atherosclerotic plaques have been proposed by some investigators. Hennig et al. showed that low density lipoprotein (LDL) transfer across cultured porcine pulmonary artery endothelial cells was increased in the presence of elevated NEFA levels *(55)*. The authors hypothesized that exposure of endothelium to elevated NEFA concentrations may allow excessive amounts of cholesterol-rich lipoproteins to enter arterial intima *(55)*. Another group showed that NEFA/ albumin molar ratio was strongly correlated with intracellular lipid accumulation by arterial intimal cells *(56)*.

INSULIN RESISTANCE AND ABNORMALITIES
OF FASTING LIPIDS AND LIPOPROTEINS

Effects of Impaired Insulin Suppression of NEFA
on Triglyceride and apoB Metabolism

Circulating NEFA are the major substrates for triglyceride synthesis in liver, and triglyceride synthesis and secretion are stimulated by increases in NEFA flux to the liver. Thus there is a direct relation between resistance to insulin suppression of NEFA and very low density (VLDL)-triglyceride synthesis and secretion *(40–42)*.

NEFA have also been shown to stimulate apoB release from HepG2 cells in vitro *(57–61)*, and to be correlated with apoB levels in vivo *(23,54)*. Elevated NEFA levels play therefore a key role in VLDL-triglyceride and apoB metabolism, initiating an atherogenic lipoprotein cascade *(1,62–65)*. Important steps in this cascade occur in the postprandial state and will be discussed in more detail below.

Effects of Resistance to Insulin-Stimulated Glucose Uptake
and Hyperinsulinemia on Triglyceride Synthesis
and Fasting Triglyceride Levels

Several studies have investigated the effects of resistance to insulin-mediated glucose uptake on fasting lipid and lipoprotein abnormalities *(33–37)*. Decreases in the ability of insulin to stimulate glucose uptake as measured directly by glucose clamp *(66)* or by the insulin suppression test *(67)*, have been shown to correlate strongly with hypertriglyceridemia and low high-density lipoprotein (HDL) cholesterol concentrations *(31,33,34)*. In other studies, hyperinsulinemia (a marker for insulin resistance) has been shown to correlate with increased triglyceride concentrations and decreased HDL cholesterol concentrations in normoglycemic men and women *(38,39)*.

Impaired insulin stimulation of glucose uptake has also been shown to be associated with increased levels of small, dense LDL cholesterol particles *(68–73)*, which are strongly related to CHD risk *(74)*.

Despite strong correlations of resistance to insulin-stimulated glucose uptake and hyperinsulinemia with triglyceride metabolism, the basis for the associations remain the subject of controversy. In vivo studies attempting to elucidate these relationships have been complicated by the fact that insulin also regulates NEFA concentrations. Small increases in ambient insulin concentrations can profoundly suppress NEFA levels *(53)*, thereby decreasing both NEFA flux to liver and triglyceride synthesis *(40–42,75)*. Therefore it is difficult to assess the effects of hyperinsulinemia per se on triglyceride metabolism in vivo.

In vitro studies of cultured rat *(76,77)* and human hepatocytes *(78)* and HepG2 cells *(57–59)* have consistently demonstrated that insulin inhibits VLDL triglyceride and apoB synthesis and/or release. There is evidence, however, that this may be an acute but not a chronic effect *(61,78)*. Some investigators have proposed, therefore, that hypertriglyceridemia in insulin resistant persons is a result of resistance in the liver to the inhibitory effect of insulin on VLDL triglyceride and apoB synthesis and/or release *(58,59,61)*.

On the other hand, other investigators have maintained that there is a direct stimulatory effect of hyperinsulinemia on triglyceride synthesis and secretion. There is, in fact, abundant evidence suggesting that hyperinsulinemia per se plays a direct role in hypertriglyceridemia. Insulin levels are strongly and consistently correlated with triglyceride concentrations in diverse populations *(38,39,75)*. High carbohydrate diets produce a rises in triglyceride levels that are highly correlated with increased insulin concentrations *(79,80)*. Hyperinsulinemia correlates strongly with VLDL triglyceride production rates in humans *(75,80–81)* and rats *(82–84)*. On the basis of these studies, therefore, some investigators have argued that hyperinsulinemia directly stimulates VLDL triglyceride synthesis and secretion *(1–5,12,68–73,75–84)* from liver.

Is there a metabolic pathway that would explain a stimulatory effect of insulin resistance and chronic hyperinsulinemia on VLDL-triglyceride synthesis in liver? The effect of insulin on *de novo* hepatic lipogenesis is one possible pathway.

Although the NEFA used for triglyceride synthesis in the liver during the post-absorptive state are primarily taken up from the splanchnic circulation, the liver also synthesizes fatty acids *de novo* in the postprandial state. The rate-limiting step in the pathway of fatty acid synthesis is catalyzed by acetyl CoA carboxylase (ACC). Long-term regulation of ACC depends on insulin-modulated synthesis of the enzyme *(85)*. Thus, levels of ACC are decreased in insulin-deficient states such as fasting and Type 1 diabetes, and increased by refeeding, especially with a high-carbohydrate diet *(85)*.

The other critical steps in fatty acid synthesis are catalyzed by fatty acid synthase (FAS), a multifunctional enzyme *(85,86)*. FAS is thought to be a major long-term regulator of hepatic *de novo* lipogenesis *(86)*. Like ACC, FAS concentration is highly sensitive to its nutritional and hormonal environment. Insulin has been shown to cause a marked and rapid increase in mRNA level and transcription rate of the FAS gene in mouse livers *(87)*. FAS is decreased during fasting, and increased with high-carbohydrate refeeding. That the increase in FAS with refeeding is due to the rise in insulin levels *per se*, and not to circulating glucose levels (which can themselves stimulate hepatic lipogenesis) is supported by a study in rats showing that chronic hyperinsulinemia caused dramatic increases in mRNA of glucokinase, ACC and FAS even though euglycemia was maintained *(88)*.

Based on the effects of insulin on ACC and FAS, it would be predicted that the hypertriglyceridemia caused by high carbohydrate diets (which induce hyperinsulinemia), would consist of an increased proportion of fatty acids derived from *de novo* synthesis in liver. This has in fact been demonstrated. Barter et al. *(41)* used isotopically labeled palmitic acid to determine the contribution of plasma NEFA to VLDL-TGFA. They showed that in the fasting state, the contribution of plasma NEFA to VLDL-TGA was 80–100%, whereas following prolonged carbohydrate ingestion in the form of glucose, plasma NEFA contributed only 30–60% of VLDL-triglyceride. Using ^{14}C-U-glucose, they also showed that during carbohydrate ingestion, 80% of the ^{14}C label that appeared in plasma triglyceride was in the fatty acid moiety. Thus this study confirms the expected effects of high carbohydrate diets and hyperinsulinemia on hepatic *de novo* fatty acid synthesis. Recently these findings have been confirmed in a study by Hudgins et al. *(89)*. Using palmitate enrichment of VLDL-triglyceride as a marker of *de novo* hepatic fatty acid synthesis, they showed that *de novo* hepatic lipogenesis was substantially increased on high carbohydrate compared to high fat diets *(89)*. Unfortunately, neither of these studies measured plasma insulin levels which would have confirmed that increased hepatic fatty acid synthesis correlated with plasma insulin concentration. However, the effect of high carbohydrate diets in causing hyperinsulinemia is well-documented *(21,79)*.

The effects of insulin on ACC and FAS and therefore on hepatic *de novo* fatty acid synthesis would also explain the results an elegant series of studies by Reaven et al. *(63,90)*. Comparing patients with Type 2 diabetes (who were hyperinsulinemic), Type 1 diabetes (who were insulin deficient) and controls, they showed that in the presence of equivalent levels of glucose and NEFA, the VLDL-triglyceride secretion rates and plasma triglyceride levels were increased in the hyperinsulinemic Type 2 diabetes patients, but not in the hypoinsulinemic Type 1 diabetes patients *(90)*.

Thus, a large body of epidemiologic, clinical, metabolic and molecular research supports a direct role for resistance to insulin-stimulated glucose uptake and hyperinsulinemia in increased VLDL-triglyceride synthesis and secretion.

Relations of Hypertriglyceridemia to Atherogenic Lipoprotein Particles

Hypertriglyceridemia per se increases risk for atherosclerosis through its effects on the composition of lipoproteins, specifically LDL- and HDL- cholesterol *(91,92)*. Eisenberg et al. *(92)*, examined men with hypertriglyceridemia (HTG) compared to men with normal triglyceride (NTG) levels. The HTG men were studied before and after treatment with bezafibrate which lowers plasma triglycerides levels. In untreated HTG men, VLDL particles showed low protein and triglyceride content, and high cholesterol ester and free cholesterol content compared to the NTG men. LDL and HDL_3 particles in HTG men were smaller and denser and relatively depleted of free and esterified cholesterol. They were enriched in apoprotein and triglyceride. HDL_2 levels were markedly decreased or absent among HTG men. These abnormalities in lipoproteins were strongly and significantly correlated with plasma triglyceride concentration, and reflect excessive transfer of triglyceride to LDL and HDL particles, and of cholesteryl ester to VLDL. During bezafibrate treatment, the compositional abnormalities in VLDL, LDL and HDL reverted towards normal in proportion to the amount of triglyceride lowering. This study demonstrates that hypertriglyceridemia results directly in atherogenic changes in the compositions of lipoproteins.

INSULIN RESISTANCE AND ABNORMALITIES OF POSTPRANDIAL LIPIDS AND LIPOPROTEINS: *IMPLICATIONS FOR ATHEROGENESIS*

Insulin resistance to NEFA suppression and to glucose uptake both affect a number of postprandial lipid and lipoprotein mechanisms. Persons with impaired postprandial insulin suppression of NEFA have an increased flux of NEFA to liver which, as discussed above, causes increased synthesis and secretion of VLDL-triglyceride and increased secretion of apoB. Resistance to insulin-mediated glucose uptake *(31,93)*, hyperinsulinemia *(31,93)* and insulin secretion *(94)* also correlate strongly with postprandial triglyceride levels.

In addition to stimulating VLDL-triglyceride and apoB secretion from liver, increased postprandial NEFA levels have been shown to be have other adverse effects on lipid and lipoprotein metabolism. NEFA are inversely related to postprandial lipoprotein lipase (LPL) activity, most likely via a local feedback mechanism *(95)*. LPL is essential for catabolism of triglyceride-rich lipoproteins including chylomicrons and VLDL lipoproteins. NEFA have been shown to dissociate LPL from its binding sites in humans *(96)* and in endothelial cell culture *(97)*. With lipolytic activity reduced, triglycerides accumulate in plasma.

Post-heparin plasma and muscle lipoprotein lipase activity have also been shown to be reduced in persons with resistance to insulin- stimulated glucose uptake *(98–104)*. Maheux et al. recently showed that insulin resistance is strongly inversely correlated with plasma post-heparin lipoprotein lipase activity and mass, and adipose tissue mRNA *(102)*. Insensitivity to insulin-stimulated glucose uptake also appears to be associated with an increase in hepatic lipase *(100)*.

In the postprandial period, these changes in lipases that are associated with insulin resistance result in decreased clearance of triglyceride-rich particles, including chylomicrons and endogenous VLDL-triglyceride, which compete for the same lipolytic pathway *(105,106)*. This leads to an excess of triglyceride-rich particles in the circulation, including chylomicrons and chylomicron remnants, which are highly atherogenic *(107–108)*.

The effects of resistance to insulin-mediated glucose uptake and to NEFA suppression on lipids and lipoproteins in the postprandial period can be summarized as follows (Fig. 2A): Following a meal, insulin levels rise. The increase in insulin concentration is accentuated following high carbohydrate ingestion. In insulin resistant persons, there is a concomitant decrease in postprandial insulin suppression of NEFA which leads to increased NEFA flux to liver. Increased levels of circulating insulin, glucose and NEFA then interact in liver to cause increased VLDL-triglyceride synthesis and secretion, while increased NEFA causes increased apoB secretion from liver (Fig. 2B).

In the circulation, relatively high NEFA levels in insulin resistant persons reduce the lipolytic activity of lipoprotein lipase. Increased levels of endogenous VLDL-triglyceride from liver compete with diet-derived chylomicrons for LPL. Clearance of atherogenic chylomicrons and chylomicron remnants is thereby reduced (Fig. 2C).

Postprandial hypertriglyceridemia has been shown to be strongly and independently associated with coronary artery disease *(109)*. This is likely mediated by the adverse effects of hypertriglyceridemia on concentrations and composition of lipoproteins that increase risk of atherogenesis, as discussed above.

Also during the postprandial period, neutral lipid transfer via cholesterol ester transfer protein (CETP) effects transfer of triglycerides from VLDL to HDL_2 cholesterol, with reciprocal transfer of cholesterol ester to VLDL *(110–112)* (Fig. 2D). Elevated triglyceride *(112)* and NEFA *(113)* levels amplify this process *(113)*. Triglyceride enriched HDL_2 are then converted by hepatic lipase to HDL_3, resulting in a decrease in cardioprotective HDL_2 cholesterol concentrations *(114)*.

Elevated postprandial insulin and triglyceride levels also affect HDL cholesterol concentrations via apo A-I catabolism. In humans in vivo, the primary metabolic predictor of variability in HDL cholesterol concentration is the apo A-I fractional catabolic rate (FCR) *(65,115,116)*. One study showed the apo A-I FCR alone accounted for two-thirds

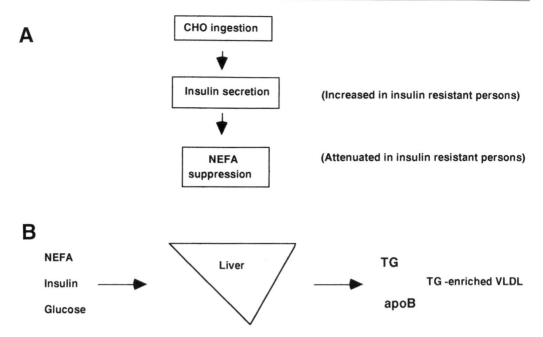

Fig. 2. Postprandial lipid and lipoprotein changes related to insulin resistance. **(A)** Carbohydrate ingestion in persons who are insulin resistant causes hyperinsulinemia. In persons resistant to NEFA suppression by insulin, postprandial NEFA levels are relatively elevated. **(B)** High insulin and NEFA levels circulate to liver where they stimulate TG production and release, and NEFA stimulates apoB release. VLDLc particles become TG-enriched in insulin resistant persons.

of the variability in HDL cholesterol *(65)*. Two of the strongest determinants of apo A-I FCR in this study were in turn plasma insulin and triglyceride concentrations *(65)*. Therefore low HDL cholesterol levels, which are well known to increase CHD risk, are caused in part by hypertriglyceridemia and insulin resistance.

Neutral lipid transfer via CETP also results in transfer of triglyceride to LDL particles, resulting in increased numbers of small, dense LDL particles *(117,118)* (Fig. 2D) Postprandial triglyceride and triglyceride-rich lipoproteins have been shown to be strong determinants of small, dense LDL cholesterol levels *(117)*. Small, dense LDL cholesterol particles have been shown to be strongly associated with incident CHD, independently of other risk factors *(74,118)*.

SUMMARY

Resistance to insulin-stimulated glucose uptake and to insulin suppression of NEFA affect numerous, interrelated steps in lipid and lipoprotein metabolism, beginning with hepatic synthesis and secretion of VLDL triglycerides and secretion of apoB. These changes result in increased triglyceride-enriched lipoproteins in the circulation, especially in the postprandial period. Insulin resistance affects lipoprotein lipase and hepatic lipase activities, resulting in competition between endogenous and exogenous triglyceride-rich particles for lipolysis. Insulin resistance is also associated with increased CETP mass and activity, and apo AI catabolic rate, leading to low HDL cholesterol concentrations. Increased triglyceride levels resulting from insulin resistance also lead to an increase

C

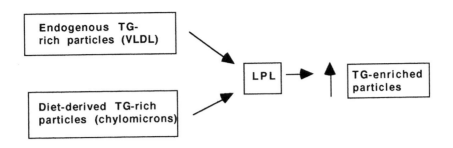

D

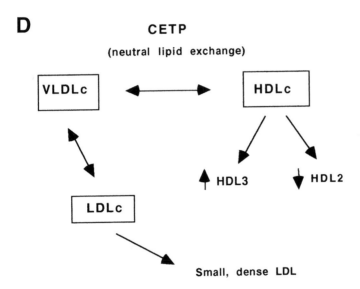

Fig. 2. (C) Diet-derived and endogenous TG-enriched particles compete for the LPL lilpolytic pathway, contributing to hypertriglyceridemia. **(D)** Neutral lipid exchange between VLDLc and HDLc via CETP results in decreases in cardioprotective HDL2. Neutral lipid exchange between VLDLc and LDLc results in elevated atheragenic, small, dense LDL particles.

in small, dense LDL particles. All of these lipid and lipoprotein changes associated with insulin resistance increase the risk for CHD.

REFERENCES

1. Reaven GM. Role of insulin resistance in human disease. Diabetes 1988;37:1595–1607.
2. Krauss RM. The tangled web of coronary risk factors. Am J Med 1991;90(Suppl 2):36S–41S.
3. Laws A, Reaven GM. Insulin resistance and coronary heart disease risk factors. Bailliere's Clin Endocrinol Metab 1993;4:1063–1078.
4. Frayn KN. Insulin resistance and lipid metabolism. Curr Opin Lipidol 1993;4:197–204.
5. Reaven GM, Laws A. Insulin resistance, compensatory hyperinsulinemia and coronary heart disease. Diabetologia 1994;37:948–952.
6. Despres J-P, Marette A. Relation of components of insulin resistance syndrome to coronary disease risk. Curr Opin Lipidol 1994;5:274–289.

7. Taskinen M-R. Insulin resistance and lipoprotein metabolism. Curr Opin Lipidol 1995;6:153–160.

8. Albrink MJ, Lavietes PH, Man EB. Vascular disease and serum lipids in diabetes mellitus: Observations over thirty years (1931–1961). Ann Intern Med 1963;58:305–323.

9. West KM, Ahuja MMS, Bennett PH, Czyzyk A, Mateo de Acosta O, Fuller JH, Grab B, Grabauskas V, Jarrett RJ, Kosake K, Keen H, Krolewski AS, Miki E, Schliak B, Teuscher A, Watkins PJ, Strober JA. The role of circulating glucose and triglyceride concentrations and their interactions with other "risk factors" as determinants of arterial disease in nine diabetic population samples from the WHO multinational study. Diabetes Care 1983;6:361–369.

10. Pyorala K, Laasko M, Uusitupa M. Diabetes and atherosclerosis: An epidemiologic view. Diabet Metab Rev 1987;3:463–524.

11. Ronnemaa T, Laakso M, Kallio V, Pyorala K, Marniemi J, Puuka P. Serum lipids, lipoproteins and apolipoproteins and the excessive occurrence of coronary heart disease in non-insulin-dependent diabetic patients. Am J Epidemiol 1989;130:632–645.

12. Steiner G. The dyslipoproteinemias of diabetes. Atherosclerosis 1994;110(Suppl):S27–S33.

13. Bergstrom RW, Leonetti DL, Newell-Morris LL, Shuman WP, Wahl PW, Fujimoto WY. Association of plasma triglyceride and C-peptide with coronary heart disease in Japanese-American men with a high prevalence of glucose intolerance. Diabetologia 1990;33,489–496.

14. Fontbonne A, Eschwege E, Cambien F, Richard J-L, Ducimetiere P, Thibult N, Warnet J-M, Claude J-R, Rosselin G-E. Hypertriglyceridaemia as a risk factor of coronary heart disease mortality in subjects with impaired glucose tolerance or diabetes: Results from the 10-year follow-up of the Paris Prospective Study. Diabetologia 1989;32,300–304.

15. Reckless JPD, Betteridge DJ, Wu P, Payne B, Galton DJ. High-density and low density lipoproteins and prevalence of vascular disease in diabetes mellitus. BMJ 1978;1:883–886.

16. Welborn TA, Knuiman M, McCann V, Stanton K, Constable IJ. Clinical macrovascular disease in Caucasoid diabetic subjects: Logistic regression analysis of risk variables. Diabetologia 1984; 27:568–573.

17. Laakso M, Vourilainen E, Pyorala K, Sarlund H. Association of low HDL and HDL$_2$ cholesterol with coronary heart disease in noninsulin-dependent diabetics. Arteriosclerosis 1985;5:653–658.

18. Laws A, Marcus EB, Grove JS, Curb JD. Lipids and lipoproteins as risk factors for coronary heart disease in men with abnormal glucose tolerance: The Honolulu Heart Program J Intern Med 1993;234:471–478.

19. Goldschmid MG, Barrett-Connor E, Edelstein SL, Wingard DL, Cohn BA, Herman WH. Dyslipidemia and ischemic heart disease mortality among men and women with diabetes. Circulation 1994;89:991–997.

20. Ferrannini E, Buzzigoli G, Bonadonna R, Giorico MA, Oleggini M, Graziadei L, Pedrinelli R, Brandi L, Bevilacqua S. Insulin resistance in essential hypertension. N Engl J Med 1987;317:350–357.

20. Laws A, Reaven GM. The effect of physical activity on age-related glucose intolerance. Clinics in Geriatric Medicine 1990;6:849–863.

21. Olefsky J, Crapo LA, Ginsberg H., Reaven GM. Metabolic effects of increased caloric intake in man. Metabolism 1975;24:495–503.

22. Byrne CD, Wareham NJ, Brown DC, Clark PMS, Cox LJ, Day NE, Palmer DR, Wang TWM, Williams DRR, Hales CN. Hypertriglyceridemia in subjects with normal and abnormal glucose tolerance: relative contributions of insulin secretion, insulin resistance and suppression of plasma non-esterified fatty acids. Diabetologia 1994;37:889–896.

23. Laws A, Hoen HM, Selby JV, Saad MF, Haffner SM, Howard BV. Differences in insulin suppression of free fatty acid levels by gender and glucose tolerance status: Relation to plasma triglyceride and apolipoprotein B concentrations. Arterioscl Thromb Vasc Biol 1997;17:64–71.

24. Laws A, Stefanick ML, Reaven GM. Insulin resistance and hypertriglyceridemia in first-degree relatives of patients with NIDDM. J Clin Endocinol Metab 1989;69:343–347.

25. Eriksson J, Franssila-Kallunki A, Ekstrand A, Saloranta C, Widen E, Schalin C, Groop L. Early metabolic defects in persons at increased risk for non-insulin dependent diabetes mellitus. N Engl J Med 1989;321:337–343.

26. Ferrannini E, Buzzigoli G, Bonadonna R. Insulin resistance in essential hypertension. N Engl J Med. 1987;317:350–357.

27. Shen D-C, Shieh S-M, Fuh MM-T, Wu D-A, Chen Y-DI., Reaven GM. Resistance to insulin-stimulated-glucose uptake in patients with hypertension. J Clin Endocrinol Metab 1988;66:580–583.

28. Haffner SM, Valdez RA, Hazuda HP, Mitchell BD, Morales PA, Stern MP. Prospective analysis of the insulin-resistance syndrome (Syndrome X). Diabetes 1992;41:715–722.

29. Lee ET, Howard BV, Savage PJ, Cowan LD, Fabsitz RR, Oopik AJ, Yeh J, Go O, Robbins DC, Welty TK. Diabetes and impaired glucose tolerance in three American Indian populations aged 45–74. The Strong Heart Study. Diabetes Care 1995;18:599–610.

30. McKeigue PM, Shah B, Marmot MG. Relation of central obesity and insulin resistance with high diabetes prevalence and cardiovascular risk in South Asians. Lancet 1991;337:382–386.

31. Laws A, Jeppesen JL, Maheux PC, Schaaf P, Chen Y-DI, Reaven GM. Resistance to insulin-stimulated glucose uptake and dyslipidemia in Asian Indians. Arterioscl Thromb 1994;14:917–922.

32. Reaven GM, Hollenbeck CB, Chen Y-DI. Relationship between glucose tolerance, insulin secretion, and insulin action in non-obese individuals with varying degrees of glucose tolerance. Diabetologia 1989;32:52–55.

33. Saad MF, Anderson RL, Laws A, Watanabe RM, et al. A comparison between the minimal model and the glucose clamp in the assessment of insulin sensitivity across the spectrum of glucose tolerance. Diabetes 1994;43:1114–1121.

34. Abbott WGH, Lillioja S, Young AA, Zawadzki JK, Yki-Jarvinen H, Christin L, Howard BV. Relationships between plasma lipoprotein concentrations and insulin action in an obese hyperinsulinemic population. Diabetes 1987;36:897–904.

35. Garg A, Helderman HJ, Koffler M, Ayuso R, Rosenstock J, Raskin P. Relationship between lipoprotein levels and in vivo insulin action in normal young white men. Metabolism 1988;37:982–987.

36. Laakso M, Sarlund H, Mykkanen L. Insulin resistance is associated with lipid and lipoprotein abnormalities in subjects with varying degrees of glucose tolerance. Arteriosclerosis 1990;10:223–231.

37. Laws A, Reaven GM. Evidence for an independent relationship between insulin resistance and fasting plasma triglyceride and HDL-cholesterol concentrations. J Intern Med 1992;23:25–30.

38. Godsland IF, Crook D, Walton C, Wynn B, Oliver MF. Influence of insulin resistance, secretion, and clearance on serum cholesterol, triglycerides, lipoprotein cholesterol, and blood pressure in healthy men. Arterioscler Thromb 1992;12:1030–1035.

39. Laws A, King A, Haskell W, Reaven GM. Relation of fasting plasma insulin concentration to high density lipoprotein cholesterol and triglyceride concentrations in men. Arterioscl Thromb 1991;11:1636–1642.

40. Laws A, King A, Haskell W, Reaven GM. Metabolic and behavioral covariates of high-density lipoprotein cholesterol and triglyceride concentrations in postmenopausal women. J Amer Geriatr Soc 1993;41:1289–1294.

41. Havel RJ, Kane JP, Balasse EO, Segel N, Basso LV. Splanchnic metabolism of free fatty acids and production of triglycerides of very low density lipoproteins in normotriglyceridemic and hypertriglyceridemic humans. J Clin Invest 1970;49:2017–2035.

42. Barter PJ, Nestel PJ, Carroll KF. Precursors of plasma triglyceride fatty acid in humans. Effects of glucose consumption, clofibrate administration and alcoholic fatty liver. Metabolism 1972;21:117–124.

43. Barter PJ, Nestel PJ. Precursors of plasma triglyceride fatty acids in obesity. Metabolism 1973;22:779–785.

44. Kissebah AH, Alfarsi S, Adams PW, Wynn V. Role of insulin resistance in adipose tissue and liver in the pathogenesis of endogenous hypertriglyceridaemia in man. Diabetologia 1976;12:563–571.

45. Coppack SW, Evans RD, Fisher RM, Frayn KN, Gibbons GF, Humphreys ML, Kirk ML, Potts JL, Hockaday TDR. Adipose tissue metabolism in obesity: Lipase action in vivo before and after a mixed meal. Metabolism 1992;41:264–272.

46. Wolfe RR, Peters EJ. Lipolytic response to glucose infusion in human subjects. Am J Physiol 1987;252:E218–E223.

47. Pei D, Chen Y-DI, Hollenbeck CB, Bhargava R, Reaven GM. Relationship between insulin-mediated glucose disposal by muscle and adipose tissue lipolysis in healthy volunteers. J Clin Endocrinol Metab 1995;80:3368–372.

48. Yki-Jarvinen H, Taskinen M-R. Interrelationships among insulin's antilipolytic and glucoregulatory effects and plasma triglycerides in nondiabetic and diabetic patients with endogenous hypertriglyceridemia. Diabetes 1988;37:1271–1278.

49. Roust LR, Jensen M. Postprandial free fatty acid kinetics are abnormal in upper body obesity. Diabetes 1993;42:1567–1573.

50. Bierman EL, Dole VP, Roberts TN. An abnormality of nonesterified fatty acid metabolism in diabetes mellitus. Diabetes 1957;6:475–479.

51. Kashyap ML, Magill F, Rojas L, Hoffman MM. Insulin and non-esterified fatty acid metabolism in asymptomatic diabetics and atherosclerotic subjects. CM Journal. 1970;102:1165–1169.

52. Kissebah AH, Adams PW, Wynn V. Inter-relationships between insulin secretion and plasma free fatty acid and triglyceride transport kinetics in maturity onset diabetes and the effect of phenethylbiguanide (phenformin). Diabetologia 1974;10:119–130.

53. Swislocki ALM, Chen Y-DI, Golay A, Chang M-O, Reaven GM. Insulin suppression of plasma-free fatty acid concentration in normal individuals and patients with Type 2 (non-insulin-dependent) diabetes. Diabetologia 1987;30:622–626.

54. McKeigue PM, Laws A, Chen Y-DI, Marmot MG, Reaven GM. Relation of plasma triglyceride and apolipoprotein B levels to insulin-mediated suppression of nonesterified fatty acids: possible explanation for sex differences in lipoprotein pattern. Arterioscl Thromb 1993;8:1187–1192.

55. Hennig B, Shasby DM, Spector AA. Exposure to fatty acid increases human low density lipoprotein transfer across cultured endothelial monolayers. Circ Res 1985;57:776–880.

56. Laughton CW, Ruddle DL, Bedord CJ, Alderman EL. Sera containing elevated nonesterified fatty acids from patients with angiographically documented coronary atherosclerosis cause marked lipid accumulation in cultured human arterial smooth muscle-derived cells. Atherosclerosis 1988;70:233–246.

57. Pullinger CR, North JD, Teng B-B, Rifici VA, Ronhild de Brito AE, Scott J. The apolipoprotein B gene is constitutively expressed in HepG2 cells: Regulation of secretion by oleic acid, albumin, and insulin, and measurement of the mRNA half-life. J Lipid Res 1989;30:1065–1077.

58. Byrne CD, Brindle NPJ, Wang TWM, Hales CN. Interaction of non esterified fatty acid and insulin in control of triacylglycerol secretion by Hep G2 cells. Biochem J 1991;280:99–104.

59. Byrne CD, Wang TWM, Hales CN. Control of Hep G2 cell triacylglycerol and apolipoprotein-B synthesis and secretion by polyunsaturated nonesterified fatty acids and insulin. Biochem J 1992;299:101–107.

60. Dixon JL, Ginsberg HN. Regulation of hepatic secretion of apolipoprotein B-containing lipoproteins: Information obtained from cultured liver cells. J Lipid Res 1993;34:167–179.

61. Sparks JD, Sparks CE. Insulin regulation of triacylglycerol-rich lipoprotein synthesis and secretion. Biochemica et Biophysica Acta 1994;1215:9–32.

62. Ginsberg HN. Lipoprotein physiology in nondiabetic and diabetic states: Relationship to atherogenesis. Diabetes 1991;14:839–855.

63. Cianflone K, Dahan S, Monge JC, Sniderman AD. Pathogenesis of carbohydrate-induced hypertriglyceridemia using HepG2 cells as a model system. Arterioscler Thromb 1992;12:271–277.

64. Brinton EA, Eisenberg S, Breslo JL. Elevated high density lipoprotein cholesterol levels correlate with decreased apoA-I and apoA-II fractional catabolic rate in women. J Clin Invest 1989;84:262–269.

65. Brinton EA, Eisenberg S, Breslow JL. Human HDL cholesterol levels are determined by ApoA-I Fractional catabolic rate, which correlates inversely with estimates of HDL particle size: Effects of gender, hepatic and lipoprotein lipases, triglyceride and insulin levels, and body fat distribution. Arterioscler Thromb 1994;14:707–720.

66. DeFronzo RA, Tobin JD, Andres R. Glucose clamp technique: A method quantifying insulin secretion and resistance. Am J Physiol 1979;237:E214–E219.

67. Shen SW, Reaven GM, Farquhar JW. Comparison of impedance to insulin-mediated glucose uptake in normal subjects and in subjects with latent diabetes. J Clin Invest 1979;49:2151–2160.

68. Barakat HA, Carpenter JW, McLendon VD, Khazanie P, Leggett N, Heath J, Marks R. Influence of obesity, impaired glucose tolerance and NIDDM on LDL structure and composition. Possible link between hyperinsulinemia and atherosclerosis. Diabetes 1990;39:1527–1533.

69. Bruce R, Godsland I, Walton C, Cook D, Wynn V. Associations between insulin sensitivity, and free fatty acid and triglyceride metabolism independent of uncomplicated obesity. Metabolism 1994;43:1275–1281.

70. Reaven GM, Chen Y-DI, Jeppesen J, Krauss RM. Insulin resistance and hyperinsulinemia in individuals with small, dense, low density lipoprotein particles. J Clin Invest 1993;92,141–146.

71. Selby JV, Austin MA, Newman B, Zhang D, Quesenberry CO, Mayer EJ, Krauss RM. LDL subclass phenotypes and the insulin resistance syndrome in women. Circulation 1993;88:381–387.

72. Katzel LI, Kraus RM, Goldberg AP. Relations of plasma TG and HDL-C concentrations to body composition and plasma insulin levels are altered in men with small LDL particles. Arterioscler Thromb 1994;14:1121–1128.

73. Tan KCB, Cooper MB, Ling KLE, Griffin BA, Freeman DJ, Packard CJ, Shepherd J, Hales CN, Betteridge DJ. Fasting and postprandial determinants for the occurrence of small dense LDL species in non-insulin-dependent diabetic patients with and without hypertriglyceridaemia: the involvement of insulin, insulin precursor species and insulin resistance. Atherosclerosis. 1995;113:273–287.

74. Austin MA, Breslow JL, Hennekens CH, Buring JE, Willet WC, Krauss RM. Low density lipoprotein subclass patterns and risk of myocardial infarction. JAMA 1988;260:1917–1921.

75. Steiner G. Hyperinsulinaemia and hypertriglyceridaemia. J Intern Med 1994;236(Suppl 736):23–26.

76. Durrington PN, Newton RS, Weinstein DB, Steinberg D. Effects of insulin and glucose on very low density lipoprotein triglyceride secretion by rat hepatocytes. J Clin Invest 1982;70:63–73.

77. Patsch W, Franz S, Schonfield G. Role of insulin in lipoprotein secretion by cultured rat hepatocytes. J Clin Invest 1983;71:1161–1174.

78. Bartlett SM, Gibbons GF. Short- and longer-term regulation of very low density lipoprotein secretion by insulin, dexamethasone and lipogenic substrates in cultured hepatocytes. A biphasic effect of insulin. Biochem J 1988;249:37–43.

79. Farquhar JW, Frank A, Gross RC, Reaven GM. Glucose, insulin and triglyceride responses to high and low carbohydrate diets in man. J Clin Invest 1966;45:1648–1656.

80. Tobey TA, Greenfield M, Kraemer F, Reaven GM. Relationship between insulin resistance, insulin secretion, very low density lipoprotein kinetics and plasma triglyceride levels in normotriglyceridemic man. Metabolism 1981;30:165–171.

81. Kazumi T, Vranic M, Steiner G. Triglyceride kinetics: effects of dietary glucose, sucrose, or fructose alone or with hyperinsulinemia. Am J Physiol 1986;250:E325–E330.

82. Steiner G, Haynes FJ, Yoshina G, Vranic M. Hyperinsulinemia and in vivo very-low-density lipoprotein-triglyceride kinetics. Am J Physiol 1982;246:E187–E192.

83. Reaven GM, Mondo CE. Effect of in vivo plasma insulin levels on the relationship between perfusate free fatty acid concentration and triglyceride secretion by perfused rat livers. Horm Metabol Res 1984;16:230–232.

84. Reaven GM, Hill DB, Gross RC, Farquhar JW. Kinetics of triglyceride turnover of very low density lipoproteins of human plasma. J Clin Invest 1965;44:1826–1832.

85. Wolf G. Nutritional and hormonal regulation of fatty acid synthase. Nutr Rev 1996;54:22–27.

86. Wakil SJ, Stoops JK, Joshi VC. Fatty acid synthesis and its regulation. Ann Rev Biochem. 1983;52:537–579.

87. Paulauskis JD, Sul HS. Hormonal regulation of mouse fatty acid synthase gene transcription in liver. J Biol Chem 1989;264:574–577.

88. Assimacopoulos-Jeannet F, Brichard S, Rencurel F, Cusin I, Jeanrenaud B. In vivo effects of hyperinsulinemia on lipogenic enzymes and glucose transporter expression in rat liver and adipose tissues. Metabolism 1995;44:228–233.

89. Hudgins LC, Hellerstein M, Seidman C, Neese R, Diakun J, Hirsch J. Human fatty acid synthesis is stimulated by a eucaloric low fat, high carbohydrate diet. J Clin Invest 1996;97:2081–2091.

90. Reaven GM, Greenfield MS. Diabetic hypertriglyceridemia: Evidence for three clinical syndromes. Diabetes 1981;30(Suppl 2):66–75.

91. Deckelbaum RJ, Granot E, Oschry Y, Rose L, Eisenberg S. Plasma triglyceride determines structure-composition in low and high density lipoproteins. Arteriosclerosis 1984;4:225–231.

92. Eisenberg S, Gavish D, Oschry Y, Fainaru M, Deckelbaum RJ. Abnormalities in very low, low, and high density lipoproteins in hypertriglyceridemia. Reversal toward normal with Bezafibrate treatment. J Clin Invest 1984;74:470–482.

93. Jeppesen J, Hollenbeck CB, Zhou M-Y, Coulston AM, Jones C, Chen Y-DI, Reaven GM. Relation between insulin resistance, hyperinsulinemia, postheparin plasma lipoprotein lipase activity and postprandial lipemia. Arterioscl Thromb Vasc Biol 1995;15:320–324.

94. Cavallero E, Dachet C, Neufcour D, Wirquin E, Math D, Jacotot B. Postprandial amplification of lipoprotein abnormalities in controlled Type II diabetic subjects: Relationship to postprandial lipemia and C-peptide/glucagon levels. Metabolism 1994;43:270–278.

95. Karpe F, Olivecrona T, Walldius G, Hamsten A. Lipoprotein lipase in plasma after an oral fat load: relation to free fatty acids. J Lipid Res 1992;33:975–984.

96. Peterson J, Bihain BE, Bengtsson-Olivecrona G, Deckelbaum RJ, Carpentier YA, Olivecrona T. Fatty acid control of lipoprotein lipase: a link between energy metabolism and lipid transport. Proc Natl Acad Sci USA 1990;87:909–913.

97. Saxena U, Witte LD, Goldberg IJ. Release of endothelial cell lipoprotein lipase by plasma lipoproteins and free fatty acids. J Biol Chem 1989;264:4349–4355.

98. Lithell H, Jacobs I, Vessby JB, Hellsing K, Karlsson J. Decrease of lipoprotein lipase activity in skeletal muscle in man during a short-term carbohydrate-rich dietary regime. With special reference to HDL-cholesterol, apolipoprotein and insulin concentrations. Metabolism 1982;31:994–998.

99. Pollare T, Vessby B, Lithell H. Lipoprotein lipase activity in skeletal muscle is related to insulin sensitivity. Arterioscl Thromb 1991;11:1192–1203.

100. Baynes C, Henderson AD, Amyaoku V, Richmond W, Hughes CL, Johnston DG, Elkeles RS. The role of insulin insensitivity and hepatic lipase in the dyslipidaemia of Type 2 diabetes. Diabetic Med 1991;8:560–566.

101. Knudsen P, Eriksson J, Lahdenpera S, Kahri J, Groop L, Taskinen M-R, and the Botnia Study Group. Changes of lipolytic enzymes cluster with insulin resistance syndrome. Diabetologia 1995;38:344–350.

102. Maheux P, Axhar S, Kern PA, Chen Y-DI, Reaven GM. Relationship between insulin-mediated glucose disposal and regulation of plasma and adipose tissue lipoprotein lipase. Diabetologia 1997;40:850–858.

103. Kiens B, Lithell H, Mikines KJ, Richter EA. Effects of insulin and exercise on muscle lipoprotein lipase activity in man and its relation to insulin action. J Clin Invest 1989;84:1124–1129.

104. Potts JL, Coppack SW, Fisher RM, Humphreys SM, Gibbons GF, Frayn KN. Impaired postprandial clearance of triacylglycerol-rich lipoproteins in adipose tissue in obese subjects. Am J Physiol 1995;268:E588–E594.

105. Brunzell JD, Hazzard WR, Porte D Jr, Bierman EL. Evidence for a common, saturable, triglyceride removal mechanism for chylomicrons and very low density lipoproteins in man. J Clin Invest 1973;52:1578–1585.

106. Karpe F, Hultin M. Endogenous triglyceride-rich lipoproteins accumulate in rat plasma when competing with a chylomicron-like triglyceride emulsion for a common lipolytic pathway. J Lipid Res 1995;36:1557–1566.

107. Zilversmit, DB. Atherogenesis: A postprandial phenomenon. Circulation 1979;60:473–485.

108. Havel RJ. Postprandial hyperlipidemia and remnant lipoproteins. Curr Opin Lipidol 1994;5:102–109.

109. Patsch JR, Miesenbock G, Hopferwieser T, Muhlberger V, Knapp E, Dunn JK, Gotto AM, Patsch W. Relation of triglyceride metabolism and coronary artery disease: Studies in the postprandial state. Arterioscl Thromb 1992;12:1336–1345.

110. Morton RE, Zilversmit DB. Inter-relationship of lipids transferred by the lipid-transfer protein isolated from human lipoprotein-deficient plasma. J Biol Chem 1989;258:11751–11757.

111. Yen FY, Deckelbaum RJ, Mann CJ, Marcel YL, Milne RW, Tall AR. Inhibition of cholesteryl ester transfer protein activity by monoclonal antibody: effects of cholesteryl ester formation an neutral lipid mass transfer in human plasma. J Clin Invest 1989;83:2018–2024.

112. Hayek T, Azrolan N, Verdery RB, Walsh A, Chajek-Shaul T, Agellon LB, Tall AR, Breslow JL. Hypertriglyceridemia and cholesterol ester transfer protein interact to dramatically alter high density lipoprotein levels, particle sizes, and metabolism: Studies in transgenic mice. J Clin Invest 1993;92:1143–1152.

113. Lagrost L, Florentin E, Guyard-Dangremont V, Athias A, Gandjini H, Lallemant C, Gambert P. Evidence for nonesterified fatty acids as modulators of neutral lipid transfers in normolipidemic human plasma. Arterioscl Thromb Vasc Biol 1995;15:1388–1396.

114. Patsch JR, Prasad S, Gotto AM, Bengtsson-Olivecrona G. Postprandial lipemia: A key for the conversion of high density lipoprotein2 into high density lipoprotein3 by hepatic lipase. J Clin Invest 1984;74:2017–2023.

115. Golay A, Zech L, Shi M-Z, Chiou Y-AM, Reaven GM, Chen Y-DI. High density lipoprotein (HDL) metabolism in non-insulin-dependent diabetes mellitus: measurement of HDL turnover using tritiated HDL J Clin Endocrinol Metab 1987;65:512–518.

116. Patsch, JR, Prasad, S, Gotto, AM, Patsch, W High density lipoprotein2: Relationship of the plasma levels of this lipoprotein species of its composition, to the magnitude of postprandial lipemia, and to the activities of lipoprotein lipase and hepatic lipase. J Clin Invest 1987;80:341–347.

117. Karpe R, Tornval P, Olivecrona T, Steiner G, Carlson LA, Hamsten A. Composition of human low density lipoprotein: effects of postprandial triglyceride-rich lipoproteins, lipoprotein lipase, hepatic lipase and cholesteryl ester transfer protein. Atherosclerosis 1993;98:33–49.

118. Griffin BA, Freeman DJ, Tait GW, Thomson J, Caslake MJ, Packard CJ, Shepherd J. Role of plasma triglyceride in the regulation of plasma low density lipoprotein (LDL) subfractions: relative contribution of small, dense LDL to coronary heart disease risk. Atherosclerosis 1994;106:241–253.

15 Insulin Resistance and Blood Pressure

Ele Ferrannini, MD

CONTENTS

INTRODUCTION
EPIDEMIOLOGY
TYPE OF DIABETES
OBESITY
PLASMA INSULIN
INSULIN RESISTANCE
MECHANISMS
CONCLUSIONS
CLINICAL AND THERAPEUTIC IMPLICATIONS
REFERENCES

INTRODUCTION

Abnormalities in carbohydrate metabolism are found more often in hypertensive individuals than in the background population. *Prima facie*, this association is readily explained. In fact, with aging blood pressure (BP) rises and glucose tolerance worsens, the former because of a stiffening vascular tree, the latter due to declining insulin secretion. Therefore, even if entirely independent of one another, hypertension and glucose intolerance would end up as companions in the late decades of life. Furthermore, patients with overt diabetes, whether insulin-dependent (IDDM or Type 1 diabetes) or noninsulin-dependent (NIDDM or Type 2 diabetes), often develop high BP as a consequence of diabetic renal damage. Finally, obesity and a sedentary lifestyle amplify the risk for both hypertension and diabetes, thereby bringing them together in the same subject. Thus, the association of hypertension with disordered carbohydrate metabolism could be largely circumstantial. However, the association has deeper roots than appears on the surface. This chapter reviews the available evidence, and indicates its clinical and therapeutic implications.

EPIDEMIOLOGY

A wealth of epidemiological data document that reduced glucose tolerance (impaired glucose tolerance [IGT] or overt diabetes) is consistently associated with high BP. This

From: *Contemporary Endocrinology: Insulin Resistance*
Edited by: G. Reaven and A. Laws © Humana Press Inc., Totowa, NJ

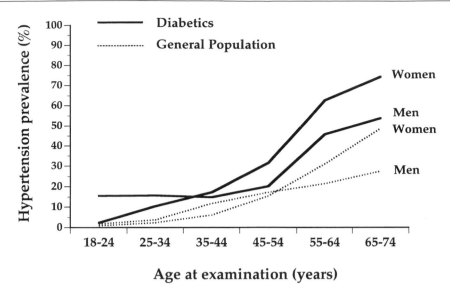

Age at examination (years)

Fig. 1. Prevalence of hypertension (defined as systolic BP≥160 mmHg and/or diastolic BP≥95 mmHg) in 702 diabetic patients and in the white US population as a function of age at examination. In diabetics, the age-adjusted prevalence is 26% in men and 36% in women, ~twofold higher than in the general population (14% in men and 20% in women). (Drawn from data in ref. *4*).

association persists beyond the confounding influence of factors that affect the value of arterial BP (arm girth, time of day, room temperature, posture, antecedent physical activity or cigarette smoking, stress, medication) as well as those factors that modulate glucose tolerance (prior diet and physical activity, glucose load, timing of glucose measurements, gastric emptying rate) *(1)*. For example, in the Framingham Study 9% of the women population presented both glucose intolerance and hypertension viz the expected 3% *(2)*. Conversely, in the United Kingdom Prospective Diabetes Study *(3)*, almost one half of patients with newly-diagnosed Type 2 diabetes were hypertensive instead of the expected 30%. When comparing the data collected at the Joslin Clinic in Boston over a period of 25 yr *(4)* to those of the Caucasian US population, the excess prevalence of hypertension in diabetics is evident in all age groups (Fig. 1). Furthermore, whereas in nondiabetic women the prevalence rate of hypertension surpasses that of men at age 45–54 yr, the corresponding lines for diabetics cross each other about one decade earlier. Thus, the presence of diabetes significantly diminishes the protection that women enjoy until menopause. Abstracting from different epidemiological surveys *(5–9)*, one finds that the excess hypertension of diabetes declines with age, and tends to disappear in men over 70 years of age. These results may be explained by the fact that many hypertensive diabetic men have died out by the time of screening (survival bias).

In both the Joslin database *(4)* and the United Kingdom Prospective Diabetes Study *(3)*, the prevalence of hypertension was higher in diabetics than in the nondiabetic population already at diagnosis or shortly thereafter, especially in women (Fig. 1). This finding suggests that factors antedating the clinical manifestation of diabetes must be responsible for its association with high BP. If hypertension antedates the clinical manifestation of diabetes, then individuals with a strong predisposition to diabetes should present high BP more often than persons at lesser risk for diabetes. This prediction has been verified in a study of Polish families *(10)*, which documented a significant surplus of hypertension in the nondiabetic relatives of diabetic probands, both for parents (34% vs 21% of the reference population) and siblings (8% vs 2%). Interestingly, the increase in hypertension prevalence was even more pronounced among relatives of lean than obese diabetic probands.

If familial diabetes co-segregates with hypertension, BP and blood glucose concentration might be related variables even in normal subjects. There is data to support this both in adults *(11)* and, more significantly, in children *(12)*, in whom the confounding influence of alcohol and drugs is negligible. In fact, both BP and blood glucose levels are tracking variables: persons in the upper range of the distribution tend to remain in the same position over time. As a consequence, the blood glucose concentration is as good a predictor of subsequent diabetes as the BP value is for future hypertension. Furthermore, there is evidence that glucose tolerance is a predictor of subsequent development of hypertension. Thus, in an 18-yr follow up of middle aged men in Finland *(13)* initially normotensive subjects in the upper tertile of baseline blood glucose levels developed significantly more hypertension than men in the lowest tertile (after adjusting for age, adiposity, alcohol consumption, and initial BP value). The converse, namely that BP predicts diabetes, has also been shown. In a 5-yr follow up of approximately 10,000 men in Israel, BP resulted to be a significant predictor of diabetes (particularly in the age group 40–49 yr) independent of age, obesity, and presence of peripheral vascular disease *(14)*.

TYPE OF DIABETES

The excess of hypertension is found in both Type 1 diabetes and Type 2 diabetes in comparison with the nondiabetic population. Type 1 diabetes patients present more hypertension once significant nephropathy has developed (as eventually happens in ~50% of them). Proteinuria, heralded by microalbuminuria, signals incipient diabetic nephropathy, and is the best predictor of progression to endstage renal failure *(15)*. High BP may also precede nephropathy. In addition, a family history of hypertension *(16)*, and a high rate of sodium-lithium countertransport activity (Na/Li CT) in red cells of Type 1 diabetes patients appear to have a negative prognostic value for diabetic nephropathy *(17)*. Which, microalbuminuria or high BP, comes first in the natural history of Type 1 diabetes may be difficult to establish in the individual patient. In either case, hypertension strongly accelerates loss of renal function. In microalbuminuric Type 1 diabetes patients, 24-h ambulatory BP is higher than in normoalbuminuric patients even when casual BP readings do not distinguish between the two groups *(18)*. Furthermore, in normoalbuminuric Type 1 diabetes patients ambulatory BP recordings are intermediate between those of microalbuminuric patients and those of nondiabetic subjects. Finally, some Type 1 diabetes patients with high BP present a cluster of abnormalities (dyslipidemia, left ventricular hypertrophy, insulin resistance) that are characteristic of insulin resistant Type 2 diabetes *(19)*.

Essential hypertension in nondiabetic individuals also can be associated with an increased rate of urinary albumin excretion *(20)*. Furthermore, in normotensive patients with proven pancreatic diabetes (secondary to chronic pancreatitis) urinary albumin excretion rates show the same distribution as in Type 1 diabetes patients with matched duration of diabetes, degree of hyperglycemia, and daily insulin dose. These findings suggests that, even in the absence of the genetic predisposition to Type 1 diabetes, high BP and hyperglycemia may each cause albumin leakage into the urine.

Diabetic nephropathy with proteinuria occurs half as often as in Type 1 diabetes, and renal failure is relatively uncommon (5–10%), in patients with Type 2 diabetes *(21)*. Whether a family history of hypertension, abnormalities in Na/Li CT, or other factors predispose Type 2 diabetes patients to nephropathy is not clear. These patients enjoy an apparent protection from progression to renal failure due to older age and premature death from cardiovascular causes. Ethnic factors also appear to be important, since in native Americans, Hispanics, and African-Americans the frequency of endstage renal failure due to diabetic nephropathy approaches that in Type 1 diabetes. In any case, even in Caucasian Type 2 diabetes patients *(4)* the presence of proteinuria is an independent correlate of both systolic and diastolic BP even after adjustment for age, obesity, and duration of diabetes.

It should be mentioned at this point that, despite their diverse etiology, Type 1 diabetes and Type 2 diabetes are not totally separate conditions. Thus, although the overall frequency of hypertension in the families of Type 1 diabetes probands is only slightly higher than in the nondiabetic population, there is definitely more diabetes (presumably, Type 2 diabetes) in parents (13%) and siblings (7%) of Type 1 diabetes patients than among their spouses (2%) or in the general population (~2%) *(4,10)*.

The excess of hypertension in diabetes is not only due to diabetic nephropathy or interstitial disease. According to a recent autopsy study, renal artery stenosis, whether hemodynamically significant or not, is very prevalent, and largely underdiagnosed, in diabetic patients *(22)*.

Recently, attention has been called to the association between a low body weight at birth and the development of hypertension in adulthood *(23)*, with the suggestion that stunted intrauterine growth may sensitize vascular tissues to pressor stimuli. Evidence is accumulating that a similar association exists between birth weight and diabetes: a low weight at birth and 1 yr later has been found to be an independent predictor of adult Type 2 diabetes, IGT, and dyslipidemia *(24,25)*. Furthermore, in healthy women plasma glucose and insulin levels during the third trimester of pregnancy have a dual, opposite influence on neonatal weight, glucose predicting a higher, and insulin a lower, birth weight *(26)*. Thus, maternal hyperinsulinemia, by interfering with intrauterine growth, might impose an enhanced risk of both hypertension and diabetes.

OBESITY

The epidemiology of the association of obesity with hypertension is abundant. The impact of overweight on BP in normal subjects is shown in Fig. 2, which compares mean BP values across quartiles of age between lean subjects (BMI $<25 \text{ kg/m}^2$) and overweight individuals (all without diabetes, glucose intolerance, hypertension, or dyslipidemia) *(27)*. It can be seen that, in men as well as in women mean BP is higher in the obese than in the lean groups at all ages. The effect of obesity is attenuated at advancing ages, and considerably more so in men than in women. From these data, it can be calculated that an average BMI difference of 6 units (=18 kg of body weight) is equivalent to a difference of 5.2 mmHg in mean BP; in women, an average BMI difference of 8 units (=22 kg) is associated with a difference of 9.1 mmHg in mean BP. Thus, these general population data indicate that a normal person responds to a weight gain of 1 kg with an increase in mean BP of 0.1–0.3 mmHg, the increment being systematically larger in women than in men.

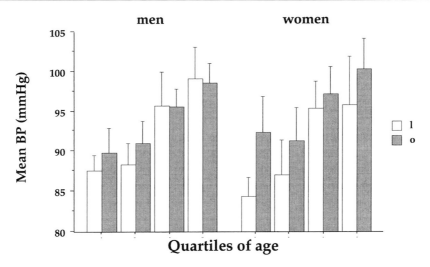

Fig. 2. Mean blood pressure values in men and women by age and body mass. Bars are mean values + 95% confidence limits. Empty bars are for lean (*l*) subjects, filled bars for obese (i.e., BMI > 25 Kg/m²) individuals (*o*). (Drawn from data in ref. *27*).

This finding is quantitatively consistent with the results of a theoretical analysis of the hemodynamics of obesity predicting the changes in mean BP induced by weight gain *(28)*. By using average hemodynamic data from the literature *(29)* and the relevant equations, it was shown that weight gain is accompanied by a fall in total peripheral vascular resistance (resulting from the addition of circulatory segments in parallel to the heart). Cardiac output, however, also rises as a function of indices of body weight *(29)*. If the increase in cardiac output were in exact proportion to the increased venous return to the heart (contributed by the new tissues), BP would remain unchanged. The fact that BP so consistently rises with weight gain indicates that cardiac output increases out of proportion to the circulatory mass. Thus, whereas raised peripheral vascular resistance is the distinctive feature of hypertension in the lean, excessive cardiac output is the hemodynamic hallmark of obesity-related hypertension. Whatever other abnormalities, structural or functional, may contribute to obesity hypertension, it seems clear that obesity is intrinsically pressogenic. The pattern of distribution of adipose mass between abdominal (particularly, visceral) and peripheral (lower body) sites (android and gynoid obesity, respectively) has received much attention as an additional disease indicator *(30–32)*. Available evidence indicates that an android fat pattern is accompanied by further hyperinsulinemia and higher BP only when obesity is present.

PLASMA INSULIN

Inappropriately high plasma insulin levels have been found in essential hypertension independently of obesity and Type 2 diabetes. In the early days of insulin radioimmunoassay, Welborn and colleagues *(33)* first reported hyperinsulinemia in a group of normotolerant hypertensive subjects (after controlling for age, body weight, and antihypertensive therapy). Subsequently, Singer et al. *(34)* reported daylong hyperinsulinemia in a group of hypertensive subjects with a normal plasma glucose response to meals, from which the authors inferred the presence of insulin resistance. In many later investigations, whether epidemiological surveys or case-control studies, an association between some measure of plasma insulin (fasting level, single postglucose reading, sum of stimulated values) and BP (more often systolic, but also diastolic or mean) has been reported. However, the strength of the association, and its persistence after adjustment for confounders (age, gender, obesity), have varied greatly, and some negative studies have been published. Clearly, the relationship is not a strong one. Furthermore, it is significantly influenced by ethnic factors. Thus, in the San Antonio Heart Study the age-, gender-, and obesity-adjusted level of plasma insulin was significantly related to the prevalence of hypertension in both Mexican-Americans and non-Hispanic Caucasians, but the regression line was shifted downwards in the former compared to the latter *(35)*. In other words, the same insulin concentration was associated with widely different rates of hypertension in different ethnic groups living in the same area. In general, whether or not one finds a statistical relationship between these two variables depends on (a) the precision of the respective measurements, (b) the sample size, (c) the number and power of common confounders, (d) the use of BP as a continuous variable or a category (hypertension), and (d) the characteristics of the population, particularly in terms of background prevalence of hypertension and glucose tolerance status. A recent meta-analysis of studies involving a total of ~6,000 nondiabetic, untreated patients with essential hypertension has concluded that high BP is positively associated with fasting plasma insulin levels independently of the effect of age, obesity, and fasting glycemia *(36)*. Several other lines of evidence weigh with an inherent link of plasma insulin with BP. Among hyperinsulinemic, normotolerant offspring of diabetic parents hypertension is almost twice as common as in matched offspring of nondiabetic parents *(37)*. In familial dyslipidemic hypertension, a subgroup of subjects have higher plasma insulin levels than can be accounted for by obesity *(38)*. In the offspring of hypertensive parents, who are at risk of developing hypertension, hyperinsulinemia is found at a stage when BP is still normal *(39)*. Finally, in a follow-up of initially normotensive people, significantly more subjects with high, as opposed to low, plasma insulin levels at baseline developed hypertension over 8 yr *(40)*. These latter observations are particularly important as they are free of any bias introduced by the presence of glucose intolerance or drug treatment.

INSULIN RESISTANCE

Several case-control studies have quantitated insulin sensitivity in patients with essential hypertension by direct methods (including the euglycemic insulin clamp and the insulin suppression test) *(41–43)*. Unlike the results obtained with plasma insulin measurements, the findings have been so far entirely consistent in showing that lean, untreated patients with essential hypertension have a variable (20–40%) reduction in whole-body insulin sensitivity. BP is inversely related to insulin sensitivity, more strongly than to plasma insulin levels when both are measured in the same subject, and 24-h BP is a better correlate of insulin sensitivity than office or occasional BP *(44)*. Importantly, while the majority of patients with Type 2 diabetes have some degree of insulin resistance, it can be estimated from available data *(42,43)* that only one-fourth to one-third of lean hypertensive patients are insulin resistant.

Insulin resistance is not prominent in renovascular hypertension *(45)* or primary hyperaldosteronism, whereas in hypertension secondary to pheochromocytoma or Cushing's disease the associated glucose intolerance and insulin insensitivity are adequately explained by the high circulating levels of catecholamines and cortisol, respectively. In contrast, the insulin resistance of essential hypertension is apparently

Table 1
The Insulin Resistance of Essential Hypertension

1. Present in one-fourth to one-third of the cases
2. Primary (not found in secondary hypertension and not explained by obesity)
3. Directly related to severity of hypertension
4. Present in normotensive offspring of hypertensive parents
5. Tissue- and pathway-specific
6. Associated with high Na/Li CT activity, salt sensitivity, or microalbuminuria (or combinations)
7. Worsened by diabetes
8. Irreversible (by acute insulin or other treatment)

primary as there is no known way of reproducing it experimentally in normotensive individuals, or means to reverse it in hypertensive subjects. Since the peripheral tissues are resistant to insulin *(46)* whereas the liver *(41)* and the heart are not *(47)*, and because glucose—but not lipid, amino acid or potassium—metabolism is involved *(41,46)*, the insulin resistance of essential hypertension is both tissue- and pathway-specific. Under euglycemic conditions, sequential infusion of progressively higher insulin doses does not overcome this insulin refractoriness at the whole-body level *(48)* or in the forearm tissues *(46)*. Finally, hypertension worsens the insulin resistance of Type 2 diabetes *(49)*.

Hypertensive patients with a high rate of Na/Li CT are more insulin resistant than similarly hypertensive patients with normal activity of the antiport *(50)*. In salt-sensitive normotensive volunteers on a high-salt diet, the plasma insulin response to glucose is higher than in salt-resistant subjects, but a low-salt diet abolishes this difference *(51)*. Microalbuminuria in hypertensive subjects is associated with further hyperinsulinemia in response to oral glucose and with insulin resistance on the insulin clamp *(52,53)*. Thus, a high rate of Na/Li CT, salt sensitivity, and microalbuminuria co-segregate with the insulin resistant variant of essential hypertension. Whether the simultaneous presence of all three traits identifies the insulin resistant hypertensive patient with more precision than each trait alone, or whether these traits circumscribe separate subgroups of resistant subjects, is not known. Insulin resistance is found in a significant number of offspring of hypertensive parents at a time when their BP is completely normal *(39)*. Whether these insulin resistant subjects also present high Na/Li CT, salt sensitivity or microalbuminuria (or combinations) has not been determined, nor is it known whether it is the insulin resistant ones among the offspring of hypertensive parents that go on to develop hypertension. At present, it is not clear that the insulin resistance of nondiabetic patients with untreated essential hypertension can be substantially corrected by antihypertensive treatment. A number of studies testing a variety of antihypertensive agents (β-blockers, calcium antagonists, angiotensin-converting enzyme inhibitors, diuretics, α-blockers) have appeared, but the results have been inconsistent and the reported effects relatively small *(54)* (Table 1).

A recent analysis of the European Group for the Study of Insulin Resistance (EGIR) database (n = 422 insulin clamp studies) has shown that, in nondiabetic normotensive Europeans BP values (systolic, diastolic, and mean BP alike) are significantly higher in insulin resistant than in insulin sensitive subjects, particularly in the lean (BMI ≤ 25 kg/m^2) group (Fig. 3). Furthermore, in the whole database insulin sensitivity was inversely associated with BP independently of gender, age, and BMI *(27)*. The results are compatible with the concept that the reciprocal association of insulin action *in vivo* and arterial

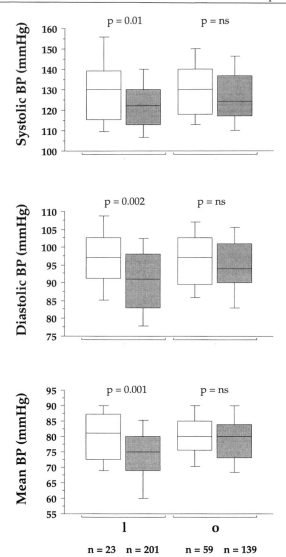

Fig. 3. Box-plots for systolic, diastolic, and mean blood pressure values by body mass (*l* = lean, *o* = obese) and insulin sensitivity (empty boxes = insulin resistant subjects, filled boxes = insulin sensitive subjects). Insulin resistance was defined as the bottom 10% of the distribution of clamp-derived insulin sensitivity values in lean, healthy individuals. P values refer to the comparison of mean values by 2-way analysis of variance. (Drawn from data in ref. *27*).

BP is inherent in the respective physiological systems; from this it follows that the hypertensive population, which represent the tail end of the BP distribution, should be enriched with insulin resistant individuals.

MECHANISMS

Theoretically, high BP could cause insulin insensitivity (hypothesis A), or insulin resistance could cause hypertension (hypothesis B), or high BP and insulin resistance could be parallel consequences of a common parent abnormality (hypothesis C).

In general, it should be borne in mind that many patients with secondary or essential hypertension show normal insulin sensitivity, and, conversely, that not all insulin resistant subjects develop hypertension. In the healthy population, the partial correlation coefficient (i.e., adjusted for gender, age, and BMI) between insulin sensitivity and mean arterial BP is only 0.15 (by comparison, that for mean BP and age is 0.43) (27). Clearly, if there are cause-effect relationships between insulin resistance and high BP, these must be indirect or relatively weak, or require special circumstances to become evident.

Hypothesis A appears to be the least likely, as secondary hypertension in humans is not associated with insulin resistance (45). Experimentally, when normal Sprague-Dawley rats are rendered severely hypertensive by transfecting them with a mouse renin gene (TGR(mREN-2)27), insulin sensitivity is preserved, both at the whole-body and tissue level (55). Hypothesis B cannot be ruled out, but is difficult to prove conclusively. In the San Antonio Heart Study (40), hyperinsulinemia preceded the development of hypertension in normotensive, nondiabetic subjects. However, even if hyperinsulinemia is taken to stand for insulin resistance, the temporal precedence of hyperinsulinemia may reflect a delayed expression of a genetic predisposition to hypertension rather than effects of insulin resistance on BP control. Experimentally, inducing insulin resistance by means of chronic exogenous insulin infusion leads to the emergence of high BP in the rat (56) but not in the dog (57), suggesting major interactions with the genetic makeup. In humans, manipulations that improve insulin sensitivity, such as weight reduction in obese subjects, also lower BP (58). Again, however, these could be parallel rather than hierarchical consequences of weight loss. To complicate the matter, hyperinsulinemia rather than insulin resistance could be the link with BP homeostasis.

Recent data in transgenic animals have provided strong evidence for common genetic determinants of insulin resistance and hypertension. Thus, mice heterozygous for the knockout of either the GLUT4 gene—encoding the expression of the insulin-regulatable glucose transporter—or the IRS-2 gene—coding for one of the major intracellular insulin signaling proteins—show both insulin resistance *and* higher BP (59,60). In humans, a polymorphism in the glycogen synthase gene (coding for the rate-limiting enzyme in the glucose storage pathway) has been found to be associated with Type 2 diabetes particularly in hypertensive patients (61).

In the following discussion, the potential physiological mechanisms linking insulin with BP will be discussed under the assumption that insulin resistance and high BP are generally parallel phenomena (hypothesis C), but that important interactions are brought about by the compensatory hyperinsulinemia that accompanies insulin resistance (Fig. 4).

Vascular Actions of Insulin

Skeletal muscle is the tissue with the highest resistance to cardiac output, and thus is the site where roughly one third of resting arterial BP is generated (62–64). Since skeletal muscle also is a quantitatively important site of insulin resistance (41), it is logical to suppose the existence of connections between vascular and insulin resistance at this level.

Structural changes in the vasculature—such as are seen in long-standing hypertension—might limit the supply of hormones and substrates to target tissues, thereby leading to insulin resistance. Thus, a raised wall-to-lumen ratio in arterioles might reduce nutritional blood flow to muscle tissues, and capillary rarefaction might lengthen the distance between the capillary axis and cell surface (65). Total blood flow to forearm or leg has

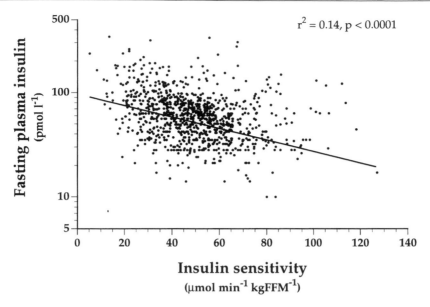

Fig. 4. Reciprocal relationship between fasting plasma insulin concentrations and insulin sensitivity (as measured by a euglycemic insulin clamp) in the nondiabetic, normotensive population of the EGIR study. (Drawn from data in ref. *27*).

generally not been found to be different in hypertensive compared to normotensive subjects *(66)*. However, it is possible that the relative distribution of blood flow to muscle and nonmuscle (subcutaneous tissue, fat, skin, and bone) tissue is altered in hypertension. Thus, if the muscle tissue of the hypertensive subject was richer in Type 2B (fast-twitch, glycolytic) fibers, which are less vascularized than Type 2A (fast-twitch, intermediate) or Type 1 (oxidative) fibers, then a larger fraction of total blood flow would be directed to nonmuscle tissues *(67)*. As a result, fewer muscle cells would be reached by arterial insulin and glucose.

There are problems with the vascular structural hypothesis. First, under conditions of constant exogenous insulin infusion interstitial insulin would eventually achieve the same level in all regions regardless of the diffusion distance. Therefore, a longer lag time between the capillary and the pericellular milieu would translate into dampened excursions of interstitial compared to plasma insulin concentrations, e.g., a flattened postprandial insulin profile, but would not produce insulin resistance under insulin clamp conditions. Second, if diffusion were flow-limited, then different substrates of similar molecular weight should be equally affected. In contrast, to the best of available evidence the insulin resistance of essential hypertension is confined to glucose uptake, FFA exchange and potassium uptake being essentially unaffected. Finally, fewer capillaries per muscle fiber (or larger fiber sections) are found in obese subjects with normal BP levels *(68)*, and, conversely, capillary rarefaction would be functionally inconsequential in the many hypertensive subjects that have normal insulin sensitivity.

In general, muscle fiber composition, with the associated differences in vascular supply and metabolic mode, can explain part of the variability of both BP and insulin sensitivity in the population. Thus, in overweight and/or physically inactive individuals skeletal muscle composition is compatible with the presence of some degree of insulin resistance and a higher BP. Conversely, weight reduction and physical training shift muscle fiber distribution towards more oxidative types, and, concomitantly, improve insulin sensitivity and lower BP *(69,70)*. The covariance of BP and insulin sensitivity with skeletal muscle composition in cross-sectional as well as longitudinal observations does indicate that a general physiological mechanism is operative. However, there is little suggestion that the marked insulin resistance of some patients with essential hypertension may be explained solely on the basis of differences in muscle composition. A corollary of this statement is that structural vascular changes in long-standing hypertension may well be a self-perpetuating mechanism of high BP *(71)* but need not result in metabolically significant changes in blood flow distribution to the limbs.

A variant of the vascular hypothesis calls upon changes in limb blood flow caused by insulin itself. Baron and his coworkers *(72–75)* have pioneered the idea that insulin is an endogenous vasodilator. Thus, in these investigators' hands the response to systemic insulin administration—either with maintenance of euglycemia or with stepped increments in plasma glucose from basal to high levels—consists in an increase in glucose uptake by leg tissues that is paralleled by a large (2–3-fold) increase in leg blood flow. The simultaneous infusion of somatostatin—to paralyze endogenous insulin release—abolishes the vasodilatory effect of hyperglycemia *(75)*. In obese or diabetic subjects with insulin resistance, insulin failed to cause leg vasodilation *(72–74)*. In healthy, insulin sensitive volunteers, insulin-mediated increments in leg blood flow correlated with both glucose utilization and BP levels *(75)*. These findings have been taken to indicate that insulin-induced vasodilation recruits muscle tissue and, in so doing, is a mechanism of insulin-mediated glucose uptake; resistance to insulin action on blood vessels therefore contributes to insulin resistance of glucose uptake.

This is an important physiological issue, which deserves detailed discussion. First of all, in reports from different laboratories the hemodynamic effect of insulin has been highly variable, ranging from robust vasodilatation to vasoconstriction *(76)*. Discrepancies have been imputed to the technique for measuring blood flow (indicator dilution, thermodilution, venous occlusion plethysmography, Doppler ultrasound, positron-emitting tomography [PET]), the limb tested (forearm vs calf), the dose and duration of insulin administration, and the selection of study subjects. As reviewed in *(76)*, insulin exposure (i.e., dose × time) and limb muscularity appear to be more important factors than the anatomical site or the experimental technique in contributing to the variability of insulin-induced vasodilatation. By pooling a number of results in the literature, the relationship between insulin exposure (with the hormone infused locally—through the brachial or femoral artery—or systemically) and changes in blood flow (forearm or calf) can be schematized as depicted in Fig. 5. On mean, it appears that within the physiological range of insulin exposure limb blood flow may rise up to 30% of its baseline value, with a rather wide scatter depending on experimental circumstances.

Second, all techniques for blood flow determination measure total blood flow, not flow distribution. Thus, the question arises whether in response to insulin blood flow only increases its linear velocity within the same metabolic units or recruits additional units (or a combination of the two). Recent PET studies *(77)* have demonstrated that blood flow is distributed in a heterogeneous pattern in leg muscle, and that glucose uptake co-localizes with higher perfusion rates in response to strong insulin stimulation. These findings, however, may simply reflect regional differences in muscle fiber composition, as oxidative Type 1 fibers are both more sensitive to insulin and more richly capillarized,

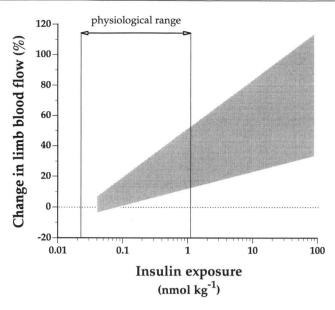

Fig. 5. Change in limb (leg or forearm) blood flow in response to insulin exposure (dose x time, regional or systemic). The shaded area includes the range of values reported by a number of different studies *(76)*.

as previously discussed. By itself, co-localization of flow and metabolism does not prove that insulin actually recruits previously unperfused areas, thereby exposing more tissue to its metabolic action. One way to address this issue is by measuring changes in tissue substrate uptake at different blood flow rates. In studies from our laboratory *(78)*, forearm glucose uptake (in response to infusion of insulin into the brachial artery) was measured in normal subjects at three different blood flow regimens: 1) basal, 2) vasoconstriction with ouabain, and 3) vasodilatation with phentolamine plus propranolol. Setting insulin-mediated glucose uptake at baseline blood flow rates at 100%, when blood flow was reduced by 35% with ouabain, glucose uptake decreased proportionally. In contrast, when blood flow was raised by 237% glucose uptake increased by only 25%. In Fig. 6, these data are plotted against the theoretical curves describing recruitment and gradient dilution (calculated by combining Renkin's model of capillary permeability of blood solutes with Fick's principle). The results are compatible with a mixed, asymmetrical model of perfusion-uptake match in the human forearm. When blood supply is acutely reduced, some tissue segments become critically underperfused (the corresponding data plot on the recruitment function). Indeed, prolonged ouabain infusions can cause ischemic muscle pain. In contrast, when blood flow is increased above baseline, the excess blood appears essentially to flow at higher speed through already perfused areas, thereby diluting tissue glucose gradients enough to stimulate metabolism by a small amount. These studies indicate that, under basal, resting conditions muscle tissue receives just enough blood flow to cover its oxygen demand. Cutting down this amount reduces the uptake of oxygen and other substrates (i.e., it induces ischemia), whereas forcing oxygen through the tissue is largely ineffectual unless metabolic demand is simultaneously increased (e.g., by contraction). This view is supported by two recent studies showing that, in normal volunteers a 20% blood flow reduction was associated

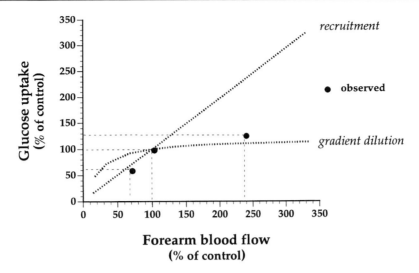

Fig. 6. Predicted (lines) and observed (black dots) changes in forearm glucose uptake as a function of changes in forearm blood flow. *See* text for explanation.

with a proportional reduction in glucose metabolism *(79)*, whereas a leg blood flow increase obtained with a local bradykinine infusion did not significantly stimulate insulin-mediated glucose uptake *(80)*. Thus, the experimental evidence agrees rather closely with the theoretical prediction, that supply through blood flow is rate-limiting for those substrates that are avidly extracted, such as oxygen in the exercising muscle (fractional extraction = 0.8), whereas muscle glucose extraction rarely exceeds 0.4. True capillary recruitment, on the other hand, does not appear to occur to any major extent in resting skeletal muscle exposed to physiological insulin stimulation.

Another observation militating against a role for insulin-mediated vasodilatation in glucose uptake is that, relative to the time-course of insulin action on glucose extraction, insulin vasodilatation is a late phenomenon, whether the hormone is infused systemically *(80)* or locally into the brachial artery *(81)*. Finally, as already mentioned, in the forearm of insulin resistant subjects insulin-mediated glucose extraction is impaired but the exchange of other substrates (lactate, pyruvate, and fatty substrates) is superimposable on that of insulin sensitive individuals *(46)*. This observation is compelling evidence against significant flow-limitation of glucose uptake during insulin stimulation. In keeping with this, several laboratories have reported that insulin vasodilatation is unaltered in native states of insulin resistance (Type 1 diabetes *[83]*, Type 2 diabetes *[77,84]*, essential hypertension *[85]*, and familial hypertension *[86]*). Moreover, in insulin resistant patients with essential hypertension the intraarterial infusion of an endogenous vasodilator, adenosine *(87)*, or of a direct nitric oxide donor, sodium nitroprusside *(88)*, was unable to overcome the insulin resistance. Dissociation between the hemodynamic and metabolic actions of insulin also emerged from recent experiments conducted by Sherrer and coworkers. These authors reported that nitric oxide (NO) synthase inhibition with N^G-monomethyl-L-arginine (L-NMMA), a competitive inhibitor of NO synthase, almost completely abolished insulin-induced calf vasodilatation but was without effect on whole-body insulin-stimulated glucose uptake *(89)*, and that acute reduction of insulin sensitivity (–39%) induced by fat infusion did not change the vascular response to insulin *(90)*.

Collectively, these observations indicate that acute pharmacologic insulinization is followed by some increase in limb blood flow, but this hemodynamic effect is of marginal consequence for insulin stimulation of glucose uptake.

Although the intrinsic vasoactive potency of insulin is weak, its mechanism is interesting. Neither adrenergic nor cholinergic blockade abolishes insulin-induced stimulation of calf blood flow *(91)*, whereas both L-NMMA—by inhibiting NO synthase *(89,92)*—and ouabain—by blocking the insulin-stimulatable Na^+-K^+-ATPase activity *(78,93)*—have been shown to antagonize insulin-induced vasodilatation. Furthermore, in both normal subjects and patients with essential hypertension local insulin infusion in physiological amounts potentiates acetylcholine-induced vasodilatation *(94)*. The exact site of this action of insulin, whether the endothelial or the smooth muscle cell, is not known. Both cell types carry insulin receptors as well as Na^+-K^+-ATPase activity in their plasma membrane *(95,96)*, and can synthetize and release NO. In cultured smooth muscle *(97)*, insulin attenuates agonist-induced increases in intracellular calcium concentrations ($[Ca^{2+}]_i$) thereby causing relaxation. This effect may be due to antagonism of inositol-triphosphate-sensitive Ca^{2+} release from intracellular stores. As L-NMMA blocks the insulin-induced decrease in $[Ca^{2+}]_i$ in smooth muscle cells, NO-mediated increases in cyclic nucleotides (both cAMP and cGMP) appear to be involved *(98)*. In turn, NO can activate Na^+-K^+-ATPase in a cGMP-independent fashion *(99)*. In endothelial cells, on the other hand, activation of Na^+-K^+-ATPase leads to a rise in $[Ca^{2+}]_i$, which would stimulate synthesis and release of NO *(100)*. Thus, insulin impacts on a regulatory system involving two tissues—the endothelium and the underlying smooth muscle—and two effectors—NO, and Na^+-K^+-ATPase—which interact in a complex fashion to elicit vasodilatation. Clearly, additional investigation is needed to understand the cellular basis of insulin-induced vasodilatation.

While the weight of evidence indicates that insulin-mediated vasodilatation is endothelium-dependent, endothelial dysfunction *per se* does not segregate either with insulin resistance of glucose metabolism or with insulin resistance of vasodilatation. Thus, both in normotensive subjects *(101)* and hypertensive patients *(102)*, acetylcholine-induced vasodilatation is similar in very insulin-resistant and insulin sensitive individuals; conversely, insulin-mediated vasodilatation is intact in obese individuals in whom bradykinin-mediated vasodilatation is impaired *(103)*.

Other Hemodynamic Effects of Insulin

Recent studies *(104)* have shown that physiological insulin administration under euglycemic conditions leads to a 3% rise in hematocrit and a 7% reduction in blood volume, compatible with hemoconcentration. Loss of intravascular water to the extravascular space could be due to redistribution of blood flow to capillary beds with higher hydrostatic or lower oncotic pressure. Alternatively, insulin could vasoconstrict postcapillary venules, thereby leading to a generalized increase of the hydrostatic pressure in the capillary bed. The latter explanation is compatible with insulin-induced activation of the adrenergic nervous system (*see* Insulin and the Sympathetic Nervous System).

During systemic insulin administration at physiological doses, cardiac output increases by 10–15% as a result of a small but consistent acceleration of heart rate coupled with an increase in stroke volume *(105)*. These hemodynamic responses also are mediated by adrenergic activation.

The overall effect of simultaneous changes in cardiac output, blood volume, and peripheral vascular resistance in response to euglycemic hyperinsulinemia is maintenance of mean arterial blood pressure. This, however, is a compound of opposite changes in systolic and diastolic blood pressure. The former, in fact, tends to increase as cardiac dynamics are excited by enhanced adrenergic discharge, while the latter decreases due to the drop in peripheral vascular resistances.

Interestingly, the effects of insulin on the cardiovascular system are mediated by both peripheral reflexes and direct central neural influences. Thus, direct relaxation of resistance arteries by insulin evokes tachycardia through the unloading of arterial baroreceptors, a reflex arch that involves central relays. In addition, insulin appears to directly desensitize the sinoatrial node to the baroreflex control of heart rate *(105)* *(see* Insulin and the Sympathetic Nervous System).

Insulin and the Sympathetic Nervous System (SNS)

Systemic insulin administration has an excitatory effect on the SNS even when hypoglycemia is prevented. Thus, exogenous insulin causes a dose-dependent increase in heart rate, systolic BP, and plasma norepinephrine levels *(106,107)*. Furthermore, in healthy subjects microneurography has documented a sustained increase in the firing rate of adrenergic fibers in the peroneal nerve (muscle sympathetic nerve activity or MSNA) in response to euglycemic hyperinsulinemia *(108)*. In accordance with the latter findings, spectral analysis of heart rate variability has shown that acute euglycemic hyperinsulinemia is promptly followed by a shift in the sympathovagal balance due to sympathetic activation and parasympathetic withdrawal *(105)*. Further information on the relationship between the SNS and insulin comes from the studies of Julius and coworkers in the Tecumseh population *(109,110)*, which have shown that: (a) the distribution of cardiac index in the population is bimodal; (b) signs of sympathetic activation (increased heart rate and cardiac output) are the earliest precursor of adult hypertension, as they can be traced back to age 5 yr, when neither overweight nor higher BP are present; and (c) hyperkinetic hypertension is associated with hyperinsulinemia. Enhanced efferent sympathetic traffic to muscle vascular beds, as reflected in MSNA, has been reported in young, borderline hypertensives *(111)*, in patients with mild hypertension *(112)*, and in patients with accelerated essential hypertension *(113)*. Furthermore, in young subjects with mild stable hypertension augmented MSNA is accompanied by increased cardiac output and calf vascular resistance *(114)*. Finally, in the forearm of hypertensive subjects insulin resistance has been found to be associated with increased release of norepinephrine *(115)*. Experimentally, infusion of epinephrine during an insulin clamp causes a profound inhibition of insulin-mediated glucose uptake, which is prevented by a concomitant infusion of propranolol *(116)*.

It has been hypothesized that enhanced central sympathetic outflow may lead to metabolic insulin resistance on one hand, and raise BP on the other *(117)*. There are, however, caveats to this attractive hypothesis. First, only a fraction (~20%) of young subjects with hyperkinetic hypertension progress to stable hypertension. Second, sympathetic traffic is highly selective, between and even within organs. For example, in response to insulin MSNA is increased in the peroneal nerve but not in the kidney; in response to mental stress, MSNA in the arm and leg are dissociated *(118)*. Third, overweight, obstructive sleep apnea, and dietary manipulations all affect MSNA, and are potential confounders in the relationship between MSNA, hemodynamics, and insulin

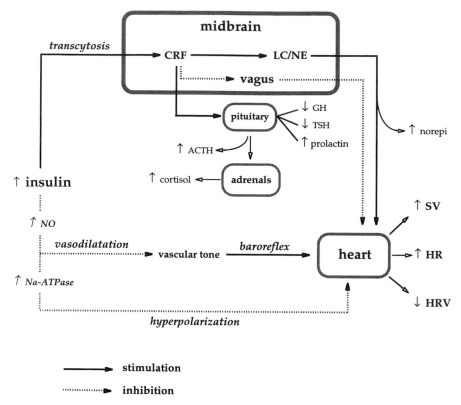

Fig. 7. Integrated scheme for the acute cardiovascular actions of insulin. *See* text for explanation (LC/NE = locus caeruleus; SV = stroke volume; HR = heart rate; HRV = heart rate variability).

resistance *(115)*. Fourth, augmented MSNA is associated with reduced blood flow in the calf *(115)* but vasodilation in the forearm *(108)*. Fifth, whereas epinephrine strongly antagonizes insulin action on glucose uptake, norepinephrine appears to be a much weaker antagonist, if at all. Indeed, chronic (10 days) in vivo norepinephrine infusion in the rat potentiates insulin-stimulated glucose uptake, the effect being partially abolished by propranolol *(119)*. Finally, angiotensin II, which activates the SNS at the level of nerve endings, sympathetic ganglia, and the central nervous system, increases glucose uptake when coinfused with insulin in healthy humans *(120)*.

At present, there is sufficient information to integrate the *acute* hemodynamic and SNS effects into a coherent view (Fig. 7). The key element of the picture is the ability of insulin to act within the central nervous system. Mounting evidence *(121)* indicates that insulin can cross the blood-brain barrier (by a process of transcytosis) in the periventricular area, thereby binding to specific receptors on neurons in the arcuate and paraventricular nuclei. These nuclei then send inhibitory impulses to the vagus and excitatory impulses to the sympathetic nuclei (in the *locus caeruleus*). This reaction is accompanied by release of corticotropin releasing hormone (CRH), which orchestrates a response including stimulation of cortisol and prolactin release, and depression of growth hormone and thyroid stimulating hormone *(105,122)*. Thus, even in the absence of hypoglycemia, the cardiovascular system responds to acute insulin administration with a moderate stress reaction. However, the full physiological significance and the possible pathophysiological implications of this response in states of *chronic* hyperinsulinemia and/or insulin resistance remain to be established.

Insulin and the Renin-Angiotensin-Aldosterone System (RAAS)

POTASSIUM

Insulin is a powerful regulator of potassium (K) metabolism. In healthy subjects, euglycemic insulin infusion causes a dose-dependent fall in plasma K concentrations *(123)*. Insulin-induced hypokalemia is due to a shift of extracellular K into the intracellular compartment mediated by stimulation of Na^+-K^+-ATPase. This effect of insulin is independent of the simultaneous enhancement of glucose uptake *(124)*, and is accompanied by hyperpolarization of the plasma membrane *(125)*. At the same time, baseline urinary K excretion decreases by about 70%, thereby saving K from renal loss *(126)*. Thus, under these conditions insulin's overall effect on K balance is to move large amounts of K from extracellular fluids into cells. If sustained, this accelerated transfer of extracellular K into cells would produce life-threatening hypokalemia. The hypokalemic action of insulin is, however, self-limiting. First, as more K is transported into cells the transmembrane chemical K gradient increases, thereby countering further decrease in extracellular K. Second, the liver, which initially responds to insulin by increasing its net K uptake from plasma, switches to a net K release as hypokalemia ensues. Under euglycemic conditions, insulin-induced hypokalemia is accompanied by a significant increase in plasma renin activity (PRA) and serum angiotensin II concentrations (in the absence of changes in the activity of the angiotensin-converting enzyme), and a pronounced fall in serum aldosterone levels *(127)*. Despite stimulation of renin production and angiotensin II release by insulin, aldosterone output drops under the overriding influence of hypokalemia. Since aldosterone promotes urinary K excretion, the fall in aldosterone potentiates the effect of insulin-induced hypokalemia, which reduces K delivery to the kidney. The overall result is a very efficient restraint on K loss through the urine.

In vitro, insulin at physiological concentrations directly stimulates renin release from rat renal cortical slices *(128)*. This effect is consensual (though weaker) with that of insulin-like growth factor I (IGF-I), and is potently antagonized by angiotensin II.

Classical observations have linked both primary and secondary hyperaldosteronism with impaired carbohydrate metabolism *(128)*. The chief mechanism is aldosterone-induced hypokalemia, which interferes with the insulin secretory response to glucose, thereby worsening glucose tolerance *(129)*. High-dose or prolonged use of thiazide diuretics impairs carbohydrate tolerance mainly through chronic hypokalemia *(130)*. In healthy humans, one week of experimental K deficiency (inducing a 5% depletion of total-body K) impairs the insulin response to steady-state hyperglycemia by ~25% *(131)*. Conversely, preventing insulin-induced hypokalemia significantly increases the insulin secretory response to oral glucose *(132)*, and chronic K supplementation corrects thiazide-induced glucose intolerance *(133)*.

Hyperglycemia opposes the hypokalemic action of insulin. In healthy volunteers, acute hyperglycemia (created by means of a hyperglycemic clamp) with the attendant endogenous insulin response causes significantly less hypokalemia than similar insulin concentrations in the presence of euglycemia *(123)*. This phenomenon is likely to be secondary to hypertonicity. A surplus of osmoles expands the extracellular fluid volume and increases urinary K excretion; simultaneously, however, it causes cellular dehydration *(134)* and an increase in intracellular K concentration, which favors passive diffusion of K out of cells *(135)*. In hyperglycemic patients, the hypokalemic effect of insulin is markedly reduced or absent *(136)*, and is restored by euglycemia *(137)*. The expected consequence of a deficient meal-related hypokalemia is an enhanced urinary K loss, which, unless compensated for by an increased K intake, may deplete total-body K stores. Indeed, in obese Type 2 diabetes patients whole-body K is reduced by 15% in comparison with lean, nondiabetic subjects, and a similar depletion is present in the *vastus lateralis* muscle *(138)*. Furthermore, in obese, glucose-intolerant subjects weight reduction is accompanied by an increase in muscle K levels, which correlates with the diet-induced amelioration of glucose tolerance *(139)*. Since K depletion downregulates Na^+-K^+-ATPase and K transport *(140)*, there is room for a vicious circle leading to progressive K loss. It is therefore expected that the diabetic population should be enriched with patients who, despite being resistant to insulin-mediated hypokalemia, are nevertheless relatively K-depleted.

Abundant evidence supports the existence of an inverse relationship between plasma K concentrations and arterial BP *(141)*. In the general population the urinary Na/K ratio is directly related to BP, both in men and in women *(142)*. Finally, among almost 900 newly diagnosed patients with Type 2 diabetes screened in the United Kingdom Prospective Diabetes Study, the hypertensive patients had significantly lower plasma K levels than the normotensive ones even when they were untreated for their high BP *(143)*.

Sodium

Following up on older observations, DeFronzo et al. *(126)* were the first to report that in healthy humans euglycemic hyperinsulinemia reduces urinary Na excretion. Antinatriuresis is related to plasma insulin in a dose-related fashion within the physiological concentration range (<70 µU/mL) *(144)*. Since insulin antinatriuresis occurs in the absence of changes in glomerular filtration rate or renal lithium clearance, the effect is thought to be exerted on distal tubules. The water co-retained with Na, by increasing the venous return to the heart, causes a rise in stroke volume. If peripheral vascular resistance is unchanged, the increased cardiac output leads to a rise in BP, which disposes of the extra Na retained (pressure natriuresis); fluid volume and BP then return to normal. Under a persistent antinatriuretic drive, the cycle is repeated, until a new steady state is reached, in which a volume-dependent form of hypertension may ensue in the absence of an increase in the total body Na pool.

It is important to distinguish between acute and chronic hyperinsulinemia. During a standard euglycemic clamp (2–4 h), the amount of water retained along with Na is quite small (30–80 mL per hour), and insufficient to cause any change in BP. Furthermore, the rise in cardiac output may be countered by a fall in total peripheral vascular resistance *(108)*. Thus, insulin-induced Na retention *per se* does not acutely raise blood pressure. Nevertheless, it is possible that a chronic antinatriuretic pressure may exert a tensiogenic effect in the long run, especially if coupled with adrenergic activation. This possibility presupposes that chronic hyperinsulinemia in humans results from insulin resistance of glucose metabolism but not natriuresis. With regard to this, obese adolescents, who are hyperinsulinemic, show profound resistance to insulin stimulation of glucose uptake but retain a normal antinatriuretic response to the hormone *(145)*; furthermore, insulin antinatriuresis is intact in patients with essential hypertension who show metabolic insulin resistance *(146)*.

Hyperinsulinemia may not only cause chronic antinatriuresis but may confer salt sensitivity to BP regulation. In fact, the obese, hyperinsulinemic adolescents studied by

Rocchini *et al.* *(147)* were salt sensitive in comparison with nonobese adolescents; such salt sensitivity was lost upon normalizing body weight and insulin levels. Conversely, Sharma et al. *(148)* have shown that in non-obese, young volunteers salt sensitivity is accompanied by a hyperinsulinemic response to oral glucose and insulin resistance. Thus, there appears to be a degree of mutual interdependence between hyperinsulinemia and salt sensitivity in man.

To the extent that pressure natriuresis is able to balance out insulin-mediated Na retention, chronic hyperinsulinemia is not expected to lead to an expansion of the body Na pool. In fact, Weidman and coworkers *(149)* found a normal body Na pool in nondiabetic patients with hypertension regardless of their body weight. In contrast, diabetes is consistently associated with a 10% increase in body Na *(150)*. In renal tubules, Na and glucose undergo coupled transport *(151)*. In diabetic subjects, Na excretion in response to a saline load or water immersion is blunted *(152)*. Therefore, the hyperglycemia of Type 2 diabetes patients is an additional, powerful mechanism of Na retention. This antinatriuretic effect of high plasma glucose levels requires insulin, however. In fact, when insulin is absolutely deficient, such as in decompensated diabetes, Na is actually wasted through the kidneys along with glucose and other electrolytes.

The plasma Na concentration has been found to be, if anything, decreased in nonazotemic diabetic subjects *(150)* in the face of a normal or slightly contracted circulatory volume. This finding, coupled with the hyperosmolarity induced by hyperglycemia and a reduction in the oncotic pressure *(152)*, indicates that diabetes may be associated with an expanded extravascular fluid volume (partly at the expense of intracellular and intravascular fluid volumes). Under these circumstances, pressure natriuresis may no longer be capable of offsetting the excess Na retained by the kidneys. When the body Na pool is expanded, its size is directly correlated with BP *(150)*. Thus, while an expanded Na pool *per se* is not sufficient to raise BP, it may nevertheless favor hypertension in interaction with other factors.

Insulin and Calcium

Cytosolic free calcium concentrations ($[Ca^{2+}]_i$) have been reported to be elevated in cells from subjects with Type 2 diabetes, obesity or hypertension, i.e., in insulin resistant states. A high $[Ca^{2+}]_i$ environment has been associated both with enhanced vascular reactivity in vitro as well as reduced insulin-mediated glucose transport. In hypertensive patients with or without diabetes, intracellular pH values have been reported to be higher than normal. Among essential hypertensives, these ion changes bear tight relations to BP, degree of adiposity, and the insulin response to oral glucose (*see [153]* for review).

These observations have led to the theory that a fundamental disturbance in intracellular calcium homeostasis is the common predecessor of both insulin resistance and hypertension *(154)*. $[Ca^{2+}]_i$ is thought to increase primarily as a result of insufficient extrusion of calcium from the cytosol through a Ca^{2+}-H^+ exchanger (calcium pump or Ca^{2+}-ATPase), which operates in the plasma membrane (calcium efflux) as well as in the endoplasmic or sarcoplasmic membrane (calcium reuptake). The Ca^{2+}-H^+ exchanger is coupled to the Na^+-H^+ antiport, which disposes of intracellular protons. The functional consequences of opposite changes in the operation of these pumps (depressed Ca^{2+}-H^+ leading to excessive Na^+-H^+ exchange) would be vasoconstriction (or enhanced sensitivity to pressor stimuli) and hypertrophy of vascular smooth muscle cells (through cellular alkalinization). Thus, one cellular defect (the triad, high $[Ca^{2+}]_i$, high Na^+-H^+ antiport activity, and higher intracellular pH) would underlie both vasoconstriction and medial hypertrophy, thereby leading to a sustained increase in peripheral vascular resistance.

Normally, insulin blunts agonist-induced increases in $[Ca^{2+}]_i$ in smooth muscle cells *(97)* and platelets *(155)*, favoring relaxation and antagonizing aggregation, respectively. In platelets from insulin resistant subjects, the effect of insulin on platelet $[Ca^{2+}]_i$ is reversed, and aggregation is favored *(155)*. It is therefore possible that resistance to insulin's action on $[Ca^{2+}]_i$ may be a substrate for enhanced vascular tone and platelet hyperaggregability.

At present, the information on $[Ca^{2+}]_i$ and insulin is insufficient or contradictory. The systems that maintain a 10,000:1 gradient between intracellular and extracellular $[Ca^{2+}]$ are as complex *(156,157)* as is the cellular machinery that transduces insulin action; in different cells the relationships between the calcium and insulin systems may be different. Information on the growth-stimulating action of insulin is still mostly based on in vitro studies *(158)*.

CONCLUSIONS

The relationship between insulin and BP is variable in strength and expression. Multiple evidence indicates that the association has a genetic component. Thus, the ethnic differences, the longitudinal observations in normotensive individuals, in prehypertensives, and in offspring of hypertensives, and the knockout experiments in mice all point to an inherent link between insulin and BP. Intrauterine exposure to common insults may also affect BP regulation and insulin sensitivity jointly.

The physiological studies here reviewed indicate that there are several effectors on each side of the association: cardiac output and vascular resistance on the cardiovascular side, plasma glucose, plasma insulin, and insulin resistance on the metabolic side. At least four categories of mechanisms (structural and/or functional changes in the vasculature, modulation by the RAAS, stimulation of the SNS, and intracellular ions) provide bridges whereby one metabolic effector can influence one or the other cardiovascular effector. In general, these mechanisms (a) appear to be operative under physiological circumstances (e.g., they intervene to integrate responses to overeating or energy restriction, to physical activity or stress); (b) are asymmetric, for there is more room for the metabolic effectors to impact on the cardiovascular variables than the other way around; and (c) are not mutually exclusive, and may in fact need to be combined to determine a quantitative shift in the cardiovascular system (e.g., capillary rarefaction plus overactive SNS in the high BP of the obese). Some mechanisms (structural vascular changes, sodium retention) have a longer time frame than others (sympathetic activation, vasodilatation, intracellular ion changes), and may therefore come into play at different stages in the natural history of 'metabolic' hypertension. None of them alone, however, appears to be strong and specific enough to explain hypertension.

CLINICAL AND THERAPEUTIC IMPLICATIONS

The finding of high plasma insulin or low insulin sensitivity in a hypertensive patient is a red flag for the presence of the cluster of abnormalities that frequently accompany insulin resistance (glucose intolerance, high serum triglycerides, low HDL-cholesterol levels, prevalence of small, dense LDL particles *(159)*, raised levels of plasminogen-activator-inhibitor 1 (PAI-1) *(160)*, microalbuminuria, and high Na/Li CT). Each of these abnormalities, and, possibly, hyperinsulinemia itself, has been shown to be a risk factor for atherosclerotic cardiovascular disease *(161,162)*. In the presence of significant co-morbidity, the diagnostic threshold for each risk factor should be lowered, and treatment of any of them should consider the impact on the others. Accordingly, a BP of 140/90 mmHg may be normal in a nondiabetic person, but may be too high in a diabetic patient, all the more so if family history is positive for hypertension, if the diabetes is of long duration, or microalbuminuria is present.

There are potential therapeutic implications to the association of insulin resistance with high BP. First, the presence of insulin resistance may weaken the BP-lowering effect of some antihypertensive agents. In one population-based study in Israel, obese, diabetic, or otherwise hyperinsulinemic patients had a higher dosage score (frequency of combined therapy or higher doses of monotherapy) of antihypertensive medication than nondiabetic, lean hypertensives *(163)*. In another study in nondiabetic hypertensives, refractoriness to antihypertensive therapy was associated with more insulin resistance, central obesity, and larger muscle fiber area *(164)*. Second, in response to physiological intervention (diet and regular physical exercise) consensual decrements in plasma insulin concentration and BP are commonly observed. In a study of obese women, these changes were more marked in those who had greater initial hyperinsulinemia *(165)*. Thus, the presence of insulin resistance may identify a subgroup of patients more likely to benefit from physiological intervention. Finally, some antihypertensive agents may negatively affect glucose tolerance and insulin sensitivity *(166)*. In particular, diuretics (thiazides at high doses) and β-blocking agents may unmask latent glucose intolerance and worsen metabolic control in known diabetics. Antihypertensive agents that do not affect glucose, insulin, or lipid metabolism (angiotensin-converting-enzyme inhibitors, α-adrenergic blockers, calcium channel blockers, angiotensin II receptor antagonists) are recommended as first-line therapy, especially in diabetic patients. Clearly, when specific clinical circumstances demand a diuretic (e.g., edema) or a β-blocker (e.g., recent MI), judicious use (in low dose, in combination, for a short time) of these drugs is warranted.

REFERENCES

1. Fuller JH. Epidemiology of hypertension associated with diabetes mellitus. Hypertension 7(Suppl II):1985;3–7.
2. Kannel, WB, McGee DL. Diabetes and glucose tolerance as risk factors for cardiovascular disease: the Framingham Study. Diabetes Care 1978;2:120–126.
3. Turner RC, Mann J, Oakes S, Nugent Z, Moore J, Peto R, Stark T, Todd L. United Kingdom Prospective Diabetes Study, a multicenter study. Hypertension 1985;7(Suppl II):8–13.
4. Krolewski AS, Warram JH, Cupples A, Gorman CK, Szabo AJ, Christlieb AR. Hypertension, orthostatic hypotension and the microvascular complications of diabetes. J Chron Dis 1985;38:319–326.
5. Haffner SM, Valdez R, Morales PA, Mitchell BD, Hazuda HP, Stern MP. Greater effect of glycemia on incidence of hypertension in women than in men. Diabetes Care 1992;15:1277–1284.
6. Sprafka JM, Bender AP, Jagger HG. Prevalence of hypertension and associated risk factors among diabetic individuals. The three-city study. Diabetes Care 1988;11:17–22.
7. Barrett-Connor E, Criqui MH, Klauber MR, Holdbrook M. Diabetes and hypertension in a community of older adults. Am J Epidemiol 1981;113:276–284.
8. Reaven PD, Barrett-Connor EL, Browner DK. Abnormal glucose tolerance and hypertension. Diabetes Care 1990;13:119–125.
9. Simpson NE. Heritabilities of liability to diabetes when sex and age at onset are considered. Ann Hum Genet 1969;32:283–303.
10. Krolewski AS, Czyzyk A, Kopczynski J, Rywik S. Prevalence of diabetes mellitus, coronary heart disease and hypertension in the families of insulin dependent and insulin independent diabetics. Diabetologia 1981;21:520–524.

11. Stamler J, Stamler R, Rhomberg P, et al. Multivariate analysis of the relationship of six variables to BP: findings from Chicago surveys, 1965–1971. J Chron Dis 1975;28:499–525.

12. Florey CduV, Uppal S, Lowy C. Relation between BP, weight, and plasma sugar and serum insulin levels in schoolchildren aged 9–12 years in Westland, Holland. BMJ 1976;1:1368–1371.

13. Salomaa VV, Strandberg TE, Vanhanen H, Naukkarinen V, Sarna S, Miettinen TA. Glucose tolerance and BP: long term follow up in middle aged men. BMJ 1991;302:493–496.

14. Medalie JH, Papier CM, Goldbourt U, Herman JB. Major factors in the development of diabetes mellitus in 10,000 men. Arch Intern Med 1975;135:811–817.

15. Mogensen CE. Prediction of clinical diabetic nephropathy in IDDM patients: alternative to microalbuminuria? Diabetes 1990;39:761–767.

16. Krolewski AS, Canessa M, Warram J, Laffel LMB, Christlieb AR, Knowler WC, Rand LI. Predisposition to hypertension and susceptibility to renal disease in insulin-dependent diabetes mellitus. N Engl J Med 1988;318:140–145.

17. Mangili R, Bending JJ, Scott G, Li LK, Gupta A, Viberti GC. Increased sodium-lithium countertransport activity in red cells of patients with insulin-dependent diabetes and nephropathy. N Engl J Med 1988;318:146–150.

18. Benhamou PY, Halimi S, De Gaudemaris R, Boizel R, Pitiot M, Siche JP, Bachelot I, Mallion JM. Early disturbances of ambulatory BP load in normotensive Type 1 diabetic patients with microalbuminuria. Diabetes Care 1992;15:1614–1619.

19. Trevisan R, Nosadini R, Fioretto P, Semplicini A, Donadon V, Doria A, Nicolosi G, Zanuttini D, Cipollina MR, Lusiani L, Avogaro A, Crepaldi G, Viberti GC. Clustering of risk factors in hypertensive insulin-dependent diabetics with high sodium-lithium countertransport. Kidney Int 1992;41:855–861.

20. Parving HH, Mogensen CE, Jensen HAE, Evrin PE. Increased urinary albumin excretion rate in benign essential hypertension. Lancet 1974;1:1190–1192.

21. Viberti GC, Walker JD, Pinto J. Diabetic nephropathy. In: Alberti KGMM, DeFronzo RA, Keen H, Zimmet P, eds. International Textbook of Diabetes Mellitus. John Wiley & Sons, Chichester, 1992, pp. 1267–1328.

22. Savicki PT, Kaiser S, Heinemann L, Frenzel H, Berger M. Prevalence of renal artery stenosis in diabetes mellitus—an autopsy study. J Intern Med 1991;229:489–492.

23. Barker DJP, Bull AR, Osmond C, Simmonds SJ. Fetal and placental size and risk of hypertension in adult life. BMJ 1990;301:259–262.

24. Hales CN, Barker DJP, Clark PMS, Cox LJ, Fall C, Osmond C, Winter PD. Fetal and infant growth and impaired glucose tolerance at age 64. BMJ 1991;303:1019–1022.

25. Valdez R, Athens M, Thompson GA, Bradshw BS, Stern M. Birth weight and adult health outcomes in a biethnic population in the US. Diabetologia 1994;37:624–631.

26. Breschi MC, Seghieri G, Bartolomei G, Sironi A, Baldi S, Ferrannini E. Relation of birth weight to maternal plasma glucose and insulin concentrations during normal pregnancy. Diabetologia 1993;36:1315–1321.

27. Ferrannini E, Natali A, Capaldo B, Lehtovirta M, Jacob S, Yki-Järvinen H. Insulin resistance, hyperinsulinemia, and blood pressure. Role of age and obesity. Hypertension 1997;30:1144–1149.

28. Ferrannini E. The hemodynamics of obesity: a theoretical analysis. J Hypertens 1992;10:1417–1423.

29. Messerli FH, Sundgaard-Riise K, Reisin E, Dreslinski G, Dunn FG, Frolich E. Disparate cardiovascular effects of obesity and arterial hypertension. Am J Med 1983;74:808–812.

30. Kissebah AH, Vydelingum N, Murray R, Evans DJ, Hartz AJ, Kalkhoff RK, Adams P. Relation of body fat distribution to metabolic complications of obesity. J Clin Endocrinol Metab 1982;54:254–260.

31. Krotkieswi M, Biörntorp P, Sjöström L, Smith U. Impact of obesity on metabolism in men and women: importance of regional adipose tissue distribution. J Clin Invest 1983;72:1150–1162.

32. Björntorp P. Visceral fat accumulation: the missing link between psychosocial factors and cardiovascular disease? J Intern Med 1991;230:195–201.

33. Welborn TA, Breckenridge A, Rubinstein AH, Dollery CT, Russel Frazer, T. Serum-insulin in essential hypertension and in peripheral vascular disease. Lancet 1966;i:1366–1367.

34. Singer CB, Lucas CP, Estigarribia JA, Darga LL, Reaven GM. Insulin and blood pressure in obesity. Hypertension 1985;7:702–706.

35. Ferrannini E, Haffner SM, Stern MP, Mitchell BD, Natali A, Hazuda HP, Patterson JK. High blood pressure and insulin resistance: influence of ethnic background. Eur J Clin Invest 1991;21:280–287.

36. Denker PS, Pollock VE. Fasting serum insulin levels in essential hypertension. A meta-analysis. Arch Intern Med 1992;152:1649–1651.

37. Haffner SM, Stern MP, Hazuda HP, Mitchell BD, Patterson JK, Ferrannini E. Parental history of diabetes is associated with increased cardiovascular risk factors. Arteriosclerosis 1989;9:928–933.

38. Hunt SC, Wu LL, Hopkins PN, Stults BM, Kuida H, Ramirez ME, Lalouel JM, Williams RR. Apolipoprotein, low density lipoprotein subfraction and insulin associations with familial combined hyperlipidemia: study of Utah patients with familial dyslipidemic hypertension. Arteriosclerosis 1989;9:335–344.

39. Ferrari P, Weidmann P, Shaw S, Giachino D, Riesen W, Allemann Y, Heynen G. Altered insulin sensitivity, hyperinsulinemia, and dyslipidemia in individuals with a hypertensive parent. Am J Med 1991;91:589–596.

40. Haffner SM, Ferrannini E, Hazuda HP, Stern MP. Clustering of cardiovascular risk factors in confirmed prehypertensive individuals. Hypertension 1992;20:38–45.

41. Ferrannini E, Buzzigoli G, Bonadonna R, Giorico MA, Oleggini M, Graziadei L, Pedrinelli R, Brandi L, Bevilacqua S. Insulin resistance in essential hypertension. N Engl J Med 1987;317:350–357.

42. Shen D-C, Shieh S-M, Fuh MM-T, Wu D-A, Chen Y-DI, Reaven GM. Resistance to insulin-stimulated glucose uptake in patients with hypertension. J Clin Endocrinol Metab 1988;66:580–583.

43. Pollare T, Lithell H, Berne C. Insulin resistance is a characteristic feature of primary hypertension indepedent of obesity. Metabolism 1990;39:167–174.

44. Lind L, Lithell H, Pollare T. Is it hyperinsulinemia or insulin resistance that is related to hypertension and other metabolic cardiovascular risk factors? J Hypertens 1993;11(Suppl 4):S11–S16.

45. Natali A, Quiñones Galvan A, Arzilli F, Taddei S, Pecori N, Frascerra S, Salvetti A, Ferrannini E. Renovascular hypertension and insulin sensitivity. Eur J Clin Invest 1996;26:556–563.

46. Natali A, Santoro D, Palombo C, Cerri M, Ghione S, Ferrannini E. Impaired insulin action on skeletal muscle metabolism in essential hypertension. Hypertension 17:170–178.

47. Nuutila P, Maki M, Laine H, Knuuti MJ, Ruotsalainen U, Luotolahti M, Haaparanta M, Salin O, Jula A, Koivisto V, et al. Insulin action on heart and skeletal muscle glucose uptake in essential hypertension. J Clin Invest 1995;96:1003–1009.

48. Salvatore T, Cozzolino D, Giunta R, Giugliano D, Torella R, D'Onofrio F. Decreased insulin clearance as a feature of essential hypertension. J Clin Endocrinol Metab 1992;74:144–149.

49. Laakso M, Sarlund H, Mykkänen I. Essential hypertension and insulin resistance in non-insulin-dependent diabetes. Eur J Clin Invest 1989;19:518–526.

50. Doria A, Fioretto P, Avogaro A, Carraro A, Morocutti A, Trevisan R, Frigato F, Crepaldi G, Viberti G, Nosadini R. Insulin resistance is associated with high sodium-lithium countertransport in essential hypertension. Am J Physiol 1991;261:E694–E691.

51. Sharma AM, Ruland K, Spies KP, et al. Salt sensitivity in young normotensive subjects is associated with a hyperinsulinemic response to oral glucose. J Hypertension 1991;9:329–335.

52. Bianchi S, Bigazzi R, Valtriani C, Chiapponi I, Sgherri S, Baldari G, Natali A, Ferrannini E, Campese VM. Hyperinsulinemia in patients with essential hypertension and microalbuminuria. Hypertension 1994;23:681–688.

53. Bianchi S, Bigazzi R, Quiñones Galvan A, Muscelli A, Pecori N, Ciociaro D, Ferrannini E, Natali A. Insulin resistance in microalbuminuric hypertension: sites and mechanisms. Hypertension 1995;26:789–796.

54. Ferrari P, Weidmann P. Insulin, insulin sensitivity and hypertension. J Hypertens 1990;8:491–500.

55. Vettor R, Cusin I, Ganten D, Rohner-Jeanrenaud F, Ferrannini E, Jeanrenaud B. Insulin resistance and hypertension: studies in transgenic hypertensive TGR(mREN-2)27 rats. Am J Physiol 1994; 267:R1503–1510.

56. Brands MW, Hildebrandt DA, Mizelle L, Hall JE. Hypertension during chronic hyperinsulinemia in rats is not salt-sensitive. Hypertension 1992;19(Suppl I):I83–I89.

57. Brands MW, Mizelle HL, Gaillard CA, Hildebrandt DA, Hall JE. The hemodynamic response to chronic hyperinsulinemia in conscious dog. Am J Hypertens 1991;4:164–168.

58. Schotte DE, Stunkard AJ The effects of weight reduction on blood pressure in 301 patients. Arch Intern Med 150:1701–1704.

59. Stenbit EA, Tsao TS, Li J, Burcelin R, Geenen DL, Factor SM, Houseknecht K, Katz EB, Charron MJ. GLUT4 heterozygous knockout mice develop muscle insulin resistance and diabetes. Nat Med 1997;10:1096–1101.

60. Whithers DJ, Gutierrez JS, Towery H, Burks DJ, Ren JM, Previs S, Zhang Y, Bernal D, Pons S, Shulman GI, Bonner-Weir S, White M. Disruption of IRS-2 causes Type 2 diabetes in mice. Nature 1988;391:900–904.

61. Groop LC,. Kankuri M, Schalin-Jantti C, Ekstrand A, Nikula-Ijas P, Widen E, Kniskanen E, Eriksson J, Franssila-Kallunki A, Saloranta C, et al. Association between polymorphism of the glycogen synthase gene and non-insulin-dependent diabetes mellitus. N Engl J Med 1993;328:10–14.

62. Greene AS, Tonellato PJ, Lui J, Lombard JH, Cowley AW Jr. Microvascular rarefaction and tissue vascular resistance in hypertension. Am J Physiol 1989;256:H126–H131.

63. Edgerton VR, Smith JL, Simpson DR. Muscle fiber type populations of human leg muscles. Histochem J 1975;7:259–266.

64. Weinsier RL, Norris DJ, Birch R, Bernstein RS, Wang J, Yang M-U, Pierson RN Jr, Van Itallie TB. The relative contribution of body fat and fat pattern to blood pressure level. Hypertension 1985; 7:578–585.

65. Ferrannini E. Insulin and blood pressure: possible role of hemodynamics. Clin Exp Hyper 1992; A14(1&2):271–284.

66. Raison JM, Safar ME, Cambien F, London GM. Forearm haemodynamics in obese normotensive and hypertensive subjects. J Hypertens 1988;6:299–303.

67. Juhlin-Dannfelt A, Frisk-Holmberg M, Karlsson J, Tesch P. Central and peripheral circulation in relation to muscle-fibre composition in normo-and hyper-tensive man. Clin Sci 1979;56:335–340.

68. Lillioja S, Young AA, Cutter CL, Ivy JL, Abbott WGH, Zawadski JK, Yki-Järvinen H, Christin L, Secomb TW, Bogardus C. Skeletal muscle capillary density and fiber type are possible determinants of in vivo insulin resistance in man. J Clin Invest 1987;80:415–424.

69. McArdle W, Katch FI, Katch VL. Exercise physiology. Energy, nutrition, and human performance, 3rd ed. Lea & Febiger, London, 1991, pp. 348–366.

70. Zeman RJ, Ludemann R, Easton TG, Etlinger JD. Slow to fast alterations in skeletal muscle fibers caused by clenbuterol, a β-2-receptor agonist. Am J Physiol 1988;254:E726–E732.

71. Lever AF. Slow pressor mechanisms in hypertension: a role for hypertrophy of resistance vessels? J Hypertension 1986;7:259–266.

72. Laakso M, Edelman SV, Brechtel G, Baron AD. Decreased effect of insulin to stimulate skeletal muscle blood flow in obese man: a novel mechanism for insulin resistance. J Clin Invest 1990;85:1844–1852.

73. Baron AD, Laakso M, Brechtel G, Edelman SV. Mechanism of insulin resistance in insulin-dependent-diabetes mellitus: a major role for reduced skeletal muscle blood flow. J Clin Endocrinol Metab 1991;73:637–643.

74. Laakso M, Edelman S, Brechtel G, Baron AD. Impaired insulin mediated skeletal muscle blood flow in patients with NIDDM Diabetes 1992;41:1076–1083.

75. Baron AD. Cardiovascular actions of insulin in humans. Implications for insulin sensitivity and vascular tone. In: Ferrannini E, ed. Insulin resistance and disease. Baillière's Clinical Endocrinology and Metabolism, LBaillière Tindall, London, vol 7, n° 4, 1993, pp. 961–988.

76. Yki-Järvinen H, Utriainen T. Insulin-induced vasodilatation: physiology or pharmacology? Diabetologia 1998;41:369–379.

77. Utriainen T, Nuutila P, Takala T, Vicini P, Ruotsalainen U, Rönnemaa T, Tolvanen T, Raitakari M, Haaparanta M, Kirvelä O, Cobelli C, Yki-Järvinen H. Intact insulin stimulation of skeletal muscle blood flow, its heterogeneity and redistribution but not of glucose uptake in non-insulin-dependent diabetes mellitus. J Clin Invest 1997;100:777–785.

78. Ferrannini E, Taddei S, Santoro D, Natali A, Boni C, Del Chiaro D, Buzzigoli G Independent stimulation of glucose metabolism and Na^+-K^+ exchange by insulin in the human forearm. Am J Physiol 255:E953–E958.

79. Jamerson K, Smith S, Amerena J, Grant E, Julius S. Vasoconstriction with norepinephrine causes less forearm insulin resistance than a reflex sympathetic vasoconstriction. Hypertension 1994;23:1006–1011.

80. Nuutila P, Raitakari M, Laine H, et al. Role of blood flow in regulating insulin-stimulated glucose uptake in humans. J Clin Invest 1996;97:1741–47.

81. Utriainen T, Malmström R, Mäkimattila S, Yki-Järvinen H. Methodological aspects, dose-response characetristics and causes of inter-individual variation in insulin stimulation of limb blood flow in normal subjects. Diabetologia 1995;38:555–564.

82. Tack CJ, Schefman AE, Willems JC, Thien T, Lutterman JA, Smits P. Direct vasodilator effects of physiological hyperinsulinaemia in human skeletal muscle. Eur J Clin Invest 1996;26:772–778.

83. Mättimakila S, Virtamäki A, Malmström R, Utriainen T, Yki-Järvinen H. Insulin resistance in type I diabetes mellitus: a major role for reduced glucose extraction. J Clin Endocrinol Metab 1996;81:707–712.

84. Tack CJJ, Smits P, Willemsen JJ, Lenders JWM, Thien T, Lutterman JA. Effects of insulin on vascular tone and sympathetic nervous system in NIDDM Diabetes 1996;45:15–22.

85. Hunter SJ, Harper R, Ennis CN, Sheridan B, Atkinson AB, Bell PM. Skeletal muscle blood flow is not a determinant of insulin resistance in essential hypertension. J Hypertens 1997;15:73–77.

86. Hulten UL, Endre T, Mattiasson I, Berglund G. Insulin and forearm vasodilatation in hypertension-prone men. Hypertension 1995;25:214–218.

87. Natali A, Bonadonna R, Santoro D, Quiñones Galvan A, Baldi S, Frascerra S, Palombo C, Ghione S, Ferrannini E. Insulin resistance and vasodilatation in essential hypertension. Studies with adenosine. J Clin Invest 1994;94:1570–1576.

88. Natali A, Quiñones Galvan A, Toschi E, Pecori N, Sanna G, Ferrannini E (1998) Vasodilation with sodium nitroprusside does not improve insulin action in essential hypertension. Hypertension 1998;31:632–636.

89. Scherrer U, Randin D, Vollender P, Vollender L, Nicod P. Nitric oxide release accounts for insulin's vascular effects in humans. J Clin Invest 1994;94:2511–2515.

90. Vollenweider L, Tappy L, Owlya R, Jéquier E, Nicod P, Scherrer U. Insulin-induced sympathetic activation and vasodilatation in skeletal muscle. Effects of insulin resistance in lean subjects. Diabetes 1995;44:641–645

91. Randin D, Vollenweider P, Tappy L, Jequier E, Nicod P, Scherrer U. Effects of adrenergic and cholinergic blockade on insulin-induced stimulation of calf blood flow in humans. Am J Physiol 1994;266:R809–R816.

92. Steinberg HO, Brechtel G, Johson A, Fireberg N, Baron AD. Insulin-mediated skeletal muscle vasodilatation is nitric oxide dependent. A novel action of insulin to increase nitric oxide release. J Clin Invest 94:1172–1179.

93. Tack CJJ, Lutterman JA, Vervoot G, Thien T, Smits P. Activation of the sodium-potassium pump contributes to insulin-induced vasodilatation in humans. Hypertension 1996;28:426–432.

94. Taddei S, Virdis A, Mattei P, Natali A, Ferrannini E, Salvetti A. Effect of insulin on acetylcholine-induced vasodilatation in normotensive subjects and patients with essential hypertension. Circulation 1995;92:2911–2918.

95. Meharg JV, McGowan-Jordan J, Charles A, Parmelee JT, Cutaia MV, Rounds S. Hydrogen peroxide stimulates sodium-potassium pump activity in cultured pulmonary arterial endothelial cells. Am J Physiol 1993;265:L613–L621.

96. Tirupattur PR, Ram JL, Tandley PR, Sowers JR. Regulation of Na^+-K^+-ATPase gene expression by insulin in vascular smooth muscle cells. Am J Hypertens 1993;6:626–629.

97. Kahn AM, Seidel CL, Allen JC, O'Neil G, Shelat H, Song T. Insulin reduces contraction and intracellular calcium concentration in vascular smooth muscle. Hypertension 1993;22:735–742.

98. Trovati M, Anfossi G. Insulin, insulin resistance and platelet function: similarities with insulin effects on cultured vascular smooth muscle cells. Diabetologia 1998;41:609–622.

99. Gupta S, McArthur C, Grady C, Ruderman NB. Stimulation of vascular Na^+-K^+-ATPase activity by nitric oxide: a cGMP-independent effect. Am J Physiol 1994;266:H2146–2151.

100. Moncada S, Palmer RMJ. The L-arginine-nitric oxide pathway in the vessel wall. In: Moncada S, Higgs B, eds. Nitric Oxide from L-arginine: A Bioregulatory System Elesevier, Amsterdam. 1990, pp. 19–33.

101. Utriainen T, Makimattila S, Virkamaki A, Bergholm R, Yki-Järvinen H. Dissociation between insulin sensitivity of glucose uptake and endothelial function in normal subjects. Diabetologia 1996;39:1477–1482.

102. Natali A, Taddei S, Quiñones Galvan A, Camastra S, Baldi S, Frascerra S, Virdis A, Sudano I, Salvetti A, Ferrannini E. Insulin sensitivity, vascular reactivity, and clamp-induced vasodilatation in essential hypertension. Circulation 96:849–855.

103. Laine H, Yki-Järvinen H, Kirvela O, Tolvanen T, Raitakari M, Solin O, Haaparanta M, Knuuti J, Nuutila P Insulin resistance of glucose uptake in skeletal muscle cannot be ameliorated by enhancing endothelium-dependent blood flow in obesity. J Clin Invest 1998;101:1156–1162.

104. Catalano C, Muscelli E, Quiñones Galvan A, Baldi S, Masoni A, Gibb I, Torffvit O, Seghieri G, Ferrannini E. Effect of insulin on systemic and renal handling of albumin in nondiabetic and NIDDM subjects. Diabetes 1997;46:868–875.

105. Muscelli E, Emdin M, Natali A, Pratali L, Camastra S, Baldi S, Carpeggiani C, Ferrannini E. Cardiac responses to insulin in vivo: influence of obesity. J Clin Endocrinol Metab 1998;83:2084–2090.

106. Rowe JR, Young JB, Minaker KL, Stevens AL, Pallotta J, Landsberg L. Effect of insulin and glucose infusions on sympathetic nervous system activity in normal man. Diabetes 1981;30:219–225.

107. Gans ROB, v d Toorn L, Bilo HJG, et al. Renal and cardiovascular effects of exogenous insulin in healthy volunteers. Clin Sci 1991;80:219–225.

108. Anderson EA, Hoffman RP, Balon TW, Sinkley CA, Mark, AL. Hyperinsulinemia produces both sympathetic neuronal activation and vasodilation in normal humans. J Clin Invest 1991;87:2246–2252.

109. Julius S, Krause L, Schork N, et al. Hyperkinetic borderline hypertension in Tecumseh, Michigan. J Hypertens 1991;9:77–84.

110. Julius S. The interconnection between sympathetics, microcirculation, and insulin resistance in hypertension. Blood Press 1992;1:9–19.

111. Anderson EA, Christine AS, Lawton WJ, Mark AL. Elevated sympathetic nerve activity in borderline hypertensive humans. Hypertension 1989;14:177–183.

112. Yamada Y, Miyajima E, Tochikubo O, Matsukawa T, Ishii M. Age-related changes in muscle sympathetic nerve activity in essential hypertension. Hypertension 1989;13:870–877.

113. Matsukawa T, Mano T, Ishii M. Elevated sympathetic nerve activity in patients with accelerated essential hypertension. J Clin Invest 1993;92:25–28.

114. Floras JS, Hara K. Sympathoneural and hemodynamic characteristics of young subjects with mild essential hypertension. J Hypertens 1993;11:647–655.

115. Lembo G, Napoli R, Capaldo B, Redina V, Iaccarino G, Volpe M, Trimarco B, Saccà L. Abnormal sympathetic overactivity evoked by insulin in the skeletal muscle of patients with essential hypertension. J Clin Invest 1992;90:24–29.

116. Deibert DC, DeFronzo RA (1980) Epinephrine-induced insulin resistance in man. J Clin Invest 65:717–721.

117. Reaven GM, Lithell H, Landsberg L. Hypertension and associated metabolic abnormalities. The role of insulin resistance and the sympathoadrenal system. N Engl J Med 1996;334:374–381.

118. Anderson EA, Wallin BG, Mark AL. Dissociation of sympathetic nerve activity in arm and leg muscle during mental stress. Hypertension 1987;9(Suppl III):III114–III119.

119. Lupien JR, Hirshman MF, Horton ES. Effects of norepinephrine infusion on in vivo insulin sensitivity and responsiveness. Am J Physiol 1990;259:E210–E215.

120. Buchanan TA, Thawani H, Kades W, Modrall JG, Weaver FA, Laurel C, Poppiti R, Xiang A, Hsueh W. Angiotensin II increases glucose utilization during acute hyperinsulinemia via a hemodynamic mechanism. J Clin Invest 92:720–726.

121. Davis SN, Colburn C, Robbins R, Nadeau S, Neal D, Williams P, Cherrington AD. Evidence that the brain of the conscious dog is insulin sensitive. J Clin Invest 1995;95:593–602

122. Schwartz MW, Figlewicz DP, Baskin DB, Woods SC, Porte D Jr. Insulin in the brain: a hormonal regulator of energy balance. Endocr Rev 1992;13:81–113

123. DeFronzo RA, Felig P, Ferrannini E, Wahren J. Effect of graded doses of insulin on splanchnic and peripheral potassium metabolism in man. Am J Physiol 1980; 238:E421–E427.

124. Andres R, Baltzan, M, Cader G, Zierler K. Effects of insulin on carbohydrate metabolism and on potassium in the forearm of man. J Clin Invest 1962;41:108–15.

125. Zierler K. Effect of insulin on membrane potential and potassium content of rat muscle. Am J Physiol 1959;197:515–523.

126. DeFronzo RA, Cooke CR, Andres R, Faloona GR, Davis PJ. The effect of insulin on renal handling of sodium, potassium, calcium, and phosphate in man. J Clin Invest 1975;55:845–855.

127. Trovati M, Massucco P, Anfossi G, Cavalot F, Mularoni E, Mattiello L, Rocca G, Emanuelli G. Insulin influences the renin-angiotensin-aldosterone system in humans. Metabolism 1989;38:501–503.

128. Jost-Vu E, Horton R, Antonipillai I. Altered regulation of renin secretion by insulin-like growth factors and angiotensin II in diabetic rats. Diabetes 1992;41:1100–1105.

129. Conn JW. Hypertension, the potassium ion and impaired carbohydrate tolerance. N Engl J Med 273:1135–1143.

130. Gorden P. Glucose intolerance with hypokalemia. Diabetes 1973;22:544–551.

131. Rowe JW, Tobin JD, Rosa RM, Andres R. Effect of experimental potassium deficiency on glucose and insulin metabolism. Metabolism 1980;29:498–502.

132. Natali A, Quiñones Galvan A, Santoro D, Taddei S, Salvetti A, Ferrannini E. Relationship between insulin release, antinatriuresis, and hypokalemia following glucose ingestion in normal and hypertensive man. Clin Sci 1993;85:327–335.

133. Helderman JH, Elahi D, Andersen DK, Raizes GS, Tobin JD, Shocken D, Andres R (1983) Prevention of the glucose intolerance of thiazide diuretics by maintenance of body potassium. Diabetes 32:106–111.

134. Feig PU, McCurdy DK. The hypertonic state. N Engl J Med 1977;297:1444–1454.
135. Sterns RH, Cox M, Feig PU, Singer I. Internal potassium balance and the control of plasma potassium concentration. Medicine 1981;60:339–354.
136. Ferrannini E, Seghieri G, Muscelli E. Insulin and the renin-angiotensin-aldosterone system: influence of ACE inhibition. J Cardiovasc Pharmacol 1994;24(Suppl 3):S61–S80.
137. Bevilacqua S, Buzzigoli G, Bonadonna R, Brandi LS, Oleggini M, Boni C, Geloni M, Ferrannini E. Operation of Randle's cycle in patients with NIDDM Diabetes 1990;39:383–389.
138. Landin K, Lindgärde F, Saltin B, Wilhelmsen L Increased skeletal muscle Na/K ratio in obese men, but not in women, with glucose intolerance. J Intern Med 225:89–94.
139. Landin K, Lindgärde F, Saltin B. Skeletal muscle potassium increases after diet and weight reduction in obese subjects with normal and impaired glucose tolerance. Acta Endocrinol 1989;121:21–26.
140. Norgaard A, Kjeldsen K, Clausen T. Potassium depletion decreases the number of 3H-ouabain binding sites and the Na-K transport in skeletal muscle. Nature 1981;293:739–741.
141. Beretta-Piccoli C, Davies DL, Boddy K, Brown JJ, Cumming AMM, East BW, Fraser R, Lever AF, Padfield PL, Semple PF, Robertson JI, Weidmann P, Williams ED. Relation of arterial pressure with body sodium, body potassium and plasma potassium in essential hypertension. Clin Sci 1982;63:257–270.
142. Khaw K-T, Barrett-Connor E. The association between blood pressure, age, and dietary sodium and potassium: a population study. Circulation 1988;77:53–61.
143. United Kingdom Prospective Diabetes Study. III. Prevalence of hypertension and antihypertensive therapy in patients with newly diagnosed diabetes: a multicenter study. Hypertension 1985;7(Suppl II):II811–II813.
144. Skott P, Hother-Nielsen O, Bruun NE, et al. Effects of insulin on kidney function and sodium excretion, in healthy subjects. Diabetologia 1989;32:694–699.
145. Rocchini AP, Katch V, Kveselis,D, et al. Insulin and renal sodium retention in obese adolescents. Hypertension 1989;14:367–374.
146. Muscelli E, Natali A, Bianchi S, Bigazzi R, Quiñones Galvan A, Sironi AM, Frascerra S, Ciociaro D, Ferrannini E. Effect of insulin on renal sodium and uric acid handling in patients with essential hypertension. Am J Hypertens 1996;9:746–752.
147. Rocchini AP, Key J, Bondie D, et al. The effect of weight loss on the sensitivity of blood pressure to sodium in obese adolescents. N Engl J Med 321:580–585.
148. Sharma AM, Ruland K, Spies KP, et al. Salt sensitivity in young normotensive subjects is associated with a hyperinsulinemic response to oral glucose. J Hypertension 1991;9:329–335.
149. Weidman P, Ferrari P. Central role of sodium in hypertension in diabetic subjects. Diabetes Care 1991;14:220–232.
150. De Chatel R, Weidmann P, Flammer J, Ziegler WH, Beretta-Piccoli C, Vetter W, Reubi FC. Sodium, renin, aldosterone, catecholamines, and blood pressure in diabetes mellitus. Kidney Int 1977;12:412–421.
151. Duling BR. The kidney. In: Berne RM, Levy MN, eds. Physiology. Mosby, St. Louis, MO, 1988, pp. 757–779.
152. O'Hare JP, Corral LJM. De natrio diabeticorum, increased exchangeable sodium in diabetes. Diabetic Med 1988;5:22–26.
153. Resnick LM. Calcium metabolism in hypertension and allied metabolic disorders. Diabetes Care 1991;14:505–520.
154. Lasker N, Aviv A. A common cellular pathway for insulin resistance in essential hypertension and NIDDM. In: Smith U, Bruun NE, Hedner T, Hökfelt B, eds. Hypertension as an insulin-resistant disorder. Excerpta Medica International Congress Series 980, Amsterdam, 1991, pp. 147–154.
155. Baldi S, Natali A, Buzzigoli G, Quiñones Galvan A, Sironi AM, Ferrannini E. In vivo effect of insulin on intracellular calcium concentrations: relation to insulin resistance. Metabolism 1996;45:1402–1407.
156. Rasmussen H. Calcium and c-AMP as synarchic messengers. John Wiley, New York, 1981.
157. Blaustein MP, Goldman WF, Fontana G, Krueger BK, Santiago EM, Steele TD, Weiss DN, Yarowsky PJ. Physiological roles of the sodium-calcium exchanger in nerve and muscle. In: Blaustein MP, DiPolo R, Reeves JP, eds. Sodium-calcium exchange. Ann NY Acad Sci 1991;639:254–274.
158. Straus DS. Growth-stimulatory actions of insulin in vitro and in vivo. Endocr Rev 1984;5:356–369.
159. Reaven GM, Chen I Y-D, Jeppesen J, Maheux P, Krauss RM. Insulin resistance and hyperinsulinemia in individuals with small, dense, low density lipoprotein particles. J Clin Invest 1993;92:141–146.

160. Juhan-Vague I, Alessi MC, Vague P. Increased plasminogen activator inhibitor 1 levels. A possible link between insulin resistance and atherothrombosis. Diabetologia 1991;34:457–462.
161. Pyorala K, Laakso M, Uusitupa M. Diabetes and atherosclerosis: an epidemiologic view. Diabetes Metab Rev 1987;3:463–524.
162. Stamler J, Vaccaro O, Neaton JD, Wentworth D. Diabetes, other risk factors, and 12-yr cardio-vascular mortality for men screened in the multiple risk factor intervention trial. Diabetes Care 1993;16:434–444.
163. Modan M, Almog S, Fuchs Z, Chetrit A, Lusky A, Halkin H. Obesity, glucose intolerance, hyperinsulinemia, and response to antihypertensive drugs. Hypertension 1991;17:565–573.
164. Isaksson H, Cederholm T, Jansson E, Nygren A, Östergren J. Therapy-resistant hypertension associated with central obesity, insulin resistance, and large muscle fibre area. Blood Pressure 1993;2:46–52.
165. Krotkiewsky M, Mandroukas K, Sjöstrom L, Sullivan L, Weterqvist P, Björntorp P. Effect of long-term physical training on body fat, metabolism, and blood pressure in obesity. Metabolism 1979;28:650–658.
166. Stein PP, Black HR. Drug treatment of hypertension in patients with diabetes mellitus. Diabetes Care 1991;14:425–448.

16

Microalbuminuria and Insulin Resistance

*Jeannie Yip, MB, BS
and Roberto Trevisan MD, PhD*

CONTENTS

INTRODUCTION
SIGNIFICANCE OF MICROALBUMINURIA
TYPE 1 INSULIN-DEPENDENT DIABETES
TYPE 2 NON-INSULIN-DEPENDENT DIABETES
ESSENTIAL HYPERTENSION
GENERAL POPULATION
CONCLUSION
REFERENCES

INTRODUCTION

Microalbuminuria has emerged in the last decade as a recognized independent cardiovascular risk factor in addition to being a predictor of diabetic kidney disease *(1,2)*. It has been described to be associated with essential hypertension *(3,4)*, elevated plasma triglycerides, total cholesterol and reduced HDL-cholesterol, endothelial dysfunction *(5–7)*: all features of the metabolic syndrome *(11,12)*. Whether microalbuminuria has a direct pathophysiological link to insulin resistance, or is related to the syndrome by sheer associations with other metabolic abnormalities is largely unknown. We shall present evidence in this chapter that connects microalbuminuria to insulin resistance/ hyperinsulinemia in the development of cardiovascular disease. In certain high risk patient groups such as those with diabetes or essential hypertension, the presence of microalbuminuria seems to add to the insulin resistant state to confer a more deleterious cardiovascular profile.

SIGNIFICANCE OF MICROALBUMINURIA

Microalbuminuria is defined as an albumin excretion rate (AER) of 30–300 mg in a 24-h urine collection, or 20–200 µg in a timed (commonly overnight) collection in the

From: *Contemporary Endocrinology: Insulin Resistance*
Edited by: G. Reaven and A. Laws © Humana Press Inc., Totowa, NJ

Table 1
Odds Ratios for Cardiovascular Mortality
in Patients with Type 1 and Type 2 Diabetes

	n	*Follow-up (yr)*	*Odds ratio (95% C.I.)*
Messent et al. *(20)*	63	23	2.9 (1.2–7.3)
Rossing et al. *(21)*	939	10	1.87 (1.03–3.40)
Neil et al. *(25)*	236	6	1.9 (0.8–4.9)
Macleod et al. *(26)*	306	8	1.7 (1.1–2.5)[a]
Niskanen et al. *(27)*	133	10	3.98 (1.04–15.2)[a]

[a]Adjusted for other risk factors.

absence of urinary tract infection *(13)*. The urinary albumin excretion in healthy individuals is approximately 4 µg/min with 10 µg/min as the 90th percentile.

The significance of microalbuminuria was first described in 1982 by Viberti et al. who showed a 24-fold increased risk of development of clinical proteinuria in Type 1 insulin-dependent diabetic patients with microalbuminuria *(14)*. This finding was later confirmed by other medium to long-term longitudinal studies, not only in patients with Type 1 diabetes *(15,16)* but in Type 2 noninsulin dependent diabetes *(17–19)*. The prevalence of microalbuminuria is approximately 5–20% and 20–40% in the Type 1 and Type 2 diabetes. Microalbuminuria is also a predictor of total and cardiovascular morbidity and mortality in diabetes *(10,17–27)* (Table 1). Similar observation in nondiabetic individuals has also been reported in population studies *(28–33)*. Although microalbuminuria is rarely seen in the absence of elevated blood pressure (BP) and dyslipidemia, it was possible to calculate in some of these studies that statistically, the predictive value of microalbuminuria was independent of conventional athersclerotic risk factors such as age, male gender, BP or cholesterol. Therefore in theory the link between microalbuminuria and cardiovascular disease needs to be explained by other pathophysiological processes not previously investigated, insulin resistance/hyperinsulinemia being one possible candidate.

Albumin excretion rate is partly BP dependent although there is no consistent correlation between the levels of BP and AER *(34,35)*. It is present in 20–40% of patients with essential hypertension *(36)*. The lowering of BP causes a reduction but not always normalization in AER *(37)*. Whether the presence of microalbuminuria in patients with essential hypertension denotes a more adverse outcome in terms of glomerular function and cardiovasular morbidity and mortality remains speculative and prospective data are lacking. However, the finding of elevated AER in a sample of well characterized patients with essential hypertension and atherosclerotic peripheral vascular disease compared to those with uncomplicated hypertension, plus the positive correlation between AER and ultrasonographic carotid thickness suggest that microalbuminuria may reflect widespread atherosclerosis in essential hypertension as well *(38)*.

TYPE 1 INSULIN-DEPENDENT DIABETES

Two recent studies have shown the association between microalbuminuria and insulin resistance measured by the euglycemic hyperinsulinemic clamp technique in patients with Type 1 diabetes *(39,40)*. Furthermore, the nondiabetic first degree relatives of diabetic patients with microalbuminuria were found to have a more atherogenic lipid profile and higher fasting insulin levels than relatives of normoalbuminuric diabetic patients *(41)*. Additional evidence that insulin resistance may play a primary role in the pathogenesis of diabetic kidney complication came from a recent study from Italy when parents of diabetic patients with nephropathy were shown to be more insulin resistant (evaluated by insulin tolerance test) than parents of those without renal disease *(42)*. All these findings suggest that insulin resistance and/or its accompanying metabolic/hemo-dynamic disturbances may be a risk factor for microalbuminuria.

TYPE 2 NON-INSULIN-DEPENDENT DIABETES

Type 2 diabetes is characterized by insulin resistance and at the beginning of the disease hyperinsulinemia. Recently two separate groups of investigators showed that Type 2 diabetic patients with hypertension and/or microalbuminuria were more insulin resistant than those with normal BP and albumin excretion rate *(43,44)*. One of these studies also reported that insulin resistant microalbuminuric patients had more coronary ischemic events over a 6-yr follow-up period compared to normoalbuminuric diabetics *(43)*. It was observed in a case-control study that C-peptide levels were higher in Type 2 microalbuminuric diabetic patients compared to those with normalbuminuria *(45)*. Since metabolic control was similar in the two group of patients, a greater degree of insulin resistance was probably associated with the abnormal albumin excretion. Yet in several other studies, diabetic patients with microalbuminuria and normoalbuminuria were equally insulin resistant *(46–49)*. In all the studies when insulin sensitivity was measured directly, the sample size tended to be small. In a 10-yr prospective study based in Finland with 133 newly diagnosed Type 2 diabetic patients, the risk of cardiovascular death was greatly augmented by the simultaneous occurrence of hyperinsulinemia and albuminuria *(27)*. In another Finnish report, baseline microalbuminuria predicted the development of Type 2 diabetes independent of BP *(50)*. There was an unusually high prevalence of microalbuminuria of 30% amongst the nondiabetic subjects in this study. After adjustment for baseline glucose and insulin levels, the prevalence of micro-albuminuria between converters to diabetes and nonconverters became statistically non-significant. These findings nonetheless suggest that microalbuminuria and insulin resistance/hyperinsulinemia are closely intertwined. While Type 2 diabetic patients are by the nature of their disease more insulin resistant than nondiabetic individuals, the presence of microalbuminuria may have an additional adverse effect in terms of cardio-vascular complications.

ESSENTIAL HYPERTENSION

Whether microalbuminuria has any prognostic significance in terms of renal and cardiovascular morbidity/mortality in essential hypertension is under investigation. It has been shown in small cross-sectional studies that hypertensive patients with microalbuminuria are less insulin sensitive and have greater left ventricular thickness than their normoalbuminuric counterparts *(51–55)*. In one case-control study, 25 hyper-tensive microalbuminuric patients were compared to 25 aged, sex and body-mass index (BMI) matched hypertensive normoalbuminuric controls *(56)*. The microalbuminuric group was found to have higher fasting and the 2-h insulin concentration postoral glucose tolerance test insulin. By the same group of investigators, it was also reported that insulin-

Table 2
Prospective Studies on Microalbuminuria and Other Associated Risk Factors
in Total or Cardiovascular Mortality in Nondiabetic Populations

	n	Age (yr)	Follow-up (yr)	Risk factors
Yudkin et al. (28)	167	>40	3.5	BP, male gender, DM/IGT
Damsgaard et al. (29)	216	60–74	10	Elevated Cr, male gender, BP, IHD
Kuusisto et al. (32)	1069	65–76	3.5	BP, WHR, smoking, HDL-choles- terol insulin

BP = blood pressure; DM = diabetes mellitus; IGT = impaired glucose tolerance Cr = serum creatinine; IHD = ischemic heart disease; WHR = waist-hip ratio.

mediated glucose disposal was 25% lower in the microalbuminuric than the normo-albuminuric hypertensive patients (57). The difference was accounted for by a 40% reduction in glycogen synthesis whereas glucose oxidation and suppression of hepatic glucose production were similar between the two groups. Yet in another study when insulin sensitivity was measured by the insulin tolerance test, insulin resistance was demonstrated in both normoalbuminuric and microalbuminuric hypertensive subjects alike (58). The role of insulin resistance in essential hypertension is still hotly debated. While patients with essential hypertension as a group is known to be more insulin resistant, only half of the non-obese subjects with hypertension are affected (59,60). Other factors may contribute to the reduced tissue sensitivity to insulin action. Salt-sensitive subjects have been found to be not only more insulin resistant (61–63), but also to have elevated intraglomerular capillary pressure and higher urinary albumin excretion compared to those who were salt-resistant (63,64). It is therefore possible that when essential hypertension is associated with salt-sensitivity, the attendant hyperinsulinemia and sodium retention may lead to an altered glomerular permeability and intrarenal hemodynamics favoring an increase of urinary albumin excretion.

GENERAL POPULATION

The association between microalbuminuria and cardiovascular disease in middle-aged nondiabetic population was first described by Yudkin et al. 10 yr ago and subsequently confirmed by both cross-sectional and prospective studies (28–33,65). Microalbuminuria is present in around 5–10% of the nondiabetic population the incidence of which increases with age. It is commonly accompanied by other metabolic risk factors (Table 2). Direct infusion of insulin to attain a supraphysiological concentration of plasma insulin had been demonstrated in a group of five healthy volunteers to increase transcapillary escape rate of albumin (66). One may speculate that hyperinsulinemia may result in a generalized vascular leak by rendering the endothelial wall more permeable, thus promoting the escape of lipoproteins into the microvasculature and at the glomeruli giving rise to microalbuminuria. In other words microalbuminuria represents widespread vascular damage (67). Both fasting and post-glucose loading hyperinsulinemia have been reported to be higher in microalbuminuric than normoalbuminuric individuals (27,32,33,65). On the other hand, some have found either no or a negative relationship between insulin level and albuminuria (7,48,68). When peripheral insulin sensitivity was measured directly in a group of healthy middle-aged men, total body glucose disposal rate was similar between the microalbuminuric subjects and the normoalbuminuric controls

(69). Two recent reports from Finland aimed to address this issue specifically. A group of 1069 elderly nondiabetic subjects were followed-up for 3.5 years *(61)*. The concurrence of microalbuminuria and hyperinsulinemia was found to be strongly predictive of coronary heart disease events (Odds Ratio 7.91) and coronary deaths (Odds Ratio 2.95) after adjusting for conventional risk factors such as waist-hip ratio (WHR), BP and HDL-cholesterol. In a second report, 144 nondiabetic subjects were assessed serially over a 10-yr follow-up period. At baseline 1.4% had microalbuminuria which increased to 12% by 10 years. A high baseline fasting insulin level was associated with the development of microalbuminuria *(27)*. In other words, in clinically healthy young individuals the isolated occurrence of microalbuminuria without other accompanying metabolic or hemodynamic abnormalities is rare. However, in those who are hyperinsulinemic or insulin resistant, the presence of microalbuminuria amplifies the risk of coronary heart disease with increasing age.

CONCLUSION

Microalbuminuria is an independent cardiovascular risk factor, the pathophysiology of which may be related to insulin resistance or hyperinsulinemia. It is probable that insulin resistance and microalbuminuria are both manifestations of a central mechanism yet to be identified which causes the clustering of metabolic/hemodynamic derangements in cardiovascular disease. In essential hypertension or diabetes, insulin resistance can be found in the absence of microalbuminuria but the reverse is uncommon. Therefore, the presence of microalbuminuria in these patients should serve as a warning signal for the insulin resistance syndrome.

REFERENCES

1. Mogensen CE. Epidemiology of microalbuminuria in diabetes and in the background population. Curr Nephrol Hypert 1994;3:248–256.
2. Dinneen S, Gerstein H. The association of microalbuminuria and mortality in non-insulin-dependent diabetes mellitus. A systemic overview of literature. Arch Intern Med 1997;157:1413–1418.
3. Parving HH, Jensen HE, Mogensen CE, Evrin PE. Increased urinary albumin excretion in benign essential hypertension. Lancet 1974;1:231–237.
4. Christensen CK, Krusell LR, Mogensen CE. Increased blood pressure in diabetes: essential hypertension or diabetic nephropathy? Scand J Clin Lab Invest 1987;47:363–370.
5. Jones SL, Close CF, Mattock MB, Jarrett RJ, Keen H, Viberti GC. Plasma lipids and coagulation factor concentrations in insulin dependent diabetics with microalbuminuria. BMJ 1989;298:487–490.
6. Jensen T, Stender S, Deckert T. Abnormalities in plasma concentrations of lioproteins and fibrinogen in Type 1 (insulin-dependent) diabetic patients with increased urinary albumin excretion. Diabetologia 1988; 31:142–145.
7. Winocour PH, Harland JOE, Millar JP, Laker MF, Alberti KGMM. Microalbuminuria and associated cardiovascular risk factors in the community. Athersclerosis 1992;93:71–81.
8. Feldt-Rasmussen B. Increased transcapillary escape rate of albumin in Type 1 (insulin-dependent) diabetic patients with microalbuminuria. Diabetologia 1986;29:282–286.
9. Jensen T, Bjerre-Knudsen J, Feldt-Rasmussen B, Deckert T. Features of endothelial dysfunction in early diabteic nephropathy. Lancet 1989;1:461–464.
10. Stehouwer, CDA, Nauta JJP, Zeldenrust GC, Hackeng WHL, Donker AJM, Den Ottolander GJH. Urinary albumin excretion, cardiovascular disease and endothelial dysfunction in non-insulin dependent diabetes mellitus. Lancet 1992;340:319–323.
11. Reaven GM. Role of insulin resistance in human disease. Diabetes 1988;37:1595–1607.
12. DeFronzo RA, Ferrannini E. Insulin resistance- a multifaceted syndrome responsible for NIDDM, obesity, hypertension, dyslipidemia, and athersclerotic cardiovascular disease. Diabetes Care 1991;14:173–94.

13. Consensus Statement. Am J Kidney Dis 1989;13:2–6.

14. Viberti GC, Hill RD, Jarrett RJ, Argyropoulos A, Mahmud U, Keen H. Microalbuminuria as a predictor of clinical proteinuria in insulin-dependent diabetes mellitus. Lancet 1992; i:1430–1432.

15. Mogensen CE, Christensen CK. Predicting diabetic nephropathy in insulin-dependent patients. N Engl J Med 1984;311:89–93.

16. Mathiesen ER, Oxenboll B, Johansen K, Svedsen PAA, Deckert T. Incipient nephropathy in Type 1 (insulin-dependent) diabetes. Diabetologia 1984;26:406–410.

17. Mogensen CE. Microalbuminuria predicts clinical proteinuria and early mortality in maturity-onset diabetes. New Engl J Med 1984;310:356–360.

18. Jarrett RJ, Viberti GC, Argyropoulos A, Hill RD, Mahmud U, Murrells TJ. Microalbuminuria predicts mortality in non-insulin-dependent diabetes. Diabetic Med 1984;1:17–19.

19. Schmitz A, Vaeth M. Microalbuminuria: A major risk factor in non-insulin-dependent diabetes: a 10-year follow-up study of 503 patients. Diabetic Med 1988;5:126–134.

20. Messent JWC, Elliott TG, Hill RD, Jarrett RJ, Keen H Viberti GC. Prognostic significance of microalbuminuria in insulin-dependent diabetes mellitus: a twenty-three year follow-up. Kidney Int 1992;41:836–839.

21. Rossing P, Hougaard P, Borch-Johnsen K, Parving HH. Predictors of mortality in insulin dependent diabetes: 10-year observational follow up study. BMJ 1996;313:779–784.

22. Deckert T, Yokoyama H, Mathiesen E, Ronn B, Jensen T, Feldt-Rasmussen B, Borch-Johnsen K, Jensen JS. Cohort study of predictive value of urinary albumin excretion for atherosclerotic vascular disease in patients with insulin dependent diabetes. BMJ 1996;312:871–874.

23. Mattock MB, Morrish NJ, Viberti GC, Keen H, Fitzgerald AP, Jackson G. Prospective study of microalbuminuria as predictor of mortality in NIDDM. Diabetes 1992;41:736–741.

24. Patrick AW, Leslie PJ, Clarke BF, Frier BM. The natural history and associations of microalbuminuria in Type 2 diabetes during the first year after diagnosis. Diabetic Med 1990;7:902–908.

25. Neil A, Hawkins M, Potok M, Thorogood M, Cohen D, Mann J. A prospective population-based study of microalbuminuria as a predictor of mortality of NIDDM. Diabetes Care 1993;16:996–1003.

26. Macleod JM, Lutale J, Marshall SM. Albumin excretion and vascular deaths in NIDDM. Diabetologia 1995;38:610–616.

26. Niskanen LK, Parviainen M, Penttila I, Uusitupa M. Evolution, risk factors, and prognostic implications of albuminuria in NIDDM. Diabetes Care 1996;19: 491–493.

28. Yudkin JS, Forrest RD, Jackson CA. Microalbuminuria as a predictor of vascular disease in nondiabetic subjects. Lancet 1988;2:530–533.

29. Damsgaard EM, Froland A, Jorgensen OD, Mogensen CE. Prognostic value of urinary albumin excretion rate and other risk factors in elderly diabetic and nondiabetic control subjects surviving the first five years after assessment. Diabetologia 1993;36:1175–1184.

30. Metcalf P, Baker J, Scott A, Wild C, Scragg R, Dryson E. Albuminuria in people at least 40 years old: Effect of obesity, hypertension, and hyperlipidemia. Clin Chem 1992;38:1802-1808.

31. Woo J, Cockram CS, Swaminathan R, Lau E, Chan A, Cheung K. Microalbuminuria and other cardiovascular risk factors in nondiabetic subjects. Int J Cardiol 1992;325–350.

32. Kuusisto J, Mykkanen L, Pyorala K, Laakso M. Hyperinsulinemic microalbuminuria: A new risk indicator for coronary heart disease. Circulation 1995;91; 831–837.

33. Haffner SM, Stern MP, Gruber MK, Hazuda HP, Mitchell BD, Patterson JK. Microalbuminuria. Potential marker for increased cardiovascular risk factors in nondiabetic subjects? Arteriosclerosis 1990;10:727–731.

34. Gosling P, Beevers DG. Urinary albumin excretion rate and blood pressure in the general population. Clin Sci 1989;76:39–42.

35. Hoegholm A, Bang LE, Kristensen KS, Nielsen JW, Holm J. Microalbuminuria in 411 untreated individuals with established hypertension, white coat hypertension, and normotension. Hypertension 1994;24:101–105.

36. Bigazzi R, Bianchi S, Campese VM, Baldari G. Prevalence of microalbuminuria in a large population of patients with mild to moderate essential hypertension. Nephron 1992;61:94–97.

37. Bianchi S, Biggazi R, Baldari G, Campese VM. Microalbuminuria in patients with essential hypertension: effect of several antihypertensive drugs. Am J Med 1992;93:525–528.

38. Pedrinelli R, Lindpaintner K, Dell'Omo G, Napoli V, Di Bello V, De Caterina R, Petrucci R. Urinary albumin excretion and atherosclerosis in essential hypertension. Clin Sci 1997;92:45–50.

39. Yip J, Mattock MB, Morocutti A, Sethi M, Trevisan R, Viberti GC. Impaired insulin-sensitivity: part of a metabolic syndrome in insulin-dependent diabetic patients with microalbuminuria. Lancet 1993;342:883–887.

40. Trevisan R, Nosadini R, Fioretto P, Semplicini A, Donadon V, Doria A, Nicolosi G, Zanuttini D, Cipollina MR, Lusiani L, Avogaro A, Crepaldi G, Viberti GC. Clustering of risk factors in hypertensive insulin-dependent-diabetics with high sodium-lithium countertransport. Kidney Int 1992:41:855–861.

41. Yip J, Mattock M, Sethi M, Morocutti A, Viberti GC. Insulin resistance in family members of insulin-dependent-diabetic patients with microalbuminuria. Lancet 1993;34:369–370.

42. De Cosmo S, Bacci S, Piras GP, Cignarelli M, Placentino G, Margaglione M, Colaizzo D, Di Minno G, Giogino R, Liuzzi A, Viberti GC. High prevalence of risk factors for cardiovascular disease in parents of IDDM patients with albuminuria. Diabetologia 1997;40:1191–1196.

43. Nosadini R, Cipollina MR, Solini A, Sambotaro M, Morocutti A, Doria A, Fioretto P, Brocco E, Muollo B, Frigato F. Close relationship between microalbuminuria and insulin resistance in essentail hypertension and non-insulin-dependent diabetes mellitus. J Am Soc Nephrol 1992;3:356–363.

44. Groop L, Ekstrand A, Forsblom G, Widen E, Groop PH, Teppo AM, Eriksson J. Insulin resistance, hypertension and microalbuminuria in type 2 (noninsulin dependent) diabetes mellitus. Diabetologia 1993;32:642–647.

45. Trevisan R, Orrasch M, Jori E, Tiengo A. Hyperinsulinemia in type 2 diabetic patients with microalbuminuria. Diabetes Care 1993;16:1211.

46. Nielsen S, Schmitz O, Orskov H, Mogensen CE. Similar insulin sensitivity in NIDDM patients with normo- and microalbuminuria. Diabetes Care 1995;6:834–842.

47. Hodge AM, Dowse GK, Zimmet PZ. Microalbuminuria, cardiovascular risk factors, and insulin resistance in two populations with a high risk of type 2 diabetes mellitus. Diabetic Med 1996;13:441–449.

48. Sheu W, Jeng CY, Fuh M, Chen YD, Reaven GM. Resistance to insulin-mediated glucose disposal in patients with non-insulin-dependent diabetes mellitus in the absence of obesity or microalbuminuria—a Clinical Research Center Study. J Clin Endocrinol Metab 1996;81:1156–1159.

49. Rizvi A, Varasteh B, Chen YD, Reaven GM. Lack of a relationship between urinary albumin excretion rate and insulin resistance in patients with non-insulin dependent diabetes mellitus. Meta: Clin Exp 1996;45:1062–1064.

50. Mykkanen L, Haffner S, Kuusisto J, Pyorala K, Laakso M. Microalbuminuria precedes the development of NIDDM. Diabetes 1994;43:552–557.

51. Agewell, Fagerberg B, Attvall S, Ljungman S, Urbanvicius V, Tengborn L, Wilkstrand J. Microalbuminuria, insulin sensitivity and haemostatic factors in nondiabetic treated hypertensive men. J Int Med 1995:237:195–203.

52. Agewell S, Persson B, Samuelsson O, Ljungman S, Herlitz H, Fagerberg B. Microalbuminuria in treated hypertensive men at high risk of coronary disease. The Risk Factor Intervention Study Group. J Hypertens 1993;11:461–469.

53. Redon J, Miralles A, Pascual J, Baldo E, Robles RG, Carmena R. Hyperinsulinemia as a determinant of microalbuminuria in essential hypertension. J Hypertens 1997;15:79–86.

54. Redon J, Liao Y, Lozano JV, Miralles A, Baldo E, Cooper RS. Factors related to the presence of microalbuminuria in essential hypertension. Am J Hypertens 1994;7:801–807.

55. Pedrinelli R, di bello V, Catapano G, Talarico L, Materazi F, Santoro G, Giusti C, Mosca F, Melillo E, Ferrari M. Microalbuminuria is a marker of left ventricular hypertrophy but not hyperinsulinemia in nondiabetic atherisclerotic patients. Arterioscl Thromb 1993;13: 900–906.

56. Bianchi S, Bigazzi R, Valtriani C, Chiapponi I, Sgherri G, Baldari G, Natali A, Ferrannini E, Campese VM. Elevated serum insulin levels in patients with essential hypertension and micraolbuminuria. Hypertension 1994;23:681–687.

57. Bianchi S, Bigazi R, Quinones GA, Muscelli E, Baldari G, Percori N, Ciociaro D, Ferrannini E, Natali A. Insulin resistance in microalbuminuric hypertension. Sites and mechanisms. Hypertension 1995;26:789–795.

58. Yip JW, Jones C, Facchini F, Chen I, Reaven RM. Insulin resistance i patients with essential hypertension can occur in the absence of microalbuminuria. Am J Hypertens 1996;9:959–963.

59. Pollare T, Lithell H, Berne C. Insulin resistance is a characteristic feature of primary hypertension independent of obesity. Metabolism 1990;39:167–174.

60. Zavaroni I, Mozza S, Dall'Aglio E, Gasparini P, Passeri M, Reaven GM. Prevalence of hyperinsulinemia in patients with high blood pressure. J Intern Med 1992;231:235–240.

61 Zavaroni I, Coruzzi P, Bonini L, Mossini GL, Musiari L, Gasparini P, Fantuzzi M, Reaven GM. Association between salt sensitivity and insulin concentrations in patients with hypertension. Am J Hypertens 1995;8:855–858.

62. Sharma AM, Schorr U, Distler A. Insulin resistance in young salt-sensitive normotensive subjects. Hypertension 1994;23:195–199.

63. Bigazzi R, Bianchi S, Baldari G, Campese VM. Clustering of cardiovascular risk factors in salt-sensitive patients with essential hypertension: role of insulin. Am J Hypertens 1996;9:24–32.
64. Bigazzi R, Bianchi S, Baldari D, Sgherri G, Baldari G, Campese VM. Microalbuminuria in salt-sensitive patients: a marker for renal and cardiovascular risk factors. Hypertension 1994;23:195–199.
65. Jensen JS, Borch-Johnsen K, Jensen G, Feldt-Rasmussen B. Athersclerostic risk factors are increased in clinically healthy subjects with microalbuminuria. Athersclerosis 1995;11:245–52.
66. Nestler JE, Barlascini O, Tetrault GA, Fratkin MJ, Clore JN, Blackard WG. Increased transcapillary escape rate of albumin in nondiabetic men in response to hyperinsulinemia. Diabetes 1990;39:1212–1217.
67. Deckert T, Feldt-Rasmussen B, Borch-Johnsen K, Kofoed-Enevoldsen A. Albuminuria reflects widespread vascular damage. The Steno Hypothesis. Diabetologia 1989;32:219–226.
68. Zavaroni I, Bonini L, Gasoparini P, Zuccarelli A, Dall'Aglio E, Barilli L, Cioni F, Strata A, Reaven GM. Dissociation between urinary albumin excretion and variables associated with insulin resistance in a healthy population. J Intern Med 1996;240:151–156.
69. Jensen JS, Borch-Johnsen K, Jensen G, Feldt-Rasmussen. Insulin sensitivity in clinically healthy individuals with microalbuminuria. Athersclerosis 1996;119:69–76.

17 PAI-1, Obesity, and Insulin Resistance

Irène Juhan-Vague, MD, PhD,
Marie-Christine Alessi, MD, PhD,
and Pierre E. Morange, MD

CONTENTS

INTRODUCTION
THE FIBRINOLYTIC SYSTEM
PAI-1 AND CARDIOVASCULAR RISK
PAI-1 AND INSULIN RESISTANCE
MODULATION OF PLASMA PAI-1 ACTIVITY
CONCLUSION
REFERENCES

INTRODUCTION

Thrombosis favors the development of vascular damage and is responsible for many complications of atherosclerosis. It occurs primarily at the site of a ruptured atherosclerotic plaque and can be incorporated into the vascular wall. This event is partly determined by the thrombotic/thrombolytic equilibrium at the time of plaque rupture. Thrombolytic potential is mainly under the control of an inhibitor of plasminogen activation (PAI-1), whose modulation has been shown to influence fibrin and extracellular matrix accumulation. Elevated PAI-1 concentration in plasma is presently considered a risk factor for coronary vascular events *(1,2)*. Moreover, an elevation of circulating PAI-1 has been shown to be associated with insulin-resistance with obesity and noninsulin dependent diabetes *(3)*. It has thus been postulated *(3)* that PAI-1 could contribute to increased susceptibility to atherothrombosis in insulin-resistant patients *(4–9)*. The elucidation of the regulation of PAI-1 synthesis and the identification of factors responsible for increased plasma PAI-1 concentration in the insulin resistance states might lead to therapeutic concepts for prevention of vascular lesions.

THE FIBRINOLYTIC SYSTEM

Fibrinolysis (Fig. 1) is a proteolytic system in which plasmin is the main enzyme. Plasmin is formed from its inactive precursor plasminogen by the action of the tissue-type

From: *Contemporary Endocrinology: Insulin Resistance*
Edited by: G. Reaven and A. Laws © Humana Press Inc., Totowa, NJ

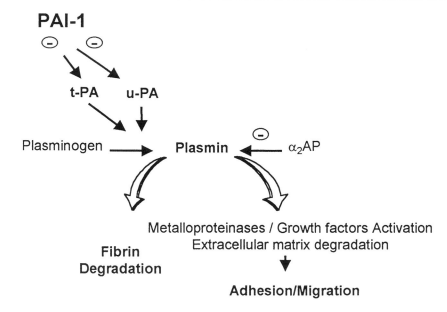

Fig. 1. The fibrinolytic system. (PAI-1 = plasminogen activator inhibitor type 1; t-PA = tissue-type plasminogen activator; uPA = urokinase; α2 AP = α2 antiplasmin.)

and urokinase-type plasminogen activators (t-PA and u-PA). Plasmin activity is inhibited by α2-antiplasmin, whereas that of t-PA and u-PA are inhibited by PAI-1 which is considered to be the predominant regulator of plasminogen activation, since its expression is actively regulated.

Plasmin is a broadly acting trypsin-like enzyme that not only degrades fibrin and a variety of extracellular matrix proteins, but may activate metalloproteinases and prourokinase, bind to receptors, localizing plasmin activity to the cell surface and can then be employed by migrating cells to degrade and/or modify tissue barriers during a variety of normal and pathological processes such as angiogenesis, tumor progression and inflammatory reaction *(10,11)*.

PAI-1 *(12)* is a single chain glycoprotein of 50 kd which belongs to the serpin superfamily. The amino acids arginine and methionine in position 358 and 359 form the active center which inactivates t-PA and u-PA by forming a 1:1 complex. PAI-1 is synthesized in an active form, and is rapidly converted into an inactive (latent) form. This inactivation is avoided if PAI-1 binds to vitronectin which results in stabilization of the inhibitor. Interaction of PAI-1 with vitronectin occurs with high affinity in plasma and in matrices of several cells. Synthesis of PAI-1 is increased by several stimuli including endotoxin, cytokines (IL1,TNFα), growth factors (TGFβ) and hormones (insulin, glucocorticoids) and decreased by a rise in AMPc. Till now a constitutive production of PAI-1 has not been precisely attributed to a particular cell type, although endothelial cells are usually proposed as good candidates. In blood, PAI-1 is found in plasma (*10–20* ng/mL) and in platelets (*100–200* ng/mL serum) stored in the α granules mainly in an inactive form. PAI-1 concentration in plasma exhibits a circadian rhythm with maximal activity in the early morning and a nadir in the afternoon *(13,14)*.

PAI-1 has several functions. Apart from its capacity to decrease fibrin degradation, it appears to be capable of directly influencing cell adhesion and migration, mainly due to

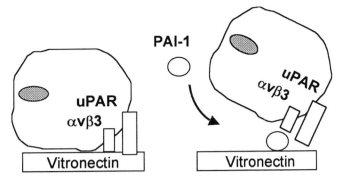

Fig. 2. PAI-1 contribution to cell adhesionl (PAI-1 = plasminogen activator inhibitor type 1; uPAR - uPA receptor; αvβ3 = vitronectin receptor.)

its effect on uPA receptors (uPAR). PAI-1 promotes uPA clearance from the uPAR thereby decreasing the interaction of this receptor with vitronectin. This disruption of uPAR-Vitronectin interactions is reinforced by the direct competition between PAI-1 and uPAR for vitronectin interactions (Fig. 2). Moreover PAI-1 may block the interaction between αv integrins and vitronectin which is another way of disrupting cell adhesion (Fig. 2) *(11,15,16)*. All these properties underline the intervention of PAI-1 in the tissue remodelling processes.

PAI-1 AND CARDIOVASCULAR RISK

The importance of PAI-1 for the regulation of the intravascular fibrinolytic system and for the development of atherothrombosis is well documented by a large number of experimental, clinical and epidemiological studies.

Increased plasma activity of PAI-1 induced by intravenous infusion of recombinant PAI-1 prevented endogenous fibrinolysis or pharmacological thrombolysis of experimental thrombi in animals *(17)*. The reduction of PAI-1 activity by anti-PAI-1 antibodies *(18)* or specific low molecular weight PAI-1 inhibitors *(19,20)* had an opposite effect, with increased thrombolysis and protection against thrombus formation. Transgenic mice which overexpress PAI-1 developed thrombotic occlusion *(21)* whereas PAI-1 deficient mice lysed clots at a higher rate and exhibited accelerated neointima formation and increased extracellular matrix degradation *(22,23)*. Moreover human atherosclerotic plaques are characterized by an increased PAI-1 expression *(24–26)*.

Clinical studies revealed a consistent association between increased plasma PAI-1 concentration and cardiovascular disease such as angina pectoris, previous myocardial infarction, extent of atherosclerosis *(27)* and restenosis after coronary angioplasty *(28)*.

In patients with acute myocardial infarction undergoing thrombolytic therapy, increased PAI-1 activity before treatment and immediately after treatment was correlated with reduced coronary patency after thrombolysis *(29–31)*.

Several longitudinal epidemiological studies have evaluated the prognostic value of fibrinolytic variables. While decreased fibrinolytic activity *(32)* and increased t-PA antigen (which mainly quantify t-PA/PAI-1 complexes) *(33–35)* have been shown to be predictive of cardiovascular events and mortality, conflicting results have been obtained for PAI-1 determination—increased PAI-1 activity being predictive in some reports *(1,2,36,37)* but not in others *(33,34)*.

We have hypothesized that the discrepancy between the studies could be attributed in part to the different choice of confounding variables controlled for, fibrinolytic parameters being strongly related to other coronary risk markers such as insulin-resistance parameters *(3)* and inflammation markers *(38,39)*. We have—in the ECAT study which is a large prospective multicenter study of approximately 3000 patients with angina—followed for 2 yr *(34)*, analyzed and compared the prognostic value of PAI-1 and t-PA antigen before and after specific adjustments for clusters of confounding variables *(2)*. Before adjustment, the 3 parameters—t-PA antigen, PAI-1 antigen and PAI-1 activity—were predictive of coronary events. The relative risks according to quintiles of distribution increased by almost fivefold from the bottom to the top quintile of t-PA antigen $(p < 0.0002)$, threefold for PAI-1 antigen $(p < 0.001)$ and twofold for PAI-1 activity $(p < 0.02)$. After adjustment with insulin-resistance parameters (body mass index (BMI), triglyceride and high-density lipoprotein (HDL) cholesterol), PAI-1 activity or PAI-1 antigen were no longer considered as risk factors, whereas adjustment for inflammation variables (fibrinogen and C reactive protein) had no effect at all on PAI-1 predictive capacity. The two different adjustments affected the prognostic value of t-PA antigen to the same extent and, when the adjustments were combined, the predictive capacity of t-PA antigen disappeared. This study has clarified the prognostic capacity of PAI-1, increased plasma PAI-1 concentration being a risk factor of cardiovascular event in the context of the insulin resistance syndrome *(2)*.

Plasma PAI-1 and t-PA antigen levels are strongly positively correlated in epidemiological studies. The reason for their association is not fully understood. It has been proposed that PAI-1 and t-PA could be triggered simultaneously. Another explanation could be that t-PA-PAI-1 complex, having a delayed clearance compared to free t-PA as we have shown recently *(40)*, t-PA antigen could accumulate in the presence of a high concentration of PAI-1, as seen in the insulin resistance state.

PAI-1 AND INSULIN RESISTANCE

Many cross-sectional studies have shown in various groups of subjects—nondiabetic subjects with various body weight *(41–45)*, subjects with android obesity *(46)*, subjects with noninsulin dependent diabetes *(47)* and subjects with angina pectoris *(48)*, that plasma PAI-1 levels measured between 8 and 10 AM were in strong correlation with the components of the insulin resistance syndrome, BMI, waist to hip ratio (WHR) , fasting plasma insulin, triglyceride and HDL cholesterol—the strongest association being seen for fasting insulin concentration (reviews in *3,49*). However in a study based on a population of normo and hypertriglyceridemic men *(50)* very low density lipoproteins (VLDL) triglyceride concentration was much more related to PAI-1 concentration than all other parameters assayed, including fasting insulin.

The basic disturbance is thought to be peripheral insulin-resistance. Apart from two exceptions *(51,52)* most of the studies found a significant correlation between different indices of peripheral insulin sensitivity and PAI-1 levels *(53-57)*. Generally the inclusion of specific measure of insulin-resistance did not provide more information with respect to hyperinsulinemia. Some investigators have pointed to plasma proinsulin as being the main determinant of plasma PAI-1. In fact conventional radio immunoassays for insulin over estimate plasma insulin concentrations due to a cross reaction with insulin precursors. By using more specific assays, it was shown in several cross sectional studies that proinsulin and other precursors were more strongly correlated with PAI-1 levels than *true* insulin levels *(58–61)*.

The relationship between increased PAI-1 levels and the metabolic disturbances of the insulin resistance syndrome differs with gender *(43,57,62)*. According to Mykkanen et al. *(57)* WHR, HDL cholesterol and 2 h insulin concentration were independently related to PAI-1 concentration in women whereas the independent determinants of PAI-1 in men were BMI and triglyceride levels. The same discordance was noticed in untreated hypertensive patients *(62)*, increased BMI and WHR were independent predictors of PAI-1 activity in women only, whereas elevated plasma glucose was independently associated with decreased fibrinolytic activity in men. Thus, the relations between WHR and plasma PAI-1 levels are more marked in women than in men. These results strongly infer a possible effect of sex hormones on PAI-1/insulin-resistance relationships. This effect has already been underlined since free testosterone is negatively associated with PAI-1 levels in men *(63,64)* and positively in women *(65)* ; the same association being observed between free testosterone and abdominal adiposity *(66)*.

Critical Appraisal of the Link Observed Between Circulating PAI-1 and Insulin-Resistance

The strong dose-response relationship between insulin-resistance and circulating PAI-1 does not necessarily imply that insulin-resistance is directly implicated in fibrinolysis dysregulation. Some arguments militate in favor and others against.

Among those in favor, interventional studies indicate that improvement of insulin sensitivity concomitantly reduced PAI-1 levels. In a 15-d double-blind placebo-controlled study using Metformin (1.7 g/d) in nondiabetic obese women, a decrease in fasting plasma insulin and triglyceride as well as PAI-1 was observed in the group treated but not in the placebo group *(67)*. The effects of Metformin on PAI-1 levels were observed by several groups *(68–70)* ; an effect being observed on t-PA antigen but not on PAI-1 in two studies *(71,72)*. Similar changes in PAI-1 have been reported after hypocaloric diets *(73–76)*. The subjects most responsive to low calorie measures were those with the highest values of PAI-1 and triglyceride *(74)*. However, dietary fat modification had a variable effect on PAI-1 values *(77–79)*. Increased intake of fiber also decreased insulin-resistance and PAI activity levels at the same time *(80)*. The beneficial effect of physical exercise on insulin-resistance is well known and it has been shown that physical training also improved fibrinolytic activity *(81)*, and decreased PAI-1 levels *(82,83)*, whereas PAI-I levels and physical activity are strongly negatively correlated in cross-sectional studies *(84)*.

The link observed between PAI-1 levels and insulin-resistance is reinforced by the notion that several of the components of the insulin-resistance cluster are able to increase the synthesis of PAI-1 by different cultured cells: Insulin *(85–94)*, proinsulin *(85,89,95)* IGF-1 *(87,91,96)* lipoproteins, mainly VLDL *(97–100)*, oxidized low density lipoproteins (LDL) *(101,102)*. In vitro studies with proinsulin have produced conflicting results *(85,89,95,103)* regarding its effect on endothelial cells. The proinsulin effect on hepatocytes was much less pronounced than that of insulin *(85,89,95)*. However induction of PAI-1 synthesis by proinsulin and insulin could be observed in rabbits in vivo; the inducers being administered intravenously over 1 h to euglycemic rabbits *(104)*. It has also been proposed that insulin-resistance *per se* could, at the cellular level, be responsible for the increased PAI-1 production *(55,57)*. In vitro, hepatocytes made insulin resistant by a downregulation of the receptors, present an enhanced PAI-1 production after insulin stimulation *(88)*. Concerning the VLDL effect, VLDL mainly from hypertriglyceridemic subjects induce a dose dependent increase in PAI-1 secretion by endothelial cells *(97–100)* and by liver cells *(98,99)*.

Besides this group of mechanisms linking PAI-1 to insulin-resistance, there are however some inconsistencies. It is interesting to observe that PAI-1 levels have not been described as elevated in all studies on Type 2 diabetes patients *(47,105–110)*. Lean Type 2 diabetes patients in particular have normal PAI-1 levels *(49,111)* whereas patients with central obesity—either diabetics or nondiabetics—have the same increase in PAI-1 levels. Normal PAI-1 levels have also been reported in Chinese *(112,113)* or Japanese *(114)* Type 2 diabetic patients. These results showing normal PAI-1 level in Type 2 diabetes without obesity as well as the normal levels of PAI-1 described in Type 1 diabetes *(105,115)* are not in favor of a direct link between insulin-resistance and circulating PAI-1 and of an important effect of glucose on endothelial production of PAI-1, as has been shown in vitro *(116,117)*.

In the same way, the link assumed between insulin or VLDL particles and circulating PAI-1 cannot easily be disentangled. Indeed the strong in vitro effect of insulin added on hepatocytes *(85–87)* could not be reproduced by induction of acute hyperinsulinemia with euglycemic hyperinsulinemic clamps or oral glucose tolerance test *(118–121)* and insulin therapy in Type 2 diabetes did not induce change in PAI-1 levels *(59,111)*. Moreover PAI-1 levels were found in the normal range not only in normal weight noninsulin dependent diabetic patients, as previously underlined, but also in nonobese patients with Cushing's disease or acromegaly in spite of hyperinsulinemia and insulin resistance *(122)*. Heterogeneity in the association between hypertriglyceridemia and increased PAI-1 levels has also been evidenced. In a study comparing PAI-1 levels in three groups of patients with hypertriglyceridemia *(123)*—one with obesity, one of normal body weight and one with alcohol induced hypertriglyceridemia—both PAI-1 activity and plasma insulin were elevated in obese hypertriglyceridemic patients, but not different from controls in normal weight hypertriglyceridemic patients. In alcoholic hypertriglyceridemic patients, PAI-1 activity was elevated but insulin was normal. In the whole group PAI-1 activity was weakly correlated with triglycerides level but strongly positively correlated with insulin levels. The lack of consistent association between triglyceride levels and PAI activity in these highly selected groups of patients does not plead for high triglyceride levels as the main cause of high PAI levels in subjects with insulin resistance. Finally the lack of effect of antioxidant therapy on PAI-1 levels is not in favor of a relationship between oxydized lipoprotein in plasma and circulating PAI-1 levels *(124)*.

To summarize, although it is established that PAI-1 and t-PA antigen levels are elevated in patients who present with the insulin resistance syndrome, namely in those who aggregate more or less excessive body weight, high WHR, hypertension, hyperinsulinemia, hypertriglyceridemia and hypo HDL cholesterolemia, the real mechanisms responsible for the dysregulation of fibrinolysis in insulin resistance have not yet been elucidated.

PAI-1 and Insulin-Resistance: New Perspectives

The participation of adipose tissue in the PAI-1 increase observed in insulin-resistant patients has attracted much attention recently. In addition to the fact that PAI-1 antigen levels were not increased in Type 2 diabetic patients without obesity *(49)*, Folsom et al. *(76)* have shown that the reduction in PAI-1 antigen levels after weight loss was more related to the degree of weight loss than to triglyceride or insulin changes. Moreover plasma levels of adipsin, a serine protease mainly produced by adipocytes, were independently and positively associated with those of PAI-1 *(125)*. Data on PAI-1 expression by adipose tissue were first provided in rodents (reviewed in Samad and Loskutoff) *(126)*. TGFβ, TNFα and endotoxin or insulin administered to mice increased PAI-1 mRNA expression in adipose tissue *(127–130)*. PAI-1 mRNA was detected in visceral as well as subcutaneous fat in obese rats but increased only in visceral fat during the development of obesity *(131)*.

   We have recently investigated PAI-1 production by human adipose tissue and its different cellular fractions *(132)*. As the relative degree of android (central) adiposity is better correlated with the risk of CHD than the absolute degree of fatness *(133,134)* and the WHR or direct measurement of visceral fat are strongly correlated with insulin resistance and plasma PAI-1 levels *(42,44,46,54,135,136)*, we were interested in studying the capacity to produce PAI-1 of human adipose tissue from different territories. PAI-1 protein detected by immunolocalization was present at the stromal and adipocyte level whatever the territories tested (omental, mammary, gluteal). In subcutaneous tissue, whereas only stromal vascular cells expressed a detectable amount of PAI-1 mRNA in the basal state, adipocyte fractions were able to express PAI-1 mRNA under incubation. Interestingly omental tissue explants produced significantly more PAI-1 antigen than subcutaneous tissue from the same individual. These results suggest that adipose tissue, in particular visceral tissue accumulation, participates in the elevated PAI-1 levels observed in insulin-resistant patients *(132)*.

   The nature of the cells responsible for PAI-1 production in adipose tissue, as well as the mechanisms related to the insulin-resistance involved, are an exciting field of investigation. There is much evidence in favor of the role of TNFα in the pathogenesis of the insulin-resistance syndrome *(137)*. Since TNFα is a potent inducer of PAI-1 synthesis one hypothesis could be that PAI-1 could be specifically triggered by TNFα. We observed that TNFα had a slight effect on PAI-1 antigen production by human adipose tissue whereas TGFβ induced a higher increase in PAI-1 expression *(132)*. These data in accordance with those obtained in mice by Samad et al. *(126)* underlined the role of TGFβ in PAI-1 production by adipose tissue. Although the role of TGFβ in adipose tissue remodelling could easily be imagined, its intervention in triggering PAI-1 in visceral obesity needs further investigation. Apart from a TGFβ induction of PAI-1 expression by adipose tissue, we have also observed that in vitro treatment of human adipose tissue explants with different types of glucocorticoids rapidly induced an increased PAI-1 expression, whereas insulin exerts only a slight effect *(138)*. These results may indicate that corticosteroids contribute to the elevated plasma PAI-1 concentrations found in obesity.

Insulin-Resistance and the PAI-1 Gene

   Different polymorphisms of the PAI-1 gene have recently been described *(139–141)* and a contribution of genetic variation to plasma PAI-1 levels has been proposed *(139,140,142–145)*. The most significant association between polymorphisms of the PAI-1 gene and plasma PAI-1 level concerns the 4G/5G polymorphism at position-675 in the promoter: subjects homozygote for the 4G allele presenting higher plasma PAI-1 activity than the others. This relationship has been observed in patients with previous myocardial infarction *(140,141)*, and obesity (unpublished data). However, discrepant results have been obtained in Type 2 diabetes or in healthy subjects, the association reaching *(143,144)* or not reaching *(140,141,145,146)* a significant level. A stronger association between triglyceride levels *(143,145)* and plasma PAI-1 activity has been observed in diabetic patients homozygous for the 4G allele than in those homozygous for the 5G allele. It has been proposed that the candidate site in the promoter could have a sequence involved in the binding of a transcriptional factor, whose level could be influenced by VLDL *(144)*. However in the large population of the ECTIM study, a case-control study of myocardial infarction, no significant difference in the relationships between PAI-1 levels and triglyceride among the three genotype classes was noted *(142)*. Interestingly in a recent study *(144)* the prevalence of the 4G allele was significantly higher in a group of 100 patients aged 35–45 years with myocardial infarction than in controls. However, this relation was not confirmed in the ECTIM study of patients aged 25–64 yr *(142)* and in the Physicians' Health Study *(147)*. Thus, a genetic control of plasma PAI-1 levels has to be considered and the influence of a gene-environment interaction needs to be evaluated. We recently performed a family study involving 228 healthy nuclear families from the Stanislas cohort of Nancy, France *(148)*. The insulin resistance variables (BMI, WHR, insulin, triglycerides, HDL cholesterol) jointly explained 48.5% and 28.1% of the variability of PAI-1 activity in fathers and mothers respectively (this difference disappears after adjustment for insulin-resistance parameters), whereas, the 4G/5G polymorphism explained 4.5% ($p = 0.008$) in mothers and 1% (NS) in fathers (in univariate and multivariate analysis) No significant difference was found between 4G and 5G alleles for the PAI-1/triglyceride relationships. The weak genetic influence on plasma PAI-1 levels was demonstrated by the comparison of correlations of PAI-1 values between family members. Correlation coefficients of PAI-1 values between spouses were of similar magnitude as parent-offspring or sib-sib correlations. This study *(148)* illustrates the relative contribution of metabolic status and PAI-1 gene polymorphisms to plasma PAI-1 concentration in healthy males and females.

MODULATION OF PLASMA PAI-1 ACTIVITY

PAI-1 levels can be modulated by prescription of hygienic and dietetic rules (hypocaloric diet and physical exercise) and by drugs such as oral antidiabetics (Metformin) *(67–71)* and some hypotensive agents *(149,150)*. Several other drugs such as ACE inhibitors *(151)*, acid nicotinic *(152)* have a moderate effect on PAI-1 levels and the fibrate Gemfibrozil gives discordant results *(153–156)*.

The specific modulation of PAI-1 activity by anti-PAI-1 inhibitors *(19,20,157,158)* also opens up a promising field of interest.

CONCLUSION

Circulating plasminogen activator inhibitor 1 (PAI-1) levels are elevated in patients with coronary heart disease and may play an important role in the development of atherothrombosis.

Many clinical studies have indicated that the insulin resistance syndrome, which is a situation predisposing to diabetes and ischemic heart disease, may be a major regulator of PAI-1 expression, especially in determining plasma PAI-1 levels. Prospective cohort studies of patients with previous myocardial infarction or angina pectoris have underlined the association between increased plasma PAI-1 levels and the risk of coronary events, but the predictive capacity of PAI-1 disappears after insulin resistance marker adjustments.

Central obesity is a characteristic of insulin resistance and is a well recognized risk factor for coronary heart disease. Recently production of PAI-1 by adipose tissue, in particular by tissue from omentum, has been evidenced and this opens up new perspectives for a better understanding of the mechanisms which lead to the elevated plasma PAI-1 levels observed in insulin-resistant patients.

REFERENCES

1. Hamsten A, de Faire U, Walldius G, Dahlen G, Szamosi A, Landou C, Blombäck M, Wiman B. Plasminogen activator inhibitor in plasma: Risk factor for recurrent myocardial infarction. Lancet 1987;II:3–9.
2. Juhan-Vague I, Pyke SDM, Alessi MC, Jespersen J, Haverkate F, Thompson SG. Fibrinolytic factors and the risk of myocardial infarction or sudden death in patients with angina pectoris. Circulation 1996;94:2057–2063.
3. Juhan-Vague I, Alessi MC, Vague P. Increased plasma plasminogen activator inhibitor 1 levels. A possible link between insulin resistance and atherothrombosis. Diabetologia 1991:34:457–462.
4. Pyorala K. Relationship of glucose tolerance and plasma insulin to the incidence of coronary heart disease: Results from two population studies in Finland. Diabetes Care 1979;2:131–141.
5. Welborn TA, Wearne K. Coronary heart disease incidence and cardiovascular mortality in Busselton with reference to glucose and insulin concentrations. Diabetes Care 1979;2:154–160.
6. Ducimetiere P, Eschwege E, Papoz L, Richard JL, Claude JR, Rosselin G. Relationship of plasma insulin levels to the incidence of myocardial infarction and coronary heart disease mortality in a middle-aged population. Diabetologia 1980;19:205–210.
7. Reaven GM. Role of insulin resistance in human disease. Diabetes 1988;37:1595–1607.
8. Desprès JP, Lamarche B, Mauriège P, Cantin B, Dagenais GR, Moorjani S, Lupien PJ. Hyperinsulinemia as an independent risk factor for ischemic heart disease. N Eng J Med 1996;334:952–957.
9. Bao W, Srinivasan R, Berenson G. Persistent elevation of plasma insulin levels is associated with increased cardiovascular risk in children and young adults: the Bogalusa Heart Study. Circulation 1996;93:54–59.
10. Collen D. On the regulation and control of fibrinolysis. Thromb Haemost 1980;43:77–89.
11. Chapman HA. Plasminogen activators, integrins, and the coordinated regulation of cell adhesion and migration. Current Opinon in Cell Biology 1997;9:714–724.
12. Van Meijer M, Pannekoek H. Structure of plasminogen activator inhibitor 1 (PAI-1) and its function in fibrinolysis: An update. Fibrinolysis 1995;9:263–276.
13. Kluft C, Jie AFH, Rijken DC, Verheijen JH. Daytime fluctuations in blood of tissue-type plasminogen activator (t-PA) and its fast acting inhibitor PAI-1. Thromb Haemost 1988;59:329–332.
14. Juhan-Vague I, Alessi MC, Raccah D, Aillaud MF, Billerey M, Ansaldi J, Philip-Joet C, Vague P. Daytime fluctuations of plasminogen activator inhibitor 1 (PAI-1) in populations with high PAI-1 levels. Thromb Haemost 1992;67:76–82.
15. Stefansson S, Lawrence DA. The serpin PAI-1 inhibits cell migration by blocking integrin $\alpha_v\beta_3$ binding to vitronectin. Nature 1996;383:441–443.
16. Waltz DA, Natkin LR, Fujita RM, Wei Y, Chapman HA. Plasmin and plasminogen activator inhibitor type 1 promote cellular motility by regulating the interaction between the urokinase receptor and vitronectin. J Clin Invest 1997;100:58–67.
17. Vaughan DE, Declerck PJ, Van Houte E, De Mol M, Collen D. Reactivated recombinant plasminogen activator inhibitor (rPAI-1) effectively prevents thrombolysis in vivo. Thromb Haemost 1992;68:60–63.
18. Biemond BJ, Levi M, Coronel R, Janse MJ, Ten Cate JW, Pannekoek H. Thrombolysis and reocclusion in experimental jugular vein and coronary artery thrombosis. Effect of plasminogen activator inhibitor type 1 neutralizing monoclonal antibody. Circulation 1995;91:1175–1181.
19. Charlton PA, Faint RW, Bent F, et al. Evaluation of a low molecular weight modulator of human plasminogen activator inhibitor-1 activity. Thromb Haemost 1996;75:808–815.
20. Friederich PW, Levi M, Bart J, Biemond BJ, Charlton P, Templeton D, Van Zonneveld AJ, Bevan P, Pannekoek H, Ten Cate JW. Novel low-molecular weight inhibitor of PAI-1 (XR5118) promotes endogenous fibrinolysis and reduces postthrombolysis thrombus growth in rabbits. Circulation 1997;96:916–921.
21. Erickson LA, Fici GJ, Lund JE, Boyle TP, Polites HG, Marotti KR. Development of venous occlusion in mice transgenic for the plasminogen activator inhibitor 1 gene. Nature 1990;346:74–76.

22. Carmeliet P, Stassen JM, Schoonjans L, Ream B, van den Oord JJ, de Mol M, Mulligan RC, Collen D. Plasminogen activator inhibitor 1 gene-deficient mice. II Effects on hemostasis, thrombosis and thrombolysis. J Clin Invest 1993;92:2756–2760.

23. Carmeliet P, Bouche A, De Clercq C et al. Biological effects of disruption of the tissue-type plasminogen activator, urokinase type plasminogen activator and plasminogen activator inhibitor-1 gene in mice. Ann NY Acad Sci 1995;748:367–382.

24. Schneiderman J, Sawdey MS, Keeton MR, Bordin GM, Bernstein EF, Dilley RB, Loskutoff DJ. Increased type 1 plasminogen activator inhibitor gene expression in atherosclerotic human arteries. Proc Natl Acad Sci USA 1992;89:6998–7002.

25. Lupu F, Bergonzelli GE, Heim DA, Cousin E, Genton CY, Bachmann F, Kruithof EKO. Localization and production of plasminogen activator inhibitor-1 in human healthy and athrosclerotic arteries. Arterioscl Thromb 1993;13:1090–1100.

26. Chomiki N, Henri M, Alessi MC, Anfosso F, Juhan-Vague I. Plasminogen activator inhibitor-1 expression in human liver and healthy or atherosclerotic vessel walls. Thromb Haemost 1994;72:44–53.

27. Salomaa V, Stinson V, Kark JD. Association of fibrinolytic parameters with early atherosclerosis. The ARIC Study. Atherosclerosis Risk in Communities Study. Circulation 1995;91:284–90.

28. Juhan-Vague I, Alessi MC. Fibrinolysis and risk of coronary artery disease: Fibrinolysis 1996; 10:127–136.

29. Barbash GI, Hod H, Roth A, Miller HI, Rath S, Har Zahav Y, Modan M, Zivelin A, Laniado S, Seligsohn U. Correlation of baseline plasminogen activator inhibitor activity with patency of the infarct artery after thrombolytic therapy in acute myocardial infarction. Am J Cardiol 1989;64:1231–1235.

30. Sane DC, Stump DC, Topol EJ, Sigmon KN, Kereiakes DJ, George BS, Mantell SJ, Macy E, Collen D, Califf RM. Correlation between baseline plasminogen activator inhibitor levels and clinical outcome during therapy with tissue plasminogen activator for acute myocardial infarction. Thromb Haemost 1991;65:275–279.

31. Paganelli F, Alessi MC, Morange P, Billerey M, Levy S, Ansaldi J, Juhan-Vague I. Plasminogen activator inhibitor 1 and thrombolytic therapy in patients with acute myocardial infarction. Thromb Haemost 1997;503(Suppl) (Abstract).

32. Meade TW, Ruddock V, Stirling Y, Chakrabarti T, Miller GJ. Fibrinolytic activity, clotting factors and long-term incidence of ischaemic heart disease in the Northwick Park Heart Study. Lancet 1993;342:1076–1079.

33. Jansson JH, Nilsson TK, Olofsson BO. Tissue plasminogen activator and other risk factors as predictors of cardiovascular events in patients with servere angina pectoris. Eur Heart J 1991;12:157–167.

34. Thompson SG, Kienast J, Pyke SKM, Haverkate F and van de Loo JCW. Hemostatic factors and the risk of myocardial infarction or sudden death in patients with angina pectoris. N Engl J Med 1995;332:635–641.

35. Ridker PM, Vaughan DE, Stampfer MJ, Manson JE, Hennekens CH. Endogenous tissue type plasminogen activator and risk of myocardial infarction. Lancet 1993;341:1165–1168.

36. Gram J, Jesperen J, Kluft C, Rijken DC. On the usefulness of fibrinolysis variables in the characterization of a risk group for myocardial infarction. Acta Med Scan 1987;221:149–153.

37. Cortellaro M, Cofrancesco E, Boschetti C, Mussoni L, Donati MB., Cardillo M, Catalano M, Gabrielli L, Lombardi B, Specchia G, Tarazzi L, Tremoli E, Pozzili E, Turri M, for the PLAT Group. Increased fibrin turnover and high PAI-1 activity as predictors of ischemic events in atherosclerotic patients: A case-control study. Arterioscl Thromb 1993;13:1412–1417.

38. Juhan-Vague I, Alessi MC, Joly P, Thirion X, Vague P, Declerck PJ, Serradimigni A, Collen D. Plasma plasminogen activator inhibitor-1 in angina pectoris. Influence of plasma insulin and acute-phase response. Arteriosclerosis 1989; 9:362–367.

39. Haverkate F, Thompson SG, Duckert F. Haemostasis factors in angina pectoris; relation to gender, age and acute-phase reaction. Thromb Haemost 1995;73:561–567.

40. Chandler WL, Alessi MC, Aillaud MF, Vague P, Henderson P, Juhan-Vague I. Clearance of t-PA and t-PA/PAI-1 complex: Relationship to elevated total t-PA antigen in patients with high PAI-1 activity levels.Circulation 1997;96:761–768.

41. Vague P, Juhan-Vague I, Aillaud MF, Badier C, Viard R, Alessi MC, Collen D. Correlation between blood fibrinolytic activity, plasminogen activator inhibitor level, plasma insulin level and relative body weight in normal and obese subjects. Metabolism 1986:35:250–253.

42. Eliasson M, Evrin PE, Lundblad D. Fibrinogen and fibrinolytic variables in relation to anthropometry, lipids and blood pressure. The Northern Sweden MONICA Study. J Clin Epidemiol 1994; 47:513–524.

43. Eliasson M, Asplund K, Evrin PE, Lindahl B, Lundblad D. Hyperinsulinemia predicts low tissue plasminogen activator activity in a healthy population: The Northern Sweden MONICA Study. Metabolism 1994;43:1579–1586.

44. Sundell IB, Nilsson TK, Ranby M, Hallmans G, Hellsten G. Fibrinolytic variables are related to age, sex, blood pressure, and body build measurements: A cross-sectional study in Norsjö, Sweden. J Clin Epidemiol 1989;42:719–723.

45. Yudkin JS, Denver AE, Mohamed-Ali V, Ramaiya KL, Nagi DK, Goubet S, McLarty DG, Swai A. The relationship of concentrations of insulin and proinsulin-like molecules with coronary heart disease prevalence and incidence. Diabetes Care 1997;20:1093–1100.

46. Vague P, Juhan-Vague I, Chabert V, Alessi MC, Atlan C. Fat distribution and plasminogen activator inhibitor activity in non diabetic obese women. Metabolism 1989;38:913–915.

47. Juhan-Vague I, Roul C, Alessi MC, Ardissone JP, Heim M, Vague P. Increased plasminogen activator inhibitor activity in non insulin dependent diabetic patients. Relationship with plasma insulin. Thromb Haemost 1989;61:370–373.

48. Juhan-Vague I, Thomson SG, Jespersen J. Involvement of the haemostatic system in the insulin resistance syndrome. A study of 1 500 patients with angina pectoris. Arterioscl Thromb 1993;13:1865–1873.

49. Mc Gill JB, Schneider DJ, Arfken CL, Lucore CL, Sobel BE. Factors responsible for impaired fibrinolysis in obese subjects and NIDDM patients. Diabetes 1994;43:104–109.

50. Asplund-Carlson A, Hamsten A, Wiman B, Carlson LA. Relationship between plasma plasminogen activator inhibitor 1 activity and VLDL triglyceride concentration, insulin levels and insulin sensivity: studies in randomly selected normo and hypertriglyceridemic men. Diabetologia 1993;36:817–825.

51. Gough SCL, Rice PJS, McCormack L, Chapman C, Grant PJ. The relation between plasminogen activator inhibitor 1 and insulin resistance in newly diagnosed type 2 diabetes mellitus. Diabetic Med 1993;10:638–642.

52. Nagi DK, Tracy R, Pratley R. Relationship of hepatic and peripheral insulin resistance with plasminogen activator inhibitor-1 in Pima Indians. Metabolism 1996;45:1243–1247.

53. Eliasson B, Attwall S, Taskinen MR, Smith U. The insulin resistance syndrome in smokers is related to smoking habits. Arterioscl Thromb 1994;14:1946–1950.

54. Landin K, Stigendal L, Eriksson E Krotkiewski M, Risberg B, Tengborn L Smith U. Abdominal obesity is associated with an impaired fibrinolytic activity and elevated plasminogen activator inhibitor-1. Metabolism 1990;39:1044–1048.

55. Potter van Loon BJ, Kluft C, Radder JK, Blankenstein MA, Meinders AE. The cardiovascular risk factor plasminogen activator inhibitor type-1 is related to insulin resistance. Metabolism 1993; 42:945–949.

56. Lindahl B, Asplund K, Eliasson M, Evrin PE. Insulin resistance syndrome and fibrinolytic activity; The Northern Sweden MONICA Study. Int J Epidemiol 1996;25:291–299.

57. Mykkänen L, Rönnemaa T, Marniemi J, Haffner SM, Bergman R, Laakso M. Insulin sensitivity is not an independent determinant of plasma plasminogen activator inhibitor-1 activity. Arterioscl Thromb 1994;14:1264–1271.

58. Bavenholm P, Proudler A, Silveira A, Crook D, Blombäck M, de Faire U, Hamsten A. Relationships of insulin and intact and split proinsulin to haemostatic function in young men with and without coronary artery disease. Thromb Haemost 1995;73:568–575.

59. Jain SK, Nagi DK, Slavin BM, Lumb PJ, Yudkin JS. Insulin therapy in type 2 diabetic subjects suppresses plasminogen activator inhibitor (PAI-1) activity and proinsulin-like molecules independently of glycaemic control. Diabetic Med 1993;10:27–32.

60. Nagi DK, Hendra TJ, Ryle AJ, Cooper TM, Temple RC, Clark PMS, Schneider AE, Hales CN, Yudkin JS. The relationships of concentrations of insulin, intact proinsulin and 32–33 split proinsulin with cardiovascular risk factors in type 2 (non insulin dependent) diabetic subjects. Diabetologia 1990;33:532–537.

61. Gray RP, Panahloo A, Mohamed - Ali V, Petterson DLH, Yudkin JS. Proinsulin like molecules and plasminogen activator inhibitor type 1 (PAI-1) activity in diabetic and non-diabetic subjects with and without myocardial infarction. Atherosclerosis 1997;130:171–178.

62. Toft I. Bonaa KH, Ingebretsen OC, Nordoy A, Birkeland KI, Jenssen T. Gender Differences in the relationships between plasma plasminogen activator inhibitor-1 activity and factors linked to the insulin resistance syndrome in essential hypertension. Arterioscl Thromb Vasc Biol 1997;17:553–559.

63. Caron P, Bennet A, Camare R, Louvet JP, Boneu B, Sie P. Plasminogen activator inhibitor in plasma is related to testosterone in men. Metabolism 1989;38:1010–1015.

64. Phillips GB, Pinkernell BH, Jing TY. The association of hypotestosteronemia with coronary artery disease in men. Arterioscl Thromb. 1994;14:701–706.

65. De Pergola G, De Mitrio V, Perricci A, Cignarelli M, Garruti G, Lomuscio S, Ferri G, Schiraldi O, Giorgino R. Influence of free testosterone on antigen levels of plasminogen activator inhibitor-1 (PAI-1) in premenopausal women with central obesity. Metabolism 1992;41:131–134.

66. Tchernof A, Labrie F, Belanger A, Despres JP. Obesity and metabolic complications: contribution of dehydroepiandrosterone and other steroid hormones. J Endocrinol 1996;150:S155–S164.

67. Vague P, Juhan-Vague I, Alessi MC, Badier C, Valadier J. Metformin decreases the high plasminogen activator inhibition capacity, plasma insulin and triglyceride levels in non diabetic obese subjects. Thromb Haemost 1987;57:326–328.

68. Grant PJ. The effects of high and medium dose metformin therapy on cardiovascular risk factors in patients with type II diabetes. Diabetes Care 1996;19:64–66.

69. Landin K, Tengborn L, Smith U. Effects of metformin and metroprolol CR on hormones and fibrinolytic variables during a hyperinsulinemic euglycemic clamp in man. Thromb Haemost 1994;71:783–787.

70. Velazquez EM, Mendoza SG, Wang P, Glueck CJ. Metformin therapy is associated with a decrease in plasma plasminogen activator Inhibitor 1, lipoprotein (a), and immunoreactive insulin levels in patients with the polycystic ovary syndrome. Metabolism 1997;46:454–457.

71. Fontbonne A, Charles MA, Juhan-Vague I, Bard JM, André P, Isnard F, Cohen JM, Grandmottet P, Vague P, Safar ME, Eschwège E, the BIGPRO Study Group. The effect of Metformin on the metabolic abnormalities associated with upper body fat distribution. Diabetes Care 1996;19:920–926.

72. Nagi DK, Yudkin JS. Effects of metformin on insulin resistance, risk factors for cardiovascular disease and plasminogen activator inhibitor in NIDDM subjects. Diabetes Care 1993;16:621–629.

73. Sundell IB, Dahlgren S, Ranby M, Lundin E, Stenling R, Nilsson TK. Reduction of elevated plasminogen activator inhibitor levels during modest weight loss. Fibrinolysis 1989;3 51–53.

74. Mehrabian M, Peter JB, Barnard RJ, Lusis AJ. Dietary regulation of fibrinolytic factors. Atherosclerosis 1990;84:25–32.

75. Huisveld IA, Leen R, VdKooy K, Hospers JEH, Seidell JC, Deurenberg P, Koppeschaar HPF, Moster WL, Bouma BN. Body composition and weight reduction in relation to antigen and activity of plasminogen activator inhibitor (PAI-1) in overweight individuals. Fibrinolysis 1990;4:184–185.

76. Folsom AR, Qamhieh HT, Wing RR, Jeffrey RW, Stinson VL, Kuller LH, Wu KK Impact of weight loss on plasminogen activator inhibitor (PAI-1) factor VII, and other hemostatic factors in moderately over weight adults. Arterioscl Thromb 1993;13:162–169.

77. Andersen P, Seljeflot I, Abdelnoor M, Arnesen H, Dale P, Lovik A, Birkeland K. Increased insulin sensitivity and fibrinolytic capacity after dietary intervention in obese women with polycystic ovary syndrome. Metabolism 1995;44:611–616.

78. Niskanen L, Schwab US, Sarkkinen ES, Krusius T, Vahtera E, Uusitupa MIJ. Effects of dietary fat modification on fibrinogen, factor VII, and plasminogen activator inhibitor 1 activity in subjects with impaired glucose tolerance. Metabolism 1997;46:666–672.

79. Lopez-Segura F, Velasco F, Lopez-Miranda J, Castro P, Lopez-Pedrera R, Blanco A, Jimenez-Pereperez J. Torres A, Trujillo J, Ordovas JM, Perez-Jimenez. Monounsaturated fatty acid-enriched diet decreases plasma plasminogen activator inhibitor type 1. Arterioscl Thromb Vasc Biol 1996;16:82–88.

80. Nilsson TK, Sundell BI, Hellsten G, Hallmans G. Reduced plasminogen activator inhibitor activity in high consumers of fruits, vegetables and root vegetables. J Intern Med 1990;227:267–271.

81. Speiser W, Langer W, Pschaick A, Selmayre E, Ibe B, Owacki PR, Muller-Bergaus G. Increased blood fibrinolytic activity after physical exercise: Comparative study in individuals with different sporting activities and in patients after myocardial infarction taking part in a rehabilitation sports program. Thromb Res 1988;51:543–555.

82. Estelles A, Aznar J, Tormo G, Sapena P, Tormo V, Espana F. Influence of a rehabilitation sports program on the fibrinolytic activity of patients after myocardial infarction. Thromb Res 1989;55:203–212.

83. Gris JC, Schved JF, Aguilar-Martinez P, Arnaud A, Sanchez N. Impact of physical training on plasminogen activator inhibitor activity in sedentary men. Fibrinolysis 1990;4:97–98.

84. Shaukat N, Douglas JT, Bennett JL, de Bono DP. Can physical activity explain the differences in insulin levels and fibrinolytic activity between young indo-origin and european relatives of patients with coronary artery disease? Fibrinolysis 1995;9:55–63.

85. Alessi MC, Juhan-Vague I, Kooistra T, Declerck PJ, Collen D. Insulin stimulates the synthesis of plasminogen activator inhibitor 1 by hepatocellular cell line Hep G2. Thromb Haemost 1988;60:491–494.

86. Kooistra T, Bosma PJ, Töns HAM, van den Berg AP, Meyer P, Princen HMG. Plasminogen activator inhibitor 1: Biosynthesis and mRNA level are increased by insulin in cultured human hepatocytes. Thromb Haemost 1989;62:723–728.

87. Schneider DJ, Sobel BE. Augmentation of synthesis of plasminogen activator inhibitor type 1 by insulin and insulin like growth factor type 1: Implications for vascular disease by hyperinsulinemic states. Proc Natl Acad Sci USA 1991;88:9959–9963.

88. Anfosso F, Chomiki N, Alessi MC, Vague P, Juhan-Vague I. Plasminogen activator inhibitor 1 synthesis in the human hepatoma cell line Hep G2. Metformin inhibits the stimulating effect of insulin. J Clin Invest 1993;91:2185–2193.

89. Alessi MC, Anfosso F, Henry M, Peiretti F, Nalbone G, Juhan-Vague I. Up-regulation of PAI-1 synthesis by insulin and proinsulin in Hep G2 cells but not in endothelial cells. Fibrinolysis 1995;9:237–242.

90. Nordt TK, Schneider DJ, Sobel BE. Augmentation of the synthesis of plasminogen activator inhibitor type 1 by precursors of insulin. A potential risk factor for vascular disease. Circulation 1994;89:321–330.

91. Anfosso F, Alessi MC, Nalbone G, Chomiki N, Henry M, Juhan-Vague I. Up-regulated expression of plasminogen activator inhibitor-1 in Hep-G2 cells: Interrelationship between insulin and insulin-like growth factor-1. Thromb Haemost1995;73:268–274.

92. Fattal PG, Schneider DJ, Sobel BE, Billadello JJ. Post-transcriptional regulation of expression of plasminogen activator inhibitor type 1 mRNA by insulin and insulin-like growth factor 1. J Biol Chem 1992;267:12412–12415.

93. Pandolfi A, Iacoviello L, Capani F. Vitacolonna E, Donati MB, Consoli A. Glucose and insulin independently reduce the fibrinolytic potential of human vascular smooth muscle cells in culture. Diabetologia 1996;39:1425–1431.

94. Schneider DJ, Sobel BE. Synergistic augmentation of expression of plasminogen activator inhibitor type 1 induced by insulin, very-low-density lipoproteins, and fatty acids. Coronary Artery Disease 1996;7:813–817.

95. Schneider DJ, Nordt TK, Sobel BE. Stimulation by proinsulin of expression of plasminogen activator inhibitor type 1 in endothelial cells. Diabetes 1992;41:890–895.

96. Padayatty SJ, Orme S, Zenobi PD, Stickland MH, Belchetz PE, Grant PJ. The effects of insulin-like growth factor-1 on plasminogen activator inhibitor-1 synthesis and secretion: Results from in vitro and in vivo studies. Thromb Haemost 1993;70:1009–1013.

97. Stiko-Rahm A, Wiman B, Hamsten A, Nilsson J. Secretion of plasminogen activator inhibitor-1 from cultured human umbilical vein endothelial cells is induced by very low density lipoprotein. Arteriosclerosis 1990;10:1067–1073.

98. Mussoni L, Mannucci L, Sirtori M, Camera M, Maderna P, Sironi L, Tremoli E. Hypertriglyceridemia and regulation of fibrinolytic activity. Arteriosl Thromb 1992;12:19–25.

99. Tremoli E, Camera M, Maderna P, Sironi L, Prati L, Colli S, Piovella F, Bernini F, Corsini A, Mussoni L. Increased synthesis of plasminogen activator inhibitor-1 by cultured human endothelial cells exposed to nature and modified LDLs. An LDL receptor-independent phenomenon. Arteriosl Thromb 1993;13:338–346.

100. Sironi L, Mussoni L, Prati L, Baldassarre D, Camera M, Banfi C, Tremoli E. Plasminogen activator inhibitor type-1 synthesis and mRNA expression in hepG2 cells are regulated by VLDL. Arterioscler. Thromb Vasc Biol 1996;16:89–96.

101. Latron Y, Chautan M, Anfosso F, Alessi MC, Nalbone G, Lafont H, Juhan-Vague I. Stimulating effect of oxidized low density lipoproteins on plasminogen activator inhibitor-1 synthesis by endothelial cells. Arteriosl Thromb 1991;11:1821–1829.

102. Chautan M, Latron Y, Anfosso F, Alessi MC, Lafont H, Juhan-Vague I, Nalbone G. Phosphatidylinositol turnover during stimulation of plasminogen activator inhibitor-1 secretion induced by oxidized low density lipoproteins in human endothalial cells. J Lipid Res 1993;34:101–110.

103. Latron Y, Alessi MC, George F, Anfosso F, Poncelet P, Juhan-Vague I. Characterization of epitheloid cells from human omentum: Comparison with endothelial cells from umbilical veins.Thromb Haemost1991;66:361–367.

104. Nordt TK, Sawa H, Fujii S, Sobel BE. Induction of plasminogen activator inhibitor type 1 (PAI-1) by proinsulin and insulin in vivo. Circulation 1995;91:764–770.

105. Auwerx J, Bouillon R, Collen D, Geboers J. Tissus-type plasminogen activator antigen and plasmino-gen activator inhibitor in diabetes mellitus. Arteriosclerosis 1988;8:68–72.

106. Joki R, Klein RL, Lopez-Virella MF, Colwell JA. Release of platelet plasminogen activator inhibitor 1 in whole blood is increased in patients with type II diabetes. Diabetes Care 1995;18:1150–1155.

107. Garcia Frade LJ, de la Calle H, Torade MC, Lara JI, Cuellar L, Garcia Avello A. Hypofibrinolysis associated with vasculopathy in non-insulin dependent diabetes mellitus. Thromb Res 1990;59:51–59.

108. Schneider DJ, Nordt TK, Sobel BE. Attenuated fibrinolysis and accelerated atherosclerosis in type II diabetic patients. Diabetes 1993;42:1–7.

109. Gray RP, David L, Patterson H, Yudkin JS. Plasminogen activator inhibitor activity in diabetic and nondiabetic survivors of myocardial infarction. Arterioscler Thromb 1993;13:415–420.

110. Gray RP, Yudkin JS, Patterson DL. Plasminogen activator inhibitor: A risk factor for myocardial infarction in diabetic patients. Br Heart J 1993;69:228–232.

111. Vukovich T, Proidl S, Knöbl P, Teufelsbauer H, Schnack C, Schernthaner G. The effect of insulin treatment on the balance between tissue plasminogen activator and plasminogen activator inhibitor 1 in type 2 diabetic patients. Thromb Haemost 1992;68:253–256.

112. Ho CH, Jap TS. Fibrinolytic activity in chinese patients with diabetes or hyperlipidemia in comparison with healthy controls. Thromb Haemost 1991;65:3–6.

113. Ho CH, Jap TS. Relationship of plasminogen activator inhibitor-1 with plasma insulin, glucose, trig-lyceride and cholesterol in chinese patients with diabetes. Thromb Res 1993;69:271–277.

114. Takada Y, Urano T, Watanabe I, Taminato A, Yoshimi T, Takada A. Changes in fibrinolytic parameters in male patients with type 2 (non-insulin-dependent) diabetes mellitus. Thromb Res 1993;71:405–415.

115. Mahmoud R, Raccah D, Alessi MC, Aillaud MF, Juhan-Vague I, Vague P. Fibrinolysis in insulin dependent diabetic patients with or without nephropathy. Fibrinolysis 1992;6:105–109.

116. Nordt TK, Klassen KJ, Schneider DJ, Sobel BE. Augmentation of synthesis of plasminogen activator inhibitor type 1 in arterial endothelial cells by glucose and its implications for local fibrinolysis. Arterioscl Thromb 1993;13:1822–1828.

117. Maiello M, Boeri D, Podesta F, Cagliero E, Vichi M, Odetti P, Adezati L, Lorenzi M. Increased expression of tissue plasminogen activator and its inhibitor and reduced fibrinolytic potential of human endothelial cells cultured in elevated glucose. Diabetes 1992;41:1009–1015.

118. Potter van Loon BJ, De Bart ACW, Radder JK, Frouch M, Kluft C, Menders AE. Acute exogenous hyperinsulinaemia does not result in elevation of plasma plasminogen activator inhibitor 1 (PAI-1) in human. Fibrinolysis 1990;4:93–94.

119. Juhan-Vague I, Vague P. Hypofibrinolysis and insulin resistance. Diabete Metab 1991;17:91–100.

120. Landin K, Tengborn L, Chmielewska J, von Schenck H, Smit U. The acute effect of insulin on tissue plasminogen activator and plasminogen activator inhibitor in man. Thromb Haemost 1991;65:130–133.

121. Grant PJ, Kruithof EKO, Felley CP, Felber JP, Bachmann F. Short-term infusions of insulin triacyglycerol and glucose do not cause acute increases in plasminogen activator inhibitor-1 concen-tration in man. Clin Sci 1990;79:513–516.

122. Scelles V, Raccah D, Alessi MC, Vialle JM, Juhan-Vague I, Vague P. Plasminogen activator inhibitor 1 and insulin levels in various insulin resistance states. Diabete Métab. 1992;18:38–42.

123. Raccah D, Alessi MC, Scelles V, Menard C, Juhan-Vague I, Vague P. Plasminogen activator inhibitor activity in various types of endogenous hypertriglyceridemia. Fibrinolysis 1993;7:171–176.

124. Rifici VA, Schneider SH, Chen Y, Khachadurian AK. Administration of antioxidant vitamins does not alter plasma fibrinolytic activity in subjects with central obesity. Thromb Haemost 1997;78:1111–1114.

125. Alessi MC, Parrot G, Guenoun E, Scelles V, Vague P, Juhan-Vague I. Relation between plasma PAI activity and Adipsin levels. Thromb Haemost 1995;74:1200–1202.

126. Samad F, Loskutoff DJ. The fat mouse: A powerful genetic model to study eleva plasminogen activator inhibitor 1 in obesity/NIDDM. Thromb Haemost 1997;78:652–655.

127. Sawdey S, Loskutoff DJ. Regulation of murine type 1 plasminogen activity inhibitor (PAI-1) gene expression in vivo. Tissue specificity and induction by lipopolysaccharide, tumor necrosis factor a and transforming growth factor b. J Clin Invest 1991;88:1346–1353.

128. Samad F, Yamamoto K, Loskutoff DJ Distribution and regulation of plasminogen activator inhibitor 1 in murine adipose tissue in vivo. J Clin Invest 1996;97:37–46.

129. Lundgren CH, Brown SL, Nordt TD, Sobel BE, Fujii S. Elaboration of type 1 plasminogen activator inhibitor from adipocytes. A potential pathogenetic link between obesity and cardiovascular disease. Circulation 1996;93:106–10.

130. Samad F, Loskutoff DJ. Tissue distribution and regulation of plasminogen activator inhibitor 1 in obese mice. Mol Med 1996;2:568–582.

131. Shimomura I, Funahashi T, Takahashi M, Maeda K, Kotani K, Nakamura T, Yamashita S, Miura M, Fukuda Y, Takemura K, Tokunaga K, Matsuzawa Y. Enhanced expression of PAI-1 in visceral fat: Possible contributor to vascular disease in obesity. Nature Medicine 1996;2:800–803.

132. Alessi MC, Peiretti F, Morange P, Henry M, Nalbone G, Juhan-Vague I. Production of plasminogen activator inhibitor 1 by human adipose tissue. Possible link between visceral fat accumulation and vascular disease. Diabetes 1997;46:860–867.

133. Björntorp P."Portal" adipose tissue as a generator of risk factors for cardiovascular disease and diabetes. Arteriosclerosis 1990;10:493–496.

134. Larsson B, Svärdsud DK, Welin L, Wilhelmsen L, Björntorp P, Tibbin G. Abdominal adipose tissue distribution, obesity and risk of cardiovascular disease and death: 13 year follow-up of participants in the study of men born in 1913. BMJ 1984;288:1401–1404.

135. Cigolini M, Targher G, Bergamo Andreis IA, Tonoli M, Agostino G, De Sandre G. Visceral fat accumulation and its relation to plasma hemostatic factors in healthy men. Arterioscl Thromb Vasc Biol 1996;16:368–74.

136. De Pergola G, De Mitrio V, Giorgino F, Sciaraffia M, Minenna A, Di Bari L, Pannacciulli N, Giorgino R. Increase in both pro-thrombotic and anti-thrombotic factors in obese premenopausal women: relationship with body fat distribution. Int J Obes 1997;21:527–535.

137. Hotamisligil GS, Shargill NS, Spiegelman BM. Adipose expression of tumor necrosis factor α: Direct role in obesity-linked insulin resistance. Science 1993;259:87–91.

138. Morange PE, Aubert J, Peiretti F, Lljnen HR, Vague P, Verdier M, Negrel R, Juhan-Vague I, Alessi MC. Glucocorticoids and insulin promote plasminogen activator inhibitor 1 production by human adipose tissue. Diabetes (in press).

139. Dawson S, Hamsten A, Wiman B, Henney A, Humphries S. Genetic variation at the plasminogen activator inhibitor-1 locus associated with altered levels of plasma plasminogen activator inhibitor-1 activity. Arterioscl Thromb 1991;11:183–90.

140. Dawson SJ, Wiman B, Hamsten A, Green F, Humphries S, Henney AM. The two allele sequences of a common polymorphism in the promoter of the plasminogen activator inhibitor-1 (PAI-1) gene respond differently to interleukin–1 in HepG2 cells. J Biol Chem 1993;268:10739–10745.

141. Henry M, Chomiki N, Scarabin PY, Alessi MC, Pereitti F, Arveiler D, Ferrieres J, Evans A, Amouyel P, Poirier O, Cambien F, Juhan-Vague I. Five frequent polymorphisms of plasminogen activator inhibitor 1 gene: Lack of association between genotypes, PAI activity and triglycerides levels in a healthy population. Arterioscl Thromb Vasc Biol 1997;17:851–858.

142. Ye S, Green FR, Scarabin PY, Nicaud V, Bara L, Dawson SJ, Humphries SE, Evans A, Luc G, Cambon JP, Arveiler D, Henney AM, Cambien F. The 4G/5G genetic polymorphism in the promoter of the plasminogen activator inhibitor-1(PAI-1) associated with differences in plasma PAI-1 activity but not with risk of myocardial infarction in the ECTIM study. Thromb Haemost 1995;74:837–841.

143. Panahloo A. Mohamed Ali V, Lane A, Green F, Humphries SE, Yudkin JS. Determinants of plasminogen activator inhibitor 1 activity in treated NIDDM and its relation to a polymorphism in the plasminogen activator inhibitor 1 gene. Diabetes. 1995;44:37–42.

144. Erickson P, Kallin B, van't Hooft FM, Bavenholm P, Hamsten A. Allele specific increase in basal transcription of the plasminogen-activator inhibitor 1 gene is associated with myocardial infarction. Proc Natl Acad Sci 1995;92:1851–1855.

145. Mansfield MW, Strickland MH, Grant PJ. Environmental and genetic factors in relation to elevated circulating levels of plasminogen activator inhibitor 1 in caucasian patients with non insulin dependent diabetes mellitus. Thromb Haemost 1995;74:842–848.

146. McCormack LJ, Nagi DK, Stickland MH, Mansfield MW, Mohamed-Ali V, Yudkin JS, Knowler WC, Grant PJ. Promoter (4G/5G) plasminogen activator inhibitor 1 genotype in Pima Indians: relationship to plasminogen activator inhibitor 1 levels and features of the insulin resistance syndrome. Diabetologia 1996;39:1512–1518.

147. Ridker PM, Hennekens CH, Lindpaintner K, Stampfer MJ, Miletich JP. Arterial and venous thrombosis is not associated with the 4G/5G polymorphism in the promoter of the plasminogen activator inhibitor gene in a large cohort of US men. Circulation 1997;95:59–62.

148. Henry M, Tregouët DA, Alessi MC, Aillaud MF, Visvikis S, Siest G, Tiret L, Juhan-Vague I. Metabolic determinants are much more important than genetic polymorphisms in determining the PAI-1 activity

and antigen plasma concentrations : A family study with part of the Stanislas cohort. Arterioscl Thromb Vasc Biol 1997, 1998;18:84–91.

149. Zehetgruber M, Beckmann R, Gabriel H, Christ G, Binder BR, Huber K. Comparative cross-over study of the effects of lisinopril and doxazosin on insulin, glucose and lipoprotein metabolism and the endogenous fibrinolytic system. Fibrinolysis and Proteolysis 1997;11:153–158.

150. Jeng JR, Sheu WH, Jeng CY, Huang SH, Shieh SM. Effect of doxazosin on fibrinolysis in hypertensive patients with and without insulin resistance. Am Heart J 1996;132:783–789.

151. Wright RA, Flapan AD, Alberti KGMN, et al. Effects of captopril therapy on endogenous fibrinolysis in men with recent, uncomplicated myocardial infarction. J Am Coll Cardiol 1994;24:67–73.

152. Brown S, Sobel B, Fujii S. Attenuation of the synthesis of plasminogen activator inhibitor type 1 by niacin: a potential link between lipid lowering and fibrinolysis. Circulation 1995;92:767–772.

153. Nordt TK, Kornas K, Peter K, Fujii S, Sobel BE, Kubler W, Bode C. Attenuation by gemfibrozil of expression of plasminogen activator type 1 induced by insulin and its precursors. Circulation 1997;95:677–683.

154. Broijersen A, Eriksson M, Wiman B, Angelin B, Hjemdahl P. Gemfibrozil treatment of combined hyperliporoteinemia. No improvement of fibrinolysis despite marked reduction of plasma triglyceride levels. Arterioscler. Thromb Vasc Biol 1996;16:511–516.

155. Jeng JR, Jeng CY, Sheu WHH, Lee MMS, Huang SH, Shieh SM. Gemfibrozil treatment of hypertriglyceridemia: improvement on fibrinolysis without change of insulin resistance. Am Heart J 1997;134:565–571.

156. Asplund-Carlson A. Effects of gemfibrozil therapy on glucose tolerance, insulin sensitivity and plasma plasminogen activator inhibitor activity in hypertriglyceridaemia. J Cardiovasc Risk 1996;3:385–90.

157. Eitzman DT, Fay WP, Lawrence DA, et al. Peptide-mediated inactivation of recombinant and platelet plasminogen activator inhibitor-1 in vitro. J Clin Invest 1995;95:2416–2420.

158. Ngo TH, Debrock S, Declerck PJ. Identification of functional synergism between monoclonal antibodies. Aplication to the enhancement of plasminogen activator inhibitor 1 neutralizing effects. FEBS Lett 1997;416:373–376.

18   Insulin Resistance and Cardiovascular Disease

Aaron R. Folsom, MD

CONTENTS

INTRODUCTION
MEASUREMENT IN EPIDEMIOLOGIC STUDIES
INSULIN RESISTANCE AND ATHEROSCLEROTIC
    CARDIOVASCULAR DISEASE
INTERPRETATION
CONCLUSIONS
REFERENCES

INTRODUCTION

Over the past two decades, researchers have devoted considerable effort to testing the hypothesis that insulin resistance and hyperinsulinemia contribute to the etiology of atherosclerotic cardiovascular diseases. There is clearly an association of insulin resistance and hyperinsulinemia with metabolic risk factors that are involved in the etiology of atherosclerotic disease. Yet, proving an etiologic role for insulin has been difficult, and differences of opinion about the evidence have sparked recent discussion (1–5). This chapter summarizes existing evidence on this topic and concludes that 1) hyperinsulinemia is a weak marker of cardiovascular risk and 2) there are insufficient data to conclude whether insulin resistance, *per se*, increases cardiovascular disease incidence.

MEASUREMENT IN EPIDEMIOLOGIC STUDIES

Part of the difficulty of testing the hypothesis that insulin resistance increases the risk of atherosclerotic cardiovascular disease is that direct measurement of insulin resistance is relatively costly and burdensome to study participants, making it largely impractical for large scale epidemiologic research. Because insulin resistance leads to hyperinsulinemia, most studies have instead measured concentrations of insulin, either fasting or one or two h after an oral glucose load. Insulin levels and insulin resistance are correlated moderately well. Laakso reported the correlations of fasting, 1-h, and 2-h

From: *Contemporary Endocrinology: Insulin Resistance*
Edited by: G. Reaven and A. Laws © Humana Press Inc., Totowa, NJ

insulin concentrations with insulin mediated glucose disposal were –0.66, –0.58, and –0.68, respectively, in people with normal glucose tolerance *(6)*. These correlations ranged from –0.47 to –0.39 in people with impaired glucose tolerance and –0.48 to –0.15 in people with non-insulin-dependent diabetes. The true correlation of fasting insulin concentration and insulin resistance in normals must be even higher than 0.6 because fasting insulin, itself, has a reliability coefficient on repeat testing of individuals of only approximately 0.8 (7).

Most epidemiologic studies have measured immunoreactive insulin concentrations using assays that cross-react with proinsulin and des-31, 32 proinsulin. In the past decade specific assays for insulin, with almost no cross-reactivity, have become available. Only a few recent epidemiologic studies have been able to use the more specific insulin assays. However, in nondiabetic populations the concentration of proinsulin molecules is low, and the correlation of immunoreactive insulin and specific insulin is high *(8)*.

INSULIN RESISTANCE AND ATHEROSCLEROTIC CARDIOVASCULAR DISEASE

Coronary Artery Disease

Evidence for an association between blood insulin concentrations and coronary artery disease was first offered by cross-sectional clinical studies almost three decades ago. Stout thoroughly reviewed this clinical evidence through 1990 *(9)*. The majority of clinical studies have reported a positive association of prevalent coronary artery disease with insulin response to oral glucose, but inconsistent associations of coronary disease with fasting insulin and insulin responses to intravenous glucose, tolbutamide, or arginine. A number of additional clinical studies have been reported since 1990, most of which have reported a positive association between some insulin measure and coronary disease *(10–23)*. However, only three small studies have directly measured insulin resistance in relation to coronary disease *(17,19,20)*. All three showed a positive association between insulin resistance and coronary disease. Clinical evidence, however, potentially suffers from biases related to patient representativeness, confounding by medications and comorbidity, and the inability to distinguish whether the hyperinsulinemia or insulin resistance preceded the onset of disease. Population-based prospective studies should offer better evidence.

Since the early 1980s, there have been nearly 20 prospective epidemiologic studies testing whether insulin concentrations in nondiabetics are associated with incidence or death from coronary artery disease (Table 1). Four of these studies had less than 50 coronary events *(24–27)* and one of these used survey ECG evidence only for defining coronary disease *(27)*. None of these four studies showed any independent association of insulin with coronary artery disease, although one found a univariate (crude) positive association *(26)*. The remaining studies are summarized in Table 1 and Fig. 1.

Care must be taken in interpreting multivariate relative risks from these epidemiologic studies. Univariate models provide an overall association between insulin concentrations and disease but may be confounded by other risk factors. Models that adjust for risk factors not believed to be on the causal path between insulin and coronary disease (e.g., age, smoking, total cholesterol) may be the most relevant. Models that include risk factors believed to be in the causal pathway (e.g., HDL cholesterol, hypertension, obesity) can be further helpful in defining possible pathways but provide "over adjusted" estimates of relative risks. Existing studies often did not model in the best ways. Thus, Table 1 and the text generally focus on the fullest multivariate models; yet, positive univariate findings are also identified in Table 1.

The first three prospective studies, completed in the late 1970s, all reported moderately large, statistically significant associations between at least one measure of insulin concentration and coronary heart disease (CHD) occurrence *(28–30)*. Welborn and Wearne *(28)* measured insulin concentrations one h post-glucose in 1634 men and 1697 women aged 21 yr and older in Brusselton, Australia. Over six yr of follow-up, the relative risk (RR) of CHD incidence for the highest quintile versus the lowest four quintiles of insulin was elevated nonsignificantly: RR of 1.50 for men (adjusted for systolic blood pressure and relative weight) and 1.28 for women (unadjusted) (both $p > 0.05$). The corresponding association for 12 yr CHD -mortality was RR= 1.67 ($p < 0.05$) in men (adjusted for systolic pressure and serum cholesterol) and 0.94 (unadjusted, $p > 0.05$) in women. At 13 yr, there was no association between insulin and CHD mortality in a subset aged 45–59 *(31)*. After 23 yr follow-up *(32)*, 1-h insulin concentration showed no association with CHD death in women, and a statistically significant U-shaped relation in men (RRs for quintiles in men of 2.11, 1.48, 1.00, 1.03, and 1.81, adjusted for age, blood pressure, total cholesterol and smoking). Thus, although this Brusselton study is often cited as supporting the insulin and CHD hypothesis, it largely does not.

Pyörälä measured insulin concentrations fasting, 1-h, and 2-h post-glucose in 1042 middle-aged Helsinki policemen *(29)*. After 5 yr of follow-up, fasting insulin was not associated with CHD but 1 h and 2-h post-glucose insulins were. The relative risk per standard deviation increment of 2-h insulin was 1.52 (95% CI= 1.18-1.97), adjusted for age, total cholesterol, 2-h glucose, triglycerides, diastolic pressure, smoking, and body mass index. This positive association was substantiated at 9 1/2 yr of follow-up (33). In a recent analysis of 22 yr of follow-up, Pyörälä (34) showed a diminution of the multivariately adjusted relative risk for the upper quintile versus the lowest four quintiles of the integrated insulin area, from RR = 2.43 at 5 yr, to 2.29 at 10 yr, 1.71 at 15 yr, and 1.30 at 22 yr. The age-adjusted relative risk was 1.57 ($p < 0.05$) at 22 yr.

Ducimetiere et al. measured fasting and 2-h post-glucose insulin in 7246 male Paris policemen aged 43–54 *(30)*. At five yr of follow-up, the relative risk of CHD incidence per SD increment of insulin was 1.46 for fasting ($p < 0.05$) and 1.20 for 2 h (>0.05), adjusted for total cholesterol, systolic pressure, smoking, and glucose. At an 11.2 year follow-up, CHD mortality was still associated significantly and independently with fasting but not 2-h insulin *(35)*, but at 15 yr, it was independently associated with 2 h and not fasting insulin *(36)*. At all follow-up points, there was a statistically significant univariate association for both 2 h and fasting insulin *(30,35,36)*.

Three studies of men reported in the early 1990s provided evidence mostly opposing an association of fasting insulin with CHD *(37–39)*. As illustrated in Fig. 1, Orchard et al. found no overall association of fasting insulin with CHD incidence in the Multiple Risk Factor Intervention Trial, although there was a significant interaction with apolipoprotein E phenotype *(37)*. Insulin showed a positive association with CHD in the apo E 3/2 subgroup. Welin et al. reported no association of fasting and 1 h insulin with CHD *(38)* and Yarnell et al. *(39)* observed a statistically significant age-adjusted relative risk of 1.2 for CHD per standard deviation of insulin, but adjustment for triglycerides, prevalent CHD, or body mass index dropped the RR close to 1.0. Another study reported only in abstract *(40)*, reported no association between fasting or post-OGTT insulin concentrations and incidence of myocardial infarction in 25–74 year-old men and women.

Table 1
Prospective Epidemiologic Studies of Blood Insulin Concentrations and Occurrence of Coronary Heart Disease (CHD)

Name (ref.)	Population, years recruited	N, sex	Age (y)	Excluded	Contrast†	Insulin‡ measure	Multivariate relative risk‖	Endpoints§	N Events	Follow-up time (y)
Welborn (28)	Brusselton, 1966 Australia	1634 M, 1697 W	≥21	?	V/I–IV	1 h	M 1.50, W 1.28	CHD-I	114 M, 111 W	6
Cullen (31)	Brusselton, 1966 Australia	840 M, 724 W	45–74	?	—	1 h	M 1.67*, W 0.94 N.S.	CHD-D CHD-D	149 M, 120 W 51 M, 18 W	12 13
Welborn (32)	Brusselton, 1966 Australia	1456 M, 1514 W	≥21	DM, IGT	Quintiles	1 h	M 2.11*, 1.48, 1.0, 1.03, 1.81* W 0.78, 1.05, 1.0, 1.34, 1.04	CHD-D	137 M, 94 W	23
Pyörälä (29)	Helsinki, 1971–2	1042 M	30–59	DM	One SD	F 1 h 2 h	N.S. Positive* 1.52*	CHD-I	36	5
Pyörälä (33)	Helsinki, 1971–2	982 M	35–64	DM	One SD	F 1 h 2 h	N.S. 1.44* 1.42*	CHD-I	63	9.5
Pyörälä (34)	Helsinki, 1971–2	974	34–64	DM	V/I–IV	Insulin area	1.30	CHD-I	165	22
Ducimetiere (30)	Paris, 1968–73	7246	43–54	DM	1 ln mU/L	F 2 h	1.46* 1.20	CHD-I	128	5
Eschwege (35)	Paris, 1968–73	6775	43–54	DM	One SD	F 2 h	2.02* 1.50	CHD-D	126	11.2
Fontbonne (36)	Paris, 1968–73	7028	43–54	Insulin Rx	>vs<452 pmol/L	2 h F	1.55* N.S.	CHD-D	178	15
Hargreaves (24)	Edinburgh, 1976	107 M	40	?	Means	F, Insulin Area	N.S.	CHD-I	11	12
Welin (38)	Gothenburg, Sweden 1963	563 M	67	DM	Quintiles	F 1 h	N.S. N.S.	CHD-I	56	8
Liu (27)	Pima Indians, 1975	589 M & W	≥25	DM	X/I	F 2 h	2.30 1.52	ECG abn	16	1–16

Study	Location, years	N	Age	DM	?	F, Insulin Area	¶ Result	§ Endpoint	Cases	Years
Rewers (40)	Colorado, 1984–88	897 M & W	25–74	DM	?		N.S.	MI–I	72	4
Yarnell (39)	Caerphilly, UK 1979–83	2,022 M	45–59	DM	One SD	F	1.04	CHD–I	113	5
Orchard (37)	MRFIT, 1973–76	622 M	35–57	DM	IV/I	F	0.94 Positive* for Apo E 3/2 Subgroup	CHD–I	114	7–10
Ferrara (25)	Rancho Bernardo, CA, 1984–87	538 M, 705W	50–89	DM	One SD	F 2 h	M N.S., W N.S. M N.S., W 0.68*	CVD–D	24 M, 21 W	5
Kuusisto (41)	Kuopio, 1986–8 Finland	1069 M & W	65–76	DM	V/I–IV	F	1.20 2.57*	CHD–I CHD–D	74 30	3.5
Møller (42)	Copenhagen, 1976	504 M, 548 W	40	?	One SD	F	1.16*	CHD–I	54	17
Perry (43)	U.K., 1978–80	5,550 M	40–59	DM	X/I–IX	NF	1.6*	CHD–I	521	11.5
Després (44)	Quebec, 1985	196 M	45–76	DM	One SD	F	1.6*	CHD–I	91	5
Yudkin (26)	Tanzania, 1986	137 M & W	>15	DM	One SD	F	0.99	CHD–I	25	6.5
Lakka (45), Lakka (46)	Kuopio, Finland 1984–9	1882 M	42–60	DM	III/I IV/I	F F	1.17 2.43	MI–I CHD–D	93 22	8 9
Folsom (47)	US, 1987–9	13,446 M & W	45–64	DM	Quintiles	F	M 1.0, 0.50, 0.65, 0.63, 0.49 W 1.0, 0.98, 2.29, 1.97, 2.06	CHD–I	209 M, 96 W	4–7

*$p < 0.05$; N.S. = nonsignificant at $p > 0.05$; M = Men, W = Women.

§CHD-I is CHD incidence; MI-I is myocardial infarction incidence; CHD-D is CHD mortality; CVD-D is cardiovascular mortality.

†Roman numerals indicate quantile groups. For example, V/I–IV is a contrast of quintile 5 versus quintiles 1–4.

‡F = Fasting; 1 h = 1 hour post glucose; 2 h = 2 hour post glucose; NF = Nonfasting.

¶Only multivariate results shown, including, in some cases, adjustment for variables potentially in the causal pathway (e.g., HDL–cholesterol, hypertension). The following studies showed at least one statistically significant univariate or minimally–adjusted positive association: 28, 29, 30, 33–36, 39, 41–47.

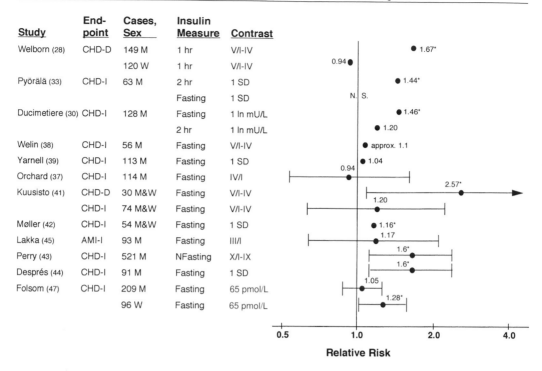

Fig. 1. Prospective studies of insulin and CHD occurrence. Figure shows multivariately-adjusted relative risks (95% confidence interval, where provided) for prospective studies with ≥50 endpoints—one publication per study. (*$p < 0.05$; N.S. = nonsignificant.)

In the late 1990s, five studies offered additional evidence for an association between insulin and CHD incidence. Each of them showed a univariate or minimally-adjusted positive association that generally weakened with adjustment for multiple other risk factors. Kuusisto et al. reported fasting insulin in the upper quintile versus the lowest four quintiles was associated with a 2.57 fold higher risk of CHD death ($p < 0.05$) but only a 1.20 higher risk of CHD incidence ($p > 0.05$) over 3.5 yr in 65–76 year-old Finns *(41)*. These estimates were adjusted for sex, smoking, waist/hip ratio, systolic pressure, total and HDL cholesterols. Møller and Jespersen reported a weak but statistically significant association between fasting insulin and CHD incidence in a cohort of Copenhagen adults (RR = 1.16 per S.D., $p = 0.002$, adjusted for multiple risk factors), although it was not clear whether these investigators excluded diabetics *(42)*. Perry et al. studied 40–59 year-old British men, including some with prevalent CHD, using a specific insulin assay and nonfasting serum *(43)*. After adjustment of insulin concentration for time of sampling, they observed an increased risk of CHD events over 11.5 yr, limited to the upper decile (RR = 1.6, 95% CI = 1.1–2.3, adjusted for multiple risk factors). The relative risk was stronger (RR = 2.1) at 5 yr of follow-up. Després et al. reported a relative risk of 1.6 (95% CI = 1.1–2.3) per SD of fasting insulin, measured by a specific assay, in a nested case-control study of 45–76 year-old men in Quebec *(44)*. This association was independent of hypertension, family history of CHD, plasma triglycerides, apo B, LDL-C, and HDL-C. A study of 42–60 year-old Finnish men found fasting insulin univariately associated with CHD incidence *(45)* and CHD mortality *(46)*, but the association disappeared with adjustment for other risk factors. Finally, there was a positive association between fasting insulin and CHD risk in middle-aged women, but not in men, in the Atherosclerosis Risk in Communities Study *(47)*. For this chapter, we recomputed the relative risks for a 65 pmol/L increment (the interquartile range) of fasting insulin, not presented in the original manuscript *(47)*. The relative risk for women was 1.30 (95% CI = 1.17–1.53) and for men was 1.13 (95% CI = 0.98–1.31), after adjustment for age, race, field center, smoking, drinking, and physical activity. The relative risks were 1.28 (1.03–1.59) and 1.05 (0.87–1.26), respectively, after further adjustment for body mass index, waist/hip ratio, total and HDL cholesterol, triglycerides, fibrinogen, and hypertension.

The studies shown in Table 1 for the most part involved people initially free of diabetes. Wingard and Barrett-Connor have pointed out that endogenous insulin concentrations in non-insulin dependent diabetics are not associated with CHD incidence *(48)*, but this might be expected given the initial rise, then fall in insulin over the course of diabetes development. Non-insulin dependent diabetics are generally insulin resistant and at high risk of CHD, but there has been no study relating the degree of their insulin resistance to CHD incidence.

Administration of exogenous insulin to diabetics has been associated with increased, decreased, and no effect on CHD occurrence *(48)*; however, it is not clear that observations of exogenous insulin are relevant to the understanding of insulin resistance in the etiology of CHD.

Peripheral Arterial Disease

Several population-based cross-sectional studies have tested the hypothesis that insulin concentration is associated positively with peripheral arterial disease assessed by a reduced ankle/brachial systolic blood pressure index. Their findings have partly supported this hypothesis. For example, Newman et al. reported that age and sex-adjusted mean fasting insulin was 47% higher in those with an ankle/brachial index of <0.8 versus those with an index ≥1.0 (p for trend <0.0001) among 3372 participants without clinical cardiovascular disease in the Cardiovascular Health Study *(49)*. There was apparently no association after accounting for other cardiovascular risk factors. The Honolulu Heart Study reported that the multivariately-adjusted odds ratio for an ankle/brachial index of <0.9 was 1.13 (95% CI = 1.06–1.21) for the highest versus lowest quintile of fasting insulin *(50)*; however, there was no association with 2 h post-glucose insulin concentration. The Edinburgh Artery Study reported a positive association of 1 h post-glucose insulin with peripheral arterial disease, defined on the basis of intermittent claudication symptoms and/or reduced ankle/brachial index, in comparison with disease-free controls *(51)*. The odds ratio was 1.86 (95% CI = 0.99–3.48) adjusted for age, sex, blood pressure, and lipids, but dropped to 1.64 (95% CI = 0.83–3.23) after adjustment for smoking.

Only one study has prospectively examined incidence of peripheral arterial disease in relation to insulin concentration. Uusitupa, et al. reported that there was an independent positive association between fasting insulin and the 5 yr incidence of intermittent claudication among newly diagnosed diabetes patients and controls from Finland *(52)*.

In the late 1980s, the availability of B-mode ultrasound technology enabled several studies to examine the association of insulin concentration and insulin resistance with atherosclerosis of superficial arteries. In cross-sectional studies, fasting insulin concentration was shown to be correlated moderately strongly and statistically significantly with carotid intima-media thickness, a marker of subclinical atherosclerosis, in diabetics *(53)*; in nondiabetics *(54)*, although one study of nondiabetics reported a U-shaped association

(55); and in people of unspecified glycemia status *(56)*. Salomaa et al. also reported that fasting insulin was positively associated with a ultrasonic measure of stiffness of the carotid artery *(57)*.

Ultrasonic assessment of atherosclerosis has also been used to study people in whom insulin resistance/sensitivity was measured directly. Laasko et al. used the euglycemic hyperinsulinemic clamp to show that 30 subjects with asymptomatic atherosclerosis in the femoral or carotid arteries had 20% lower whole-body glucose uptake than did 13 control subjects *(58)*. Agewell et al. also showed insulin sensitivity by the euglycemic hyperinsulinemic clamp to be strongly and inversely correlated with common carotid maximum intima-media thickness in 25 high-risk and 23 low-risk subjects *(59)*. Suzuki et al. used the steady-state plasma glucose method to show insulin sensitivity was inversely associated with common carotid intima-media thickness in 72 subjects with essential hypertension *(60)*. The Insulin Resistance Atherosclerosis Study (IRAS) studied 1,399 subjects and reported that insulin sensitivity, by the frequently sampled intravenous glucose tolerance test with analysis by the minimal model of Bergman, was inversely correlated with carotid intima-media thickness *(61)*. The association was apparent for Hispanic and non-Hispanic Caucasians, but not blacks, was modestly strong, and was independent of most other risk factors. In contrast with these findings, Kekäläinen et al. reported that the presence versus absence of sonographically-determined femoral plaques (in 85 and 33 Finnish young adults, respectively) was not associated with insulin sensitivity measured by the intravenous glucose tolerance test cross-sectionally, nor with fasting or 2-h insulin over approximately 9 yr of follow-up *(62)*.

Stroke

Several cross-sectional clinical studies have shown that ischemic stroke is accompanied by insulin resistance or hyperinsulinemia *(63–67)*. Surprisingly, there appears to have been only two prospective epidemiologic studies of the relation of hyperinsulinemia with stroke. Kuusisto et al. reported a statistically significant positive relation between fasting insulin and occurrence of stroke (n = 36) in 1,069 nondiabetic 65–74 year-old Finns followed 3.5 yr; however, there was no association for 2-h insulin *(68)*. Furthermore, after exclusion of participants with previous stroke, the association between fasting insulin and stroke became nonsignificant. The small number of incident strokes limited this study's power, and unfortunately estimates of relative risk were not provided. The Helsinki Policemen Study also recently reported a moderately strong association between hyperinsulinemia and stroke incidence that was mainly due to the impact of obesity on stroke risk *(81)*.

INTERPRETATION

Quality of the Evidence

Existing data provide modest support for the hypothesis that insulin resistance is a risk factor for atherosclerotic cardiovascular disease. However, it has been nearly impossible to design studies to optimally test this hypothesis. Measurement of insulin sensitivity has largely been limited to cross-sectional studies, because its measurement has generally been impractical for large prospective studies. Insulin concentration has served as a less satisfactory substitute, and existing evidence suggests that hyperinsulinemia is only a weak predictor of atherosclerotic disease risk. Reaven and Law *(3)* argued that insulin resistance and compensatory hyperinsulinemia, not all hyperinsulinemia, increases risk. While this insulin resistant subgroup with hyperinsulinemia may be at highest risk, the moderately high correlation between insulin concentration and insulin resistance *(6)* argues against a subgroup effect. The best direct evidence on insulin resistance and vascular disease are cross-sectional studies of peripheral arterial disease assessed ultrasonographically *(58–61)*. More prospective studies directly measuring insulin resistance and cardiovascular disease incidence are clearly needed.

Some have suggested that insulin resistance and hyperinsulinemia may affect atherosclerotic vascular disease risk more in some populations (e.g., populations at highest risk of CHD, like Finns; men; or younger people) than in other populations. Yet, recent data do not support these interactions with insulin effects, except perhaps for a weaker association in the elderly (Fig. 1), which is true for many cardiovascular risk factors. A potential source of bias in epidemiologic studies is that comorbid conditions, smoking, and undernutrition reduce insulin concentrations *(5)*.

Criteria for Causality

It is instructive to consider the evidence in relation to criteria for causality of epidemiologic associations:

CONSISTENCY

Existing prospective studies on insulin and atherosclerotic vascular disease are not very consistent. This is perhaps the most distracting aspect of the evidence, since true cause-effect relations should be replicable. If one discounts the small studies, only about half of the prospective investigations reported before 1995 showed a positive association of insulin with CHD, and even those that were positive tended not to demonstrate a positive association for their multiple measures of insulin for both sexes, and the associations weaken over time. (Obesity, the main determinant of insulin resistance, also shows an inconsistent association with CHD, but when present, the association appears to strengthen, not weaken, over longer follow-up time *(69)*). In contrast, most studies reported since 1995 have shown univariate associations between hyperinsulinemia and CHD that weakened but often remained statistically significant after multivariate adjustment.

STRENGTH OF ASSOCIATION

Relative risks range from near 1.0 (nonexistent) to 2.5 (moderately strong). The median relative risk is around 1.25, which is modest. A recent meta-analysis yielded a summary relative risk of 1.18 (95% CI=1.08–1.29) for a difference equivalent to that between the 75th and the 25th percentiles of the general population in the Netherlands *(82)*.

DOSE-RELATION

When any association exists, most studies show a positive dose-response between insulin and atherosclerotic disease. That is, the higher the insulin concentration, or level of insulin resistance, the greater the disease risk. However, some have reported U-shaped associations between insulin and atherosclerotic endpoints *(32,55)*.

TEMPORALITY

Prospective studies have shown that the presence of hyperinsulinemia precedes the onset of CHD, though, of course, subclinical disease may still have been present at the

Table 2
Possible Mechanisms Linking Hyperinsulinemia and Insulin Resistance
to Cardiovascular Disease

Direct effects
　　Increased vascular matrix
　　Proliferation and migration of smooth muscle
　　Decreased endothelial nitric oxide production
　　Increased LDL receptor activity in arterial smooth muscle cells and macrophages

Indirect effects
　　Elevated risk factors (Insulin Resistance Syndrome)
　　　　High blood pressure
　　　　↓ HDL; ↑ Triglycerides; small, dense LDL
　　　　Postprandial hypertriglyceridemia
　　　　↑ Plasminogen activator inhibitor-1
　　　　Impaired glucose tolerance

Noncausal role
　　Consequence of vascular disease and endothelial dysfunction
　　Coincidental with obesity

Sources: References 78–80.

time of baseline assessment. There are no prospective data on direct measures of insulin resistance and CHD incidence. There are few prospective studies relating hyperinsulinemia to peripheral arterial disease and ischemic stroke.

SPECIFICITY

Atherosclerotic cardiovascular disease has other, more important risk factors, so hyperinsulinemia is not a highly specific risk factor for vascular disease. Hyperinsulinemia obviously is a more specific risk factor for diabetes than CHD. From the point of view of other common diseases, relatively few studies have examined relations with insulin. Insulin has been associated negatively with total mortality in an elderly cohort (70). Insulin concentrations (71–73) but not C-peptide (74), were increased in endometrial cancer cases versus controls. Increased insulin has been found in association with gastrointestinal cancers (75) and increased C-peptide predicted risk of breast cancer, but not melanoma, lymphoma, and cervical cancer (76).

BIOLOGICAL PLAUSIBILITY

There are many potential direct and indirect biologic links between insulin resistance and atherothrombotic disease (Table 2). Hyperinsulinemia and insulin resistance have been linked to greater atherosclerosis (53,54,56,58–61). Many other potential mechanisms are discussed in detail in other chapters of this book. The most convincing biologic basis is the strong association of hyperinsulinemia and insulin resistance with metabolic risk factors (the "Insulin Resistance Syndrome"). The fact that insulin resistance and hyperinsulinemia are so strongly linked to dyslipidemia and elevated plasminogen activator inhibitor-1 makes it somewhat surprising that several studies did not find a univariate association of insulin with CHD (1). However, recent studies have (41–47). In these latter studies, adjustment for HDL-cholesterol, triglycerides, and obesity attenuated the associations, as would be expected if they mediate the effects of insulin.

The association between insulin and vascular disease might not be causal. Obesity and insulin resistance are tightly intertwined; however, obesity, particularly abdominal obesity, may lead to metabolic abnormalities independent of insulin resistance. Or, cardiovascular disease may, itself, lead to insulin resistance. For example, Yudkin has proposed that endothelial dysfunction could lead to impaired insulin action and the associated metabolic derangements of the insulin resistance syndrome *(77)*.

REVERSIBILITY

The strongest evidence that hyperinsulinemia or insulin resistance may be associated with atherosclerotic vascular diseases would come from a clinical trial to reverse insulin resistance. Such a trial has not been feasible, although with newer agents, such as the thiazolidinediones, such a trial might be possible. It would be difficult, however, to prove that reduction of insulin resistance, and not improvement of related cardiovascular risk factors, would be the cause of any reduction in vascular events.

CONCLUSIONS

Although insulin resistance is strongly associated with multiple metabolic abnormalities, its role in causing atherosclerotic diseases is unestablished. Additional prospective studies of insulin concentration and CHD are unlikely to clarify this theory, though studies involving other vascular diseases (e.g., stroke) would be welcome. More useful would be large prospective studies with direct measures of insulin resistance; the IRAS study *(61)* could accomplish this with extended follow-up. Further work with animal models and trials of new agents that reduce insulin resistance in humans also will be valuable. From a clinical perspective, certainly there is little justification for measuring insulin concentrations to help identify patients at high risk of cardiovascular disease.

REFERENCES

1. Jarrett RJ. Why is insulin not a risk factor for coronary heart disease? Diabetologia 1994;37:945–947.
2. Fontbonne A. Why can high insulin levels indicate a risk for coronary heart disease? Diabetologia 1994;37:953–955.
3. Reaven GM, Laws A. Insulin resistance, compensatory hyperinsulinaemia, and coronary heart disease. Diabetologia 1994;37:948–952.
4. Stern MP. The insulin resistance syndrome: the controversy is dead, long live the controversy! Diabetologia 1994;37:956–958.
5. McKeigue P, Davey G. Associations between insulin levels and cardiovascular disease are confounded by comorbidity. Diabetes Care 1995;18:1294–1298.
6. Laakso M. How good a marker is insulin level for insulin resistance? Am J Epidemiol 1993;137:959–965.
7. Eckfeldt JH, Chambless LE, Shen YL. Short-term, within-person variability in clinical chemistry test results: Experience from the Atherosclerosis Risk in Communities Study. Arch Pathol Lab Med 1994;118:496–500.
8. Mohamed-Ali V, Gould MM, Gillies S, Goubet S, Yudkin JS, Haines AP. Association of proinsulin-like molecules with lipids and fibrinogen in non-diabetic subjects - evidence against a modulating role for insulin. Diabetologia 1995;38:1110–1116.
9. Stout RW. Insulin and atheroma: 20-yr perspective. Diabetes Care 1990;13:631–654.
10. Modan M, Or J, Karasik A, Drory Y, Fuchs Z, Lusky A, Chetrit A, Halkin H. Hyperinsulinemia, sex, and risk of atherosclerotic cardiovascular disease. Circulation 1991;84:1165–1175.
11. Negri M, Sheiban I, Arigliano PL, Tonni S, Montresor G, Carlini S, Manzato F. Interrelation between angiographic severity of coronary artery disease and plasma levels of insulin, C-peptide and plasminogen activator inhibitor–1. Am J Cardiol 1993;72:397–401.

12. Solymoss BC, Marcil M, Chaour M, Gilfix BM, Poitras AM, Campeau L. Fasting hyperinsulinism, insulin resistance syndrome, and coronary artery disease in men and women. Am J Cardiol 1995;76:1152–1156.

13. Mykkänen L, Laakso M, Pyörälä K. High plasma insulin level associated with coronary heart disease in the elderly. Am J Epidemiol 1993;137:1190–1202.

14. Rönnemaa T, Laakso M, Pyörälä K, Kallio V, Puuka P. High fasting plasma insulin is an indicator of coronary heart disease in non-insulin-dependent diabetic patients and nondiabetic subjects. Arterioscler Thromb 1991;11:80–90.

15. Båvenholm P, Proudler A, Tornvall P, Godsland I, Landou C, de Faire U, Hamsten A. Insulin, intact and split proinsulin, and coronary artery disease in young men. Circulation 1995;92:1422–1429.

16. Dhawan J, Bray CL. Relationships between angiographically assessed coronary artery disease, plasma insulin levels and lipids in Asians and Caucasians. Atherosclerosis 1994;105:35–41.

17. Shinozaki K, Suzuki M, Ikebuchi M, Hara Y, Harano Y. Demonstration of insulin resistance in coronary artery disease documented with angiography. Diabetes Care 1996;19:1–7.

18. Katz RJ, Ratner RE, Cohen RM, Eisenhower E, Verme D. Are insulin and proinsulin independent risk markers for premature coronary artery disease? Diabetes 1996;45:736–741.

19. Bressler P, Bailey S, Matsuda M, DeFronzo RA. Insulin resistance and coronary artery disease. Diabetologia 1996;39:1345–1350.

20. Young MH, Jeng CY, Sheu WH, Shieh SM, Fuh MM, Chen YD, Reaven GM. Insulin resistance, glucose intolerance, hyperinsulinemia and dyslipidemia in patients with angiographically demonstrated coronary artery disease. Am J Cardiol 1993;72:458–460.

21. Zamboni M, Armellini F, Sheiban I, De Marchi M, Todesco T, Bergamo-Andreis IA, Cominacini L, Bosello O. Relation of body-fat distribution in men and degree of coronary artery narrowings in coronary artery disease. Am J Cardiol 1992;70:1135–1138.

22. Spallarossa P, Cordera R, Andraghetti G, Bertino G, Brunelli C, Caponnetto S. Association between plasma insulin and angiographically documented significant coronary artery disease. Am J Cardiol 1994;74:177–179.

23. Feskens EJM, Kromhout D. Hyperinsulinemia, risk factors and coronary heart disease, The Zutphen study. Arterioscler Thromb 1994;14:1641–1647.

24. Hargreaves AD, Logan RL, Elton RA, Buchanan KD, Oliver MF, Riemersma RA. Glucose tolerance, plasma insulin, HDL cholesterol and obesity: 12-year follow-up and development of coronary heart disease in Edinburgh men. Atherosclerosis 1992;94:61–69.

25. Ferrara A, Barrett-Connor EL, Edelstein SL. Hyperinsulinemia does not increase the risk of fatal cardiovascular disease in elderly men or women without diabetes: The Rancho Bernardo Study, 1984–1991. Am J Epidemiol 1994;140:857–869.

26. Yudkin JS, Denver AE, Mohamed-Ali V, Ramaiya KL, Nagi DK, Goubet S, McLarty DG, Swai A. The relationship of concentrations of insulin and proinsulin-like molecules with coronary heart disease prevalence and incidence. Diabetes Care 1997;20:1093–1100.

27. Liu QZ, Knowler WC, Nelson RG, Saad MF, Charles MA, Liebow IM, Bennett PH, Pettitt DJ. Insulin treatment, endogenous insulin concentration, and ECG abnormalities in diabetic Pima Indians: Cross-sectional and prospective analyses. Diabetes 1992;41:1141–1150.

28. Welborn TA, Wearne K. Cardiovascular heart disease incidence and cardiovascular mortality in Busselton with reference to glucose and insulin concentrations. Diabetes Care 1979;2:154–160.

29. Pyörälä K. Relationship of glucose tolerance and plasma insulin to the incidence of coronary heart disease: Results from two population studies in Finland. Diabetes Care 1979;2:131–141.

30. Ducimetiere P, Eschwege E, Papoz L, Richard JL, Claude JR, Rosselin G. Relationship of plasma insulin levels to the incidence of myocardial infarction and coronary heart disease mortality in a middle-aged population. Diabetologia 1980;19:205–210.

31. Cullen K, Stenhouse NS, Wearne KL, Welborn TA. Multiple regression analysis of risk factors for cardiovascular disease and cancer mortality in Busselton, Western Australia—13-year study. J Chronic Dis 1983;36:371–377.

32. Welborn TA, Knuiman MW, Ward N, Whittall DE. Serum insulin is a risk marker for coronary heart disease mortality in men but not in women. Diabetes Res 1994;26:51–59.

33. Pyörälä K, Savolainen E, Kaukola S, Haapakoski J. Plasma insulin as coronary heart disease risk factor: Relationship to other risk factors and predictive value during 9-1/2 year follow-up of the Helsinki Policemen Study population. Acta Med Scand 1985;701(Suppl):38–52.

34. Pyörälä M, Pyörälä K, Laakso M. Hyperinsulinemia as predictor of coronary heart disease risk: 22-year follow-up results of the Helsinki Policeman Study. Circulation 1996;94(Suppl):I–213.

35. Eschwege E, Richard JL, Thibult N, Ducimetiere P, Warnet JM, Claude JR, Rosselin GE. Coronary heart disease mortality in relation with diabetes, blood glucose and plasma insulin levels: The Paris Prospective Study, ten years later. Horm Metab Res Suppl 1985;15:41–46.

36. Fontbonne A, Charles MA, Thibult N, Richard JL, Claude JR, Warnet JM, Rosselin GE, Eschwege E. Hyperinsulinemia as a predictor of coronary heart disease mortality in a healthy population: the Paris Prospective Study, 15-year follow-up. Diabetologia 1991;34:356–361.

37. Orchard TJ, Eichner J, Kuller LH, Becker DJ, McCallum LM, Grandits GA. Insulin as a predictor of coronary heart disease: Interaction with apolipoprotein E phenotype: A report from Multiple Risk Factor Intervention Trial. Ann Epidemiol 1994;4:40–45.

38. Welin L, Eriksson H, Larsson B, Ohlson L-O, Svärdsudd K, Tibblin G. Hyperinsulinemia is not a major coronary risk factor in elderly men. The Study of Men Born in 1913. Diabetologia 1992;35:766–770.

39. Yarnell JWG, Sweetnam PM, Marks V, Teale JD, Bolton CH. Insulin in ischaemic heart disease: are associations explained by triglyceride concentrations? The Caerphilly prospective study. Br Heart J 1994;71:293–296.

40. Rewers M, Shetterly SM, Baxter J, Hamman RF. Insulin and cardiovascular disease in Hispanics and non-Hispanic whites (NHW): The San Luis Valley Diabetes Study [Abstract]. Circulation 1992;85:865.

41. Kuusisto J, Mykkänen L, Pyörälä K, Laakso M. Hyperinsulinemic microalbuminuria: A new risk indicator for coronary heart disease. Circulation 1995;91:831–837.

42. Møller LF, Jespersen J. Fasting serum insulin levels and coronary heart disease in a Danish cohort: 17-year follow-up. J Cardiovasc Risk 1995;2:235–240.

43. Perry IJ, Wannamethee SG, Whincup PH, Shaper AG, Walker MK, Alberti KG. Serum insulin and incident coronary heart disease in middle-aged British men. Am J Epidemiol 1996;144:224–234.

44. Després J-P, Lamarche B, Mauriège P, Cantin B, Dagenais GR, Moorjani S, Lupien P-J. Hyperinsulinemia as an independent risk factor for ischemic heart disease. N Engl J Med 1996;334:952–957.

45. Lakka TA, Lakka HM, Salonen JT. Hyperinsulinemia and the risk of coronary heart disease [Letter]. N Engl J Med 1996;335:976–977.

46. Lakka H-M, Lakka TA, Tuomilehto J, Salonen JT. Hyperinsulinemia and cardiovascular mortality. Atherosclerosis 1997;134:161.

47. Folsom AR, Szklo M, Stevens J, Liao F, Smith R, Eckfeldt JH. A prospective study of coronary heart disease in relation to fasting insulin, glucose, and diabetes: The Atherosclerosis Risk in Communities (ARIC) Study. Diabetes Care 1997;20:935–942.

48. Wingard DL, Barrett-Connor EL, Ferrara A. In insulin really a heart disease risk factor? Diabetes Care 1995;18:1299–1304.

49. Newman AB, Siscovick DS, Manolio TA, Polak J, Fried LP, Borhani NO, Wolfson SK. Ankle-arm index as a marker of atherosclerosis in the Cardiovascular Health Study. Circulation 1993;88:837–845.

50. Curb JD, Masaki K, Rodriguez BL, Abbott RD, Burchfiel CM, Chen R, Petrovitch H, Sharp D, Yano K. Peripheral artery disease and cardiovascular risk factors in the elderly: The Honolulu Heart Program. Arterioscler Thromb Vasc Biol 1995;15:1495–1500.

51. Price JF, Lee AJ, Fowkes FGR. Hyperinsulinaemia: a risk factor for peripheral arterial disease in the non-diabetic general population. J Cardiovasc Risk 1996;3:501–505.

52. Uusitupa MIJ, Niskanen LK, Siitonen O, Voutilainen E, Pyörälä K. 5-year incidence of atherosclerotic vascular disease in relation to general risk factors, insulin level, and abnormalities in lipoprotein composition in non-insulin-dependent diabetic and nondiabetic subjects. Circulation 1990;82:27–36.

53. Niskanen L, Rauramaa R, Miettinen H, Haffner SM, Mercuri M, Uusitupa M. Carotid artery intima-media thickness in elderly patients with NIDDM and in nondiabetic subjects. Stroke 1996;27:1986–1992.

54. Folsom AR, Eckfeldt JH, Weitzman S, Ma J, Chambless LE, Barnes RW, Cram KB, Hutchinson RG. Relation of carotid artery wall thickness to diabetes mellitus, fasting glucose and insulin, body size, and physical activity. Stroke 1994;25:66–73.

55. Bonora E, Willeit J, Kiechl S, Oberhollenzer F, Egger G, Bonadonna R, Muggeo M. Relationship between insulin and carotid atherosclerosis in the general population: The Bruneck Study. Stroke 1997;28:1147–1152.

56. O'Leary DH, Polak JF, Kronmal RA, Kittner SJ, Bond MG, Wolfson SK Jr, Bommer W, Price TR, Gardin JM, Savage PJ. Distribution and correlates of sonographically detected carotid artery disease in the Cardiovascular Health Study. Stroke 1992;23:1752–1760.

57. Salomaa V, Riley W, Kark JD, Nardo C, Folsom AR. Non-insulin dependent diabetes mellitus and fasting glucose and insulin concentrations are associated with arterial stiffness indexes: The ARIC Study. Circulation 1995;91:1432–1443.

58. Laakso M, Sarlund H, Salonen R, Suhonen M, Pyörälä K, Salonen JT, Karhapää P. Asymptomatic atherosclerosis and insulin resistance. Arterioscler Thromb 1991;11:1068–1076.

59. Agewall S, Fagerberg B, Attvall S, Wendelhag I, Urbanavicius V, Wikstrand J. Carotid artery wall intima-media thickness is associated with insulin-mediated glucose disposal in men at high and low coronary risk. Stroke 1995;26:956–960.

60. Suzuki M, Shinozaki K, Kanazawa A, Hara Y, Hattori Y, Tsushima M, Harano Y. Insulin resistance as an independent risk factor for carotid wall thickening. Hypertension 1996;28:593–598.

61. Howard G, O'Leary DH, Zaccaro D, Haffner S, Rewers M, Hamman R, Selby JV, Saad MF, Savage P, Bergman R. Insulin sensitivity and atherosclerosis. Circulation 1996;93:1809–1817.

62. Kekäläinen P, Sarlund H, Farin P, Kaukanen E, Yang X, Laakso M. Femoral atherosclerosis in middle-aged subjects: Association with cardiovascular risk factors and insulin resistance. Am J Epidemiol 1996;144:742–748.

63. Gertler MM, Leetma HE, Saluste E, Welsh JJ, Rusk HA, Covalt DA, Rosenberger J. Carbohydrate, insulin, and lipid interrelationship in ischemic vascular disease. Geriatrics 1970;25:134–138.

64. Gertler MM, Leetma HE, Saluste E, Covalt DA, Rosenberger JL. Covert diabetes mellitus in ischemic heart and cerebrovascular disease. Geriatrics 1972;27:105–116.

65. Gertler MM, Leetma HE, Koutrouby RJ, Johnson ED. The assessment of insulin, glucose and lipids in ischemic thrombotic cerebrovascular disease. Stroke 1975;6:77–84.

66. Shinozaki K, Naritomi H, Shimizu T, Suzuku M, Ikebuchi M, Sawada T, Harano Y. Role of insulin resistance with compensatory hyperinsulinemia in ischemic stroke. Stroke 1996;27:37–43.

67. Zunker P, Schick A, Buschmann H-C, Georgiadis D, Nabavi DG, Edelmann M, Ringelstein EB. Hyperinsulinism and cerebral microangiopathy. Stroke 1996;27:219–223.

68. Kuusisto J, Mykkänen L, Pyörälä K, Laakso M. Non-insulin-dependent diabetes and its metabolic control are important predictors of stroke in elderly subjects. Stroke 1994;25:1157–1164.

69. Hubert HB, Feinleib M, McNamara PM, Castelli WP. Obesity as an independent risk factor for cardiovascular disease: a 26-year follow-up of participants in the Framingham Heart Study. Circulation 1983;67:968–977.

70. Lindberg O, Tilvis RS, Strandberg TE, Valvanne J, Sairanen S, Ehnholm C, Tuomilehto J. Elevated fasting plasma insulin in a general aged population: An innocent companion of cardiovascular diseases. J Am Geriatr Soc 1997;45:407–412.

71. Nagamani M, Hannigan EV, Van Dinh T, Stuart CA. Hyperinsulinemia and stromal luteinization of the ovaries in postmenopausal women with endometrial cancer. J Clin Endocrinol Metab 1988;67:144–148.

72. Rutanen EM, Stenman S, Blum W, Karkkainen T, Lehtovirta P, Stenman UH. Relationship between carbohydrate metabolism and serum insulin-like growth factor system in postmenopausal women: comparison of endometrial cancer patients with healthy controls. J Clin Endocrinol Metab 1993;77:199–204.

73. Brown R. Carbohydrate metabolism in patients with endometrial carcinoma. J Obstet Gynecol Br Commonwealth 1974;81:940–946.

74. Troisi R, Potischman N, Hoover RN, Siiteri P, Brinton LA. Insulin and endometrial cancer. Am J Epidemiol 1997;146:476–482.

75. Heslin MJ, Neuman E, Wolf RF, Pisters PWT, Brennan MF. Effect of systemic hyperinsulinemia in cancer patients. Cancer Res 1992;52:3845–3850.

76. Bruning PF, Bonfrèr JM, van Noord PA, Hart AA, de Jong-Bakker M, Nooijen WJ. Insulin resistance and breast-cancer risk. Int J Cancer 1992;52:511–516.

77. Yudkin JS. Hyperinsulinaemia, insulin resistance, microalbuminuria and the risk of coronary heart disease. Ann Med 1996;28:433–438.

78. Stout RW. The impact of insulin upon atherosclerosis. Horm Metab Res 1994;26:125–128.

79. Petrie JR, Ueda S, Webb DJ, Elliott HL, Connell JM. Endothelial nitric oxide production and insulin sensitivity. A physiological link with implications for pathogenesis of cardiovascular disease. Circulation 1996;93:1331–1333.

80. Nathan DM, Meigs J, Singer DE. The epidemiology of cardiovascular disease in type 2 diabetes mellitus: how sweet it is . . . or is it? Lancet 1997;350(Suppl 1):4–9.

81. Pyörälä M, Miettinen H, Laakso M, Pyörälä K. Hyperinsulinemia and the risk of stroke in healthy middle-aged men. The 22-year follow-up results of the Helsinki Policemen Study. Stroke 1998;29:1860–1866.

82. Ruige JB, Assendelft WJJ, Dekker JM, Kostense PJ, Heine RJ, Bouter LM. Insulin and risk of cardiovascular disease. A meta-analysis. Circulation 1998;97:996–1001.

19

Insulin Resistance Effects on Sex Hormones and Ovulation in the Polycystic Ovary Syndrome

John E. Nestler, MD

Contents

INTRODUCTION
INSULIN RESISTANCE: *AN INTEGRAL FEATURE OF PCOS*
INSULIN AND OVARIAN ANDROGENS
INSULIN AND SHBG
INSULIN AND FOLLICULAR DEVELOPMENT
THERAPEUTIC AND CLINICAL IMPLICATIONS
SUMMARY
REFERENCES

INTRODUCTION

The polycystic ovary syndrome (PCOS) is a prevalent disorder affecting an estimated 6% (range, 4–10%) of women of reproductive age. It is the most common cause of female infertility in the United States, and arguably the most common endocrinopathy affecting premenopausal women. PCOS is characterized by chronic anovulation and hyperandrogenism, and its diagnosis requires the exclusion of other disorders that can mimic PCOS (e.g., congenital or nonclassical adrenal hyperplasia).

In the past decade, the realization that many women with PCOS also manifest insulin resistance accompanied by compensatory hyperinsulinemia has significantly influenced the manner in which such women are evaluated and, most recently, treated. The reason for this change in clinical practice is due to the following: 1) It has been recognized that women with PCOS frequently develop other disorders likely related to insulin resistance (Type 2 diabetes mellitus, hypertension, dyslipidemia, atherosclerosis), and 2) it has been demonstrated that hyperinsulinemia plays an important role in the pathogenesis of PCOS. Specifically, hyperinsulinemia both increases serum androgens and impedes ovulation in a substantial number of obese and lean women with PCOS.

The aim of this chapter is to briefly review some of the evidence that supports the pathogenic role of hyperinsulinemia in PCOS, and to detail how the relationship between

From: *Contemporary Endocrinology: Insulin Resistance*
Edited by: G. Reaven and A. Laws © Humana Press Inc., Totowa, NJ

insulin resistance and PCOS influences the evaluation and treatment of women with the disorder.

INSULIN RESISTANCE: *AN INTEGRAL FEATURE OF PCOS*

Numerous studies have shown that many—likely the majority—of women with PCOS manifest insulin resistance accompanied by compensatory hyperinsulinemia (which may be termed "*hyper*insulinemic insulin resistance" to distinguish it from the insulin resistance of Type 2 diabetes mellitus, which is characterized by relative hypoinsulinemia). This applies to both obese and nonobese (normal weight or thin) women with PCOS, and was demonstrated in studies in which affected women were age- and weight-matched to healthy women *(1–12)*.

Hyperinsulinemic insulin resistance is a feature of PCOS not only in the United States, but in other societies as well. Women with PCOS from the United States, Japan and Italy have been compared to healthy counterparts in their respective countries *(13)*. Although clinical differences existed among the women (e.g., women with PCOS from the United States were more obese than Japanese women with PCOS, and women with PCOS from the United States and Italy were hirsute whereas Japanese women with PCOS were not), women with PCOS from all three countries manifested insulin resistance. This common finding across multiple ethnic groups suggests that hyperinsulinemic insulin resistance represents a relatively universal and fundamental feature of PCOS that crosses ethnic boundaries.

Elevated serum androgens may at times cause mild insulin resistance *(14)*, but it is unlikely that the insulin resistance of PCOS occurs as a result of hyperandrogenism. Insulin resistance persists in women with PCOS in whom both ovaries have been removed surgically, or in whom ovarian androgen production has been suppressed with the use of a long-acting gonadotropin hormone-releasing hormone (GnRH) agonist. Prepubertal women with acanthosis nigricans are hyperinsulinemic, yet elevated serum androgen levels do not appear until several years following the diagnosis of insulin resistance *(15)*. Some women with point mutations in the insulin receptor gene causing hyperinsulinemic insulin resistance have been shown to have PCOS *(16)*. Collectively, these observations support the idea that the hyperinsulinemia of PCOS is a causal factor in the accompanying hyperandrogenism. In addition, the observation that hyperinsulinemic insulin resistance is a salient feature of adolescent girls with hyperandrogenism *(12)* suggests that hyperinsulinemia likely plays an early and central role in the pathogenesis of PCOS.

There is a form of insulin resistance intrinsic to PCOS that appears to be unique and is not well understood *(7,10,17)*. This form of "PCOS-specific" insulin resistance affects both nonobese and obese women with PCOS. In addition, since 50–80% of women with PCOS are obese, obese women with the disorder additionally possess a form of insulin resistance that is directly related to the obesity *(18)*. To what degree the "PCOS-specific" form of insulin resistance is sufficient to initiate the processes involved in the pathogenesis of PCOS is unknown, but it is instructive to note that many women with PCOS relate a history of weight gain immediately prior to the onset of clinical PCOS symptoms, thereby suggesting that obesity's contribution to the disorder is at times substantial.

The "PCOS-specific" form of insulin resistance that is intrinsic to the disorder does not appear to be related to an abnormality in insulin itself, or to the quantity or affinity of insulin receptors on classical target tissues. Rather, it appears to reside at the postreceptor level. In a study of a limited number of women with PCOS, Dunaif and colleagues demonstrated in a small subset of PCOS women a defect characterized by increased serine phosphorylation of the insulin receptor in cultured fibroblasts *(10)*. However, cells from the majority of women did not demonstrate the abnormality, indicating that this is not the sole explanation for the insulin resistance of PCOS. Intringuingly, Miller and colleagues have demonstrated that serine phosphorylation of human P450c17α increases 17,20-lyase activity *(19)*, a key enzyme in androgen biosynthesis. Therefore, it has been suggested that a genetically determined defect increasing serine phosphorylation could explain both the insulin resistance and hyperandrogenism of PCOS. While this may be so in some women, the absence of a fibroblast serine phosphorylation defect in the majority of women with PCOS *(10)* and the failure of this unifying theory to explain the apparent ability of insulin to modulate (i.e., *stimulate*) ovarian androgen production in women with PCOS makes the speculation less attractive.

INSULIN AND OVARIAN ANDROGENS

Effects of Insulin on Circulating Ovarian Androgens

In Vitro Studies

Human ovaries possess insulin receptors, suggesting a role for insulin in the regulation of ovarian function. In vitro studies have demonstrated that insulin can directly stimulate androgen production by ovarian stroma obtained from women with PCOS *(20,21)*, and a recent study suggests that this effect of insulin is mediated by activation of the insulin receptor *(22)*. In addition, insulin and insulin-like growth factor I (IGF-I) augment LH-stimulated androgen biosynthesis in rat ovarian theca cells *(23,24)*.

Insulin Infusion Studies in Women

It has been difficult to demonstrate in vivo an acute effect of insulin on ovarian androgens in women. Multiple studies have been conducted where serum testosterone was monitored in women during a short-term elevation of circulating insulin, and the results in women with PCOS appear confusing and conflicting. Serum testosterone either rose, did not change, or fell. This was most likely related to several problems associated with insulin infusion studies—namely, 1) the very nature of these studies dictates that the duration of insulin elevation be brief, lasting only a few hours, 2) in many studies the degree of insulin elevation was far above the physiologic range, and 3) several of these studies did not control for the volume of fluids infused, diurnal and day-to-day variations in sex steroid concentrations, or for unmeasured perturbations (such as the increase in catecholamines) that accompany insulin infusions.

Perhaps the single situation in which investigators induced *long-term* hyperinsulinemia while monitoring serum androgen levels was the case study reported by DeClue and coworkers *(25)*. These investigators cared for a young woman with PCOS who was diabetic and manifested a high degree of insulin resistance. High-dose insulin therapy was started, and marked hyperinsulinemia was maintained over several months. During this period of insulin elevation, circulating testosterone levels progressively rose and ovarian volume, as measured by ultrasound, increased twofold. The insulin resistance then abated, and the insulin infusion was discontinued. As a result, serum insulin levels decreased. Notably, serum testosterone levels decreased in parallel, eventually falling into the normal range. A clear concordance existed between serum insulin and testosterone levels, consistent with a cause-and-effect relationship. These findings strongly suggested that insulin stimulated ovarian androgen production in this woman, and was directly responsible for the hyperandrogenism.

DIAZOXIDE-INDUCED SUPPRESSION OF INSULIN RELEASE IN WOMEN

In order to study the role of chronic physiologic elevations of insulin in PCOS while avoiding problems associated with insulin infusions, we utilized the drug diazoxide to directly inhibit pancreatic insulin release in women with PCOS (26). Five obese women with PCOS were administered diazoxide for 10 days. As a result, fasting and glucose-stimulated serum insulin levels decreased markedly, and fasting serum glucose and glycemic excursion during an oral glucose challenge increased into the diabetic range. Notably, serum total testosterone levels fell in all five women with PCOS during this period of insulin suppression by diazoxide, whereas serum sex hormone binding globulin (SHBG) levels rose in each woman. Because of the simultaneous decrease in serum total testosterone and increase in SHBG levels, serum free (i.e., non-SHBG-bound) testosterone levels decreased significantly by 28%.

This study did not exclude the possibility that the decline in circulating free testosterone was due to diazoxide itself. Therefore, a subsequent study was performed in identical fashion in five healthy women of normal weight (27). In contrast to the obese women with PCOS, diazoxide treatment altered neither serum testosterone nor SHBG in this group of lean women with normal levels of circulating insulin, indicating that diazoxide does not influence ovarian steroidogenic function independently of its action to inhibit insulin release.

An important conclusion that can be drawn from the above studies is that hyperinsulinemia is the culprit that stimulates ovarian androgen production in PCOS. That is, it is not insulin resistance at the ovarian level that is pathogenic—rather it is the elevation in circulating insulin. This is evident because diazoxide specifically inhibits insulin release, and is not known to influence insulin sensitivity in human beings.

STIMULATION OF OVARIAN CYTOCHROME P450c17α BY INSULIN

P450c17α is a key enzyme in the biosynthesis of ovarian androgens, and is a bifunctional enzyme that possesses both 17α-hydroxylase and 17,20-lyase activities. In the theca cell of the ovary, P450c17α converts progesterone to 17α-hydroxyprogesterone via its 17α-hydroxylase activity, and then converts 17α-hydroxyprogesterone to androstenedione via its 17,20-lyase action. Androstenedione is converted to testosterone by the enzyme 17β-reductase.

Many women with PCOS manifest increased ovarian cytochrome P450c17α activity (28,29), as evidenced by increased 17α-hydroxylase and, to a lesser extent, increased 17,20-lyase activities, and this presumably results in excessive ovarian androgen production. In these women, a hallmark of increased ovarian P450c17α activity is an exaggerated serum 17α-hydroxyprogesterone response to stimulation by GnRH agonists such as nafarelin (28–30), buserelin (31) or leuprolide (32).

It was initially presumed that the increased activity of ovarian P450c17α in women with PCOS represented an inherited and fixed phenomenon, and that it was directly responsible for the pathogenesis of PCOS. As detailed following Effects of Metformin on Ovarian P450c17α Activity in Obese Women with PCOS, more recent evidence suggests that increased ovarian P450c17α activity in PCOS results from stimulation by insulin and is at least partially reversible.

The hypothesis that hyperinsulinemia stimulates ovarian P450c17α activity in PCOS was recently tested in three separate studies. In none of the studies were the women screened

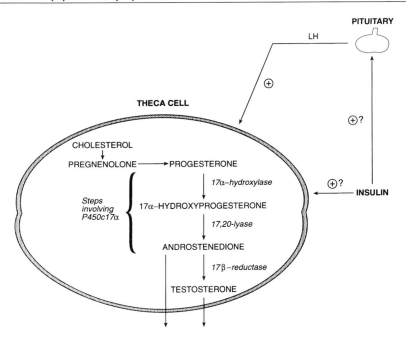

Fig. 1. Postulated schema of how insulin might stimulate ovarian androgen production. In the theca cell, insulin may directly stimulate (plus signs) ovarian cytochrome P450c17α, resulting in increased 17α-hydroxylase and, to a lesser extent, 17,20-lyase activities. This would lead to increased production of androstenedione, which is then converted to testosterone by the enzyme 17α-reductase. Alternatively or in conjunction, insulin may stimulate ovarian androgen production indirectly by enhancing the amplitude of serum luteinizing hormone pulses, and luteinizing hormone then stimulating ovarian cytochrome P450c17α activity. LH denotes luteinizing hormone. (From ref. *39*. Copyright © 1989 Massachusetts Medical Society. All rights reserved.)

for the presence of insulin resistance or exaggerated ovarian P450c17α activity. Thus, the results of these studies can likely be generalized to the PCOS population at large.

Effects of Metformin on Ovarian P450c17α Activity in Obese Women with PCOS. In the first of these studies, 24 obese women with PCOS were studied in randomized, single-blind, and placebo-controlled fashion. Oral glucose tolerance tests and 24-h GnRH agonist (leuprolide) stimulation tests were performed before and after oral administration of either metformin 500 mg (N = 11) or placebo (N = 13) three times daily for 4–8 weeks. Metformin treatment reduced serum fasting and glucose-stimulated insulin. Amelioration of hyperinsulinemia by metformin was also associated with decreased ovarian P450c17α enzyme activity, as demonstrated by substantial reductions in the leuprolide-stimulated serum 17α- hydroxyprogesterone response. Moreover, metformin treatment was associated with a decrease in basal and leuprolide-stimulated luteinizing hormone (LH), a 44% decrease in serum free testosterone, and a threefold rise in SHBG. None of these variables changed in the placebo group. As illustrated in Fig. 1, these findings suggest that hyperinsulinemia increases P450c17α activity in obese women with PCOS either by directly stimulating ovarian steroidogenesis and/or indirectly by stimulating gonadotropin release.

Effects of Weight Loss on ovarian P450c17α activity in obese women with PCOS. The possibility that the decrease in ovarian P450c17α activity may have been related to a direct action of metformin was addressed by subsequently assessing the effects of dietary weight loss on the enzyme's activity, since it is known that weight loss is accompanied by improved insulin sensitivity and reduction in circulating insulin. Twelve obese women with PCOS and 11 obese but otherwise healthy women were studied in a fashion similar to the metformin protocol before and after 8 wk of a hypocaloric (1000–1200 kcal) diet. In the PCOS group, basal serum 17α-hydroxyprogesterone concentrations and leuprolide- stimulated peak serum 17α-hydroxyprogesterone concentrations decreased. Simultaneously, serum concentrations of total and free testosterone decreased. None of these values changed in the control group of healthy obese women.

These findings indicate that dietary weight loss decreases ovarian P450c17α activity and reduces serum free testosterone concentrations in obese PCOS women, but not in obese ovulatory women. The effects of weight loss in PCOS women were most likely related to a reduction in serum insulin, and are consistent with the hypothesis that hyperinsulinemia stimulates human ovarian P450c17α activity.

Effects of Metformin on Ovarian P450c17α Activity in Normal Weight and Thin Women with PCOS. Of note, not all women with PCOS are obese. Between 20–50% of women with PCOS are normal weight or thin, and the pathophysiology of the disorder in these women may differ from that in obese women. It has been suggested that PCOS develops in nonobese women because of a hypothalamic-pituitary defect that results in increased release of luteinizing hormone, and that insulin plays no role in the disorder *(33–36)*.

We believed that this concept ignored the fact that nonobese women with PCOS demonstrate an intrinsic form of insulin resistance that is unique to the disorder *(1,3,4)* and are hyperinsulinemic compared to their healthy counterparts *(37)*. Nonobese women with PCOS also exhibit increased ovarian P450c17α activity *(28,29,38)*. Since hyperinsulinemia stimulates P450c17α activity in obese women with PCOS *(39,40)*, it seemed likely that it should do so in nonobese affected women as well. Therefore, to test the hypothesis that hyperinsulinemia stimulates ovarian cytochrome P450c17α activity in normal weight and thin women with PCOS, we measured the basal serum 17α-hydroxyprogesterone concentration and the serum 17α-hydroxyprogesterone response to administration of a GnRH agonist in nonobese women with PCOS, who ranged in body weight from normal to thin, before and after administration of metformin (N = 19) or placebo (N = 12).

In the metformin group, the mean area under the serum insulin curve after oral glucose administration decreased by 45%. The reduction in serum insulin was accompanied by significant decreases in basal serum 17α-hydroxyprogesterone, GnRH-stimulated peak serum 17α-hydroxyprogesterone, and basal serum total testosterone and free testosterone; in contrast, serum SHBG increased. None of these values changed in the placebo group. These findings strongly suggest that hyperinsulinemia stimulates ovarian P450c17α activity in nonobese women with PCOS.

Summary of In Vivo Human P450c17α Studies. Collectively, these studies indicate that a reduction in serum insulin, accomplished by improving insulin sensitivity, is accompanied by a decrease in ovarian cytochrome P450c17α activity and, hence, circulating, androgens. This is applicable to nonobese as well as to obese women with PCOS, and the method for improving insulin sensitivity is immaterial (i.e., drug vs weight loss). This conclusion is also consonant with the results of other studies assessing effects of metformin *(41–43)* or another insulin-sensitizing agent, troglitazone *(44,45)*, in PCOS.

Although ovarian P450c17α activity was not determined in these studies, serum androgens decreased as insulin sensitivity was enhanced (and insulin release decreased). These findings are important from a clinical standpoint because they demonstrate that the hyperandrogenism of PCOS can be substantially ameliorated by reducing serum insulin.

A PCOS Gene and Its Relationship to Insulin Resistance

The administration of diazoxide to inhibit insulin release is associated with a reduction in free testosterone in women with PCOS (26) but not in normal women (27). At least two possible interpretations exist for these disparate results. At the simplest level, insulin levels are not elevated in normal women; therefore, serum insulin may not be sufficiently high in those women to stimulate ovarian androgen biosynthesis. In other words, insulin may not regulate ovarian androgens under normal physiologic conditions.

However, an alternate and more attractive explanation is that normal women lack a genetic predisposition to insulin's stimulatory action on ovarian androgens. That is, it seems likely that there exists a PCOS gene or combination of genes that makes the ovaries of a woman with PCOS either absolutely susceptible to or more sensitive and/or responsive to insulin stimulation of androgen production. In support of this idea, in vitro studies have demonstrated that insulin stimulates testosterone release by ovarian stroma of women with PCOS but exerts either no effect (20) or a much attenuated effect in ovarian stroma of normal women (22). Furthermore, there is familial clustering of PCOS, which suggests genetic inheritance, and insulin sensitivity appears to be under significant genetic influence in PCOS (17). Importantly, this "PCOS gene hypothesis" would also explain why every woman who is obese, and is therefore by definition hyperinsulinemic, does not develop PCOS. Therefore, as with many pathologic conditions associated with insulin resistance, it appears that a genetic "hit" is required that predisposes the individual to respond to the effects of hyperinsulinemia and/or insulin resistance.

Cellular Mechanisms for Insulin's Stimulation of Ovarian Androgen Production

DIRECT EFFECTS OF INSULIN ON OVARIAN ANDROGEN PRODUCTION

On the surface it seems paradoxical that insulin should stimulate ovarian androgen production in a woman who is otherwise "resistant" to insulin. However, several theoretical mechanisms exist to explain how a woman resistant to insulin's effects on glucose metabolism could nonetheless remain fully sensitive to insulin's stimulation of ovarian androgenic pathways.

The most often cited possibilities propose that insulin could stimulate ovarian androgen production either by cross-associating with the ovarian insulin-like growth factor-I (IGF-I) receptor or by binding to ovarian hybrid insulin receptors (46). These explanations seem unlikely because 1) the elevation in circulating insulin in women with PCOS is usually modest and insulin would not be expected to cross-associate appreciably with the IGF-I receptor, and 2) hybrid insulin receptors have not been identified on human ovaries. It has also been suggested that insulin could act indirectly by reducing intrafollicular levels of IGF-binding protein 1 (IGFBP-1), thereby increasing intrafollicular concentrations of free IGF-I. IGF-I is a potent stimulator of LH-induced androgen synthesis by ovarian interstitial cells, which may in part be due to an induction of LH receptors on these cells by IGF-I. However, as reviewed elsewhere (47), this explanation also seems unlikely in view of evidence which suggests that *total* intrafollicular IGF-binding capacity in PCOS may be increased rather than reduced.

It seems most likely that the cellular mechanism for insulin's stimulation of ovarian androgen production involves activation of a novel signal transduction system that is distinct and separate from the insulin activated tyrosine phosphate cascade used to enhance glucose utilization. Some actions of insulin involve low molecular weight inositolglycan mediators (also known as putative insulin mediators or second messengers) *(48–50)*, and this putative mediator system is a prime candidate for the alternate signaling mechanism. Two studies, one conducted in human placental cytotrophoblasts *(51)* and the other in swine ovarian granulosa cells *(52)*, support this idea by having shown that the inositolphosphoglycan "second messenger" system serves as the signal transduction pathway for insulin's effects on steroidogenesis in these tissues. Notably, evidence was recently reported indicating that insulin stimulates testosterone production by cultured human theca cells isolated from PCOS women by activating its homologous receptor and by utilizing the inositolglycan second messenger system *(22)*. When the inositolglycan system was inactivated by a blocking antibody, insulin could no longer stimulate thecal testosterone production.

The importance of these observations is that the inositolphosphoglycan signal transduction system may remain intact and fully functional in conditions otherwise characterized by insulin resistance in terms of a defective tyrosine kinase cascade system leading to impaired glucose transport and utilization. By utilizing the alternate inositolglycan signal transduction pathway, insulin's stimulation of ovarian androgen biosynthesis is preserved even in the face of glucose intolerance. Therefore, these findings yield an explanation for the seeming clinical paradox that hyperinsulinemia stimulates ovarian androgen production in women with PCOS, even while these women are resistant to insulin's enhancement of peripheral glucose transport or utilization.

INDIRECT EFFECTS OF INSULIN ON OVARIAN ANDROGEN PRODUCTION

PCOS is often characterized by abnormalities in LH secretion by the pituitary. Some studies have found that LH pulse frequency is increased in PCOS *(37,53–56)*, while other studies have found no difference in LH pulse frequency between PCOS women and eumenorrheic women *(57–59)*. In general, however, LH pulse amplitude appears to be increased in most (but not necessarily all *[37]*) women with PCOS compared to healthy age- and weight-matched control women *(56)*. It is possible that some of the defects in LH secretory dynamics are caused or aggravated by hyperinsulinemia *(60)*.

In support of this notion, insulin receptors have been identified in the human pituitary, and insulin has been shown to augment pituitary release of gonadotropins by cultured rat pituitary cells *(61)*. Moreover, LH release appears to be increased in women with PCOS *(56)*, and there is general concordance of the diurnal pattern of serum LH and that of serum insulin in PCOS women *(62)*. As noted previously, we recently observed that treatment of PCOS women with metformin for 4–8 weeks reduced circulating insulin and both the basal serum LH concentration and the LH response to stimulation by the GnRH agonist leuprolide *(39,63)*. Similar decreases in serum LH have been noted in studies that utilized troglitazone to decrease circulating insulin *(44,64)*. This suggests that some of insulin's stimulation of ovarian androgen production may be mediated by alterations in LH secretory dynamics.

As a caveat, however, it should be noted that the effects of fasting or weight loss on LH pulse dynamics have been less consistent. In general, they have demonstrated either a decrease in serum LH concentrations *(40)* or no change *(65)*. Interpretation of these studies is complicated because weight loss leads not only to an improvement in insulin sensitivity, but also to changes in other metabolic factors—free fatty acids and leptin being just two of these. Theoretically, some of these factors may independently affect gonadotropin release and obscure changes related to changes in circulating insulin.

INSULIN AND SHBG

Regulation of SHBG by Insulin in PCOS

Insulin influences the clinical androgenic state not only by directly affecting the metabolism (production rate and/or metabolic clearance rate) of ovarian androgens, but also indirectly by regulating circulating levels of the steroid-binding protein, SHBG. SHBG binds testosterone with high affinity, and it is commonly held that it is the unbound fraction of testosterone, and not the SHBG-bound fraction, that is bioavailable to tissues. Regulation of circulating SHBG by insulin constitutes an important additional mechanism by which insulin promotes hyperandrogenism. By directly reducing circulating SHBG under conditions of stimulated ovarian androgen production (as is the case in PCOS), insulin increases the delivery of testosterone to tissues because more testosterone is unbound and bioavailable.

To determine whether insulin can directly influence SHBG metabolism in vivo, the effect of insulin suppression by diazoxide on serum SHBG levels was examined under conditions where serum androgen and estrogen levels remained unchanged (66). To accomplish this, ovarian steroidogenesis was suppressed in six obese women with PCOS for two months by the administration of the long-acting GnRH agonist leuprolide. Despite substantial reductions in both serum androgens (serum testosterone levels fell by 82%) and estrogens, serum SHBG levels did not change. In contrast, when diazoxide was administered for 10 days to inhibit insulin release, while concurrently continuing GnRH treatment, serum SHBG concentrations rose uniformly and significantly by 32%. This occurred despite no change in serum androgens or estrogens because of simultaneous suppression of ovarian steroidogenesis. Diazoxide does not affect SHBG production by cultured HepG2 cells (Stephen R. Plymate, personal communication). Thus, these observations suggest that the rise in serum SHBG levels following the administration of diazoxide was due to suppression of insulin release, and that hyperinsulinemia can reduce serum SHBG levels in obese women with PCOS independently of any effect on serum sex steroids.

More recently, as commented on elsewhere (67), results of in vivo studies suggest that insulin regulates SHBG not only in obese women with PCOS but in normal men and women as well. The results of these studies suggest that regulation of SHBG metabolism by insulin may be a generalized physiologic phenomenon, and that SHBG may serve as a biological marker for hyperinsulinemic insulin resistance in humans (67).

Decreased SHBG and Type 2 Diabetes Mellitus

It is interesting to note that a decreased serum SHBG concentration has been identified as a risk factor for the development of Type 2 diabetes mellitus in both women and men (68,69). Given the above observations in women with PCOS, it is reasonable to assume that this association is related to the fact that a decreased serum SHBG level likely reflects a subclinical and early state of subtle insulin resistance and compensatory hyperinsulinemia in otherwise healthy individuals (67).

INSULIN AND FOLLICULAR DEVELOPMENT

Anovulation is a sine qua non of PCOS, and evidence suggests that hyperinsulinemia may contribute to the ovulatory dysfunction of some women with PCOS. Insulin may disrupt normal folliculogenesis and the orderly flow to ovulation by increasing intraovarian androgens or perturbing gonadotropin release, and may also do so by directly affecting ovarian follicular development. Insulin can act as a mitogenic factor, can stimulate tissue production of other growth factors such as IGF-I and IGF-II *(70)* and, on occasion, can potentiate the effects of growth factors *(71)*. In any of these ways, insulin could directly cause the development of multiple ovarian cysts and ovarian enlargement *(72)*.

As outlined in an excellent review by Nobels and Dewailly *(72)*, evidence suggests that insulin may indeed stimulate folliculogenesis. Clinical studies have shown that at the time of puberty, girls become increasingly insulin-resistant and hyperinsulinemic. At the same time, if these girls are studied by ultrasonography, multicystic ovaries are frequently present. In many of these girls, the multicystic ovaries resolve spontaneously. Nonetheless, it seems reasonable to assume that in some of these girls the multicystic ovaries persist, and that some of these girls go on to develop PCOS. It would be instructive to ascertain whether in the girls who demonstrate resolution of the multicystic ovaries insulin resistance regresses, whereas perhaps insulin resistance persists or worsens in those girls who progress to PCOS.

The idea that insulin acts to promote folliculogenesis is further supported by the findings of Filicori and colleagues *(73)*, who studied three groups of women: women with PCOS, women with multifollicular ovaries (MFO) and normal androgen levels, and normal women. The MFO women manifested hyperinsulinemic insulin resistance compared to the normal women. Moreover, circulating insulin levels correlated with ovarian volume in both PCOS and MFO women. Based on these findings, the authors suggested that elevated insulin levels may contribute to multiple folliculogenesis and ovarian enlargement in women with PCOS and MFO. The results of this study are consistent with the idea that insulin may exert effects on folliculogenesis that are independent of its actions on ovarian androgen production and, possibly, do not require the presence of a "PCOS gene."

THERAPEUTIC AND CLINICAL IMPLICATIONS

Consistent with the observation that women with PCOS are insulin-resistant, women with PCOS have also been shown to have a high prevalence of other disorders associated with insulin resistance and hyperinsulinemia—namely, impaired glucose tolerance or Type 2 diabetes mellitus *(11,74)*, dyslipidemia (increased triglycerides and decreased HDL cholesterol) *(75–77)*, hypertension *(77,78)* and atherosclerosis *(76,78,79)*. The clustering of these disorders suggests that PCOS should be considered a new component of the putative disorder termed "Syndrome X" *(80,81)*. It also indicates that PCOS is not just a gynecological or dermatological disorder, but rather a metabolic disorder that affects multiple systems and whose key pathogenic element is insulin resistance and/or hyperinsulinemia. Therefore, every woman with PCOS should have her blood pressure and serum lipid profile checked, and should be evaluated for risk factors for heart disease (e.g., smoking). If the woman is overweight, an oral glucose tolerance test should be performed, since >25% of obese women with PCOS will develop impaired glucose tolerance or Type 2 diabetes mellitus by the age of 30. Furthermore, the comprehensive evaluation of a woman with PCOS should be performed not only once at the time of diagnosis, but longitudinally thereafter since the risk for developing these associated disorders likely increases with time.

Not only is the evaluation of the woman with PCOS influenced by the association between PCOS and insulin resistance, treatment is as well. Given the strong evidence that hyperinsulinemia plays a pivotal pathogenic role in the development of PCOS, it is reasonable to assume that interventions that reduce circulating insulin levels in women with PCOS should decrease serum androgens and, perhaps, beneficially influence reproductive function. For example, one such intervention is weight loss, which both improves peripheral insulin sensitivity and reduces circulating insulin. Several studies have shown that when women with PCOS lose weight serum free testosterone falls and reproductive function improves *(40,65,82,83)*. Hence, one could cogently argue that the first line of treatment for obese women with PCOS should be diet and weight loss.

Nonetheless, it is well recognized that it is difficult to lose weight by dieting and even more difficult to maintain weight loss. Therefore, pharmacological interventions that reduce serum insulin concentrations may prove useful in the clinical management of women with PCOS. It is probable that the use of some of these agents, particularly those classified as "insulin-sensitizing," may become standard (and perhaps second-line after diet) therapy of PCOS.

Goals of Therapy

The association of hyperinsulinemic insulin resistance with PCOS suggests several therapeutic goals of pharmacologic intervention aimed at improving insulin sensitivity:

Hyperinsulinemia appears to play a key pathogenic role in the hyperandrogenism in many women with PCOS, regardless of whether they are obese (39) or lean (63). Hence, reducing serum insulin may alleviate the hyperandrogenism (and, therefore, the hirsutism and acne) of these women.

Hyperinsulinemic insulin resistance may act at several levels (pituitary, ovary, peripheral androgen metabolism) to contribute to the anovulation and infertility of PCOS. Pharmacologic treatment that improves insulin sensitivity and lowers circulating insulin may allow for spontaneous ovulation (42,84) or, alternatively, for greater success of standard ovulation induction measures, as has already been reported (84).

Women with PCOS are at heightened risk for the development of impaired glucose tolerance or Type 2 diabetes mellitus, dyslipidemia (reduced HDL cholesterol, high triglycerides), hypertension, and atherosclerosis. Some, if not all, of these potential complications are likely related to the presence of hyperinsulinemia or insulin resistance. Therefore, the use of insulin-sensitizing drugs may be indicated for the prevention or treatment of these associated disorders. In this vein, it is notable that the administration of either metformin (43) or troglitazone (64) to PCOS women has been reported to decrease plasma PAI-1 concentrations.

It remains an unresolved issue whether insulin resistance *per se* can lead to obesity in some individuals. It is known that the use of some insulin-sensitizing agents, such as metformin, is associated with weight loss in Type 2 diabetic subjects. Were the same to hold true for nondiabetic subjects, one could argue for the use of insulin-sensitizing agents in obese women with PCOS in order to promote weight loss and reduce obesity-related health risks.

With these discrete treatment goals in mind, let us now review some of the studies that have used pharmacologic agents to reduce serum insulin in women with PCOS. The drugs used in these studies could be broadly classified as those which 1) *directly* inhibit pancreatic insulin release or 2) improve peripheral insulin sensitivity and thereby *indirectly* reduce insulin secretion (i.e., "insulin-sensitizing" drugs).

Drugs that Directly Inhibit Pancreatic Insulin Secretion

Diazoxide inhibits pancreatic insulin release, most likely by exerting an α-adrenergic-like action on the β-cell of the pancreas (85). It is used clinically to suppress insulin release by insulin-secreting islet cell tumors. Acutely it may stimulate the release of catecholamines (86), but it remains unknown whether it does so when administered chronically.

Administration of diazoxide to women with PCOS is associated with a reduction in serum free testosterone, due to a concurrent decrease in serum total testosterone and increase in serum SHBG concentrations (26). However, the use of diazoxide is also associated with aggravation of glucose intolerance or the induction of overt diabetes mellitus, as well as with intolerable bloating and swelling in many women. Therefore, it is not useful in the day-to-day management of PCOS.

Similarly, the long-acting somatostatin analogue octreotide has been used to inhibit insulin secretion in women with PCOS (87,88). In these studies, suppression of insulin release was accompanied by decreases in serum testosterone—but, again, the women also developed worsened glucose tolerance.

Drugs that Improve Peripheral Insulin Sensitivity

An intimate balance exists between insulin sensitivity and serum insulin in nondiabetic but insulin-resistant women, such as those with PCOS. Any intervention that improves peripheral insulin sensitivity will be accompanied by a reduction in circulating insulin. The net result of these changes is that glucose tolerance remains stable or may even improve slightly while tissue exposure to insulin decreases. Therefore, insulin-sensitizing agents might prove beneficial in reducing serum insulin in women with PCOS. Several studies have examined this possibility, and the results seem promising.

METFORMIN

Obese women with PCOS. Metformin is a biguanide that both enhances peripheral tissue sensitivity to insulin (89) and inhibits hepatic glucose production (90), the latter likely being the predominant action. Metformin does not produce hypoglycemia and can be administered safely to insulin-resistant but nondiabetic individuals (91). Metformin has been administered to women with PCOS as primary therapy in five independent studies (39,41,43,63,64). The first was reported by Velazquez et al. (41), and was an uncontrolled trial in which 26 women with PCOS were treated with metformin for 8 wk. Metformin treatment reduced circulating insulin in the women, and was also associated with concurrent decreases in both total and free testosterone, a rise in SHBG, and a reduction in serum LH. Moreover, 7 women experienced resumption of normal menses, and 3 additional women became pregnant. Hence, 38% of the women experienced improved reproductive function during treatment with metformin.

In a follow-up study *(43)*, now placebo controlled, the same investigators demonstrated that 8 wk of metformin therapy was associated with a decrease in circulating PAI-1 concentrations, in addition to the previously reported beneficial effects on serum insulin and androgens. This suggested that insulin reduction with metformin may reduce the risk of atherogenesis in PCOS as well as favorably affect the hyperandrogenism.

As noted previously, we conducted a randomized, single-blind, and placebo-controlled study to test the hypothesis that the increased ovarian P450c17α activity reported in obese women with PCOS was due to stimulation by hyperinsulinemia *(39)*. The study demonstrated that 4–8 wk of metformin treatment reduced both fasting serum insulin and the insulin response to a glucose challenge, and was also associated with 1) a reduction in basal and GnRH agonist-stimulated LH release, 2) decreased ovarian androgen production (i.e., decreased P450c17α activity), 3) an increase in serum SHBG concentrations, and 4) a marked decrease (–44%) in serum free testosterone concentrations. None of these variables changed in the placebo group.

These findings were consistent with the idea that hyperinsulinemia increases ovarian P450c17α activity in obese women with PCOS either by directly stimulating ovarian steroidogenesis and/or indirectly by stimulating gonadotropin release. They also demonstrated that the hyperandrogenism of PCOS can be substantially ameliorated by reducing serum insulin with metformin.

It was notable that 5 of 12 women treated with metformin for 4 wk ovulated, and that one of these women became pregnant. This improvement in reproductive function was similar to that reported earlier by Velazquez and colleagues *(41)*. Of note, several of the women were continued on metformin and subsequently became pregnant with either no other intervention or adjuvant clomiphene treatment (Personal communication: Daniela J. Jakubowicz).

There was a notable lack of efficacy of metformin in one report by Ehrmann and colleagues *(92)*. In this study, metformin had no effect on the insulin or androgen status of obese women with PCOS. This observation does not refute the "insulin hypothesis of PCOS," because serum insulin did not change. It is noteworthy that the mean body mass index (BMI) of the women was approximately 40 kg/m^2, with some women having a BMI as high as 50 kg/m^2. Therefore, these women represented an extreme of PCOS—i.e., women with morbid obesity. It is conceivable that metformin loses efficacy in women with morbid obesity, and that other agents such as troglitazone *(see under* Troglitazone) are preferred in this particular subset of women.

Lean Women with PCOS. Most recently, we had the opportunity to test the hypothesis that lean women with PCOS also respond to insulin reduction with a decrease in circulating androgens. This was a pivotal study *(63)*, because it highlighted the fact that hyperinsulinemic insulin resistance plays a key pathogenic role even in lean and normal weight women with PCOS.

Between 20–50% of women with PCOS are normal weight or thin, and it had been postulated that the pathophysiology of the disorder in those women differs from that in obese women—i.e., that PCOS develops in non-obese women because of a hypothalamic-pituitary defect that results in increased release of LH, and that insulin plays no role in the disorder *(33–36)*.

However, this concept ignored the fact that nonobese women with PCOS demonstrate an intrinsic form of insulin resistance that is unique to the disorder *(1,3,4)* and are hyperinsulinemic compared to their healthy counterparts *(37)*. Non-obese women with PCOS also exhibit increased ovarian P450c17α activity *(28,29,38)*. Since hyperinsulinemia stimulates P450c17α activity in obese women with PCOS *(39,40)*, it seemed likely that it should do so in nonobese affected women as well.

Therefore, we assessed lean (BMI, 18–24 kg/m^2) women with PCOS before and after treatment with metformin *(63)*. Similar to our observations in obese PCOS women, metformin treatment 1) decreased fasting and glucose-stimulated insulin levels, 2) decreased basal and GnRH-stimulated LH release, 3) decreased ovarian androgen production (i.e., decreased P450c17α activity), and 4) decreased both serum total and free testosterone concentrations. In these lean women, serum androstenedione and DHEA-sulfate levels decreased as well.

To our knowledge, drugs to improve insulin sensitivity or reduce insulin release had not been administered previously to lean women with PCOS. The findings demonstrated that women with PCOS who are normal weight or thin respond to a reduction in insulin release with decreases in ovarian P450c17α activity and serum ovarian androgens. This is consistent with the observation that, although these women are not obese, they nonetheless tend to have an increased waist-to-hip ratio *(77,93)* and are insulin-resistant and hyperinsulinemic compared to their normal counterparts *(1,3,4,37)*. Moreover, contrary to the postulate that the pathophysiology of the PCOS differs between obese and nonobese women *(33–36)*, these findings support the idea that the pathophysiology is similar in both groups.

Weight loss is first-line therapy for obese women with PCOS, but is not a therapeutic option for non-obese women with the disorder. The clinical importance of the above findings is that they suggest that even normal weight and thin women with PCOS should respond to pharmacologic measures to improve insulin sensitivity—such as administration of agents like metformin—with decreases in ovarian androgen production and serum androgens.

TROGLITAZONE

Troglitazone belongs to the thiazolidinedione class of insulin-sensitizing agents. Although its mechanism of action is incompletely understood, trials in Type 2 diabetic subjects suggest that troglitazone primarily improves peripheral insulin sensitivity and may decrease hepatic glucose production as well. Of note, troglitazone has also been shown to improve insulin sensitivity and glucose tolerance and to decrease circulating insulin in nondiabetic obese (and therefore insulin-resistant) subjects with either impaired or normal glucose tolerance *(94)*.

There have been only two uncontrolled studies of troglitazone in women with PCOS, and only obese women have been studied *(44,64)*. In these studies, troglitazone treatment reduced serum insulin, decreased serum LH, decreased circulating androgens, and improved reproductive status. It is notable that one of these studies was performed in morbidly obese women with PCOS who were selected on the basis of their impaired glucose tolerance *(64)*. Despite the obstacle of morbid obesity and BMI's averaging 40 kg/m^2, troglitazone was effective in reducing serum insulin and thereby decreasing serum ovarian androgens.

SUMMARY

PCOS is an excellent example of the importance of clinical research and of how a simple clinical observation can pave the way for new scientific discoveries. It was just

17 years ago that Burghen, Givens and Kitabchi made the seminal observation of a correlation between serum insulin and testosterone in women with PCOS (95). This led to a series of primarily clinical studies which examined both the nature of the insulin resistance of women with PCOS and the possible pathogenetic role of insulin in producing the hyperandrogenism (and, possibly, ovulatory dysfunction) of PCOS. The resulting findings, in turn, have influenced the manner in which women with PCOS are presently evaluated and treated.

Hyperinsulinemia produces hyperandrogenism in women with PCOS via two distinct and independent mechanisms: 1) by stimulating ovarian androgen production, and 2) by directly and independently reducing serum SHBG levels. The net result of these actions is to increase circulating free testosterone concentrations. It appears likely that an inherent (genetically determined) ovarian defect need be present in women with PCOS, which makes the ovary either susceptible to or more sensitive to insulin's stimulation of androgen production. Limited evidence suggests that hyperinsulinemia might also promote ovarian androgen production by influencing pituitary release of gonadotropins. This latter possibility, however, has not been critically evaluated.

The relationship of hyperinsulinemia to PCOS is important from a clinical standpoint for two reasons. Firstly, women with PCOS have been shown to have a higher prevalence of other disorders associated with insulin resistance, such as impaired glucose tolerance or Type 2 diabetes mellitus, hypertension, dyslipidemia, and atherosclerosis. Hence, women with PCOS suffer from a systemic metabolic disorder, and need to be evaluated comprehensively and longitudinally for these associated disorders. Secondly, medications that reduce circulating insulin might prove to be effective therapies for PCOS. Indeed, insulin reduction, whether achieved by inhibition of pancreatic insulin release or improvement in peripheral insulin sensitivity, is associated with a reduction in circulating androgens in women with PCOS. Moreover, in several studies, the accentuated LH release characteristic of PCOS appeared to be muted and reproductive function improved.

Notably, there was a clinically important disparity between agents that inhibited insulin release (diazoxide and octreotide) and those that improved insulin sensitivity (metformin and troglitazone), in that the former agents induced marked glucose intolerance whereas the latter agents did not. Moreover, insulin-sensitizing agents have the added theoretical advantage of perhaps favorably affecting those complications of PCOS that may be attributable in part to hyperinsulinemic insulin resistance—namely glucose intolerance, dyslipidemia, hypertension and atherosclerosis. Whether this will prove to be the case, however, remains to be demonstrated.

Thus, in the past 17 years, progress in characterizing the relationship between insulin resistance and PCOS has been substantial, pointing the way to new and novel therapy of PCOS. While many questions remain, clearly sufficient evidence has accumulated to justify large-scale trials of insulin-sensitizing agents in the clinical management of women with PCOS.

REFERENCES

1. Chang RJ, Nakamura RM, Judd HL, Kaplan SA. Insulin resistance in nonobese patients with polycystic ovarian disease. J Clin Endocrinol Metab 1983;57:356–359.
2. Geffner ME, Kaplan SA, Bersch N, Golde DW, Landaw EM, Chang RZ. Persistence of insulin resistance in polycystic ovarian disease after inhibition of ovarian steroid secretion. Fertil Steril. 1986;45:327–333.

3. Dunaif A, Graf M, Mandeli J, Laumas V, Dobrjansky A. Characterization of groups of hyper-androgenemic women with acanthosis nigricans, impaired glucose tolerance, and/or hyperinsulinemia. J Clin Endocrinol Metab. 1987;65:499–507.

4. Dunaif A, Segal KR, Futterweit W, Dobrjansky A. Profound peripheral insulin resistance, independent of obesity, in polycystic ovary syndrome. Diabetes. 1989;38:1165–1174.

5. Dunaif A, Green G, Futterweit W, Dobrjansky A. Suppression of hyperandrogenism does not improve peripheral or hepatic insulin resistance in the polycystic ovary syndrome. J Clin Endocrinol Metab. 1990;70:699–704.

6. Carmina E, Ditkoff EC, Malizia G, Vijod AG, Janni A, Lobo RA. Increased circulating levels of immunoreactive beta-endorphin in polycystic ovary syndrome is not caused by increased pituitary secretion. Am J Obstet Gynecol. 1992;167:1819–1824.

7. Ciaraldi TP, el Roeiy A, Madar Z, Reichart D, Olefsky JM, Yen SSC. Cellular mechanisms of insulin resistance in polycystic ovarian syndrome. J Clin Endocrinol Metab. 1992;75:577–583.

8. Dunaif A, Segal KR, Shelley DR, Green G, Dobrjansky A, Licholai T. Evidence for distinctive and intrinsic defects in insulin action in polycystic ovary syndrome. Diabetes 1992;41:1257–1266.

9. Rosenbaum D, Haber RS, Dunaif A. Insulin resistance in polycystic ovary syndrome: decreased expression of GLUT–4 glucose transporters in adipocytes. Am J Physiol 1993;264:E197–E202.

10. Dunaif A, Xia J, Book CB, Schenker E, Tang Z. Excessive insulin receptor serine phosphorylation in cultured fibroblasts and in skeletal muscle. A potential mechanism for insulin resistance in the polycystic ovary syndrome. J Clin Invest 1995;96:801–810.

11. Ehrmann DA, Sturis J, Byrne MM, Karrison T, Rosenfield RL, Polonsky KS. Insulin secretory defects in polycystic ovary syndrome. Relationship to insulin sensitivity and family history of non-insulin-dependent diabetes mellitus. J Clin Invest 1995;96:520–527.

12. Apter D, Butzow T, Laughlin GA, Yen SS. Metabolic features of polycystic ovary syndrome are found in adolescent girls with hyperandrogenism. J Clin Endocrinol Metab 1995;80:2966–2973.

13. Carmina E, Koyama T, Chang L, Stanczyk FZ, Lobo RA. Does ethnicity influence the prevalence of adrenal hyperandrogenism and insulin resistance in polycystic ovary syndrome? Am J Obstet Gynecol 1992;167:1807–1812.

14. Speiser PW, Serrat J, New MI, Gertner JM. Insulin insensitivity in adrenal hyperplasia due to nonclassical steroid 21-hydroxylase deficiency. J Clin Endocrinol Metab 1992;75:1421–1424.

15. Richards GE, Cavallo A, Meyer WJ III, Prince MJ, Peters EJ, Stuart CA, Smith ER. Obesity, acanthosis nigricans, insulin resistance, and hyperandrogenemia: pediatric perspective and natural history. J Pediatr 1985;107:893–897.

16. Moller DE, Flier JS. Detection of an alteration in the insulin-receptor gene in a patient with insulin resistance, acanthosis nigricans, and the polycystic ovary syndrome (Type A insulin resistance). N Engl J Med 1988;319:1526–1529.

17. Jahanfar S, Eden JA, Warren P, Seppala M, Nguyen TV. A twin study of polycystic ovary syndrome. Fertil Steril 1995;63:478–486.

18. Campbell PJ, Gerich JE. Impact of obesity on insulin action in volunteers with normal glucose tolerance: demonstration of a threshold for the adverse effect of obesity. J Clin Endocrinol Metab 1990;70:1114–1118.

19. Zhang LH, Rodriguez H, Ohno S, Miller WL. Serine phosphorylation of human P450c17 increases 17,20-lyase activity: implications for adrenarche and the polycystic ovary syndrome. Proc Natl Acad Sci USA 1995;92:10619–10623.

20. Barbieri RL, Makris A, Randall RW, Daniels G, Kristner RW, Ryan KJ. Insulin stimulates androgen accumulation in incubations of ovarian stroma obtained from women with hyperandrogenism. J Clin Endocrinol Metab 1986;62:904–910.

21. Bergh C, Carlsson B, Olsson JH, Selleskog U, Hillensjo T. Regulation of androgen production in cultured human thecal cells by insulin-like growth factor I and insulin. Fertil Steril 1993;59:323–331.

22. Nestler JE, Jakubowicz DJ, de Vargas AF, Brik C, Quintero N, Medina F. Insulin stimulates testosterone biosynthesis by human thecal cells from women with polycystic ovary syndrome by activating its own receptor and using inositolglycan mediators as the signal transduction system. J Clin Endocrinol Metab 1998;83:2001–2005.

23. Cara JF, Rosenfield RL. Insulin-like growth factor I and insulin potentiate luteinizing hormone-induced androgen synthesis by rat ovarian thecal-interstitial cells. Endocrinology 1988;123:733–739.

24. Cara JF, Fan J, Azzarello J, Rosenfield RL. Insulin-like growth factor-I enhances luteinizing hormone binding to rat ovarian theca-interstitial cells. J Clin Invest 1990;86:560–565.

25. DeClue TJ, Shah SC, Marchese M, Malone JI. Insulin resistance and hyperinsulinemia induce hyperandrogenism in a young Type B insulin-resistant female. J Clin Endocrinol Metab 1991;72:1308–1311.

26. Nestler JE, Barlascini CO, Matt DW, Steingold KA, Plymate SR, Clore JN, Blackard WG. Suppression of serum insulin by diazoxide reduces serum testosterone levels in obese women with polycystic ovary syndrome. J Clin Endocrinol Metab 1989;68:1027–1032.

27. Nestler JE, Singh R, Matt DW, Clore JN, Blackard WG. Suppression of serum insulin by diazoxide does not alter serum testosterone or sex hormone-binding globulin levels in healthy non-obese women. Am J Obstet Gynecol 1990;163:1243–1246.

28. Ehrmann DA, Rosenfield RL, Barnes RB, Brigell DF, Sheikh Z. Detection of functional ovarian hyperandrogenism in women with androgen excess. N Engl J Med 1992;327:157–162.

29. Rosenfield RL, Barnes RB, Ehrmann DA. Studies of the nature of 17- hydroxyprogesterone hyperresonsiveness to gonadotropin-releasing hormone agonist challenge in functional ovarian hyperandrogenism. J Clin Endocrinol Metab 1994;79:1686–1692.

30. Luppa P, Muller B, Jacob K, Kimmig R, Strowitzki T, Hoss C, Weber MM, Engelhardt D, Lobo RA. Variations of steroid hormone metabolites in serum and urine in polycystic ovary syndrome after nafarelin stimulation: evidence for an altered corticoid excretion. J Clin Endocrinol Metab 1995;80:280- 288.

31. White D, Leigh A, Wilson C, Donaldson A, Franks S. Gonadotrophin and gonadal steroid response to a single dose of a long-acting agonist of gonadotrophin-releasing hormone in ovulatory and anovulatory women with polycystic ovary syndrome. Clin Endocrinol (Oxf) 1995;42:475–481.

32. Ibanez L, Potau N, Zampolli M, Prat N, Gussinye M, Saenger P, Vicens-Calvet E, Carrascosa A. Source localization of androgen excess in adolescent girls. J Clin Endocrinol Metab 1994;79:1778–1784.

33. Grulet H, Hecart AC, Delemer B, Gross A, Sulmont V, Leutenegger M, Caron J. Roles of LH and insulin resistance in lean and obese polycystic ovary syndrome. Clin Endocrinol (Oxf) 1993; 38:621–626.

34. Holte J, Bergh T, Gennarelli G, Wide L. The independent effects of polycystic ovary syndrome and obesity on serum concentrations of gonadotrophins and sex steroids in premenopausal women. Clin Endocrinol (Oxf) 1994;41:473–481.

35. Dale PO, Tanbo T, Vaaler S, Abyholm T. Body weight, hyperinsulinemia, and gonadotropin levels in the polycystic ovarian syndrome: evidence of two distinct populations. Fertil Steril 1992;58:487–491.

36. Jacobs HS. Polycystic ovary syndrome: aetiology and management. Curr Opin Obstet Gynecol 1995;7:203–208.

37. Morales AJ, Laughlin GA, Butzow T, Maheshwari H, Bauman G, Yen SSC, Baumann G, Yen SS. Insulin, somatotropic, and luteinizing hormone axes in lean and obese women with polycystic ovary syndrome: common and distinct features. J Clin Endocrinol Metab 1996;81:2854–2864.

38. Barnes RB, Rosenfield RL. Pituitary-ovarian responses to nafarelin testing in the polycystic ovary syndrome. N Engl J Med 1989;320:559–565.

39. Nestler JE, Jakubowicz DJ. Decreases in ovarian cytochrome P450c17α activity and serum free testosterone after reduction in insulin secretion in women with polycystic ovary syndrome. N Engl J Med 1996;335:617–623.

40. Jakubowicz DJ, Nestler JE. 17α-Hydroxyprogesterone response to leuprolide and serum androgens in obese women with and without polycystic ovary syndrome after dietary weight loss. J Clin Endocrinol Metab 1997;82:556- 560.

41. Velazquez EM, Mendoza S, Hamer T, Sosa F, Glueck CJ. Metformin therapy in polycystic ovary syndrome reduces hyperinsulinemia, insulin resistance, hyperandrogenemia, and systolic blood pressure, while facilitating normal menses and pregnancy. Metabolism 1994;43:647–654.

42. Velazquez E, Acosta A, Mendoza SG. Menstrual cyclicity after metformin therapy in polycystic ovary syndrome. Obstet Gynecol 1997;90:392- 395.

43. Velazquez EM, Mendoza SG, Wang P, Glueck CJ. Metformin therapy is associated with a decrease in plasma plasminogen activator inhibitor-1, lipoprotein(a), and immunoreactive insulin levels in patients with the polycystic ovary syndrome. Metabolism 1997;46:454–457.

44. Dunaif A, Scott D, Finegood D, Quintana B, Whitcomb R. The insulin- sensitizing agent troglitazone improves metabolic and reproductive abnormalities in the polycystic ovary syndrome The insulin-sensitizing agent troglitazone improves metabolic and reproductive abnormalities in the polycystic ovary syndrome. J Clin Endocrinol Metab 1996;81:3299–3306.

45. Everett RB, Porter JC, MacDonald PC, Gant NF. Relationship of maternal placental blood flow to the placental clearance of maternal plasma dehydroepiandrosterone sulfate through placental estradiol formation. Am J Obstet Gynecol 1980;136:435–439.

46. Poretsky L. On the paradox of insulin-induced hyperandrogenism in insulin-resistant states. Endocr Rev 1991;12:3–13.
47. Buyalos RP. Insulin-like growth factor binding proteins in disorders of androgen excess. Sem Reprod Endocrinol 1994;12:21–25.
48. Saltiel AR. Second messengers of insulin action. Diabetes Care 1990;13:244–256.
49. Larner J. Insulin-signaling mechanisms: lessons from the old testament of glycogen metabolism and the new testament of molecular biology. Diabetes 1988;37:262–275.
50. Larner J. Mediators of postreceptor action of insulin. Am J Med 1983;74:38–51.
51. Nestler JE, Romero G, Huang LC, Zhang C, Larner J. Insulin mediators are the signal transduction system responsible for insulin's actions on human placental steroidogenesis. Endocrinology 1991;129:2951–2956.
52. Romero G, Garmey JC, Veldhuis JD. The involvement of inositol phosphoglycan mediators in the modulation of steroidogenesis by insulin and insulin-like growth factor-I. Endocrinology 1993; 132:1561–1568.
53. Burger CW, Korsen T, van Kessel H, van Dop PA, Caron FJM, Schoemaker J. Pulsatile luteinizing hormone patterns in the follicular phase of the menstrual cycle, polycystic ovarian disease (PCOD) and non-PCOD secondary amenorrhea. J Clin Endocrinol Metab 1985;61:1126–1132.
54. Waldstreicher J, Santoro NF, Hall JE, Filicori M, Crowley WF Jr. Hyperfunction of the hypothalamic-pituitary axis in women with polycystic ovarian disease: indirect evidence for partial gonadotroph desensitization. J Clin Endocrinol Metab 1988;66:165–172.
55. Imse V, Holzapfel G, Hinney B, Kuhn W, Wuttke W. Comparison of luteinizing hormone pulsatility in the serum of women suffering from polycystic ovarian disease using a bioassay and five different immunoassays. J Clin Endocrinol Metab 1992;74:1053–1061.
56. Berga SL, Guzick DS, Winters SJ. Increased luteinizing hormone and a-subunit secretion in women with hyperandrogenic anovulation. J Clin Endocrinol Metab 1993;77:895–901.
57. Couzinet B, Brailly S, Thomas G, Schaison G, Thalabard JC. Effects of a pure antiandrogen on gonadotropin secretion in normal women and in polycystic ovarian disease. Fertil Steril 1989;52:42–50.
58. Kazer RR, Kessel B, Yen SSC. Circulating luteinizing hormone pulse frequency in women with polycystic ovary syndrome. J Clin Endocrinol Metab 1987;65:233–236.
59. Dunaif A, Mandeli J, Fluhr H, Dobrjansky A. The impact of obesity and chronic hyperinsulinemia on gonadotropin release and gonadal steroid secretion in the polycystic ovary syndrome. J Clin Endocrinol Metab 1988;66:131-139.
60. Nestler JE. Role of obesity and insulin in the development of anovulation. In: Filicori M, Flamigni C, eds. Ovulation Induction: Basic Science and Clinical Advances. Elsevier, Amsterdam, 1994, pp. 103–114.
61. Adashi EY, Hsueh AJW, Yen SSC. Insulin enhancement of luteinizing hormone and follicle-stimulating hormone release by cultured pituitary cells. Endocrinology 1981;108:1441–1449.
62. Yen SS, Laughlin GA, Morales AJ. Interface between extra- and intraovarian factors in polycystic ovarian syndrome. Ann NY Acad Sci 1993;687:98–111.
63. Nestler JE, Jakubowicz DJ. Lean women with polycystic ovary syndrome respond to insulin reduction with decreases in ovarian P450c17α activity and serum androgens. J Clin Endocrinol Metab 1997;82:4075–4079.
64. Ehrmann DA, Schneider DJ, Sobel BE, Cavaghan MK, Imperial J, Rosenfield RL, Polonsky KS. Troglitazone improves defects in insulin action, insulin secretion, ovarian steroidogenesis, and fibrinolysis in women with polycystic ovary syndrome. J Clin Endocrinol Metab 1997;82:2108–2116.
65. Guzick DS, Wing R, Smith D, Berga SL, Winters SJ. Endocrine consequences of weight loss in obese, hyperandrogenic, anovulatory women. Fertil Steril 1994;61:598–604.
66. Nestler JE, Powers LP, Matt DW, Steingold KA, Plymate SR, Rittmaster RS, Clore JN, Blackard WG. A direct effect of hyperinsulinemia on serum sex hormone-binding globulin levels in obese women with the polycystic ovary syndrome. J Clin Endocrinol Metab 1991;72:83–89.
67. Nestler JE. Editorial: Sex hormone-binding globulin: a marker for hyperinsulinemia and/or insulin resistance? J Clin Endocrinol Metab 1993;76:273–274.
68. Lindstedt G, Lundberg P-A, Lapidus L, Lundgren H, Bengtsson C, Bjorntorp P. Low sex hormone-binding globulin concentration as independent risk factor for development of NIDDM. 12-yr follow-up of population study of women in Gothenburg, Sweden. Diabetes 1991;40:123–128.
69. Haffner SM, Valdez RA, Morales PA, Hazuda HP, Stern MP. Decreased sex hormone-binding globulin predicts non-insulin-dependent diabetes mellitus in women but not in men. J Clin Endocrinol Metab 1993;77:56–60.
70. Giudice LC. Insulin-like growth factors and ovarian follicular development. Endocr Rev 1992; 13:641–669.

71. Poretsky L, Glover B, Laumas V, Kalin M, Dunaif A. 1988 The effects of experimental hyperinsulinemia on steroid secretion, ovarian [^{125}I]insulin binding, and ovarian ['25I)insulin-like growth factor I binding in the rat. Endocrinology. 122:581–585.

72. Nobels F, Dewailly D. Puberty and polycystic ovarian syndrome: the insulin/insulin-like growth factor I hypothesis. Fertil Steril 1992;58:655–666.

73. Filicori M, Flamigni C, Cognigni G, Dellai P, Michelacci L, Arnone R. Increased insulin secretion in patients with multifollicular and polycystic ovaries and its impact on ovulation induction. Fertil Steril 1994;62:279–285.

74. Dahlgren E, Janson PO, Johansson S, Mattson L-Å, Lindstedt G, Crona N, Knutsson F, Lundberg P-A, Oden A. Women with polycystic ovary syndrome wedge resected in 1956 to 1965: a long-term follow-up focusing on natural history and circulating hormones. Fertil Steril 1992;57:505–513.

75. Wild RA, Alaupovic P, Parker IJ. Lipid and apolipoprotein abnormalities in hirsute women. I. The association with insulin resistance. Am J Obstet Gynecol 1992;166:1191–1196.

76. Wild RA. Obesity, lipids, cardiovascular risk, and androgen excess. Am J Med 1995;98:275–325.

77. Rebuffe-Scrive M, Cullberg G, Lundberg P-A, Lindstedt G, Bjorntorp P. Anthropometric variables and metabolism in polycystic ovarian disease. Horm Metab Res 1989;21:391–397.

78. Bjorntorp P. 1996 The android woman—a risky condition. J Intern Med. 239:105–110.

79. Dahlgren E, Janson PO, Johansson S, Lapidus L, Oden A. Polycystic ovary syndrome and risk for myocardial infarction. Evaluated from a risk factor model based on a prospective population study of women. Acta Obstet Gynecol Scand 1992;71:599–604.

80. Reaven GM. Banting lecture 1988. Role of insulin resistance in human disease. Diabetes 1988; 37:1595–1607.

81. Nestler JE. Assessment of insulin resistance. Sci Med 1994;1:58–67.

82. Kiddy DS, Hamilton Fairley D, Seppala M, Koistinen R, James VH, Reed MJ, Franks S. Diet-induced changes in sex hormone binding globulin and free testosterone in women with normal or polycystic ovaries: correlation with serum insulin and insulin-like growth factor-I. Clin Endocrinol (Oxf) 1989;31:757–763.

83. Kiddy DS, Hamilton Fairley D, Bush A, Short F, Anyaoku V, Reed MJ, Franks S. Improvement in endocrine and ovarian function during dietary treatment of obese women with polycystic ovary syndrome. Clin Endocrinol (Oxf) 1992;36:105–111.

84. Nestler JE, Jakubowicz DJ, Evans WS, Pasquali R. Effects of metformin on spontaneous and clomiphene-induced ovulation in the polycystic ovary syndrome. N Engl J Med 1998;338:1876–1880.

85. Zarday Z, Viktora J, Wolff FW. The effect of diazoxide on catecholamines. Metabolism 1966;15:257–261.

86. Belisle S, Osathanondh R, Tulchinsky D. The effect of constant infusion of unlabeled dehydro-epiandrosterone sulfate on maternal plasma androgens and estrogens. J Clin Endocrinol Metab 1977;45:544–550.

87. Prelevic GM, Wurzburger MI, Balint-Peric L, Nesic JS. Inhibitory effect of sandostatin on secretion of luteinising hormone and ovarian steroids in polycystic ovary syndrome. Lancet 1990;336:900–903.

88. Fulghesu AM, Lanzone A, Andreani CL, Pierro E, Caruso A, Mancuso S. Effectiveness of a somatostatin analogue in lowering luteinizing hormone and insulin-stimulated secretion in hyperinsulinemic women with polycystic ovary disease. Fertil Steril 1995;64:703–708.

89. Nagi DK, Yudkin JS. Effects of metformin on insulin resistance, risk factors for cardiovascular disease, and plasminogen activator inhibitor in NIDDM subjects: A study of two ethnic groups. Diabetes Care 1993;16:621–629.

90. DeFronzo RA, Barzilai N, Simonson DC. Mechanism of metformin action in obese and lean noninsulin-dependent diabetic subjects. J Clin Endocrinol Metab 1991;73:1294–1301.

91. Nestler JE, Beer NA, Jakubowicz DJ, Beer RM. Effects of a reduction in circulating insulin by metformin on serum dehydroepiandrosterone sulfate in nondiabetic men. J Clin Endocrinol Metab 1994;78:549–554.

92. Ehrmann DA, Cavaghan MK, Imperial J, Sturis J, Rosenfield RL, Polonsky KS. Effects of metformin on insulin secretion, insulin action, and ovarian steroidogenesis in women with polycystic ovary syndrome. J Clin Endocrinol Metab 1997;82:524–530.

93. Bringer J, Lefebvre P, Boulet F, Grigorescu F, Renard E, Hedon B, Orsetti A, Jaffiol C. Body composition and regional fat distribution in polycystic ovarian syndrome. Relationship to hormonal and metabolic profiles. Ann NY Acad Sci 1993;687:115–123.

94. Nolan JJ, Ludvik B, Beerdsen P, Joyce M, Olefsky J. Improvement in glucose tolerance and insulin resistance in obese subjects treated with troglitazone. N Engl J Med 1994;331:1188–1193.

95. Burghen GA, Givens JR, Kitabchi AE. 1980 Correlation of hyperandrogenism with hyperinsulinism in polycystic ovarian disease. J Clin Endocrinol Metab 1980;50:113–116.

INDEX

A

ACE, *see* Angiotensin I-converting enzyme
Acetyl CoA carboxylase, insulin effects, 271-272
Adipose tissue, *see also* Body fat distribution;
        Obesity
  basal lipolysis, 86
  catecholamine-induced lipolysis, 86, 88
  classification, 85
  free fatty acid release and insulin effects, 234,
      237-244
  functions, 85, 233
  hormone sensitive lipase,
    expression in adipose tissue types, 88
    regulation of lipolysis, 86-88
  hypertriglyceridemia,
    insulin effects, 240-241
    insulin resistant, hyperinsulinemic indi-
      viduals, 243, 270-272
    insulin resistant, hypoinsulinemic individu-
      als, 241-242
    insulin resistant, normoinsulinemic indi-
      viduals, 242-243
  insulin resistance,
    evidence, 233-235
    hyperglycemia, 143, 236-238
    mediators, 56-58
  insulin-mediated inhibition of lipolysis, 87
  lipoprotein lipase activity and triglyceride
      synthesis, 88
  metabolic heterogeneity, 85-89
  plasminogen activator inhibitor 1 production,
      322-323, 325
  steroid hormones and lipolysis, 87-88
β3-Adrenergic receptor, candidate gene in insulin
      resistance, 11, 58
Aging,
  hypertension association, 281
  physical activity and adaptations of insulin
      action and secretion, 105-107
Alcohol, moderate consumption and cardiovascu-
      lar benefits, 130
Angiotensin I-converting enzyme (ACE), candi-
      date gene in insulin resistance, 11
Apo A-I, postprandial free fatty acid effects, 273-
    274
ApoB, insulin resistance effects on metabolism,
    270, 272-273

B

β-cell,
  adaptation to training, 104
  free fatty acid effects on function, 238
Birth size, glucose intolerance and type 2 diabetes
      with small birth size,
  correlations in different populations, 35-36,
      44-45
  ethnic difference and diabetes prevalence, 43-
      44
  glucose levels in young adults and children,
      38-39
  insulin resistance and secretion, 39-43
  malnutrition in early life, experimental stud-
      ies, 41-42
  physiological basis, 36, 42-44
  studies, 36-38
Blood pressure, *see* Hypertension
BMI, *see* Body mass index
Body fat distribution, *see also* Obesity,
  android versus gynoid, 83
  congenital generalized lipodystrophy patients,
      85
  magnetic resonance imaging studies of ab-
      dominal fat, 89-94
  sex differences, 89
  smokers, 122-123
  visceral adipose tissue accumulation, 53
Body mass index (BMI),
  blood pressure correlation, 284
  determination, 68
  ethnic variation, 70-71
  obesity-linked insulin resistance marker, 68-
      70
  smokers, 123, 128, 131

C

Calcium, insulin effects, 294, 299-300
Cardiac output, insulin effects, 294-295
Cardiovascular disease,
  alcohol, moderate consumption and cardiovas-
      cular benefits, 130
  epidemiologic studies with insulin resistance,
    coronary heart disease, 334-339
    criteria for causality,
      biological plausibility, 342-343

Cardiovascular disease(cont.)
    epidemiologic studies with insulin resistance
        (cont.)
        criteria for causality (cont.)
            consistency, 341
            dose relation, 341
            reversibility, 343
            specificity, 342
            strength of association, 341
            temporality, 341-342
        measures, 333-334
        peripheral arterial disease, 339-340
        quality of evidence, 340-341
        stroke, 340
    free fatty acids and atherosclerosis, 269-270
    hypertension risk factor, 272-273
    insulin resistance risk relationship in South
        Asians, 23-24
    microalbuminuria as risk marker, 309-310,
        312-313
    nitric oxide protection, 260
    obesity-linked insulin resistance dyslipidemia,
        65-67
    obesity risk factor and type 2 diabetes, 53-55,
        65-67
    plasminogen activator inhibitor 1 risk factor,
        317, 319-320, 324
    type 2 diabetes association, 53-54, 267-268
CETP, *see* Cholesterol ester transfer protein
CHD, *see* Coronary heart disease
Cholesterol ester transfer protein (CETP), post-
        prandial free fatty acid effects, 273-
        274
Chronic renal failure, physical activity and adap-
        tations of insulin action and secre-
        tion, 113
Cigaret smoking, *see* Smoking
CIGMA, *see* Continuous infusion of glucose with
        model assessment
Computed tomography (CT), body fat, 70, 84, 89-
        90
Continuous infusion of glucose with model as-
        sessment (CIGMA), insulin resis-
        tance measurement, 8
Coronary heart disease (CHD), *see* Cardiovascu-
        lar disease
C-peptide, training effects, 104, 110
CT, *see* Computed tomography

D

Diazoxide,
    polycystic ovary syndrome treatment, 358,
        361
    suppression of insulin release, 350
Dyslipidemia, *see* Free fatty acid; Lipid profile

E

Endothelium,
    dysfunction and insulin resistance,
        clinical implications, 259-260
        mechanisms,
            altered insulin signaling, 254-255
            fatty acids, 253-254
    free fatty acids and atherosclerosis, 269-270
    functions, 247
    insulin effects,
        insulin sensitivity and endothelial function,
            252-253
        vasodilation of skeletal muscle vasculature,
            dose response, 248-249
            insulin receptors and signaling path-
            ways, 255-256, 258-259
            nitric oxide mediation, 250-252
    nitric oxide synthase, 255
Epidemiologic studies, criteria for causality,
    biological plausibility, 342-343
    consistency, 341
    dose relation, 341
    reversibility, 343
    specificity, 342
    strength of association, 341
    temporality, 341-342
Ethnic variation,
    body mass index, 70-71
    insulin resistance and type 2 diabetes risk,
        Mexican Americans, 25
        Native Americans, 24-25
        Native Australians, 25-26
        overview, 19-20, 28-29
        Peninsular Arabs, 24
        relation to insulin resistance and obesity,
            20-21
        South Asians, 21-24
        West Africans, 26-28
    small birth size and insulin resistance, 39-43
Euglycemic insulin clamp, insulin resistance
        measurement, 6, 97, 218
Exercise, *see* Physical activity

F

FABP2, *see* Fatty acid binding protein 2
Familial hypercholesterolemia (FH), obesity and
        ischemic heart disease, 67
Family clustering, insulin resistance, 8-9
Fatty acid, *see* Free fatty acid,
Fatty acid binding protein 2 (FABP2), candidate
        gene in insulin resistance, 11-12
Fatty acid synthase, insulin effects, 271-272
FH, *see* Familial hypercholesterolemia
Fibrinolysis, overview, 317-319
Folliculogenesis, promotion by insulin, 356

Free fatty acid,
   atherosclerosis role, 269-270
   β-cell function effects, 238
   endothelial dysfunction role with insulin
      resistance, 253-254
   hepatic glucose production effects, 239-240
   hypertriglyceridemia response, 240-244, 270
   insulin effects,
      adipose tissue, 234, 237-244
      liver, 203-204, 212, 215-216, 218
      mechanisms of suppression, 268-270
      sex differences, 269
   insulin uptake induction in liver, 219
   muscle glucose uptake effects, 238-239
   postprandial effects in insulin resistance,
      apo A-I metabolism, 273-274
      cholesterol ester transfer protein, 273-274
      lipoprotein lipase inhibition, 273
      triglyceride clearance, 273
   skeletal muscle metabolism, 171-173
   triglyceride synthesis, 268, 270

G

Gastric inhibitor peptide (GIP), training effects on
      secretion, 104
Gestational diabetes, physical activity and adapta-
      tions of insulin action and secretion,
      111, 113
GIP, see Gastric inhibitor peptide
Gluconeogenesis, insulin effects in liver, 210-213
Glucose oxidation, defects in type 2 diabetes,
      188-189
Glucose-6-phosphate, muscle concentration in
      type 2 diabetics and offspring, 163-
      167, 169, 185-186
Glucose tolerance test, insulin resistance mea-
      surement, 6
Glucose transporter, see GLUT4
GLUT4,
   abnormalities in obesity-linked insulin resis-
      tance,
      expression, 63-64
      translocation, 64-65
   glucose inhibition of translocation, 185
   hypertension in knockout mice, 289
   immunostaining, 184
   insulin effects, 167
   insulin resistance role, 143-144
   measurement,
      glucose transport, 183-184
      translocation, 184
   phosphatidylinositol-3-kinase, translocation
      role, 59-61, 142
   training effects, 103, 106, 108
   vesicle trafficking, 65, 183

Glycogen synthase,
   gene mutations, 188
   insulin stimulation and defects in resistance,
      187-188
   muscle activity in type 2 diabetics and off-
      spring, 161-163, 165-169, 172, 187-
      188
   training effects, 103
Glycolysis, insulin effects in liver, 210-213

H

Heritability, insulin resistance and insulinemia, 9-
      10, 15, 179-1890
Hexokinase,
   activity in type 2 diabetics and offspring, 165,
      167, 185-186
   insulin induction, 185, 207
   isoforms, 185
   mitochondria association, 186
   mutations in insulin resistance, 186
Hormone sensitive lipase,
   expression in adipose tissue types, 88
   regulation of lipolysis, 86-88, 268
Hyperglycemia, adipose tissue insulin resistance,
      143, 236-238
Hyperinsulinemia, see Insulinemia
Hypertension,
   aging effects, 281
   epidemiology with impaired glucose toler-
      ance, 281-283
   etiology in diabetes types, 283-284
   hyperinsulinemia association, 285-286
   insulin mechanisms,
      blood flow and metabolism, 291-294
      calcium regulation, 294, 299-300
      cardiac output increase, 294-295
      potassium metabolism, 297-298
      sodium metabolism, 298-299
      sympathetic nervous system effects, 295-
      296
      vascular structural hypothesis, 289-291
      vasodilation, 293-294
   insulin resistance,
      cause and effect relationships with hyper-
      tension, 288-289
      characteristics, 286-288
      clinical implications, 300-301
      prevalence, 286-287
   microalbuminuria, 310-312
   obesity association, 284-285
Hypertriglyceridemia,
   atherosclerosis risk, 272-273
   insulin effects, 240-241
   insulin resistant, hyperinsulinemic individuals,
      243, 270-272

Hypertriglyceridemia (cont.)
  insulin resistant, hypoinsulinemic individuals,
      241-242
  insulin resistant, normoinsulinemic individu-
      als, 242-243

I

IDDM, *see* Insulin-dependent diabetes mellitus
IGF-1, *see* Insulin-like growth factor 1
IGT, *see* Impaired glucose tolerance,
Impaired glucose tolerance (IGT), *see also* Insu-
      lin resistance,
  bed rest effects, 97-98
  definition, 268
  hypertension epidemiologic association, 281-
      283
  relatives of type 2 diabetics, 6-7
Incretin, training effects on secretion, 104,
      110
Insulin,
  blood-brain barrier permeability, 296
  candidate gene in insulin resistance, 11
  exercise effects on secretion, *see* Physical
      activity,
  hepatic clearance, 217-219
  secretory respone to glucose, phases, 197
Insulin receptor,
  abnormalities in obesity-linked insulin resis-
      tance, 61-62
  autophosphorylation, 141, 144, 180-181
  endothelial cell signaling pathways for nitric
      oxide production, 255-256, 258-259
  gene,
      messenger RNA splicing variants, 148
      mutations, 4-5, 180
      structure, 4
  insulin binding, 180
  nicotine interactions, 129
  SH2 domains in signal transduction, 141, 182
  signaling pathway activation, 182
  subunits, 140
  tyrosine kinase,
      defects in insulin resistance, 144-146, 182-
          183
      insulin receptor substrate phosphorylation,
          141, 182
      knockout mice, 146
      PC-1 inhibition, 148-152, 154-155
      serine phosphorylation and inhibition, 146,
          181
      tumor necrosis factor-a and serine phos-
          phorylation induction of IRS-1, 146,
          148, 181
Insulin-dependent diabetes mellitus (IDDM), *see*
      Type 1 diabetes

Insulinemia,
  blood pressure correlation, 285-286
  hepatic clearance defects, 217-219
  heritability, 9-10, 15
  mode of inheritance, 10-11
  polycystic ovary syndrome and
      hyperinsulinemia, 347-348, 361
  small birth size relationship, 39-43
  variability within and between families, 8-9
Insulin-like growth factor 1 (IGF-1), endothelial
      cell receptors, 258
Insulin receptor substrates,
  abnormalities in obesity-linked insulin resis-
      tance, 62-63
  hypertension in insulin receptor substrate 2
      knockout mice, 289
  insulin receptor substrate 1,
      candidate gene in insulin resistance, 11
      phosphatidylinositol-3-kinase complex,
          141, 144
      phosphorylation, 141, 144, 182
      tumor necrosis factor-a, serine phosphory-
          lation induction, 146, 148
  mutation in type 2 diabetes, 183
  phosphorylation, 62-63
  types, 59
Insulin resistance,
  adipose tissue, *see* Adipose tissue
  candidate genes, 11-12
  cardiovascular disease association, *see* Cardio-
      vascular disease
  chromosomal linkage analysis, 12
  coronary risk relationship in South Asians, 23-
      24
  definition,
      impaired free fatty acid suppression, 268-
          270
      impaired glucose uptake, 268
  endothelium dysfunction, *see* Endothelium
  ethnic variation,
      Mexican Americans, 25
      Native Americans, 24-25, 145-146
      Native Australians, 25-26
      overview, 19-20, 28-29
      Peninsular Arabs, 24
      relation to diabetes risk and obesity, 20-21
      South Asians, 21-24
      West Africans, 26-28
  exercise effects, *see* Physical activity
  heritability, 9-10, 15
  hypertension association, *see* Hypertension
  mode of inheritance, 10-11
  muscle, *see* Muscle, skeletal
  obesity-linked insulin resistance, *see* Obesity
  plasminogen activator inhibitor 1 association,
      adipose tissue role, 322-323, 325

Insulin resistance (cont.)
   plasminogen activator inhibitor 1 association
      (cont.),
      cause and effect relationships, 321-322
      gene mutations, 323-324
      measurement, 320
      sex differences, 321
   polycystic ovary syndrome association, *see*
      Polycystic ovary syndrome
   relatives of type 2 diabetics, 6-8
   variability within and between families, 8-9
Insulin resistance syndrome (IRS),
   analysis of clusters, 13-14, 140
   major gene effects, 15
   obesity-linked insulin resistance, *see* Obesity
   pleiotropy, 14
   quantitative genetic studies, 14-15
   small baby syndrome, 44
   smoking risk, 121, 131
   traits, 13, 16, 259
   troglitazone therapy, 259
IRS, *see* Insulin resistance syndrome

L

Leprechaunism,
   incidence, 5
   insulin receptor gene mutations, 4-5
Leptin, mediation of obesity-related insulin resis-
      tance, 58-59
LH, *see* Luteinizing hormone
Lipid profile, *see also* Free fatty acid,
   ethnic variation and type 2 diabetes risk,
      Mexican Americans, 25
      Native Americans, 24-25, 145-146
      Native Australians, 25-26
      overview, 19-20, 28-29
      Peninsular Arabs, 24
      relation to insulin resistance and obesity,
         20-21
      South Asians, 21-24
      West Africans, 26-28
   obesity-linked insulin resistance dyslipidemia,
      ischemic heart disease, 65-67
      clinical markers, 71-72
   small birth size relationship, 39-43
   smoking effects, 122, 124-126
   Syndrome X, 54-55
Lipolysis, *see* Adipose tissue
Lipoprotein lipase (LPL),
   activity and triglyceride synthesis, 88
   candidate gene in insulin resistance, 11
   postprandial free fatty acid effects, 273
Liver,
   glucose metabolism,
      free fatty acid effects on glucose produc-
         tion, 239-240

Liver (cont.)
   glucose metabolism (cont.)
      glycogen synthesis pathways, 200-202
      measurement of glucose production, 214
      overview, 199, 202
      uptake on first pass, 199-200
   insulin effects,
      direct versus indirect effects, 203-205
      free fatty acid levels, 203-204, 212, 215-
         216
      glucose fluxes,
         gluconeogenesis, 210-213
         glycogen metabolism, 207-210
         glycolysis, 210-213
         overview, 205-206
         uptake/output, 206-207
      importance, 202-203
   insulin resistance and type 2 diabetes, 213-214
   lipid and carbohydrate metabolism, 199, 215
   modulation of insulin action, 216-220
   obesity-linked insulin resistance pathogenesis,
      58-59, 84-85
   sensitivity to portal insulin, 213
Liver nucleotide pyrophosphatase/alkaline phos-
      phodiesterase I, *see* PC-1
LPL, *see* Lipoprotein lipase
Luteinizing hormone (LH), pulse dynamics in
      polycystic ovary syndrome, 354-355

M

Magnetic resonance imaging (MRI), body fat, 70,
      84, 89-94
Maturity-onset diabetes of the young (MODY),
   glucokinase mutations, 198, 207
   peripheral insulin resistance, 213-214
Metformin,
   effects on P450c17a stimulation by insulin,
      normal weight and thin women, 352
      obese women, 351
   polycystic ovary syndrome treatment,
      lean women, 359-360
      obese women, 358-359
Microalbuminuria,
   blood pressure dependence, 310-312
   cardiovascular disease risk, 309-310, 312-313
   clinical definition, 309-310
   diabetes association,
      prevalence, 309-310
      type 1 diabetes, 310-311
      type 2 diabetes, 311
MODY, *see* Maturity-onset diabetes of the young
MRI, *see* Magnetic resonance imaging
MSNA, *see* Muscle sympathetic nerve activity
Muscle, skeletal,
   composition in hypertensive individuals, 290-
      291

Muscle, skeletal (cont.)
   endothelium,
     insulin effects on vasodilation,
       dose response, 248-249
         insulin receptors and signaling path-
           ways, 255-256, 258-259
         nitric oxide mediation, 250-252
     insulin sensitivity and endothelial function,
       252-253
   free fatty acid effects on glucose uptake, 238-
     239
   glucose disposal and insulin resistance, 143
   insulin resistance,
     glucose oxidation, 188-189
     glucose transport, 183-185
     glycogen synthesis, 186-188
     hexokinase activity, 185-186
     insulin receptor binding, 180-181
     mediators, 56-58
     post receptor signaling, 181-183
   nuclear magnetic resonance studies,
     free fatty acid metabolism, 171-173
     offspring of type 2 diabetics,
       exercise effect studies, 167-169
       glucose-6-phosphate concentration,
         165-167, 169
       glycogen synthesis, 165-169
       hexokinase activity, 165, 167
     type 2 diabetics,
       glucose-6-phosphate concentration,
         163-165
       glycogen synthesis, 161-163
Muscle sympathetic nerve activity (MSNA),
     insulin effects, 295-296

N

Nicotine, *see also* Smoking,
   insulin receptor interactions, 129
   nicotine gum and insulin sensitivity, 126-127,
     132
   smoke-free tobacco effects, 126-127
NIDDM, *see* Type 2 diabetes
Nitric oxide (NO),
   atherosclerosis protection, 260
   guanylate cyclase induction, 250, 294
   insulin-dependent vasodilation,
     endothelial cell insulin receptors and sig-
       naling pathways, 255-256, 258-259
     evidence, 250-251
     insulin sensitivity, 251-252, 293-294
   synthesis, 249-250, 255
NMR, *see* Nuclear magnetic resonance
NO, *see* Nitric oxide
Nonesterified fatty acid, *see* Free fatty acid

Noninsulin-dependent diabetes mellitus
     (NIDDM), *see* Type 2 diabetes
Nuclear magnetic resonance (NMR), *see also*
     Magnetic resonance imaging,
   advantages in metabolism studies, 159
   nuclei and abundance, 160-161
   principle, 160-161
   skeletal muscle studies,
     free fatty acid metabolism, 171-173
     offspring of type 2 diabetics,
       exercise effect studies, 167-169
       glucose-6-phosphate concentration,
         165-167, 169
       glycogen synthesis, 165-169
       hexokinase activity, 165, 167
     type 2 diabetics,
       glucose-6-phosphate concentration,
         163-165
       glycogen synthesis, 161-163

O

Obesity, *see also* Adipose tissue; Body fat distri-
     bution,
   cardiovascular disease risk and type 2 diabe-
     tes, 53-55, 65-67
   health risks and mortality, 51-52
   hypertension association, 284-285
   imaging of visceral fat, 70
   independence as a risk factor, 52
   obesity-linked insulin resistance,
     anthropometric markers,
       body mass index, 68-70
       sagittal diameter, 70
       skinfold assessment, 68-69
       waist circumference, 69-70
     dyslipidemia,
       clinical markers, 71-72
       ischemic heart disease, 65-67
     magnetic resonance imaging studies of
       abdominal fat, 89-94
     molecular defects of insulin action,
       GLUT4, 63-65
       insulin receptor substrates, 62-63
       insulin receptor, 61-62
       overview, 59-61
       phosphatidylinositol-3-kinase, 62-63
     pathogenesis,
       liver mechanisms, 58-59, 84-85
       mediators in skeletal muscle and fat,
         56-58
       tissue variability, 55-56
   physical activity and adaptations of insulin
     action and secretion, 107
   prevalence in type 2 diabetes, 139
Octreotide, polycystic ovary syndrome treatment,
     358, 361

P

P450c17a,
  functions, 350
  phosphorylation and androgen synthesis, 349
  stimulation by insulin,
    overview, 350-353
    polycystic ovary syndrome patients,
      metformin effects in normal weight and
        thin women, 352
      metformin effects in obese women, 351
      weight loss effects, 351-352
PAI-1, *see* Plasminogen activator inhibitor 1
PC-1,
  functions, 151
  insulin receptor tyrosine kinase inhibition,
    148-149, 151-152, 154
  overexpression in insulin resistance, 151
  posttranslational processing, 151
  structure, 150-151
  tissue distribution, 150-151
PCOS, *see* Polycystic ovary syndrome
PDH, *see* Pyruvate dehydrogenase
PEPCK, *see* Phosphoenolpyruvate carboxykinase
Phosphatidylinositol-3-kinase,
  abnormalities in obesity-linked insulin resis-
    tance, 62-63
  activation by insulin, 59-60, 62
  GLUT4 translocation role, 59-61
  insulin receptor substrate 1 complex, 141
  insulin signaling for nitric oxide production,
    258-259
Phosphoenolpyruvate carboxykinase (PEPCK),
    downregulation by leptin, 59
Physical activity,
  adaptations of insulin action and secretion in
    insulin resistant groups,
    aging people, 105-107
    chronic renal failure patients, 113
    first-degree relatives of type 2 diabetes
      patients, 113
    gestational diabetes patients, 111, 113
    obese people, 107
    type 2 diabetes patients, 107-111
  bed rest and impaired glucose tolerance, 97-98
  exercise modality effects on insulin action and
    secretion, 104-105
  insulin secretion effects, overview, 97-98
  mechanisms of adaptations in insulin action
    and secretion,
    β-cell adaptation, 104
    blood flow, 102-103, 108
    C-peptide response, 104, 110
    gastric inhibitor peptide secretion, 104
    GLUT4 content, 103, 106, 108
    glycogen synthase, 103
    incretin secretion, 104, 110

Physical activity (cont.)
    site of exercise-induced increase in insulin
      effect, 102
    training effects on insulin resistance,
      comparison to acute exercise, 100, 102
      overview, 97-100
Plasmin, fibrinolysis, 318
Plasminogen activator inhibitor 1 (PAI-1),
  activation, 318
  atherosclerosis risk with elevated levels, 317,
    319-320, 324
  functions, 318-319
  insulin resistance association,
    adipose tissue role, 322-323, 325
    cause and effect relationships, 321-322
    gene mutations, 323-324
    measurement, 320
    sex differences, 321
  modulation of activity, 324
  structure, 318
Polycystic ovary syndrome (PCOS),
  folliculogenesis promotion by insulin, 356
  gene hypothesis, 353
  insulin effects on circulating ovarian androgens,
    diazoxide-induced suppression of insulin
      release, 350
    direct effects, 353-354
    indirect effects, 354-355
    insulin infusion studies, 349-350
    P450c17a stimulation by insulin,
      metformin effects in normal weight and
        thin women, 352
      metformin effects in obese women, 351
      overview, 350-353
      weight loss effects, 351-352
    sex hormone binding globulin, 350, 355
  insulin resistance association,
    clinical implications,
      overview, 347, 356-357
      patient evaluation, 356-357
    epidemiology, 348
    hyperinsulinemia, 347-348, 361
    obesity role, 348
  luteinizing hormone pulse dynamics, 354-355
  prevalence, 347
  treatment,
    diazoxide, 358, 361
    goals of therapy, 357-358
    metformin,
      lean women, 359-360
      obese women, 358-359
    octreotide, 358, 361
    *troglit*azone, 360-361
Potassium, insulin effects, 297-298
Protein kinase C, inhibition of insulin receptor,
    146, 181

Pyruvate dehydrogenase (PDH),
    defects in type 2 diabetes, 188-189
    regulation, 188-189

R

Rabson-Mendenhall syndrome, insulin receptor
        gene mutations, 4-5

S

Sagittal diameter, obesity-linked insulin resis-
        tance marker, 70
Segregation analysis, insulin resistance mode of
        inheritance, 10-11
Sex hormone binding globulin (SHBG), insulin
        effects on levels,
    overview, 350
    polycystic ovary syndrome, 355
    type 2 diabetes, 355
SHBG, see Sex hormone binding globulin
Skeletal muscle, see Muscle, skeletal
Skinfold assessment, obesity-linked insulin resis-
        tance, 68-69, 84
Smoking,
    body mass index of smokers, 123, 128, 131
    catecholamine induction, 128-129
    cessation effects, 127-128, 130-131
    confounding factors in health risks, 129-130
    diabetic complications, 129
    health risks, 122
    insulin sensitivity in type 1 versus type 2
        diabetics, 123-124, 132
    intravenous glucose tolerance test effects, 123
    lipid profiles, 122, 124-128
    nicotine replacement therapy, see Nicotine
    oral glucose tolerance test effects, 123
    prevalence, 121-122
SNAP receptors (SNAREs), GLUT4 vesicle
        trafficking, 65, 183
SNAREs, see SNAP receptors
Sodium, insulin effects, 298-299
SSPG, see Steady state plasma glucose
Steady state plasma glucose (SSPG), insulin
        resistance measurement, 6
Stroke, insulin resistance association, 340
Sympathetic nervous system, insulin effects, 295-
        296
Syndrome X, see also Insulin resistance syn-
        drome,
    lipid profiles, 54-55

Syndrome X (cont.)
    polycystic ovary syndrome, 356
    small birth size and insulin resistance, 36, 44

T

TNF-α, see Tumor necrosis factor-α
Troglitazone,
    insulin resistance syndrome therapy, 259
    polycystic ovary syndrome treatment, 360-361
Tumor necrosis factor-α (TNF-α),
    candidate gene in insulin resistance, 11, 56-58
    inhibition of insulin receptor
        autophosphorylation, 181
    serine phosphorylation induction of IRS-1,
        146, 148
Type 1 diabetes,
    hypertension, 281, 283-284
    microalbuminuria, 310-311
    smoking, insulin sensitivity versus type 2
        diabetics, 123-124, 132
Type 2 diabetes,
    cardiovascular disease association, 53-54,
        267-268
    ethnic variation in risk,
        Mexican Americans, 25
        Native Americans, 24-25, 145-146
        Native Australians, 25-26
        overview, 19-20, 28-29
        Peninsular Arabs, 24
        relation to insulin resistance and obesity,
            20-21
        South Asians, 21-24
        West Africans, 26-28
    hypertension, 281, 283-284
    insulin resistance in development, 3, 6-8
    microalbuminuria, 311
    physical activity and adaptations of insulin
        action and secretion
        first-degree relatives of patients, 113
        patients, 107-111
    prevalence, 139
Type A insulin resistance, insulin receptor gene
        mutations, 4-5
Tyrosine kinase, see Insulin receptor

W

Waist circumference,
    obesity-linked insulin resistance marker, 69-
        71, 84
    smokers, 122